MEDICAL RADIOLOGY

Diagnostic Imaging and Radiation Oncology

Springer
Berlin
Heidelberg
New York
Barcelona
Budapest
Hong Kong
London
Milan
Paris
Santa Clara
Singapore
Tokyo

Z. Petrovich · L. Baert · L.W. Brady (Eds.)

Carcinoma of the Bladder

Innovations in Management

With Contributions by

A.F. Althausen · H. Aziz · L. Baert · C.M. Bender · J.E. Binard · S. Birkenhake
B.H. Bochner · C. Bouffioux · S.D. Boyd · L.W. Brady · M.Brausi · F. Calabrò · J. Cirrone
K. Choi · B.J. Costleigh · R.J. Cote · N.De Graeve · D.J.M.K. De Ridder
M.-A. D'Hallewin · J. Dunst · A.-A. Elgamal · F. Farzin · S.C. Formenti · F.S. Freiha
J.E. Freire · H. Goethuys · H.P. Heilmann · N.M. Heney · W. Höltl · W. IJzermann
G. Jakse · P.A. Jones · P. Jung · D.S. Kaufman · R. Kühn · K.-H. Kurth · G. Lieskovsky
Y. Lievens · W.A. Longton · R. Macchia · D. Mack · P. Martus · B. Micaily
C.T. Miyamoto · E.C. M. Ooms · R.H. Oyen · Z. Petrovich · R.K. Ross · M. Rotman
R. Sauer · K.M. Schrott · A. Schulsinger · D. Schwartz · W.U. Shipley · E.C. Skinner
D.G. Skinner · T.A.W. Splinter · J.P. Stein · C.N. Sternberg · R. Sylvester
W. Van den Bogaert · M. Van den Heuvel · A.P.M. Van der Meijden · C.C.D. Van der Rijt
H. Van Herzeele · E. Van Limbergen · H. Van Poppel · L. Vanuytsel · R. Van Velthoven
R.W. Veldhuizen · C. Wittekind · M.C. Yu · A.L. Zietman

Foreword by

L.W. Brady and H.-P. Heilmann

Preface by

D.G. Skinner

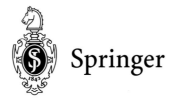

Springer

ZBIGNIEW PETROVICH, MD, FACR
Professor and Chairman
Department of Radiation Oncology
University of Southern California, USC/Norris Cancer Center
1441 Eastlake Avenue
Los Angeles, CA 90033, USA

LUC BAERT, MD, PhD
Professor and Chairman
Department of Urology, UZ Gasthuisberg, University of Leuven
Herestraat 49
B-3000 Leuven, Belgium

LUTHER W. BRADY, MD
Professor, Department of Radiation Oncology and Nuclear Medicine
Allegheny University Hospitals, Center City
Mail Stop 200, Broad & Vine Sts.
Philadelphia, PA 19102-1192, USA

MEDICAL RADIOLOGY · Diagnostic Imaging and Radiation Oncology

Continuation of
Handbuch der medizinischen Radiologie
Encyclopedia of Medical Radiology

With 82 Figures in 123 Separate Illustrations, Some in Color

ISSN 0942-5373
ISBN 3-540-60885-0 Springer-Verlag Berlin Heidelberg New York

Library of Congress Cataloging-in-Publication Data. Carcinoma of the bladder : innovations in management / Z. Petrovich, L. Baert, L.W. Brady (eds.) ; with contributions by A. F. Althausen ... [et al.] ; foreword by L. W. Brady and H.-P. Heilmann ; preface by D.G. Skinner. p. cm. -- (Medical radiology) Includes bibliographical references and index. ISBN 3-540-60885-0 (alk. paper) 1. Bladder--Cancer--Treatment. I. Petrovich, Zbigniew. II. Baert, L. (Luc) III. Brady, Luther W., 1925- . IV. Althausen, A. F. (Alex F.) V. Series [DNLM: 1. Bladder Neoplasms--therapy. 2. Carcinoma--therapy. WJ 504 C2652 1997] RC280.B5C343 1997 616.99'262--dc21 DNLM/DLC for Library of Congress 97-11285 CIP

Cover design: de'blik, Berlin

Typesetting: Best-set Typesetter Ltd., Hong Kong

SPIN: 10524941   21/3155/SPS – 5 4 3 2 1 0 – Printed on acid-free paper

This book is dedicated to

Zofia Petrovich, MD and Mrs. Bea Baert

Foreword

Bladder cancer represents a major challenge to the oncologist. In spite of new techniques for early diagnosis and innovative imaging procedures for staging, the outcome in terms of cure has not improved during the past ten years. Fortunately, about 74% of the patients present with localized disease, with 18% presenting with localized and regional disease, and 3% with distant metastases at diagnosis.

In accordance with the stage at presentation, 94% of patients with localized disease are controlled at 5 years, as are 50% of patients with local and regional disease but unfortunately only 7% of those with distant disease. The survival data for Afro-Americans are more grave, with only 79% of patients with localized disease surviving at 5 years, 38% with local and regional disease, and 4% with disseminated disease. Even after 5 years, however, patients continue to fail not only locally and regionally but also with disseminated disease, thereby creating enigmas as to the continued influence of basic molecular changes, basic etiologic agents, and unsuspected more advanced disease, as well as demonstrating the inadequacies of local surgical treatment programs. These factors have led to braoder programs of combined integrated multimodal treatment earlier in the course of the disease process. Clearly, these newer innovative programs have placed increasing emphasis on the combination of surgery with radiation therapy and chemotherapy.

This volume addresses these issues in a highly scientific manner; in addition to offering new data relating to molecular and etiologic factors it outlines appropriate treatment programs with emphasis on efficacy, outcome, survival data, and risk of complications.

Philadelphia

L. W. Brady

Hamburg

H.-P. Heilmann

Preface

Urology and urologists along with medical oncologists, radiation oncologists, pathologists, epidemiologists, and more recently basic scientists have shared in the veritable explosion of scientific knowledge of bladder cancer that has occurred over the past fifteen years. This expansion has included the progressive development of improved and innovative surgical techniques, bladder replacement strategies, evolution of chemotherapy from single agent to innovative combinations with newer and hopefully better drugs on the horizon, a better understanding of the etiology and possible causative factors leading to the development of bladder cancer, and most recently the use of molecular biologic tools that allow us to better understand basic genetic differences that will predict progression and differentiate behavior between histologically similar appearing cancers.

Although the bladder site of origin of this malignancy is within the traditional domain of the urologist, it is clear that a single modality oriented approach to therapy – surgery versus chemotherapy versus irradiation – is outmoded. It is essential that the clinician caring for a patient diagnosed with bladder cancer be thoroughly familiar with current therapeutic options as they relate to outcome and quality of life. In addition, recent advances in molecular biology may yield important new information that will significantly affect future treatment decisions. We are entering an era of what we call translational research, where important basic science discoveries in the laboratory can immediately impact on patient care and become the focus for future clinical trials.

It is only natural at this time to update and summarize our current knowledge of bladder cancer. Drs. Petrovich, Baert, and Brady have assembled an impressive list of contributors and organized this book in an attempt to bring into focus, within a single authoritative volume, the various components of medical information covering all aspects of bladder cancer. It may be anticipated that this volume will have clinical relevance for any and all physicians concerned with the diagnosis and management of bladder cancer.

Los Angeles   DONALD G. SKINNER

Contents

1 Epidemiology of Bladder Cancer

M.C. Yu and R.K. Ross

CONTENTS

1.1
Introduction

Bladder cancer is the 11th most common cancer on a worldwide basis, accounting for 3%–4% of all malignancies. Annually, about 220 000 new cases are being diagnosed; three-fourths of the patients are men and a disproportional (two-thirds) number of cases occur in developed (as opposed to developing) countries (PARKIN et al. 1988).

The two most established etiologic risk factors for bladder cancer are cigarette smoking and occupational exposure to selected arylamines. Smoking is believed to account for at least 50% of all cases diagnosed among men in the United States today. Through regulatory standards established decades ago, occupational exposure to arylamines contributes minimally to current disease burden in developed countries, including the United States.

M.C. Yu, PhD, University of Southern California, USC/Norris Comprehensive Cancer Center, 1441 Eastlake Avenue, Los Angeles, CA 90033-0800, USA
R.K. Ross, MD, University of Southern California, USC/Norris Comprehensive Cancer Center, 1441 Eastlake Avenue, Los Angeles, CA 90033-0800, USA

Recent epidemiologic research on bladder cancer has focused on the role of tobacco-metabolizing genes in modifying the risk of smoking-induced bladder cancer. This emerging topic is reviewed in some detail, followed by a description of other proposed risk factors, including those that have been subsequently found to be minimally related or unrelated to human bladder cancer.

1.2
Demographic Patterns

1.2.1
Histopathology

The uroepithelial lining of the human bladder can become transformed to tumor cells with markedly different histopathologies. Approximately 90% of tumors of the urinary bladder in the United States are of transitional cell type, 7% are squamous, 2% are glandular, and 1% are undifferentiated (MOSTOFI et al. 1988). In contrast, in Egypt and parts of the Middle East, where infection with *Schistosoma haematobium* is endemic, squamous cell carcinomas of the bladder constitute 55%–80% of all bladder cancer diagnoses (BADAWI et al. 1995b).

Transitional cell carcinomas occur in at least three distinct morphological forms which have different natural histories and prognoses. Almost 80% of transitional cell bladder cancers diagnosed in the Western world are papillary noninfiltrating tumors. Another 3%–5% are nonpapillary and noninfiltrating (i.e., carcinoma in situ, CIS). The remaining transitional cell carcinomas invade into the underlying stroma of the bladder (MOSTOFI et al. 1988).

1.2.2
International Variation

Bladder cancer shows an almost tenfold international variation in incidence. High-risk populations include non-Latino whites in the United States and most Western Europeans with age-standardized rates in men clustering around 25/100 000 population per year. Asians (including Chinese, Japanese, and Indians) are at low risk for this malignancy, with annual age-standardized rates in men around 3–6 per 100 000 population (PARKIN et al. 1992).

1.2.3
Sex, Age, and Race

In nearly all populations, men are 2.5–5.0 times more likely to develop bladder cancer than women. Incidence of bladder cancer rises monotonically with age. The disease is rare prior to age 35, and two-thirds of the cases occur in people aged 65 or older (PARKIN et al. 1992; LIU et al. 1996).

There is marked racial-ethnic variation in bladder cancer incidence. In the United States, non-Latino white men possess the highest incidence of bladder cancer among all races. Their rate is twice those in Latino and African-American men, and 2.5 times higher than those in Chinese- and Japanese-American men. A similar pattern is observed in women although within race, the male rate is about 3–4 times higher than the female rate (LIU et al. 1996).

1.2.4
Time Trends

In the United States, bladder cancer incidence has been steadily increasing in both men and women during the past two decades. Between 1973 and 1992, male rates increased by 11% while female rates increased by 15%. On the other hand, mortality rates in both sexes declined during the same time period, by 22% in men and by 20% in women (KOSARY et al. 1995). The observed increase in incidence is suggested to be at least partly due to the increasing tendency by pathologists to classify noninvasive papillary transitional cell tumors as malignant (HANKEY et al. 1991). These noninvasive papillary tumors, however, share the same important risk factors with the invasive cancers (STURGEON et al. 1994). The decline in mortality rates is consistent with improved survival rates over the same period (HANKEY et al. 1991).

1.3
Genetic/Environmental Risk Factors

1.3.1
Occupational Exposures

The first known cause of human bladder cancer was occupational exposure to a class of chemicals known as the arylamines, which include the now established bladder carcinogens 2-naphthylamine, 4-aminobiphenyl, and benzidine. A comprehensive historical perspective on the association between human bladder cancer and arylamine exposure has been described by LOWER (1982). A century ago there was already anecdotal evidence that these chemicals might cause bladder cancer, with published case reports of bladder cancer occurring in workers in the textile dye industry, first in Europe and by the early 1900s in the United States as well. In the late 1930s, HUEPER et al. (1938) demonstrated that oral administration of the industrial arylamine used extensively in the textile dye industry, 2-naphthylamine, could induce bladder carcinomas in dogs. More than a decade would elapse, however, before the definitive epidemiologic study on this relationship was conducted by Case and colleagues in England. Using a traditional epidemiologic cohort study design, they showed that workers in the textile dye industry had a 20-fold excess risk of bladder cancer compared with the general population (CASE et al. 1954). Concurrently, these investigators demonstrated that workers in the rubber tire industry, in which 2-naphthylamine and benzidine were widely used, also were at substantially elevated risk of bladder cancer (CASE and HOSKER 1954). In the United States and most developed countries, industrial use of 2-napthylamine has been banned for over 40 years, and use of other established or suspected carcinogenic arylamines is under strict regulatory guidelines (The Baus Subcommittee on Industrial Bladder Cancer 1988). Thus, these potent causes of bladder cancer are not an important contributor to bladder cancer occurring today, at least in developed countries.

Several other occupational groups have been consistently shown to exhibit an elevated risk of bladder cancer, including truck drivers, leather workers, painters, and aluminum smelters (SILVERMAN et al. 1992). The causes of the enhanced bladder cancer risk among these workers are not known.

1.3.2
Cigarette Smoking

The epidemiologic literature on cigarette smoking and bladder cancer has been summarized in detail (Ross et al. 1988). Although new studies are regularly added to this already extensive database, the major conclusion has remained unaltered since the original observations of Lillienfeld et al. (1956). Cigarette smokers overall have an approximately twofold higher risk of bladder cancer than nonsmokers and risk increases with an increasing number of cigarettes smoked on a regular basis. This twofold excess risk and dose-responsive relationship with number of cigarettes smoked per day is consistently observed among both men and women and among populations characterized by either high or low population risk of bladder cancer. Prospective studies in which a large group of healthy individuals are characterized according to their smoking habits and then followed for various health outcomes have been particularly consistent in the magnitude of the elevated risk observed in smokers compared with nonsmokers (Hammond and Horn 1958; Kahn 1966; Hammond 1966; Weir and Dunn 1970; Doll and Peto 1976). All have found almost precisely a twofold risk elevation in smokers. Risk among ex-smokers is lower than among current smokers for a given duration and dose of smoking, but like other smoking-related cancers, risk does not appear to ever return to the baseline risk of lifetime nonsmokers (Weir and Dunn 1970). Bladder cancer risk is only weakly linked to pipe and cigar smoking and not at all to use of smokeless tobacco (Morrison et al. 1984).

An important unresolved issue is the mechanism by which cigarettes induce bladder cancer. Aromatic amines, including 2-naphthylamine and 4-aminobiphenyl, are present in tobacco smoke in small quantities and are the leading candidates as the specific etiologic agents (Patrianakos and Hoffmann 1979). Also tobacco tars can induce bladder papillomas and carcinomas in mice (Holsti and Ermala 1955).

While it is widely recognized that cigarette smoking is by far the most important contributor to bladder cancer development on a population basis and that roughly one-half of all bladder cancers occurring in U.S. men are due to this single cause (Doll and Peto 1981), a number of epidemiologic observations have suggested that one or several additional factors must play a role in modifying the risk of smoking-related bladder cancer. For example, lung cancer and bladder cancer mortality rates are only weakly correlated on an international basis in either men or women, a rather surprising observation considering that the major cause of both diseases is known to be cigarette smoking. Moreover, there exist populations around the world with very high smoking rates but relatively low bladder cancer rates. An outstanding illustration of this phenomenon is Polynesian men (including native Hawaiians and New Zealand Maoris) who have one of the lowest bladder cancer rates in the world despite a rather high prevalence of smoking. Maori men in New Zealand have a 50% higher smoking rate and thus, not surprisingly, twice the lung cancer rate relative to European men living there; yet the latter have over 3 times the rate of bladder cancer relative to the Maoris (Foster 1979). Similar examples can be found in the United States. In Los Angeles, African-American men have a slightly higher rate of smoking than non-Latino white, Japanese-American, or Chinese-American men, all of whom have a very similar smoking prevalence. However, non-Latino white men exhibit a bladder cancer rate that is twice that of African-Americans and 2.5 times those of the two Asian-American groups (Yu et al. 1994).

These seemingly disparate observations suggest one or a combination of the following possibilities: (1) that differences exist among populations in the metabolism of smoking-related carcinogens and that these differences may substantially alter risk of smoking-related bladder cancer; (2) that other exogenous agents (e.g., dietary factors) may modify susceptibility to smoking-induced bladder cancer; or (3) that there exist other, as yet unidentified, major causes of bladder cancer in the United States and elsewhere.

1.3.3
Alterations in Metabolism of Tobacco Carcinogens

Mommsen et al. (1982) first proposed that genetic factors might be involved in chemical-induced bladder cancer, through either cigarette smoking or occupational exposures. The carcinogenic arylamines present in cigarette smoke (or in the workplace) require metabolic activation to transform into fully carcinogenic agents. The first step in this process is N-oxidation which is catalyzed by the hepatic cytochrome P4501A2 isoenzyme (CYP1A2) (Butler et al. 1989). This enzyme system is inducible by a number of environmental factors, including cigarette smoking itself, so that there is tremendous individual and population variability in the activity of this enzyme (KALOW and TANG 1991). Urine-based assays, which employ caffeine as the test compound, are available to assess N-oxidation phenotype (TANG et al. 1994; BUTLER et al. 1992). Although there are no case-control data on CYP1A2 activity and bladder cancer risk, there is indirect evidence that CYP1A2 phenotype may be a risk factor for bladder cancer. KADERLIK and KADLUBAR (1995) analyzed aminobiphenyl (ABP) hemoglobin adduct levels in 47 cigarette smokers and 53 nonsmokers according to their N-acetyltransferase 2 (NAT2, see below) and CYP1A2 phenotypic profiles. Mean ABP-hemoglobin adduct levels were highest among individuals possessing the slow NAT2/rapid CYP1A2 phenotype, and lowest among those with the rapid NAT2/slow CYP1A2 profile. These data are suggestive of an N-oxidation effect on ABP-hemoglobin adduct levels that is independent of NAT2 phenotype.

Several case-control studies have examined the possible association between phenotype/genotype of other P450 enzymes and bladder cancer risk, as other such enzymes might be involved in the metabolic activation of bladder carcinogens. Using debrisoquine as a probe, KAISARY et al. (1987) reported a significant, positive association between high CYP2D6 activity and stage III bladder cancer; no such association was present in stage I/II bladder cancer. These authors later confirmed their results in a second case-control study conducted within the same target population (BRANCH et al. 1995). GOUGH et al. (1990) performed *CYP2D6* genotyping on 117 bladder cancer patients and 90 race-matched controls and reported a significant excess of extensive metabolizers among cases as compared to controls. On the other hand, CARTWRIGHT et al. (1984) had previously observed no relationship between debrisoquine oxidation phenotype and bladder cancer in their case-control study; tumor staging was not considered in this earlier study.

CYP3A4 activity (using dapsone as a probe) also has been studied in two case-control studies, and both noted a significant, negative association between high enzymatic activity and high-stage bladder cancer but no relationship with lower-stage tumors (BRANCH et al. 1995; FLEMING et al. 1994). In the same two studies, the relation between CYP2C19 activity (using mephenytoin as a probe) and bladder cancer risk was investigated and no association was observed.

The metabolically active form of the arylamines (the hydroxylamines) are electrophilic and can form adducts with hemoglobin and/or circulate freely or as their glucuronide conjugates and be excreted through the kidney (BRYANT et al. 1988). These latter compounds are hydrolyzed in the acidic environment of the bladder lumen, and with or without further bioactivation by N-acetyltransferase 1 (NAT1, see below) to form a highly electrophilic N-acetoxy derivative, can covalently bind to urothelial DNA. Misrepair of the damage to DNA induced by these adducts can lead to mutations in proto-oncogenes and/or tumor suppressor genes, a critical step in the process of changing a normal cell to a malignant phenotype (KADERLIK and KADLUBAR 1995). An examination of ABP hemoglobin adducts versus DNA adducts in exfoliated urothelial cells of cigarette smokers and nonsmokers has shown a close correlation between levels of the two adducts, thus establishing the former as a valid biomarker for ABP exposure in human studies (KADERLIK and KADLUBAR 1995).

Alternatively, arylamines can be catalyzed by competing detoxification pathways. The best established of these enzymatic pathways is N-acetylation, which is regulated by N-acetyltransferase activity in the liver. N-Acetyltransferase in humans is coded by two distinct genes, *NAT1* and *NAT2*. *NAT2*, a totally genetically regulated system, has long been known to exhibit polymorphism, and the NAT2 phenotype (rapid or slow acetylator) primarily reflects enzyme activity in the liver. A number of "mutant" alleles at the *NAT2* locus have been identified, and it has been shown that individuals possessing any two of these mutant alleles display a slow acetylator phenotype (and, therefore, detoxify carcinogenic arylamines less efficiently) (BELL et al. 1993a). A number of assays exist for NAT2 phenotypic determination, including two urine-based tests both of which employ caffeine as the test compound (BUTLER et al. 1992; TANG et al. 1991).

A number of case-control studies of bladder cancer have investigated the relationship between NAT2 phenotype and/or genotype and bladder cancer risk. HEIN (1988) combined data from 12 such studies and reported a statistically significant relative risk for bladder cancer of 1.5 in slow versus rapid acetylators. When the analysis was confined to patients with documented exposure to arylamines, the summary relative risk increased to 2.2. These results were confirmed by several more recent case-control studies which evaluated either NAT2 genotype or phenotype (BRANCH et al. 1995; RISCH et al. 1995). Not all studies have found such a relationship, however. One exception, for example, was a small case-control study of bladder cancer conducted among benzidine -exposed workers in China (HAYES et al. 1993). There was no difference in either the genotypic or the phenotypic prevalence of slow acetylators between 38 male bladder cancer cases and 43 age-matched male controls in this study. These negative results could be a chance finding due to the small study sample size. Alternatively, NAT2 may not be a risk factor in benzidine-induced bladder cancer. There is, in fact, some experimental evidence that N-acetylation is not a detoxification pathway for benzidine with regard to bladder carcinogenesis (HAYES et al. 1993).

It is relatively recently that NAT1 was shown to be polymorphic, and at least two selective probes have been identified (GRANT et al. 1992; WEBER and VATSIS 1993). Appreciable NAT1 but low NAT2 activities have been observed in bladder tissues or cells (KIRLIN et al. 1989; FREDERICKSON et al. 1994). Since O-acetylation of N-hydroxy arylamine in the bladder can lead to the highly electrophilic N-acetoxy derivative that covalently binds to urothelial DNA, rapid NAT1 genotype could be associated with an increased bladder cancer risk. BADAWI et al. (1995a) examined 26 human bladder mucosa and noted significant differences in NAT1 enzymatic activity and DNA adduct levels between individuals with varying alleles as defined by a sequence polymorphism in the 3' untranslated region of NAT1. Individuals positive for the variant NAT1*10 allele exhibited a twofold increase in both NAT1 enzyme activity and DNA adduct levels in their bladder mucosa relative to those who were homozygous for the putative wild-type NAT1*4 allele. Thus, available evidence suggests that individuals who inherit the slow NAT2 and rapid NAT1 genotypes are at an increased risk for bladder cancer.

As noted above, in Los Angeles, non-Latino white, African-American, and Asian men exhibit comparable smoking habits, but substantially different risks of bladder cancer. We have suggested that the varying prevalence of slow NAT2 acetylators in these racial-ethnic groups might be partly responsible for their disparate bladder cancer risk. We determined the NAT2 phenotype and levels of 3- and 4-ABP hemoglobin adducts in 133 male smokers and nonsmokers drawn from these various racial-ethnic groups in Los Angeles. Mean 3- and 4-ABP hemoglobin adduct levels were significantly higher in cigarette smokers relative to nonsmokers, and levels increased with increasing number of cigarettes

smoked per day. Importantly, this study found substantial variation in the prevalence rates of slow NAT2 acetylator phenotype among the races, which were as predicted by the varying incidence rates of bladder cancer among these populations (54% of whites were slow NAT2 acetylators as compared with 34% of African-Americans, and 14% of Asians). Slow NAT2 acetylators consistently exhibited higher mean levels of ABP-hemoglobin adducts relative to rapid NAT2 acetylators regardless of race and level of cigarette smoking (YU et al. 1994).

Glutathione S-transferase M1 (GSTM1) is part of a family of enzymes that detoxify reactive chemical entities by promoting their conjugation to glutathione (BOARD et al. 1990). GSTM1 is polymorphic in humans; about half of the non-Latino white population of the United States lack both copies of the gene and hence exhibit no GSTM1 enzymatic activity (BELL et al. 1993b; YU et al. 1995). Metabolites of several polycyclic aromatic hydrocarbons that are present in cigarette smoke are known substrates for GSTM1. Metabolites of other carcinogenic compounds in cigarette smoke, including the arylamines and nitrosamines, are also potential substrates (BOARD et al. 1990; BELL et al. 1993b). We expanded our earlier multiethnic survey in Los Angeles to investigate whether GSTM1 genotype influences ABP-hemoglobin adduct levels in smokers and nonsmokers, and whether the polymorphic GSTM1 is partly responsible for the differential bladder cancer risk among non-Latino white, African-American, and Asian-American men in Los Angeles. The findings were compatible with the hypothesis that GSTM1 is involved in the detoxification of ABP, and may contribute to the observed racial variation in the bladder cancer incidence in Los Angeles. There was a tenfold difference in the prevalence of the high-risk profile (slow NAT2, null GSTM1) among whites, blacks, and Asians: 27% in high-risk whites versus 15% in intermediate-risk blacks and 2.7% in low-risk Asians. Whites also had less than half the prevalence of the "protective" profile (rapid NAT2, non-null GSTM1) relative to blacks and Asians (23% versus 57%). Furthermore, irrespective of smoking status, mean ABP-hemoglobin adduct levels were highest in subjects possessing the high-risk profile and lowest in those with the "protective" profile, and the differences were statistically significant (Table 1.1) (YU et al. 1995).

A number of case-control studies conducted in U.S. and Western European populations have examined the possible protective role of GSTM1 in bladder cancer development. Most have reported a

Table 1.1. Geometric mean levels of 3- and 4-ABP hemoglobin adducts in nonsmokers and smokers by acetylator phenotype/*GSTM1* genotype[a]

Acetylator phenotype/ *GSTM1* genotype	Mean level (pg/g Hb)	95% Confidence interval
4-ABP Hb Adducts		
Smokers[b]		
Slow/null	125.0	(86.4, 180.8)
Slow/non-null or rapid/null	79.1	(62.6, 99.9)
Rapid/non-null	60.7	(46.9, 78.5)
Nonsmokers		
Slow/null	29.8	(22.0, 40.3)
Slow/non-null or rapid/null	24.1	(19.4, 29.9)
Rapid/non-null	19.6	(16.0, 24.0)
3-ABP Hb Adducts		
Smokers[b]		
Slow/null	12.3	(7.0, 21.1)
Slow/non-null or rapid/null	5.0	(3.4, 7.3)
Rapid/non-null	2.9	(1.7, 4.5)
Nonsmokers		
Slow/null	0.7	(0.5, 1.1)
Slow/non-null or rapid/null	0.2	(0.1, 0.4)
Rapid/non-null	0.1	(0.0, 0.3)

[a] With adjustment for race.
[b] Further adjusted for number of cigarettes smoked/day.

significant excess of GSTM1 null genotype/phenotype among bladder cancer cases relative to controls, with the larger studies consistently observing a relative risk for bladder cancer of about 1.5–1.7 in GSTM1 null individuals (BRANCH et al. 1995; BELL et al. 1993b; BROCKMOLLER et al. 1994; DALY et al. 1993; LAFUENTE et al. 1993; LIN et al. 1994).

1.3.4
Dietary Factors

1.3.4.1
Artificial Sweeteners

In the 1970s, a number of laboratory experiments showed that saccharin, a combination of cyclamate and saccharin, and a cyclamate metabolite can each induce bladder tumors in rats when given in very high doses (ARNOLD et al. 1977; U.S. Food and Drug Administration 1973; Wisconsin Alumni Research Foundation 1973; PRICE et al. 1970). Later studies showed that these compounds are also capable of promoting the effects of other animal carcinogens (HICKS and CHOWANIEC 1977; COHEN et al. 1979).

These experimental observations raised concerns that human exposure to these chemicals, although at levels many folds lower than those administered to experimental animals, may lead to bladder cancer development. A multicenter case-control study involving about 3000 bladder cancer patients and twice as many control subjects was initiated to specifically address this important public health question (HOOVER and STRASSER 1980). Altogether, a total of 15 case-control studies have examined the possible bladder cancer risk associated with intake of artificial sweeteners and the overall evidence does not indicate that such exposure is related to human bladder cancer (the meta-analysis-based combined relative risk from all studies is 0.98 for individuals reporting regular intake versus nonusers) (ELCOCK and MORGAN 1993).

1.3.4.2
Coffee

Caffeine is a mutagen in some in vitro systems and can increase the transformation rate of cells treated with chemical carcinogens (DONOVAN and DiPAOLO 1974). Whether coffee consumption is causally related to bladder cancer development has been intensely studied for the past 25 years. Ever since COLE (1971) reported an excess of daily coffee drinkers among bladder cancer patients (especially among women) relative to population controls of similar age and sex, close to 40 case-control and five cohort studies have examined this relationship. Some (HARTGE et al. 1983; D'AVANZO et al. 1992; VENA et al. 1993) but not all (JENSEN et al. 1986; MORGAN and JAIN 1974; MORRISON et al. 1982) subsequent studies show an increased risk for bladder cancer among daily coffee drinkers. However, even among the positive studies (which generally show only modest overall increased risks), most fail to observe consistent results between men and women and/or a clear dose-response relationship. VISCOLI et al. (1993) conducted a critical review of all published case-control studies with a summary analysis of all studies that met a standard set of design criteria. The authors reported a smoking-adjusted relative risk of 0.91 in women and 1.07 in men associated with daily coffee drinking. For drinkers of four or more cups per day, the relative risks were 0.94 and 1.16 in women and men, respectively. Results of cohort studies generally are in agreement with a lack of association between coffee drinking and bladder cancer in either sex. In a cohort of Seventh-Day Adventists, SNOWDON and

PHILLIPS (1984) observed a statistically non-significant 1.9-fold increased risk for fatal bladder cancer among those who drank two or more cups of coffee per day relative to non-daily drinkers, after adjustment for confounders. However, a later cohort study conducted in the same religious group failed to confirm this earlier finding – after adjustment for confounding factors, daily coffee drinkers had a relative risk of bladder cancer of 0.94 (MILLS et al. 1991). None of three other cohort studies reported a significant association between coffee consumption and bladder cancer incidence (NOMURA et al. 1986; JACOBSEN et al. 1986; STENSVOLD and JACOBSEN 1994).

1.3.4.3
Other Beverages

Other caffeine-containing beverages, including tea and cola, have been examined for their potential role in bladder cancer development. The data on tea are largely negative. JENSEN et al. (1986) noted a marginally significant association between tea drinking and bladder cancer in men but no such relationship in women. SLATTERY et al. (1988) reported a twofold increased risk for bladder cancer among daily tea drinkers versus non-tea drinkers, which was restricted to nonsmokers. No other study has found a relationship between tea consumption and bladder cancer risk, irrespective of cigarette smoking status (D'AVANZO et al. 1992; KUNZE et al. 1992; HOWE et al. 1980; SIMON et al. 1975; MORGAN and JAIN 1974). None of the studies which have examined a cola/bladder cancer link have reported a significant association between exposure and disease risk (MORGAN and JAIN 1974; HOWE et al. 1980; D'AVANZO et al. 1992; SLATTERY et al. 1988; JENSEN et al. 1986).

A number of studies have investigated the possible role of alcohol in human bladder cancer development (HOWE et al. 1980; HARRIS et al. 1990; NOMURA et al. 1989; THOMAS et al. 1983; BRAVO et al. 1987; SLATTERY et al. 1988; KUNZE et al. 1992). The overall evidence does not support a direct role of alcohol in human bladder carcinogenesis.

1.3.4.4
Other Dietary Factors

It has been hypothesized that vitamin A and the vitamin A precursor beta-carotene (or other carotenoids) may reduce the risk of epithelial cancers, including bladder cancer (PETO et al. 1981). In rodents, vitamin A analogs can prevent the induction of bladder cancer by chemical carcinogens, including N-nitrosamines (BECCI et al. 1978). Results of epidemiologic studies have been mixed. Some studies have found an increased risk of bladder cancer among individuals with a low intake of vitamin A and beta-carotene (METTLIN and GRAHAM 1979; PAGANINI-HILL et al. 1987) while others have observed no such associations (RISCH et al. 1988; NOMURA et al. 1991; RIBOLI et al. 1991).

N-nitrosamines are chemicals that can produce bladder cancer in rodents (MAGEE and BARNES 1967). Nitrosamines can be formed in vivo from ingested nitrates and secondary amines by nitrate-reducing bacteria in the human bladder, and vitamin C can block this in vivo nitrosamine formation. Again, results of epidemiologic studies have been mixed. WILKENS et al. (1996) compared dietary sources of nitrites and nitrosamines between bladder cancer cases and controls drawn from four race-gender groups in Hawaii (Japanese and Caucasian men and women), but noted a positive association between nitrite/nitrosamine intake and bladder cancer risk only in Japanese men. Several studies have examined the possible protective effect of dietary and supplemental vitamin C intake on bladder cancer risk. Results are mostly negative (RIBOLI et al. 1991; VENA et al. 1992; RISCH et al. 1988) or the inverse association has been present only in women and not men (NOMURA et al. 1991), or has been restricted to supplemental and not dietary intake (SHIBATA et al. 1992).

1.3.5
Drinking Water Contaminants

1.3.5.1
Chloroform/Other Chlorination By-products

Chlorine has been the method of choice for water purification since the early 1900s, and is currently added to approximately 75% of the drinking water supply in the U.S. (CANTOR 1983; MORRIS et al. 1992). The presence of chlorine and organic contaminants in water can lead to the formation of halogenated organic compounds such as chloroform and bromodichloromethane, which are rodent carcinogens (PAGE and SAFFIOTTI 1976; National Toxicology Program 1986). Due to a higher level of organic precursors in surface water that also is subjected to more intense chlorination, the content of such chlorination by-products is more than 60-fold higher in treated surface water relative to treated groundwater (CANTOR 1983), raising the possibility that individuals with long-term exposure to chlorinated surface water may experience an elevated bladder cancer risk. MORRIS et al. (1992) conducted a meta-analysis on results of the seven case-control studies of bladder cancer that have examined this relationship. Overall, there was a statistically significant 15% increase in bladder cancer risk associated with exposure to chlorinated surface water. There was a dose-response relationship between level of cumulative exposure and disease risk, with individuals in the highest exposure level possessing a 40% increase in bladder cancer risk relative to those in the lowest exposure category. A subsequent case-control study conducted in Colorado, where chloramination (addition of both ammonia and chlorine, which minimizes the formation of chlorination by-products) is also practiced, further confirmed the meta-analysis findings. Individuals with more than 30 years of exposure to chlorinated surface water were found to have an 80% higher risk for bladder cancer relative to those with no exposure (MCGEEHIN et al. 1993).

1.3.5.2
Inorganic Arsenic

Arsenic is a naturally occurring element whose inorganic form has long been known to cause lung (via inhalation) and skin (via ingestion) cancers in humans (IARC 1980). In the 1980s, a series of cancer mortality surveys conducted in an area of Taiwan known to have a very high prevalence (about 4 per 1000 population) of black foot disease, a peripheral vascular disorder that can result from chronic arsenic exposure, documented the high incidence of bladder cancer in this area (5–30 times higher than the rate for the general population of Taiwan). These residents also exhibit elevated rates of cancers of the lung, skin, liver, kidney, and prostate (CHEN et al. 1985, 1988). Many of the residents in this black foot disease-endemic area receive their drinking water supply from artesian wells with arsenic contents of 350–1140 µg per liter (CHEN et al. 1985). As a comparison, the U.S. Environmental Protection Agency standard for arsenic in drinking water is 50 µg/liter, and most drinking water supplies in the United States have levels that are below 5 µg/liter (SMITH et al. 1992). Subsequent case-control and cohort studies conducted in this high-risk population have consistently demonstrated a dose- and duration-

dependent association between consumption of artesian well water and bladder cancer risk, independent of cigarette smoking status (CHEN et al. 1986; CHIOU et al. 1995). There is no evidence that the relatively low level of arsenic in drinking water in the United States is associated with bladder cancer development (BATES et al. 1995).

Other populations have provided further support that inorganic arsenic is a human bladder carcinogen. TSUDA et al. (1995) followed residents of a Japanese town with known exposure to contaminated well water for 33 years and noted a 30-fold increased risk of bladder cancer among those in the highest exposure category. CUZICK et al. (1992) conducted a long-term follow-up of a cohort of English patients who had been treated with Fowler's solution (potassium arsenite) and observed a significant, threefold excess risk for bladder cancer in these patients. High levels of arsenic have been found in well water in certain regions of Argentina, and the degree of contamination of the local water supply has been shown to correlate closely with the rate of bladder cancer deaths in the population (HOPENHAYN-RICH et al. 1996).

1.3.6
Iatrogenic Factors

1.3.6.1
Analgesics

A series of case reports (BENGTSSON et al. 1968; ANGERVALL et al. 1969; HOYBYE and NIELSEN 1971) followed by several case-control studies (MCLAUGHLIN et al. 1983; MCCREDIE and STEWART 1988; ROSS et al. 1989) have linked heavy use of over-the-counter analgesics, especially those containing phenacetin, to cancer of the renal pelvis, which is histologically similar to most bladder cancers. Four case-control studies (FOKKENS 1979; HOWE et al. 1980; MCCREDIE et al. 1983; PIPER et al. 1985) have investigated the relationship between long-term use of analgesics and bladder cancer risk, with special reference to the major active ingredients of analgesics – aspirin, phenacetin, which has been banned from most Western countries since the late 1970s because of its carcinogenic potential to the lower urinary tract, and acetaminophen, which served as the phenacetin substitute in many analgesic brands after the ban but is itself a major metabolite of phenacetin in humans (BRODIE and AXELROD 1949). Three of these studies noted a statistically significant increased risk of 2.6- to 6.5-fold for bladder cancer among regular users of phenacetin-containing analgesics, but observed no association with usage of nonphenacetin products, including acetaminophen (FOKKENS 1979; McCREDIE et al. 1983; PIPER et al. 1985). HOWE et al. (1980) found no increase in bladder cancer risk among Canadian subjects who regularly used phenacetin-containing analgesics but did note a marginally significant 50% elevation in risk among men who regularly used aspirin-containing products. However, no parallel increase in bladder cancer risk was observed in female regular users of aspirin-containing products. We recently completed a case-control study of bladder cancer in Los Angeles which was specifically designed to address the analgesic/bladder cancer association and involved over 1200 patient-control pairs. We found no relationship between regular use of analgesics of any kind and bladder cancer risk in this large-scale study (YU and Ross, unpublished data). Thus, present evidence does not implicate nonphenacetin analgesic use as an important risk factor for human bladder cancer development.

1.3.6.2
Cyclophosphamide/Chlornaphazine

Cyclophosphamide and chlornaphazine are alkylating agents that have been used to treat malignant as well as nonmalignant diseases. Both agents are experimental tumorigens. Follow-up studies of patients treated with these two agents have definitively linked them to human bladder cancer development (IARC 1982).

1.3.7
Schistosoma haematobium

In many animal systems, including primates, chronic infection with S. haematobium can lead to bladder cancer that is morphologically similar to that seen in humans (BADAWI et al. 1995b). Schistosomiasis is hyperendemic in Egypt and parts of the Middle East, where bladder cancer is among the top three most frequently diagnosed cancers. The histologic profile of the disease in these regions is distinct in that over two-thirds of the cases are squamous cell carcinomas (as compared to 5% in the United States). Cases are mainly diagnosed between ages 40 and 49 years, considerably younger than those occurring in schistosomiasis-free areas

(BADAWI et al. 1995b). Case-control studies conducted in high infection areas have consistently shown a significant positive association between a history of infection and bladder cancer risk in both men and women, with relative risks ranging from about 4.5 to 23.5 (VIZCAINO et al. 1994). Recently, it was found that levels of nitrate, nitrite, and N-nitrosamines are significantly higher in the urine of infected versus uninfected individuals, raising the possibility that N-nitroso compounds (which, as noted above, are bladder carcinogens in rodents) may be involved in schistosomiasis-associated bladder cancer (MOSTAFA et al. 1994).

1.3.8
Hair Dyes

A number of active ingredients in the two main types of hair dyes, the permanent and semi-permanent dyes, are mutagens (AMES et al. 1975) and animal carcinogens (IARC 1993). These observations became especially relevant when it was noted that individuals with occupational exposure to these chemicals (hairdressers, barbers, and beauticians) are at an elevated risk for bladder cancer (DUNHAM et al. 1968; ANTHONY and THOMAS 1970; LA VECCHIA and TAVANI 1995). However, results of several epidemiologic studies examining personal use of hair dyes and bladder cancer, including one involving nearly 3000 cases and 5800 controls, have failed to demonstrate an increased risk among users (HARTGE et al. 1982; LA VECCHIA and TAVANI 1995).

References

Ames BN, Kammen HO, Yamasaki E (1975) Hair dyes are mutagenic: identification of a variety of mutagenic ingredients. Proc Natl Acad Sci USA 72:2423–2427

Angervall L, Bengtsson U, Zetterlund CG, Zsigmond M (1969) Renal pelvic carcinoma in a Swedish district with abuse of a phenacetin-containing drug. Br J Urol 41:401–405

Anthony HM, Thomas GM (1970) Tumors of the urinary bladder: an analysis of the occupations of 1,030 patients in Leeds, England. J Natl Cancer Inst 45:879–895

Arnold DL, Moodie CA, Grice HC, et al. (1977) Long-term toxicity of ortho-toluene sulfonamide and sodium saccharin in the rat: an interim report. Toxicology Research Division, Health Protection Branch, National Health and Welfare Ministry, Ottawa, Canada

Badawi AF, Hirvonen A, Bell DA, Lang NP, Kadlubar FF (1995a) Role of aromatic amine acetyltransferases, NAT1 and NAT2, in carcinogen-DNA adduct formation in the human urinary bladder. Cancer Res 55:5230–5237

Badawi AF, Mostafa MH, Probert A, O'Connor PJ (1995b) Role of schistosomiasis in human bladder cancer: evidence of association, aetiological factors, and basic mechanisms of carcinogenesis. Eur J Cancer Prev 4:45–59

Bates MN, Smith AH, Cantor KP (1995) Case-control study of bladder cancer and arsenic in drinking water. Am J Epidemiol 141:523–530

Bell DA, Taylor JA, Butler MA, et al. (1993a) Genotype/phenotype discordance for human arylamine N-acetyltransferase (NAT2) reveals a new slow-acetylator allele common in African-Americans. Carcinogenesis 14:1689–1692

Bell DA, Taylor JA, Paulson DF, Robertson CN, Mohler JL, Lucier GW (1993b) Genetic risk and carcinogen exposure: a common inherited defect of the carcinogen-metabolism gene glutathione S-transferase M1 (GSTM1) that increases susceptibility to bladder cancer. J Natl Cancer Inst 85:1159–1164

Bengtsson U, Angervall L, Ekman H, Lehmann L (1968) Transitional cell tumors of the renal pelvis in analgesic abusers. Scand J Urol Nephrol 2:145–150

Board P, Coggan M, Johnston P, Ross V, Suzuki T, Webb G (1990) Genetic heterogeneity of the human glutathione transferases: a complex of gene families. Pharmacol Ther 48:357–369

Branch RA, Chern HD, Adedoyin A, et al. (1995) The procarcinogen hypothesis for bladder cancer: activities of individual drug metabolizing enzymes as risk factors. Pharmacogenetics 5:S97–S102

Bravo MP, Del Rey Calero J, Conde M (1987) Bladder cancer and the consumption of alcoholic beverages in Spain. Eur J Epidemiol 3:365–369

Brockmoller J, Kerb R, Drakoulis N, Staffeldt B, Roots I (1994) Glutathione S-transferase M1 and its variants A and B as host factors of bladder cancer susceptibility: a case-control study. Cancer Res 54:4103–4111

Brodie BB, Axelrod J (1949) The fate of acetophenetidin (phenacetin) in man and methods for the estimation of acetophenetidin and its metabolites in biological material. J Pharmacol Exp Ther 97:58–67

Bryant MS, Vineis P, Skipper PL, Tannenbaum SR (1988) Hemoglobin adducts of aromatic amines: associations with smoking status and type of tobacco. Proc Natl Acad Sci USA 85:9788–9791

Butler MA, Iwasaki M, Guengerich FP, Kadlubar FF (1989) Human cytochrome P450PA (P4501A2), the phenacetin O-deethylase, is primarily responsible for the hepatic 3-demethylation of caffeine and N-oxidation of carcinogenic arylamines. Proc Natl Acad Sci USA 86:7696–7700

Butler MA, Lang NP, Young JF, et al. (1992) Determination of CYP1A2 and NAT2 phenotypes in human populations by analysis of caffeine urinary metabolites. Pharmacogenetics 2:116–127

Cantor KP (1983) Epidemiologic studies of chlorination by-products in drinking water: an overview. In: Jolly RL (ed) Water chlorination: environmental impact and health effects, 4th edn. Ann Arbor Scientific Publishers, Ann Arbor, Michigan, p 1381

Cartwright RA, Philip PA, Rogers HJ, Glashan RW (1984) Genetically determined debrisoquine oxidation capacity in bladder cancer. Carcinogenesis 5:1191–1192

Case RAM, Hosker ME (1954) Tumour of the urinary bladder as an occupational disease in the rubber industry in England and Wales. Br J Prev Soc Med 8:39–50

Case RAM, Hosker ME, McDonald DB, Pearson JT (1954) Tumours of the urinary bladder in workmen engaged in the manufacture and use of certain dyestuff intermediates in the British chemical industry. I. The role of aniline, benzidine, alpha-naphthylamine, and beta-naphthylamine. Br J Ind Med 11:75–104

Chen C-J, Chuang Y-C, Lin T-M, Wu H-Y (1985) Malignant neoplasms among residents of a blackfoot disease-endemic area in Taiwan: high-arsenic artesian well water and cancers. Cancer Res 45:5895–5899

Chen C-J, Chuang Y-C, You S-L, Lin T-M, Wu H-Y (1986) A retrospective study on malignant neoplasms of bladder, lung and liver in blackfoot disease endemic area in Taiwan. Br J Cancer 53:399–405

Chen C-J, Kuo T-L, Wu M-M (1988) Arsenic and cancers. Lancet I:414–415

Chiou H-Y, Hsueh Y-M, Liaw K-F, et al. (1995) Incidence of internal cancers and ingested inorganic arsenic: a seven-year follow-up study in Taiwan. Cancer Res 55:1296–1300

Cohen SM, Arai M, Jacobs JB, Friedell GH (1979) Promoting effect of saccharin and DL-tryptophan in urinary bladder carcinogenesis. Cancer Res 39:1207–1217

Cole P (1971) Coffee-drinking and cancer of the lower urinary tract. Lancet 1:1335–1337

Cuzick J, Sasieni P, Evans S (1992) Ingested arsenic, keratoses, and bladder cancer. Am J Epidemiol 136:417–421

Daly AK, Thomas DJ, Cooper J, Pearson WR, Neal DE, Idle JR (1993) Homozygous deletion of gene for glutathione S-transferase M1 in bladder cancer. BMJ 307:481–482

D'Avanzo B, La Vecchia C, Franceschi S, Negri E, Talamini R, Buttino I (1992) Coffee consumption and bladder cancer risk. Eur J Cancer 28A:1480–1484

Doll R, Peto R (1976) Mortality in relation to smoking: 20 years' observations on male British doctors. BMJ 2:1525–1536

Doll R, Peto R (1981) The causes of cancer: quantitative estimates of avoidable risks of cancer in the United States today. J Natl Cancer Inst 66:1191–1308

Donovan PJ, DiPaolo JA (1974) Caffeine enhancement of chemical carcinogen-induced transformation of cultured Syrian hamster cells. Cancer Res 34:2720–2727

Dunham LJ, Rabson AS, Stewart HL, Frank AS (1968) Rates, interview, and pathology study of cancer of the urinary bladder in New Orleans, Louisiana. J Natl Cancer Inst 41:683–709

Elcock M, Morgan RW (1993) Update on artificial sweeteners and bladder cancer. Regul Toxicol Pharmacol 17:35–43

Fleming CM, Persad R, Kaisary A, et al. (1994) Low activity of dapsone N-hydroxylation as a susceptibility risk factor in aggressive bladder cancer. Pharmacogenetics 4:199–207

Fokkens W (1979) Phenacetin abuse related to bladder cancer. Environ Res 20:192–198

Foster F (1979) New Zealand cancer registry report. Natl Cancer Inst Monogr 53:79–80

Frederickson SM, Messing EM, Reznikoff CA, Swaminathan S (1994) Relationship between in vivo acetylator phenotypes and cytosolic N-acetyltransferase and O-acetyltransferase activities in human urothelial cells. Cancer Epidemiol Biomarkers Prev 3:25–32

Gough AC, Miles JS, Spurr NK, Moss JE, Gaedigk A, Eichelbaum M, Wolf CR (1990) Identification of the primary gene defect at the cytochrome P450 CYP2D locus. Nature 347:773–776

Grant DM, Vohra P, Avis Y, Ima A (1992) Detection of a new polymorphism of human arylamine N-acetyltransferase NAT1 using p-aminosalicylic acid as an in vivo probe. J Basic Clin Physiol Pharmacol (Suppl) 3:244

Hammond EC (1966) Smoking in relation to the death rates of one million men and women. Natl Cancer Inst Monogr 19:127–204

Hammond EC, Horn D (1958) Smoking and death rates – report on forty-four months of follow-up of 187,783 men. II. Death rates by cause. JAMA 166:1294–1308

Hankey BF, Edwards BK, Ries LA, Percy CL, Shambaugh E (1991) Problems in cancer surveillance: delineating in situ and invasive bladder cancer. J Natl Cancer Inst 83:384–385

Harris RE, Chen-Backlund J-Y, Wynder EL (1990) Cancer of the urinary bladder in blacks and whites: a case-control study. Cancer 66:2673–2680

Hartge P, Hoover R, Altman R, et al. (1982) Use of hair dyes and risk of bladder cancer. Cancer Res 42:4784–4787

Hartge P, Hoover R, West DW, Lyon JL (1983) Coffee drinking and risk of bladder cancer. J Natl Cancer Inst 70:1021–1026

Hayes RB, Bi W, Rothman N, et al. (1993) N-acetylation phenotype and genotype and risk of bladder cancer in benzidine-exposed workers. Carcinogenesis 14:675–678

Hein DW (1988) Acetylator genotype and arylamine-induced carcinogenesis. Biochim Biophys Acta 948:37–66

Hicks RM, Chowaniec J (1977) The importance of synergy between weak carcinogens in the induction of bladder cancer in experimental animals and humans. Cancer Res 37:2943–2949

Holsti LR, Ermala P (1955) Papillary carcinoma of the bladder in mice, obtained after peroral administration of tobacco tar. Cancer 8:679–682

Hoover RN, Strasser PH (1980) Artificial sweeteners and human bladder cancer: preliminary results. Lancet I:837–840

Hopenhayn-Rich C, Biggs ML, Fuchs A, Bergoglio R, Tello EE, Nicolli H, Smith AH (1996) Bladder cancer mortality associated with arsenic in drinking water in Argentina. Epidemiology 7:117–124

Howe GR, Burch JD, Miller AB, et al. (1980) Tobacco use, occupation, coffee, various nutrients, and bladder cancer. J Natl Cancer Inst 64:701–713

Hoybye G, Nielsen OE (1971) Renal pelvic carcinoma in phenacetin abusers. Scand J Urol Nephrol 5:190–192

Hueper WC, Wiley FH, Wolfe HD (1938) Experimental production of bladder tumors in dogs by administration of beta-naphthylamine. J Industr Hyg Toxicol 20:46–84

IARC Monographs on the Evaluation of Carcinogenic Risks to Humans, vol 23 (1980) Some metals and metallic compounds. International Agency for Research on Cancer, Lyon

IARC Monographs on the Evaluation of Carcinogenic Risks to Humans (Suppl no. 4) (1982) Chemicals, industrial processes and industries associated with cancer in humans. International Agency for Research on Cancer, Lyon

IARC Monographs on the Evaluation of Carcinogenic Risks to Humans, vol 57 (1993) Occupational exposures of hairdressers and barbers and personal use of hair colourants; some hair dyes, cosmetic colourants, industrial dyestuffs and aromatic amines. International Agency for Research on Cancer, Lyon

Jacobsen BK, Bjelke E, Kvale G, Heuch I (1986) Coffee drinking, mortality, and cancer incidence: results from a Norwegian prospective study. J Natl Cancer Inst 76:823–831

Jensen OM, Wahrendorf J, Knudsen JB, Sorensen BL (1986) The Copenhagen case-control study of bladder cancer. II. Effect of coffee and other beverages. Int J Cancer 37:651–657

Kaderlik KR, Kadlubar FF (1995) Metabolic polymorphisms and carcinogen-DNA adduct formation in human populations. Pharmacogenetics 5:S108–S117

Kahn HA (1966) The Dorn study of smoking and mortality among U.S. veterans: report on eight and one-half years of observation. Natl Cancer Inst Monogr 19:1–125

Kaisary A, Smith P, Jacqz E, McAllister CB, Wilkinson GR, Ray WA, Branch RA (1987) Genetic predisposition to bladder cancer: ability to hydroxylate debrisoquine and mephenytoin as risk factors. Cancer Res 47:5488–5493

Kalow W, Tang BK (1991) Caffeine as a metabolic probe: exploration of the enzyme-inducing effect of cigarette smoking. Clin Pharmacol Ther 49:44–48

Kirlin WG, Trinidad A, Yerokun T, et al. (1989) Polymorphic expression of acetyl coenzyme A-dependent O-acetyltransferase-mediated activation of N-hydroxyarylamines by human bladder cytosols. Cancer Res 49:2448–2454

Kosary CL, Ries LAG, Miller BA, Hankey BF, Harras A, Edwards BK (1995) SEER cancer statistics review, 1973–1992: tables and graphs. NIH Pub No 96–2789. National Cancer Institute, Bethesda, Maryland

Kunze E, Chang-Claude J, Frentzel-Beyme R (1992) Life style and occupational risk factors for bladder cancer in Germany. Cancer 69:1776–1790

La Vecchia C, Tavani A (1995) Epidemiological evidence on hair dyes and the risk of cancer in humans. Eur J Cancer Prev 4:31–43

Lafuente A, Pujol F, Carretero P, Villa JP, Cuchi A (1993) Human glutathione S-transferase u (GSTu) deficiency as a marker for the susceptibility to bladder and larynx cancer among smokers. Cancer Lett 68:49–54

Lillienfeld AM, Levin ML, Moore GE (1956) The association of smoking with cancer of the urinary bladder in humans. Arch Intern Med 98:129–135

Lin HJ, Han C-Y, Bernstein DA, Hsiao W, Lin BK, Hardy S (1994) Ethnic distribution of the glutathione transferase mu 1-1 (GSTM1) null genotype in 1473 individuals and application to bladder cancer susceptibility. Carcinogenesis 15:1077–1081

Liu L, Deapen D, Bernstein L, Ross R (1996) Cancer incidence in Los Angeles County by race/ethnicity, 1988–1993. Los Angeles County Cancer Surveillance Program, University of Southern California, Los Angeles

Lower GM (1982) Concepts in causality: chemically induced human urinary bladder cancer. Cancer 49:1056–1066

Magee PN, Barnes JM (1967) Carcinogenic nitroso compounds. Adv Cancer Res 10:163–246

McCredie M, Stewart JH (1988) Does paracetamol cause urothelial cancer or renal papillary necrosis? Nephron 49:296–300

McCredie M, Stewart JH, Ford JM, MacLennan RA (1983) Phenacetin-containing analgesics and cancer of the bladder or renal pelvis in women. Br J Urol 55:220–224

McGeehin MA, Reif JS, Becher JC, Mangione EJ (1993) Case-control study of bladder cancer and water disinfection methods in Colorado. Am J Epidemiol 138:492–501

McLaughlin JK, Blot WJ, Mandel JS, Schuman LM, Mehl ES, Fraumeni JF (1983) Etiology of cancer of the renal pelvis. J Natl Cancer Inst 71:287–291

Mettlin C, Graham S (1979) Dietary risk factors in human bladder cancer. Am J Epidemiol 110:255–263

Mills PK, Beeson WL, Phillips RL, Fraser GE (1991) Bladder cancer in a low risk population: results from the Adventist Health Study. Am J Epidemiol 133:230–239

Mommsen S, Sell A, Barfod N (1982) N-Acetyltransferase phenotypes of bladder cancer patients in a low risk population. Lancet II:1228

Morgan RW, Jain MG (1974) Bladder cancer: smoking, beverages and artificial sweeteners. J Can Med Assoc 111:1067–1070

Morris RD, Audet A-M, Angelillo IF, Chalmers TC, Mosteller F (1992) Chlorination, chlorination by-products, and cancer: a meta-analysis. Am J Public Health 82:955–963

Morrison AS, Buring JE, Verhoek WG, Aoki K, Leck I, Ohno Y, Obata K (1982) Coffee drinking and cancer of the lower urinary tract. J Natl Cancer Inst 68:91–94

Morrison AS, Buring JE, Verhoek WG, Aoki K, Leck I, Ohno Y, Obata K (1984) An international study of smoking and bladder cancer. J Urol 131:650–654

Mostafa MH, Helmi S, Badawi AF, Tricker AR, Spiegelhalder B, Preussmann R (1994) Nitrate, nitrite and volatile N-nitroso compounds in the urine of Schistosoma haematobium and Schistosoma mansoni infected patients. Carcinogenesis 15:619–625

Mostofi FK, Davis CJ, Sesterhenn IA (1988) Pathology of tumors of the urinary tract. In: Skinner DG, Lieskovsky G (eds) Diagnosis and management of genitourinary cancer. Saunders Philadelphia, pp 83–117

National Toxicology Program (1986) Technical report on the toxicology and carcinogenesis studies of bromodichloromethane. NIH Publication No. 86-2577. National Toxicology Program, National Institutes of Health, Research Triangle Park, North Carolina

Nomura A, Heilbrun LK, Stemmermann GN (1986) Prospective study of coffee consumption and the risk of cancer. J Natl Cancer Inst 76:587–590

Nomura A, Kolonel LN, Yoshizawa CN (1989) Smoking, alcohol, occupation, and hair dye use in cancer of the lower urinary tract. Am J Epidemiol 130:1159–1163

Nomura AMY, Kolonel LN, Hankin JH, Yoshizawa CN (1991) Dietary factors in cancer of the lower urinary tract. Int J Cancer 48:199–205

Paganini-Hill A, Chao A, Ross RK, Henderson BE (1987) Vitamin A, β-carotene, and the risk of cancer: a prospective study. J Natl Cancer Inst 79:443–448

Page NP, Saffiotti U (1976) Report on the carcinogenesis bioassay of chloroform. PB-264-018. Division of Cancer Cause and Prevention, National Cancer Institute, Bethesda, Maryland

Parkin DM, Laara E, Muir CS (1988) Estimates of the worldwide frequency of sixteen major cancers in 1980. Int J Cancer 41:184–197

Parkin DM, Muir CS, Whelan SL, Gao Y-T, Ferlay J, Powell J (1992) Cancer incidence in five continents, vol VI. IARC Scientific Publications no. 120, International Agency for Research on Cancer, Lyon

Patrianakos C, Hoffmann D (1979) Chemical studies on tobacco smoke LXIV: on the analysis of aromatic amines in cigarette smoke. J Anal Toxicol 3:150–154

Peto R, Doll R, Buckley JD, Sporn MB (1981) Can dietary beta-carotene materially reduce human cancer rates? Nature 290:201–208

Piper JM, Tonascia J, Matanoski GM (1985) Heavy phenacetin use and bladder cancer in women aged 20 to 49 years. N Engl J Med 313:292–295

Price JM, Biava CG, Oser BL, Vogin EE, Steinfeld J, Ley HL (1970) Bladder tumors in rats fed cyclohexylamine or high doses of a mixture of cyclamate and saccharin. Science 167:1131–1132

Riboli E, Gonzalez CA, Lopez-Abente G, et al. (1991) Diet and bladder cancer in Spain: a multi-centre case-control study. Int J Cancer 49:214–219

Risch A, Wallace DMA, Bathers S, Sim E (1995) Slow N-acetylation genotype is a susceptibility factor in occupational and smoking related bladder cancer. Hum Mol Genet 4:231–236

Risch HA, Burch JD, Miller AB, Hill GB, Steele R, Howe GR (1988) Dietary factors and the incidence of cancer of the urinary bladder. Am J Epidemiol 127:1179–1191

Ross RK, Paganini-Hill A, Henderson BE (1988) Epidemiology of bladder cancer. In: Skinner DG, Lieskovsky G (eds) Diagnosis and management of genitourinary cancer. Saunders Philadelphia, pp 23–31

Ross RK, Paganini-Hill A, Landolph J, Gerkins V, Henderson BE (1989) Analgesics, cigarette smoking, and other risk factors for cancer of the renal pelvis and ureter. Cancer Res 49:1045–1048

Shibata A, Paganini-Hill A, Ross RK, Henderson BE (1992) Intake of vegetables, fruits, beta-carotene, vitamin C and vitamin supplements and cancer incidence among the elderly: a prospective study. Br J Cancer 66:673–679

Silverman DT, Hartge P, Morrison AS, Devesa SS (1992) Epidemiology of bladder cancer. Hematol Oncol Clin North Am 6:1–30

Simon D, Yen S, Cole P (1975) Coffee drinking and cancer of the lower urinary tract. J Natl Cancer Inst 54:587–591

Slattery ML, West DW, Robison LM (1988) Fluid intake and bladder cancer in Utah. Int J Cancer 42:17–22

Smith AH, Hopenhayn-Rich C, Bates MN, et al. (1992) Cancer risks from arsenic in drinking water. Environ Health Perspect 97:259–267

Snowdon DA, Phillips RL (1984) Coffee consumption and risk of fatal cancers. Am J Public Health 74:820–823

Stensvold I, Jacobsen BK (1994) Coffee and cancer: a prospective study of 43,000 Norwegian men and women. Cancer Causes Control 5:401–408

Sturgeon SR, Hartge P, Silverman DT, Kantor AF, Linehan WM, Lynch C, Hoover RN (1994) Associations between bladder cancer risk factors and tumor stage and grade at diagnosis. Epidemiology 5:218–225

Tang BK, Kadar D, Qian L, Iriah J, Yip J, Kalow W (1991) Caffeine as a metabolic probe: validation of its use for acetylator phenotyping. Clin Pharmacol Ther 49:648–657

Tang BK, Zhou Y, Kadar D, Kalow W (1994) Caffeine as a probe for CYP1A2 activity: potential influence of renal factors on urinary phenotypic trait measurements. Pharmacogenetics 4:117–124

The Baus Subcommittee on Industrial Bladder Cancer (1988) Occupational bladder cancer: a guide for clinicians. Br J Urol 61:183–191

Thomas DB, Uhl CN, Hartge P (1983) Bladder cancer and alcoholic beverage consumption. Am J Epidemiol 118:720–727

Tsuda T, Babazono A, Yamamoto E, et al. (1995) Ingested arsenic and internal cancer: a historical cohort study followed for 33 years. Am J Epidemiol 141:198–209

U.S. Food and Drug Administration (1973) Histopathologic evaluation of tissues from rats following continuous dietary intake of sodium saccharin and calcium cyclamate for a maximum period of two years: final report. Project P-169-170. U.S. Department of Health, Education and Welfare, Washington, D.C.

Vena JE, Graham S, Freudenheim J, Marshall J, Zielezny M, Swanson M, Sufrin G (1992) Diet in the epidemiology of bladder cancer in western New York. Nutr Cancer 18:255–264

Vena JE, Freudenheim J, Graham S, Marshall J, Zielezny M, Swanson M, Sufrin G (1993) Coffee, cigarette smoking, and bladder cancer in western New York. Ann Epidemiol 3:586–591

Viscoli CM, Lachs MS, Horwitz RI (1993) Bladder cancer and coffee drinking: a summary of case-control research. Lancet 341:1432–1437

Vizcaino AP, Parkin DM, Boffetta P, Skinner MEG (1994) Bladder cancer: epidemiology and risk factors in Bulawayo, Zimbabwe. Cancer Causes Control 5:517–522

Weber WW, Vatsis KP (1993) Individual variability in p-aminobenzoic acid N-acetylation by human N-acetyltransferase (NAT1) of peripheral blood. Pharmacogenetics 3:209–212

Weir JM, Dunn JE (1970) Smoking and mortality: a prospective study. Cancer 25:105–112

Wilkens LR, Kadir MM, Kolonel LN, Nomura AMY, Hankin JH (1996) Risk factors for lower urinary tract cancer: the role of total fluid consumption, nitrites and nitrosamines, and selected foods. Cancer Epidemiol Biomarkers Prev 5:161–166

Wisconsin Alumni Research Foundation (1973) Long term saccharin feeding in rats: final report. WARF, Madison, Wisconsin

Yu MC, Skipper PL, Taghizadeh K, Tannenbaum SR, Chan KK, Henderson BE, Ross RK (1994) Acetylator phenotype, aminobiphenyl-hemoglobin adduct levels, and bladder cancer risk in white, black, and Asian men in Los Angeles, California. J Natl Cancer Inst 86:712–716

Yu MC, Ross RK, Chan KK, Henderson BE, Skipper PL, Tannenbaum SR, Coetzee GA (1995) Glutathione S-transferase M1 genotype affects aminobiphenyl-hemoglobin adduct levels in white, black, and Asian smokers and non-smokers. Cancer Epidemiol Biomarkers Prev 4:861–864

2 Natural History of Bladder Carcinoma

Z. Petrovich and L. Baert

CONTENTS

2.1 Introduction

Carcinoma of the bladder is a common malignancy of the genitourinary tract. In the United States in 1996, this cancer is expected to be the second genitourinary tumor in incidence and the third in mortality (Tables 2.1, 2.2) (Parker et al. 1996). The incidence of bladder cancer has been relatively stable in the United States, with only about a 7% increase since 1990 (Silverberg et al. 1990). In the past 30 years, however, a sharp increase has been observed in the incidence of survival for this disease. In the U.S. Caucasian population, the 5-year survival rate in the early 1960s was 53%, while it was 82% in 1991 (Parker et al. 1996). Much lower survival rates were recorded in patients with muscle invasive disease. Similar incidence and mortality statistics for bladder cancer have been seen in the European Community. In the United Kingdom, however, there was a 31% increase in the overall incidence of bladder cancer between 1971 and 1984 and a 22% increase in mortality (Office of Population Consensus and Studies 1987).

Carcinoma of the bladder is one of the few tumors where a strong link to environmental and occupational factors was identified more than 100 years ago (Rehn 1895). Recognition of this link and the identification of these environmental and occupational factors is of major importance since it permits appropriate preventive measures to be applied. There is, however, a problem with the application of preventive measures since in 75% of patients with carcinoma of the bladder no occupational or environmental causative factors can be identified. In this group of patients, no apparent carcinogens can be identified (Branch et al. 1995). An additional factor which complicates the introduction of preventive measures is a very long latent period between exposure to carcinogen(s) and the development of carcinoma of the bladder. This period of latency may extend to up to 40 years (Cohen and Johansson 1992) (see Chap. 1 for details).

2.2 Causative Factors

Since the publication of a classic paper late in the nineteenth century postulating a higher incidence of bladder cancer among aniline dye workers, multiple occupational, environmental, and genetic factors have been identified (Rhen 1895). These factors include the following: chemical dye exposure, 2-naphthylamine, 4-aminobiphenyl, benzidine, environmental arylamines, cigarette smoke, caffeine in male patients and parous women, inorganic arsenic,

Z. Petrovich, MD, FACR, Professor and Chairman, Department of Radiation Oncology, University of Southern California, USC/Norris Comprehensive Cancer Center, 1441 Eastlake Avenue, Los Angeles, CA 90033, USA
L. Baert, MD, PhD, Professor and Chairman, Department of Urology, UZ Gasthuisberg, University Hospitals of Leuven, Herestraat 49, B-3000 Leuven, Belgium and Clinical Professor, Department of Urology and Radiation Oncology, University of Southern California, USC/Norris Comprehensive Cancer Center, 1441 Eastlake Avenue, Los Angeles, CA 90033, USA

Table 2.1. Expected incidence of genitourinary cancer in 1996

Site	Female	Male	Total
Prostate	–	317 100	317 100
Bladder	14 600	38 300	*52 900*
Kidney	12 100	18 500	30 600
Testis	–	8 600	8 600
Total	26 700	382 500	409 200

Table 2.2. Expected genitourinary cancer mortality in 1996

Site	Female	Male	Total
Prostate	–	41 400	41 400
Kidney	4 700	7 300	12 000
Bladder	*3 900*	*7 800*	*11 700*
Testis	–	590	590
Total	8 600	57 090	65 690

end-stage analgesic nephropathy, carcinoma of the colon, and many others (CHIOU et al. 1995; HORN et al. 1995; RISCH et al. 1995; SLATTERY et al. 1995; THON et al. 1995).

Cigarette smoking has been shown to be a highly significant factor in the induction of carcinoma of the bladder. There is a good correlation between duration and severity of exposure to smoking and the incidence of this tumor (MOMAS et al. 1994). At the present time, cigarette smoking has been identified as the single most important cause of carcinoma of the bladder (WYNDER and GOLDSMITH 1977).

In a recent epidemiologic study in the United States, the incidence of bladder cancer was 7 per 100 000 population, while the incidence for the state of New Jersey was 10 per 100 000, and for Salem County in the same state, 16 per 100 000 (MASON 1995). Further analysis demonstrated that 25% of the work force in New Jersey was employed in the chemical industry. Based on the above study, carcinoma of the bladder has become a reportable disease in that state, which in turn helped to identify a higher incidence of this tumor in those with exposure to saccharin and cyclamates. In a report from Italy studying multiple occupational and environmental factors, however, only employment in the construction industry was associated with a higher incidence of bladder cancer (PORRU et al. 1996). Chronic irritation caused by chronic infection or urolithiasis is a well-known factor predisposing patients to carcinoma of the bladder. This predisposition is particu-

larly apparent in patients with neurogenic bladder who have a need for a chronic indwelling catheter (KAUFMAN et al. 1977; STONEHILL et al. 1996; DOLIN et al. 1994).

An interesting causative factor for the induction of carcinoma of the bladder in North and East Africa and the Middle East is schistosomiasis (VIZCAINO et al. 1994; WARREN et al. 1995). These patients present more frequently with squamous cell carcinoma and are genetically different from those with transitional cell carcinoma as seen in European and North American patients.

2.3 Pathology

2.3.1 Bladder Cancer in Europe and North America

An overwhelming majority (90%) of patients with carcinoma of the bladder in Europe and North America are diagnosed with transitional cell carcinoma (ROZANSKI and GROSSMAN 1994). Squamous cell carcinoma is found in about 8%, while 2% of patients present with adenocarcinoma or some other rare tumor. On the other hand, squamous cell carcinoma is more common in patients with neurogenic bladder; in this group it is seen in up to 60% of patients, while transitional cell carcinoma occurs in 30% and the remaining patients are diagnosed with adenocarcinoma or other uncommon tumors (STONEHILL et al. 1996; KAUFMAN et al. 1977). A great majority of patients diagnosed with bladder cancer are males, with a male to female ratio of up to 4:1 commonly being reported in the literature. (See Chap. 5 for details on pathology.)

2.3.2 Bladder Cancer in Africa

In contrast to Europe and North America, in some regions of Africa where schisostomiasis is endemic, bladder cancer is the most frequent tumor, with the majority of patients being diagnosed with squamous cell carcinoma and one-third giving a history of bilharziasis (VIZCAINO et al. 1994; WARREN et al. 1995).

In a recently published interesting report from Zimbabwe, a total of 697 patients with bladder cancer were studied (VIZCAINO et al. 1994). Of these 697 patients, 373 (54%) had a diagnosis of squamous

Table 2.3. Distribution of patients by histological diagnosis and sex (modified from Vizcaino et al. 1994)

Histology	Males	%	Females	%	Total	%
Sq. cell ca.	261	70	112	30	373	54
TCC	89	75	29	25	118	17
Adenocarcinoma	17	65	9	35	26	4
Sarcoma	5	71	2	29	7	1
Not well defined	75	74	27	26	102	15
Not available	52	73	19	27	71	10
Total	499	72	198	28	697	100

Sq. cell ca., Squamous cell carcinoma; TCC, transitional cell carcinoma.

cell carcinoma, while 17% had transitional cell carcinoma and most (72%) patients were males (Table 2.3).

2.4
Signs and Symptoms

2.4.1
Signs and Symptoms in the General Population

Painless gross hematuria in a middle- or past middle-aged male patient is a well-described sign of bladder cancer. The presence of such hematuria requires appropriate studies, including cystoscopy, to identify the source of bleeding and random biopsies of the bladder if no apparent lesion can be identified. Bladder cancer does not infrequently, however, present as painless microscopic hematuria. Common symptoms of early bladder cancer may be nonspecific, such as irritative symptoms similar to those seen in patients with prostatism caused by the presence of benign prostatic hyperplasia. These symptoms include frequency, dysuria, and urgency and, being nonspecific, can be ignored by patients and physicians and are frequently responsible for delays in diagnosis and timely application of appropriate therapy.

Muscle invasive disease in the late stages may produce symptoms and signs of uremia caused by ureteric obstruction. Pelvic pain is a frequent symptom of advanced locoregional disease. This pain is difficult to control with analgesic medications. Tumor spread to regional lymph nodes ultimately may also lead to pelvic pain and peripheral edema. Metastatic disease to bone, lung, liver, and multiple other organs can produce frequently distressing signs and symptoms. Clinicians should be alert and diagnose early metastatic disease in order to administer timely appropriate palliative therapy.

2.4.2
Signs and Symptoms in Patients with Neurogenic Bladder

Painless gross hematuria is also a cardinal sign of bladder carcinoma in spinal cord injury, multiple sclerosis, and other neurogenic bladder patients. In addition, the presence of chronic bladder infection, bladder calculi, long-term immunosuppression, and particularly prolonged administration of cyclophosphimide should make clinicians alert to search for bladder carcinoma. An early diagnosis in these patients is imperative. Diagnostic measures should include cystoscopy and random biopsies, but even then it may be difficult to obtain a diagnosis due to the presence of changes frequently seen in the bladder of these patients (see Chap. 26 for details).

2.4.3
Signs and Symptoms in Patients with Schistosomiasis

The symptoms and signs of bladder cancer in patients with schistosomiasis are similar to those seen in other patients. Again, painless hematuria is a cardinal sign of cancer. Due to the presence of larvae in the bladder, there are common symptoms of bladder inflammation. Additionally, patients tend to frequently develop signs and symptoms of obstruction of the ureters (Warren et al. 1995; Vizcaino et al. 1994).

2.5
Behavior of Bladder Cancer

The majority of bladder tumors are superficial and, frequently, multiple low-grade papillary lesions. Tumor recurrence of superficial bladder tumor following local resection is common, occurring in 50%–70% of patients (Kurth et al. 1992). The incidence of recurrence is particularly high in patients with multiple and/or high-grade superficial lesions (Rozanski and Grossman et al. 1994). Tumor progression to muscle invasive disease has been reported in up to 15% of these patients (Kurth et al. 1992). These features, commonly seen in patients with superficial bladder tumors, support a theory that a carcinogenic effect(s) is predisposing the entire urothelium to develop tumors rather than stimulating the tumor development in one small focus (Badalament et al. 1992, Sidransky et al. 1992).

A study of risk factors for tumor progression to muscle invasive disease has helped to identify a group of about 20% of patients with superficial tumors who have particularly aggressive lesions and require more intensive therapy (Lamm et al. 1995). The risk factors for muscle invasive disease, as would be expected, include: (a) tumor grade, (b) tumor size, and (c) prior recurrence(s).

2.5.1
Carcinoma In Situ

Intraepithelial carcinoma or carcinoma in situ (CIS) can be present in association with papillary tumors, which is by far the most common presentation, or may arise de novo from the otherwise normal-appearing epithelium. CIS arising de novo is a more aggressive disease and has a greater propensity for recurrence and/or progression to muscle invasive tumor than CIS which is associated with papillary lesions. Local resection is the treatment of choice but recurrences are common, which has stimulated the interest in the use of adjuvant intravesical therapy (see Chap. 11).

An important study on the behavior of CIS was recently reported from Denmark (Wolf et al. 1994). A total of 31 CIS patients, including 28 males and three females, were followed for up to 14 years. Follow-up to tumor progression or to death from other causes extended from 15 to 115 months, with a mean of 64 months. Of these 31 patients, 26 (84%) had CIS associated with papillary lesions, while five (16%) had de novo CIS. A history of invasive bladder carcinoma or concomitant invasive tumor was seen in 19 (61%) patients, while seven (23%) had prior or concomitant TA lesions. All study patients had grade III CIS. Patient age at the time of entry into this study ranged from 52 to 82 years, with a mean age of 65 years. No definitive treatment was given, but the patients were carefully followed.

The work-up at each follow-up visit (visits took place 3–4 times each year) included:

1. Cystoscopy
2. Eight preselected systematic biopsies
3. Urine cytology performed on two samples taken during each follow-up visit
4. In the case of positive cytology and no identifiable CIS in the bladder, intravenous urography to exclude the presence of upper tract carcinoma

Recurrence of TA or T1 tumors was not considered a failure since these lesions could be easily resected transurethrally. Definite evidence of tumor progression in this study consisted of: (a) presence of muscle invasive disease, and/or (b) presence of metastatic disease, or (c) presence of upper tract tumor.

During the period of observation, 16 (52%) patients had evidence of tumor progression, with a mean time to this progression of 59 months. Stable disease was reported in 15 (48%) patients. Among the 16 patients who showed tumor progression, the following tumor extent was found: T3 and T4 disease in six, T2 disease in five, upper tract tumor in four, and distant metastases in one. All of these patients required surgical or radiation treatment and only six survived for an unspecified period of time. It is of interest to note that in the group of patients with "stable" disease, only three had no local tumor recurrence, while five had TA and seven had T1 recurrent tumors.

This means that, of the 31 patients who were carefully followed with regular cystoscopies and multiple biopsies, only three (10%) did not show evidence of tumor recurrence during the period of observation. It is apparent that CIS is not a benign disease but a relatively aggressive tumor, since 90% of patients are expected to have significant progressive disease and only six patients with progressive disease in the above-mentioned study survived the treatment. In view of the above data, it is strongly believed that CIS patients require appropriate timely therapy once the diagnosis has been made. The administration of appropriate therapy modifies the natural history of this disease, resulting in a sharp reduction in the tumor recurrence rate and a reduction in the incidence of muscle invasive disease.

2.5.2
Superficial (TA and T1) Tumors

In a recently reported study from Sweden, the outcome in patients with TA and T1 disease was examined (Holmang et al. 1995). A total of 176 patients were treated and followed for 20 years or longer. Most (70%) patients died of intercurrent disease and 39 (22%) died of bladder cancer, while 13 (7%) had no evidence of recurrent bladder carcinoma. Death due to bladder cancer was stage related. Of the 77 TA patients, nine (12%) died of their tumor, while of the 99 T1 patients, 30 (30%) died of bladder cancer. Local recurrences were found on ten or more cystoscopies in 16 (9%) patients, of whom ten died of bladder carcinoma. This suggests that multiple recurrences were not well controlled with conservative treatment and eventually led to death. Patients with superficial bladder carcinoma need careful follow-up in order to treat tumor recurrences in a timely fashion.

An important study in patients with TA and T1 disease, using meta-analysis of multiple prospective randomized trials conducted by the European Organization for Research and Treatment of Cancer (EORTC) and the Medical Research Council (MRC), was reported by GELBER and GOLDHIRSCH (1991). A total of 2535 patients were treated in six trials. Patients were randomized to receive transurethral resection only or transurethral resection followed by adjuvant intravesical or oral therapy. Median follow-up was approaching 8 years. Natural history of the study TA and T1 patients was modified in that the disease-free interval was increased in patients who received adjuvant therapy when compared with those treated with transurethral resection alone. The adjuvant treatment, however, failed to significantly increase patient survival and failed to increase the time to the occurrence of muscle invasive disease. Although this meta-analysis does not provide definitive proof of a lack of efficacy of adjuvant therapy in patients with superficial bladder carcinoma, it does introduce caution to the interpretation of outcomes of prospective randomized trials with a limited number of patients and a relatively short period of follow-up (see Chap. 11).

From the available published data, one may draw the conclusion that patients with superficial bladder carcinoma should be studied carefully, prior to the administration of definitive therapy, with the use of recently developed important tumor markers such as p53 and p21. Such an approach could help to identify a group of patients with more aggressive disease who may not be suitable for conservative therapy (see Chaps. 3 and 4).

2.5.3
Invasive (T2, T3, and T4) Tumors

In patients with invasive carcinoma of the bladder, tumor spread initially tends to be local, with a gradual increase in tumor bulk eventually leading to transmural infiltration. This may be followed by invasion of the adjacent structures such as the prostate in male and the vagina in female patients. The involvement of regional lymphatics may occur early in the course of disease and depends on the depth of tumor invasion in the bladder (SKINNER 1982;

SKINNER and LIESKOVSKY 1988). This orderly tumor spread pattern, while useful as a model, is not always observed in patients with carcinoma of the bladder.

Radical cystectomy and pelvic lymphadenectomy is the treatment which has dramatically modified the natural history of bladder cancer (SKINNER and LIESKOVSKY 1988; SCHOENBERG et al. 1996; BRENDLER et al. 1990; WISHNOW et al. 1992). In a series of 101 patients treated with radical prostatectomy, the 10-year disease-specific survival rate and free of local relapse survival rate were 69% and 94%, respectively (SCHOENBERG et al. 1996). Similar data have been reported by other investigators (SKINNER and LIESKOVSKY 1988). There has also been a dramatic reduction in treatment-related toxicity and a major improvement in the quality of life of the treated patients (see Chaps. 12, 14, and 16).

It is of interest to note that radical cystectomy and pelvic lymphadenectomy modified the natural history of patients with pelvic lymph node metastases (LERNER et al. 1993). In a group of 591 patients treated with this procedure at the University of Southern California School of Medicine, 132 (22%) were found to have pelvic lymphadenopathy. There was a good correlation between pathologic stage and the incidence of lymph node metastases. This incidence ranged from a low of 13% for P1 tumors, to a high of 45% for P4 tumors. The incidence of local recurrence among these patients was low, at 11%. The 5- and 10-year actuarial survival rates for these 132 patients were 29% and 20%, respectively.

It is apparent that more effective systemic agents need to be developed to control the systemic aspect of this disease as locoregional disease is well controlled with radical cystectomy and pelvic lymphadenectomy.

2.5.4
Metastatic Disease

Metastatic disease is a common occurrence in patients with carcinoma of the bladder. In a study of 150 patients treated with radical cystectomy, 50 (33%) developed metastatic disease, initially in lung and bone (PROUT et al. 1979). Development of metastases is usually seen early (within 12 months) in the course of disease. Tumor characteristics in patients at high risk of developing metastatic disease include the following:

1. Depth of penetration into the bladder wall (P3b)
2. Direct extension into the prostate (P4)
3. Pelvic lymph node involvement (SKINNER and LIESKOVSKY 1988)

In a recently published report on 240 cystectomy-treated patients, local failure was found to be of major importance in the development of metastatic disease (POLLACK et al. 1995). Distant tumor spread was reported in 56% of patients with local failure.

Patients with metastatic disease have a very poor prognosis, with a reported median survival in untreated patients of about 3 months (BABAIAN et al. 1980; DIMOPOULOS et al. 1994; YAGODA 1985). Treatment of these patients with metastatic disease is necessary due to the frequently present distressing signs and symptoms caused by the distant tumor spread. This is particularly true in patients with bone metastases who suffer from pain, which is difficult to control, and those with spinal cord compression syndrome. There are no prospective randomized trials comparing the management of patients with chemotherapy to supportive care alone. At the present time, however, the standard of care in patients with metastatic bladder carcinoma requires the administration of cisplatin-based combination chemotherapy (see Chap. 28). This combination chemotherapy has become a potent palliative weapon in the management of patients with metastatic carcinoma. There is, however, no conclusive evidence that the present-day chemotherapy modifies the natural history of this disease. Following the administration of contemporary combination chemotherapy, long-term (>3 years) survival was reported in about 10% of patients (STERNBERG et al. 1989; SAXMAN et al. 1996). This long-term survival is obtainable in carefully selected patients such as:

1. Younger patients
2. Those with a low tumor burden
3. Those with a good Karnofsky performance status
4. Those with no significant loss of weight

Unfortunately, good responses and long-term survivals are not commonly obtained in patients with bone and liver metastases. Nevertheless, major progress has been made in chemotherapy of patients with metastatic bladder cancer, with the majority of patients demonstrating a short-term tumor response which is followed by a relapse. Relapse usually occurs at the site of the original bulky tumor involvement (DIMOPOULOS et al. 1994). New therapeutic strategies are needed to modify the natural history of metastatic carcinoma of the bladder.

2.6
Conclusions

Transitional cell carcinoma of the bladder is a common and aggressive disease. It is characterized by locoregional spread with invasion through the bladder wall and spread to the neighboring structures. Pelvic lymph node involvement and early distant metastatic disease are common. Radical cystectomy and pelvic lymphadenectomy represent the treatment of choice for this tumor. Contemporary surgical treatment results for patients with superficial lesions are excellent and the aforementioned surgical techniques are responsible for modifying the natural history of this disease. It will be relevant at this point in time to introduce to the clinic the routine use of tumor markers such as p53 and p21 to help identify prior to therapy more aggressive tumors and manage them appropriately.

There has also been a major improvement in treatment results for muscle invasive disease. New treatment strategies, however, need to be developed to manage more effectively metastatic tumor spread, which is a common feature of this disease process.

References

Babaian RJ, Johnson DE, Llamas L, Ayala AG (1980) Metastases from transitional cell carcinoma of the urinary bladder. Urology 16:142–144

Badalament RA, Ortolano V, Burgers JK (1992) Recurrent or aggressive bladder cancer: indications for adjuvant intravesical therapy. Urol Clin North Am 19:485–498

Branch RA, Chern HD, Adedoyin A, et al. (1995) The precarcinogen hypothesis for bladder cancer: activities of individual drug metabolizing enzymes as risk factors. Pharmacogen 5:S97–S102

Brendler CB, Steinberg GD, Marshall FF, Mostwin JL, Walsh PC (1990) Local recurrence and survival following nerve-sparing radical prostatectomy. J Urol 144:1137–1141

Chiou HY, Hsueh YM, Liaw KF, et al. (1995) Incidence of internal cancers and ingested inorganic arsenic: a seven-year follow-up study in Taiwan. Cancer Res 55:1296–1300

Cohen SM, Johansson SL (1992) Epidemiology and etiology of bladder cancer. Urol Clin North Am 19:421–428

Dimopoulos MA, Finn L, Logothetis CJ (1994) Pattern of failure and survival of patients with metastatic urothelial tumors relapsing after cisplatinum-based chemotherapy. J Urol 151:598–601

Dolin PJ, Darby SC, Beral V (1994) Paraplegia and squamous cell carcinoma of the bladder in young women: findings from a case-control study. Br J Cancer 70:167–168

Gelber RD, Goldhirsch A (1991) Meta-analysis: the fashion of summing-up evidence. Ann Oncol 2:461–468

Holmang S, Hedelin H, Anderstrom C, Johansson SL (1995) The relationship among multiple recurrences, progression and prognosis of patients with stages Ta and T1 transitional cell cancer of the bladder followed for at least 20 years. J Urol 153:1823–1827

Horn EP, Tucker MA, Lambert G, et al. (1995) A study of gender-based cytochrome P4501A2 variability: a possible mechanism for the male excess of bladder cancer. Cancer Epidemiol Biomarkers Prev 4:529–533

Kaufman JM, Fam B, Jacobs SC, et al. (1977) Bladder cancer and squamous metaplasia in spinal cord injury patients. J Urol 118:967–971

Kurth KH, Denis L, Sylvester R, et al. (1992) Prognostic factors in superficial bladder tumors. In: Soloway MS (ed) Problems in urology: transitional cell malignancy. J.B. Lippincott, Philadelphia, pp 471–483

Lamm DL, Van Der Meijden APM, Akaza H, et al. (1995) Intravesical chemo- and immunotherapy: how do we assess their effectiveness and what are their limitations and uses? Proceedings of the Fourth International Bladder Cancer Consensus Conference. J Urol 2(Suppl 2):23–25

Lerner SP, Skinner DG, Lieskovsky G, et al. (1993) The rationale for en bloc pelvic lymph node dissection for bladder cancer patients with nodal metastases: longterm results. J Urol 149:758–765

Mason TJ (1995) The development of the series of U.S. cancer atlases: implications for future epidemiologic research. Stat Med 14:473–479

Momas I, Daures JP, Festy B, Bontoux J, Gremy F (1994) Bladder cancer and black tobacco cigarette smoking. Some results from a French case-control study. Eur J Epidemiol 10:599–604

Office of Population Consensus and Studies (1987) D.H. 1. Cancer statistics. HMSO, London, 1969–1987

Parker SL, Tong T, Bolden S, Wingo PA (1996) Cancer statistics, 1996. Ca Cancer J Clin 65:5–26

Pollack Z, Zagars GK, Cole CG, Dinney CPN, Swanson DA, Grossman HB (1995) The relationship of local control to distant metastasis in muscle-invasive bladder cancer. J Urol 154:2059–2064

Porru S, Aulenti V, Donato F, et al. (1996) Bladder cancer and occupation: a case-control study in northern Italy. Occup Environm Med 53:6–10

Prout GR, Griffin PP, Shipley WU (1979) Bladder carcinoma as a systemic disease. Cancer 43:2532–2539

Rehn L (1895) Blasengeschwuelste bei Fuchsin-Arbeitern. Arch Klin Chir 50:588–600

Risch A, Wallace DMA, Bathers S, Sim E (1995) Slow N-acetylation genotype is a susceptibility factor in occupational and smoking related bladder cancer. Human Mol Genet 4:231–236

Rozanski TA, Grossman HB (1994) Recent developments in pathophysiology of bladder cancer. AJR 163:789–792

Saxman SB, Loehrer PJ, Propert K, et al. (1996) Long term follow-up of phase III intergroup study of M-VAC vs cisplatin in metastatic urothelial carcinoma. Proc Am Soc Clin Oncol (abstr) 15:248

Schoenberg MP, Walsh PC, Breazeale DR, Marshall FF, Mostwin JL, Brendler CB (1996) Local recurrence and survival following nerve sparing radical prostatectomy for bladder cancer: 10-year followup. J Urol 155:490–494

Sidransky D, Frost P, Von Eschenbach A, Oyasu R, Preisinger A, Vogelstein B (1992) Clonal origin of bladder cancer. N Engl J Med 326:737–740

Silverberg E, Boring CC, Squires TS (1990) Cancer statistics, 1990. Ca Cancer J Clin 40:9–28

Skinner DG (1982) Management of invasive bladder cancer: a meticulous pelvic node dissection can make a difference. J Urol 128:34–38

Skinner DG, Lieskovsky G (1988) Management of invasive and high-grade bladder cancer. In: Skinner DG, Lieskovsky G (eds) Diagnosis and management of genitourinary cancer. Saunders, Philadelphia, pp 295–312

Slattery ML, Mori M, Gao R, Kerber RA (1995) Impact of family history of colon cancer on development of multiple primaries after diagnosis of colon cancer. Dis Colon Rectum 38:1053–1058

Sternberg CN, Yagoda A, Scher HI, et al. (1989) Metotrexate, vinblastine, doxorubicin, and cisplatin for advanced transitional cell carcinoma of the urothelium. Efficacy and patterns of response and relapse. Cancer 64:2448–2458

Stonehill WH, Dmochowski RR, Patterson AL, Cox CE (1996) Risk factors for bladder tumors in spinal cord injury patients. J Urol 155:1248–1250

Thon WF, Kliem V, Truss MC, Anton P, Kuczyk M, Stief CG, Brunkhorst R (1995) Denovo urothelial carcinoma of the upper and lower urinary tract in kidney transplant patients with end-stage analgesic nephropathy. World J Urol 13: 254–261

Vizcaino AP, Parkin DM, Boffetta P, Skinner MEG (1994) Bladder cancer: epidemiology and risk factors in Bulawayo, Zimbabwe. Cancer Causes Control 5:517–522

Warren W, Biggs PJ, El-Baz M, Ghneim MA, Stratton MR, Venitt S (1995) Mutations in the p53 gene in schistosomal bladder cancer: a study of 92 tumours from Egyptian patients and comparison between mutational spectra from schistosomal and non-schistosomal urothelial tumours. Carcinogenesis 16:1181–1189

Wishnow KI, Levinson AK, Johnson DE, et al. (1992) Stage B (P2/3A/N0) transitional cell carcinoma of bladder highly curable by radical cystectomy. Urology 39:12–16

Wolf H, Melsen F, Pedersen SE, Nielsen KT (1994) Natural history of carcinoma in situ of the urinary bladder. Scand J Urol Nephrol (Suppl) 157:147–151

Wynder EL, Goldsmith R (1977) The epidemiology of bladder cancer: a second look. Cancer 40:1246–1268

Yagoda A (1985) Progress of treatment of advanced urothelial tract tumors. J Clin Oncol 3:1448–1452

3 Prognostic Factors in Bladder Cancer: Emphasis on Immunohistochemical Analysis

J.P. STEIN and R.J. COTE

CONTENTS

3.1 Introduction

Transitional cell carcinoma of the bladder is the second most common malignancy of the genitourinary tract, and the second most common cause of death among all genitourinary tumors. In 1996, it is estimated that 52 900 new cases of the disease will be diagnosed, with 11 700 of these patients projected to die from the disease (PARKER et al. 1996). Approximately 80% of patients with primary bladder cancer present with low-grade tumors confined to the superficial mucosa. The risk of superficial recurrence in patients with bladder tumors confined to the mucosa is 70%, with the majority of cancers amenable to

initial transurethral resection and selected administration of intravesical immuno- or chemotherapy (CRAWFORD and DAVIS 1987; SKINNER and LIESKOVSKY 1988; DROLLER 1990). Unfortunately, as many as 30% of these recurrent tumors demonstrate tumor progression with higher grade and/or stage disease. Furthermore, nearly 30% of all patients with bladder cancer initially present muscle invasive tumors; 50% of these patients who are treated locally for their invasive tumors will relapse with metastatic disease within 2 years (SKINNER and LIESKOVSKY 1988). These data clearly underscore the heterogeneous nature and malignant capabilities of transitional cell carcinoma of the bladder.

The optimal management of invasive bladder cancer requires the detection and accurate assessment of the tumor's biologic potential. Currently, tumor grade and stage, as evaluated histologically, are the primary prognostic variables of bladder cancer which dictate treatment strategies. Although these two conventional histopathologic variables provide a certain degree of stratification of the tumor's biologic potential, there remains a significant degree of tumor heterogeneity even within various prognostic subgroups. This hampers the accurate and reliable prediction of the tumor's aggressiveness. The ability to predict an individual tumor's true biologic potential would in turn facilitate treatment selection decisions for patients who may benefit from adjuvant therapy, and the selection of patients who may require less aggressive treatment strategies.

Intense research efforts are being made to identify and characterize the different types of bladder cancer and their varying biologic potential. The desire to predict which superficial tumors will recur or progress, and which invasive tumors will metastasize, has spurred the development of a variety of bladder cancer prognostic markers. In this chapter we will provide a contemporary review of bladder tumor prognostic markers as determined by immunohistochemical techniques and comment on the potential clinical application of these tumor markers.

J.P. STEIN, MD, Assistant Professor, Department of Urology, University of Southern California, USC/Norris Comprehensive Cancer Center, 1441 Eastlake Avenue, Los Angeles, CA 90033, USA

R.J. COTE, MD, Associate Professor of Pathology and Urology, Department of Pathology, University of Southern California, USC/Norris Comprehensive Cancer Center, 1441 Eastlake Avenue, Los Angeles, CA 90033, USA

3.2
Blood Group Antigens

On the surface of all cells there exist a variety of antigenic substances which include glycoproteins and glycolipids. The specific assembly, maturation, and expression of these cell surface antigens reflect the individual's normal cellular differentiation. These surface molecules are associated with various cellular activities, including cell adhesion, cell recognition, and cell signaling. Changes in cellular morphology, differentiation, or proliferation in certain epithelial cells are often characterized by alterations in the expression of these cell surface molecules (HAKOMORI 1985). Loss of these cell surface antigens may indicate cellular dedifferentiation characteristic of cells that have undergone neoplastic transformation. With the advent of hybridoma techniques it has become possible to generate monoclonal antibodies specific to these cell surface epitopes (KOHLER and MILSTEIN 1975). This technology allows the study of cellular surface antigens which may provide a better understanding of the cell's malignant potential. These antibodies provide a powerful tool in the biologic research into bladder cancer and have been employed to characterize antigenic expression in exfoliated cells and in tissue sections with the use of immunohistochemical techniques.

Blood group-related antigens are a group of carbohydrate determinants carried on membrane lipids and proteins (LLOYD 1987). These antigens were first described on the cell surface of erythrocytes and have been identified on various epithelial tissues, including transitional urothelium. The ABH and Lewis antigens ($Le^{a,b,x,y}$) are blood group antigens that differ only in sugar residues. The majority of individuals (75%–80%) are secretors and express the ABH, Le^b, and Le^y antigens in normal urothelium, whereas nonsecretors do not express these antigens.

In 1975, DECENZO and associates first studied the expression of ABH antigens in 22 patients with superficial bladder cancer. They found that the loss of ABH blood group antigen expression in these superficial bladder cancers correlated with the development of invasive tumors, with increased recurrence, and with tumor progression. In the largest reported series, NEWMAN et al. (1980) evaluated 322 patients with superficial bladder tumors for the same blood group antigens. They found that 88% of these superficial tumors that progressed to muscle invasion lacked ABH antigen expression in the original tumor. In addition, 90% of the tumors which recurred superficially expressed the appropriate blood group antigen in the original tumor. In another study, WEINSTEIN et al. (1979) evaluated cystectomy specimens with carcinoma in situ, and found that half of these specimens demonstrated areas of normal histologic urothelium that lacked ABH antigen expression, suggesting that this field change associated with bladder cancer may occur prior to the histologic changes.

These initial observations of ABH antigen expression were confirmed by several other investigators (D'EILA et al. 1982; LANGE et al. 1978; YOUNG et al. 1979; WILEY et al. 1982; LIMAS et al. 1979; CORDON-CARDO et al. 1986). However, certain problems precluded the clinical application of blood group antigen determination in bladder cancer including: (a) lack of prospective evaluation, (b) technical problems employing polyclonal antibodies, and (c) the fact that the secretory status of the individual was not well appreciated. Improved immunohistochemical techniques with monoclonal antibodies have been found to be more sensitive and consistent than techniques using polyclonal antibodies. In addition, it has been discovered that the individual's secretory status influences the expression of the blood group antigens in normal urothelium (SARKIS et al. 1994). In most individuals (75%–80%), normal urothelium is rich in ABH, Le^b, and Le^y blood group antigens (secretors), while 20% of individuals with normal urothelium lack expression of these antigens (nonsecretors). Therefore, the deletion of ABH antigen expression can only be reliably determined in secretory individuals. Despite the use of newer detection methods and specific monoclonal antibodies, the results of the early studies in respect of loss of ABH antigen expression could not be duplicated in a large well-controlled study (CORDON-CARDO et al. 1988).

The focus of studies on blood group antigens subsequently shifted to the evaluation of the related Lewis antigens ($Le^{a,b,x,y}$). With the exception of the Lewis X (Le^x), these antigen have provided limited clinical benefit. Similar to ABH expression, the problem with the Lewis ($Le^{a,b,y}$) antigens is their absence in 20% of normal urothelium, which limits their prognostic application. Currently, Le^x remains the only blood group antigen with potential prognostic value. Immunohistochemical evaluation of Le^x on fresh frozen and formalin-fixed bladder tissues has demonstrated that most tumors (90%) and only an occasional umbrella cell of normal urothelium express this blood group antigen (CORDON-CARDO et al. 1988).

SHEINFELD et al. (1990) evaluated the ability of Le^x immunocytology on bladder barbotage specimens to improve tumor detection compared with routine cytologic evaluation. They found the overall sensitivity of Le^x immunocytology to be 85%, compared to 61% with routine conventional cytology alone. Combining a positive cytology and a positive immunocytology, the sensitivity of detection was increased to 93%. In addition, Le^x immunocytology was found to be particularly sensitive in detecting low-grade bladder tumors which are generally not detected on routine cytology. Most recent studies have confirmed that the diagnostic accuracy is improved when Le^x evaluation is combined with routine urinary cytologic evaluation for noninvasive bladder cancer (GOLIJANIN et al. 1995). Currently, the data suggest that immunocytologic evaluation of the Le^x antigen on exfoliated bladder cells enhances the detection of tumor cells, particularly from low-grade and low-stage cancers. Furthermore, expression of Le^x may be a useful clinical marker in predicting tumor recurrence or progression in patients with a history of superficial bladder cancer who are high-risk disease-free patients (SHEINFELD et al. 1992).

3.3
Tumor-Associated Antigens

Although a number of monoclonal antibodies specific to transitional cell carcinoma of the bladder have been generated (DALBAGNI et al. 1992), only three antigens (M344, 19A211, and T138) appear to possess any proven prognostic clinical application (FRADET and CORDON-CARDO 1993). The monoclonal antibodies M344 and 19A211 are reactive to antigens of superficial bladder tumors and are absent in normal transitional epithelium. The M344 antigen is a cytoplasmic mucin-like antigen that is expressed in 70% of superficial (Ta, T1) bladder tumors, 25% of carcinoma in situ (Tis) tumors, and approximately 15% of invasive bladder tumors. In general, M344 expression decreases with increasing grade of bladder cancers and is rarely positive in poorly differentiated, aneuploid bladder tumors (FRADET and CORDON-CARDO 1993). The 19A211 antigen is a sialoglycoprotein cell-surface antigen that is expressed in 70% of Ta and T1 tumors, 60% of Tis tumors, and approximately 50% of invasive tumors (FRADET and CORDON-CARDO 1993). In a prospective study evaluating M344 and 19A211 expression, 260 bladder irrigations from 140 patients with a history of bladder cancer were analyzed

(FRADET et al. 1991). Overall, 95% of Ta and T1 tumors with positive urinary cytology, and 85% of those with negative urine cytology were positive for these antibodies. In addition, 30% of patients with a normal cystoscopic examination and a previous history of a bladder tumor demonstrated a positive antibody test. Those patients with a positive test had a 75% recurrence rate, compared with a rate of only 20% among those without M344 or 19A211 expression. These data suggest a potential role for these antibodies in detecting and monitoring superficial bladder cancer.

The T138 antigen is a surface glycoprotein that is expressed in 15% of superficial Ta and T1 bladder tumors and 60% of muscle invasive bladder cancers (FRADET and CORDON-CARDO 1993). This antigen is not expressed in normal transitional epithelium; however, reactive urothelium may be positive for it. The expression of T138 in patients with bladder cancer was found to be associated with an ominous prognosis of metastatic disease in two independent studies (FRADET et al. 1990; BRETTON et al. 1990). Fradet and associates evaluated 68 patients with bladder cancer and found that cancer-specific death occurred in 35% of those with diploid, T138-positive tumors, in none with diploid, T138-negative tumors, and in 65% of those with aneuploid, T138 positive tumors (FRADET et al. 1990). Furthermore, 80% of patients with Ta or T1, T138-positive tumors demonstrated progressive disease in this study. The T138 antigen appears to be a promising bladder cancer marker and will require further evaluation to define its true role as a prognostic marker.

Recently, a urine antibody test for bladder tumor antigen (BTA) (Bard Diagnostic Sciences, Redmond, Wash.) has been developed. The BTA is an assay for the qualitative detection of bladder tumor antigen in the urine (SAROSDY et al. 1995). The antigen is composed of basement membrane complexes that have been isolated and characterized from the urine of patients with bladder cancer. In a well-designed, blinded, large, prospective, multicenter trial involving 499 patients, the BTA test was found to be more sensitive than urine cytology studies alone in detecting recurrent cancer in patients with low-grade, low-stage tumors (SAROSDY et al. 1995). The BTA had an overall sensitivity of 40%, compared with only 16% for urine cytology, and a specificity of 96%. The BTA test is a simple, rapid, and inexpensive adjunct to cystoscopy and appears to be an attractive method for surveillance purposes in patients with a history of superficial bladder cancer.

3.4
Proliferating Antigens

The fraction of proliferating cells (the growth fraction) of a tumor is an important prognostic feature of any malignancy and helps define the cancer's biologic potential. Markers used to assess cellular proliferation of a tumor have included: mitotic count, silver-stained nucleolar organizer regions (AgNORs), Ki-67, and the proliferating cell nuclear antigen (PCNA). The two most promising immunohistochemical markers of cellular proliferation are Ki-67 and PCNA. Increased expression of these antigens suggests a higher level of proliferative activity in cells and is associated with tumors of more aggressive biologic potential with an increased propensity for progression and metastasis (FRADET and CORDON-CARDO 1993).

Ki-67 is a murine monoclonal antibody found to react with a nuclear antigen expressed in proliferating cells (GERDES et al. 1983). The exact nature of this antigen has not been well characterized; however, it is thought that Ki-67 recognizes a nuclear protein involved in a portion of the DNA replicase complex (LOKE et al. 1987). Since the discovery of this antibody in 1983, it has been extensively evaluated in a variety of human malignancies (BROWN and GATTER 1990). OKAMURA et al. (1990) evaluated 55 bladder cancers with Ki-67 immunostaining and found a correlation between increased expression and tumor grade and stage. Several other studies have confirmed this relationship and have found a significantly higher recurrence rate in bladder cancer patients with tumors demonstrating a higher proliferative index as determined by increased Ki-67 immunoreactivity (FONTANA et al. 1992; COHEN et al. 1993; TSUJIHASHI et al. 1991; MULDER et al. 1992; BUSH et al. 1991; KING et al. 1996). Overall, there is sufficient evidence to suggest that determination of the proliferative index, by immunohistochemical staining for Ki-67, may supplement the routine histologic grade and stage in assessing a bladder tumor's aggressiveness and metastatic potential.

Proliferating cell nuclear antigen is a well-characterized antigen critical to DNA polymerase delta activity (OGATA et al. 1987; ROBBINS et al. 1987). This antigen is present in all proliferating eukaryotic cells and plays an important role in the cell cycle. Recently developed techniques allow the immunohistochemical evaluation of PCNA expression in formalin-fixed tissues. COHEN and associates (1993) studied 25 transitional cell carcinomas of the bladder for PCNA and found a strong correlation between tumor grade and stage and PCNA immunoexpression. With further investigation PCNA may become a more widely employed prognostic tumor marker for bladder cancer. Nonetheless, before any marker of proliferative activity can be applied in clinical practice, its prognostic ability must be evaluated in larger groups of patients.

3.5
Oncogenes

Oncogenes are normal cellular genes which can become altered by either mutations or gene amplification, resulting in deregulation of cellular growth control mechanisms. Oncogenes thought to be involved in human malignancies include: c-myc, c-ras, and c-erbB2. Of these, the proto-oncogene c-erbB-2 (also known as HER-2/neu) has been extensively studied and implicated in a number of tumors, including breast, prostate, and bladder cancer (UNDERWOOD et al. 1995). The c-erbB-2 oncogene encodes a transmembrane glycoprotein similar to the epidermal growth factor receptor. Accumulating evidence suggests that the c-erbB-2 protein is a growth factor receptor possessing similar structural homology (BARGMANN et al. 1986; YAMAMOTO et al. 1986), tyrosine kinase activity (STERN et al. 1986; AKIYAMA et al. 1986), and the ability to stimulate cellular growth (LEE et al. 1989).

Initial studies of c-erbB-2 conducted in breast carcinoma demonstrated a significant relationship between gene expression, tumor progression, and overall survival (SLAMON et al. 1989; BORG et al. 1991). Subsequently, several studies have reported that c-erbB-2 expression, as determined by immunohistochemical methods, in patients with bladder cancer is associated with higher stage tumors (GORGOULIS et al. 1995; SATO et al. 1992; MOCH et al. 1993; MORIYAMA et al. 1991), increased tumor progression (UNDERWOOD et al. 1995), increased incidence of metastasis (MOCH et al. 1993; MORIYAMA et al. 1991), and worse overall survival (SATO et al. 1992). Although these studies suggest a prognostic value of c-erbB-2 expression in human bladder cancer, other studies have reported conflicting results, stating that immunohistochemical evaluation of c-erbB-2 provides no additional prognostic value over previously established predictors for transitional cell carcinoma of the bladder (LIPPONEN 1993a; MELLON et al. 1996; LIPPONEN and ESKELINEN 1994). In view of these discrepant results, further evaluation will be required to accurately determine the prognostic value of c-erbB-2 in bladder cancer.

3.6
Epidermal Growth Factor Receptor

The epidermal growth factor (EGF) signals through the epidermal growth factor receptor (EGFR). This receptor is the product of the c-erbB-1 gene and is a 17-kDa transmembrane glycoprotein with an intracellular tyrosine kinase component which signals intracellular events by phosphorylating tyrosine residues (PARTANEN 1990). The EGFR is found on most epithelial cells, including transitional epithelium. In the normal bladder, EGFR is located only in the basal cells (LIEBERT 1995; MESSING 1990). When malignant transformation occurs in transitional epithelium, EGFR can be found throughout the urothelial layers and may be expressed at high levels (NEAL et al. 1990; SAUTER et al. 1994; BERGER et al. 1987; NEAL et al. 1985; MESSING et al. 1987). It has been suggested that this receptor is involved in mediating the events of various growth factors and may contribute to neoplastic transformation (YAMAMOTO et al. 1986).

The immunohistochemical evaluation of EGFR has been as a prognostic marker for transitional cell carcinoma of the bladder. Clinically, a good correlation between EGFR overexpression and higher grade and stage of bladder cancer has been demonstrated (LIEBERT 1995; MESSING 1990; NEAL et al. 1990; SAUTER et al. 1994; BERGER et al. 1987; NEAL et al. 1985; MESSING et al. 1987). The correlation between EGFR expression as determined by immunohistochemistry and clinical outcome was evaluated in a large group of patients with bladder cancer (NEAL et al. 1990). Overexpression of EGFR in this study correlated with higher stage invasive tumors and an increase in cancer-specific death. Furthermore, patients with superficial bladder tumors with an increase in EGFR immunostaining demonstrated a significantly shorter interval to recurrence, a higher rate of recurrence, and an increased rate of progression. Interestingly, the difference in survival observed between EGFR-positive and EGFR-negative tumors was not significant when the data were analyzed separately from patients with muscle invasive bladder cancers. These findings, coupled with the fact that high levels of EGFR are found in normal transitional epithelium distant from the tumor (MESSING 1990), suggest that increased EGFR expression may be an early event in bladder cancer tumorigenesis.

3.7
Peptide Growth Factors

Peptide growth factors provide the basic communication between cells in the microenvironment. In general, peptide growth factors mediate the cellular response to infection or injury and regulate the events of embryogenesis. In addition, these factors are intimately involved in cellular growth, differentiation, and death. Alterations in the expression of these peptide growth factors may contribute to uncontrolled cell growth. While three major families of peptide growth factors exist [epidermal growth factor (EGF), fibroblast growth factor (FGF), and transforming growth factor β (TGFβ)], EGF has been subjected to the most extensive immunohistochemical evaluation in bladder cancer.

In 1981, CHODAK and associates demonstrated that biopsies of bladder cancer stimulated capillary proliferation of rabbit irises. In addition, they found that urine from patients with bladder tumors stimulated capillary endothelial cell migration, suggesting that transitional cell carcinoma may produce an FGF-like angiogenic factor. Other studies have been done to support this notion. Bladder cancer cell lines exposed to FGF in vitro have demonstrated an increase in motility, higher metastatic potential, and definite changes in cellular morphology, all of which are properties of tumorigenesis (VALLES et al. 1990; JOUANNEAU et al. 1991).

Acidic and basic FGFs are thought to be the angiogenic factors found in the urine from patients with bladder cancer. CHOPIN and associates (1993) have demonstrated a tenfold increase in tissue acidic FGF in transitional cell carcinoma compared with normal transitional epithelium. In addition, acidic FGF immunoreactivity was found to be elevated in urine from patients with bladder cancer and to be correlated with tumor stage and the presence of metastases (CHOPIN et al. 1993). Similar results have been found with the detection of basic FGF (NGUYEN et al. 1993). These results suggest that FGF may be used as a noninvasive method to follow patients with bladder cancer.

3.8
Cell Adherence Molecules

For cancer cells to metastasize, they must be released into the blood or lymphatic stream. Loss of intercellular adhesive properties favors the detachment of cancer cells and may play a role in the development of metastatic disease.

3.8.1
E-cadherin

E-cadherin is an epithelial cell adhesion molecule associated with cellular differentiation and is lost in many types of cancer (SHIOZAKI et al. 1991). The binding function of E-cadherin is homotypic; that is, the receptors bind to each other on neighboring cells, thereby performing a tumor suppressor function (FRIXEN et al. 1991). Several studies have demonstrated an association between loss of E-cadherin expression as determined by immunohistochemical methods and an increase in bladder cancer stage. In one study, loss of E-cadherin expression, analyzed in 49 bladder tumors, correlated with increase grade and stage of tumors and poorer overall survival (BRINGUIER et al. 1993). These results were confirmed by other studies (OTTO et al. 1994; LIPPONEN and ESKELINEN 1995). Further studies will be required to evaluate precisely the usefulness of this cellular adhesion marker.

3.8.2
Integrins

Integrins are a family of transmembrane heterodimers that function as receptors for each other and the extracellular matrix (ALBEDA 1993; LARJAVA et al. 1990; SYMINGTON et al. 1993). It is thought that they play an important role in cell-to-cell adhesion. Recently, immunohistochemical evaluation has been performed to evaluate the expression of certain integrins and their role as a prognostic marker in bladder cancer. Immunohistochemical study of alpha-$2\beta1$ and alpha-$3\beta1$ integrin expression demonstrated a progressive loss of alpha-$2\beta1$ immunoreactivity with increasing bladder tumor stage, while alpha-$3\beta1$ immunoexpression was maintained in these tumors (LIEBERT et al. 1994a). The expression of another integrin (alpha-$6B4$) has also been evaluated through immunohistochemical techniques in bladder cancer. In general, the alpha-$6B4$ integrin is associated with the basal anchoring structure in normal epithelial tissues, including the bladder (LIEBERT et al. 1994b). Interestingly, this anchoring structure is lost with the development of invasive bladder cancer and subsequently becomes overexpressed, which may suggest that the tumor

cells incorporate this receptor to move through the basement membrane (LIEBERT et al. 1993, 1994b).

3.9
Angiogenesis
and Angiogenesis Inhibitors

3.9.1
Tumor Angiogenesis

Substantial evidence exists to support the notion that tumor growth and metastatic potential require induction of neovascular response (FOLKMAN et al. 1966; SUTHERLAND et al. 1971; GIMBRONE et al. 1972, 1974). The formation of new microvessel growth within and around a tumor is stimulated by angiogenic factors produced by tumor cells and/or recruited inflammatory cells, or by tumor-initiated release of angiogenic factors bound in the extracellular matrix (BLOOD and ZETTER 1990; POLVERINI and LEIBOVICH 1984; FOLKMAN and KLAGSBRUN 1987). This process is known as angiogenesis.

Angiogenesis is the ability to induce new blood vessel growth. Most neoplastic cells that compose a tumor already possess the capability of uncontrolled cell growth, and the ability to induce a well-vascularized environment only strengthens the growth and metastatic potential of the tumor. In an attempt to better define a tumor's malignant potential, immunohistochemical methods have been developed to evaluate this angiogenic phase in a particular cancer. This allows the determination of the microvessel density within and adjacent to the tumor. The microvessel density is a measure of the tumor's angiogenic development and has been found to be a useful prognostic indicator of tumor progression and malignancy in a variety of tumor systems, including cutaneous melanoma (SRIVASTAVA et al. 1988; BARNHILL and LEVY 1992), breast cancer (WEIDNER et al. 1992; HORAK et al. 1992), and prostate cancer (SRIVASTAVA et al. 1988; BARNHILL and LEVY 1992; WEIDNER et al. 1992; HORAK et al. 1992; WEIDNER et al. 1993; BRAWER et al. 1994). In general, tumor angiogenesis as determined by immunohistochemical methods with increasing microvessel counts is associated with tumor progression and worsening prognosis (WEIDNER et al. 1993; BRAWER et al. 1994).

Recently, several investigators have explored the relationship of tumor-associated angiogenesis and tumor progression in bladder cancer (BOCHNER et al. 1995; JAEGER et al. 1995; DICKINSON et al. 1994;

O'BRIEN et al. 1995; CAMBELL and BOUCK 1996). Our group evaluated the extent of angiogenesis in 164 patients with primary transitional cell carcinoma of the bladder by immunohistochemical techniques (BOCHNER et al. 1995). We found that microvessel density, a measure of the degree of angiogenesis within a tumor, was strongly associated with disease recurrence and overall survival in patients with invasive bladder cancers. Elevated microvessel counts were associated with an increased risk of disease recurrence and worse overall cancer-specific survival. Statistically significant differences in disease progression were observed in organ-confined tumors (P1, P2, P3a), tumors extending beyond the bladder wall (P3b, P4), and tumors with pathologic evidence of regional lymph node involvement. Although not associated with histologic grade or pathologic stage, microvessel density was found to be a highly significant and an independent predictor of disease recurrence and overall survival.

These findings were consistent, and confirmed data from other investigators who demonstrated significant angiogenic activity in bladder cancer and the prognostic importance of this tumor marker (JAEGER et al. 1995; DICKINSON et al. 1994; O'BRIEN et al. 1995). JAEGER and associates (1995) found a strong correlation between microvessel counts as determined by immunohistochemistry and lymph node involvement in 41 invasive bladder cancers. Furthermore, DICKINSON and associates (1994) evaluated a series of 45 patients with invasive bladder tumors (median follow-up of 37 months) and found that microvessel density was an independent prognostic indicator, conveying a 2.5 times greater risk of dying for those patients with elevated microvessel counts.

It appears that angiogenesis, as determined by immunohistochemical microvessel density, is an important prognostic factor in bladder cancer progression. Although additional studies are warranted, bladder cancers which exhibit an angiogenic phenotype appear to be more malignant and may benefit from an aggressive treatment program.

3.9.2
Angiogenesis Inhibitors

Just as angiogenesis, and the evaluation of microvessel density, has become an increasingly important predictor of bladder cancer progression, so inhibitors of this angiogenic process may also provide prognostic information. Many inhibitors of

angiogenesis exist (CAMBELL and BOUCK 1996). Thrombospondin-1 is a 450-kDa glycoprotein that is an important part of the extracellular matrix in many human tissues (WALZ 1992), and a known potent inhibitor of angiogenesis (DAMERON et al. 1994; GOOD et al. 1990; LAWLER et al. 1985). This protein has been evaluated as a prognostic factor in bladder cancer progression (GROSSFELD et al. 1996a).

Recently, we showed that the immunohistochemical evaluation of thrombospondin-1 can be performed on formalin-fixed, paraffin-embedded tissue sections (GROSSFELD et al. 1996b). Employing this technique, we then evaluated 163 patients, who underwent radical cystectomy for invasive bladder cancer, for thrombospondin-1 expression (GROSSFELD et al. 1996a). A highly significant association was found between thrombospondin-1 expression and tumor recurrence and overall survival in this group. Patients with low thrombospondin-1 expression exhibited increased microvessel density counts and poorer overall survival compared to patients with moderate or high thrombospondin-1 expression. In a multivariate analysis, thrombospondin-1 expression was an independent predictor of disease recurrence and overall survival compared with tumor stage and grade. In addition, thrombospondin-1 expression was significantly associated with microvessel density counts. Tumors with low thrombospondin expression were significantly more likely to demonstrate high microvessel density counts.

Inhibitors of angiogenesis, such as thrombospondin-1, therefore appear to be promising prognostic bladder cancer markers, though further investigation will be required to confirm this. The data suggest that inhibitors of angiogenesis may help predict bladder cancer progression which may act in part through the regulation of tumor neovascularity.

3.10
Cell Cycle-Regulatory Proteins

In general, malignant diseases are characterized by uncoordinated cell growth. Cellular proliferation occurs through an orderly progression through the cell cycle which is regulated by cell-cycle-associated protein complexes composed of cyclins and cyclin-dependent kinases (CORDON-CARDO 1995). These complexes exert their control mechanism by phosphorylating key proteins involved in cell cycle transition such as the protein encoded by the retinoblastoma gene (pRB) or the p53 protein. Loss of this cell cycle control appears to be an early step in the development of carcinogenesis and ultimately cancer progression. Recent investigative efforts have explored several genes and their protein products involved in cell cycle regulation, to determine their prognostic significance in bladder cancer progression.

3.10.1
Retinoblastoma Tumor Suppressor Gene

The retinoblastoma (*RB*) tumor suppressor gene was the first tumor suppressor gene to be identified. The *RB* gene is located on chromosome 13q14 and encodes for a 110-kDa nuclear phosphoprotein (FUNG et al. 1987). Although initially discovered to be mutated in patients with inherited retinoblastoma, altered *RB* gene expression has been reported in various human tumors, including transitional cell carcinoma of the bladder (CAIRNS et al. 1991; CORDON-CARDO et al. 1992; LOGOTHETIS et al. 1992; PRESTI et al. 1991). In its physiologic active hypophosphorylated form, pRB acts by inhibiting cell cycle progression at the G_1-S phase by binding to a number of cellular proteins including the transcription factor E2F (BAGCHI et al. 1991; WANG et al. 1994). The pRB is phosphorylated in a cell cycle-dependent manner, underphosphorylated pRB being the predominant form in G_1, resulting in a tumor suppresser effect. With entry into the S phase, pRB becomes phosphorylated.

Inactivation of the *RB* gene is thought to be an important step in bladder cancer progression. Several monoclonal and polyclonal antibodies have been discovered which allow the reliable evaluation of pRB expression through immunohistochemical methods (GERADTS et al. 1994). With a combination of immunohistochemical techniques and molecular analysis, several groups have demonstrated that the proportion of bladder cancers demonstrating *RB* alterations increases with higher tumor grade and stage (XU et al. 1993; ISHIKAWA et al. 1991). The results of these studies suggest that loss of pRB expression may be an important prognostic factor in transitional cell carcinoma of the bladder. CORDON-CARDO and associates (1992) reported that patients with muscle invasive bladder tumors that had lost *RB* immunoexpression had a statistically significant shorter 5-year survival ($P = 0.001$) than those patients with normal RB protein expression. Similarly, LOGOTHESIS and associates (1992) studied 43 pa-

tients with invasive bladder cancer and demonstrated that *RB* alterations were more common in advanced tumors, and that patients whose tumors had lost pRB expression had a worse overall survival than patients whose tumors had maintained RB immunoexpression. Based on the aforementioned data, it appears that pRB expression is an important prognostic factor in patients with invasive bladder cancer.

3.10.2
p53 Tumor Suppressor Gene

Mutations in the *p53* gene are the most common genetic defect in human tumors (HOLLSTEIN et al. 1991). The *p53* gene is located on chromosome 17p13 and encodes for a 53-kDa protein. The *p53* gene functions as a tumor suppressor gene. Specifically, the p53 protein plays a vital role in the regulation of the cell cycle (LANE 1992). When DNA damage occurs, the level of p53 protein increases, causing cell cycle arrest and allowing time for the repair of the DNA. This prevents propagation of the DNA defect. Mutations of the *p53* gene result in the production of an abnormal and usually dysfunctional protein product with a prolonged half-life compared with the wild-type protein. Consequently, this abnormal protein accumulates in the cell nucleus and can be detected by immunohistochemical staining. Several studies have demonstrated that nuclear accumulation of p53 protein as determined by immunohistochemical staining correlates with gene mutations detected by DNA sequence analysis (ESRIG et al. 1993; DALBAGNI et al. 1995).

Several studies have shown that *p53* alterations, as determined by immunohistochemical techniques, are an important prognostic marker for bladder cancer progression (ESRIG et al. 1994; CORDON-CARDO et al. 1994; LIPPONEN 1993b; SARKIS et al. 1993). Increased p53 immunoreactivity has been found in higher grade and stage bladder cancers and is associated with disease progression and worse overall disease-specific survival. Our group evaluated the nuclear reactivity of p53 in 243 patients with invasive bladder cancer who were uniformly treated with radical cystectomy (ESRIG et al. 1994). We found that the immunohistochemical detection of p53 protein in tumor nuclei provided important prognostic information in this group of patients. Patients with an increase in p53 expression were found to have a significantly increased risk of recurrence and decreased overall survival. This association was independent of tumor grade, pathologic stage, and lymph node status, and was most marked in patients with organ-confined tumors (P1, P2, P3a). Furthermore, nuclear accumulation of p53 immunoreactivity was found to be the only independent predictor of disease progression in a multivariate comparison of p53 status, histologic grade, and pathologic stage.

LIPPONEN (1993b) reported the findings in 212 patients with primary bladder cancer who were evaluated for p53 immunoreactivity. Increased p53 nuclear reactivity was found to be a significant adverse prognostic factor in patients with muscle invasive bladder cancers. Increased tumor grade and progression were associated with increased p53 expression. In another study, SARKIS and associates (1993) evaluated p53 expression in 11 patients with muscle invasive bladder tumors treated with neoadjuvant chemotherapy. They found that patients with increased p53 nuclear reactivity had higher rates of disease progression and cancer-specific death compared with patients who did not demonstrate increased p53 expression.

The accumulating evidence from a number of independent studies suggests that p53 immunoreactivity is a reliable and consistent prognostic marker for bladder cancer progression. Increased expression of p53 as determined by immunohistochemical methods is generally seen in bladder tumors with increase grade and advanced pathologic stage. In addition, increased p53 immunoreactivity is associated with a higher likelihood of disease progression and cancer-specific death.

3.10.3
Combination of *RB* and *p53* Tumor Suppressor Genes

Two independent studies have evaluated the prognostic significance of combining the *RB* and *p53* status of bladder cancers as determined by immunohistochemical techniques. Preliminary data from these studies support the concept that bladder tumors with alterations in *p53* and *RB* confer a worse prognosis and survival than tumors with normal *p53* and *RB*. Tumors with an alteration of only one of these genes as determined by immunohistochemical methods behave in an intermediate fashion. These data suggest that the status of both *p53* and *RB* is important, and that these genes behave in an independent yet synergistic manner in patients with bladder cancer.

3.10.4
p21 Tumor Suppressor Gene

Although p53 nuclear accumulation, as detected by immunohistochemical methods, is a significant predictor of bladder cancer progression, not all *p53*-altered bladder tumors recur (ESRIG et al. 1993; SARKIS et al. 1993). One of the primary functions of p53 is as a cell cycle regulatory protein (CORDON-CARDO 1995; LANE 1992). p53 mediates its effects on the cell cycle through the regulation of $p21^{WAF1/CIP1}$ expression (CORDON-CARDO 1995). Alterations in *p53* result in loss of p21 expression, which leads to unregulated cell growth. This is thought to be one of the mechanisms through which *p53* alterations may influence tumor progression. However, it has recently been demonstrated that p21 expression may also be mediated through p53-independent pathways (MICHIELI et al. 1994; BOND et al. 1995; PARKER et al. 1995). This important finding suggests that despite the presence of a *p53* alteration, p21 expression (and therefore cell cycle control) can be maintained.

With a better understanding of cell-cycle regulation, including the interactions of p53 and p21 and cell-cycle control, we sought to determine whether the presence or absence of p21 expression in bladder tumors demonstrating *p53* alterations might be an important factor in predicting clinical behavior. We reasoned that the expression of p21 through p53-independent pathways might abrogate the deleterious effects of *p53* alterations by resulting in the maintenance of cell cycle control.

We evaluated bladder tumors from 101 patients who underwent radical cystectomy for invasive bladder cancer, for p21 expression by immunohistochemical techniques. All patients had been previously determined to have *p53* altered tumors. We found that immunohistochemical detection of p21 protein in the nuclei of bladder cancers which show *p53* alterations (*p53*-altered) provides important prognostic information in patients with bladder cancer. Patients with *p53*-altered transitional cell carcinomas of the bladder that were p21-negative demonstrated a significantly increased probability of recurrence and decreased probability of overall survival compared with *p53*-altered tumors that maintained expression of p21 (p21-positive). The association of p21 status and prognosis in *p53*-altered bladder tumors was independent of tumor grade, pathologic stage and lymph node status. The strongest association between p21 status and tumor progression was observed in patients with organ-

confined (Pis, P1, P2, P3a) and extravesical disease (P3b, P4) without evidence of lymph node
metastases. Loss of p21 expression was strongly associated with an increased probability of recurrence
and decreased overall probability of survival in patients with lymph node-negative organ-confined disease and extravesical disease. In fact, p21 was the
only independent predictor of disease progression in
p53-altered bladder tumors in a multivariable analysis comparing p21 status, histologic grade, and
pathologic stage. These findings suggest that p21 expression through p53 independent pathways exist,
and that patients with *p53* altered tumors that lose
p21 expression have a worse prognosis and should
be considered for adjuvant treatment.

3.11
Conclusion

It is clear that at the present time conventional
histopathologic evaluation of bladder cancer, including tumor grade and stage, is inadequate to accurately predict the behavior of most bladder cancers.
Tumor heterogeneity, even within the same subgroups of patients, prevents the determination of a
bladder cancer's biologic potential. Dedicated efforts
have been made to identify other potential prognostic markers that may better stratify and identify a
tumor's true malignant potential. With a better understanding of the cell cycle and cell-to-cell interactions, along with improved diagnostic techniques
(immunohistochemistry), progress is being made in
characterizing other potential prognostic markers. It
is safe to say that standard analysis is inadequate to
accurately predict the course of a particular bladder
tumor, and is thus inadequate for the determination
of patient-specific treatment. It will soon be possible
to use immunohistochemical techniques to help in
the differentiation between patients who require
more aggressive treatment schemes and those who
require potentially less aggressive regimens.

References

Akiyama T, Sudo C, Ogawara H, Toyoshima K, Yamamoto T
  (1986) The product of the human c-*erb*B-2 gene: a 185–
  kilodalton glycoprotein with tyrosine kinase activity. Science 232:1644–1646
Albeda SM (1993) Biology of disease: role of integrins and
  other cell adhesion molecules in tumor progression and
  metastasis. Lab Invest 68:4–17
Bagchi S, Weinman R, Raychaudhuri P (1991) The
  retinoblastoma protein copurifies with E2F-1, an E1A-

regulated inhibitor of the transcription factor E2F. Cell
  65:1063–1072
Bargmann CI, Hung M-C, Weinberg RA (1986) The *neu*
  oncogene encodes an epidermal growth factor receptor-
  related protein. Nature 319:226–229
Barnhill RL, Levy MA (1992) Regressing thin cutaneous
  malignant melanomas (≤1.0mm) are associated
  with angiogenesis. Am J Pathol 143:99–104
Berger MS, Greenfield C, Gullick WJ, et al. (1987) Evaluation
  of epidermal growth factor receptors in bladder tumors. Br
  J Cancer 56:533–537
Blood CH, Zetter BR (1990) Tumor interactions with the vasculature: angiogenesis and tumor metastasis. Biochem
  Biophys Acta 1032:89–118
Bochner BH, Cote RJ, Weidner N, Groshen S, Chen S-C,
  Skinner DG, Nichols PW (1995) Angiogenesis in bladder
  cancer: relationship between microvessel density and
  tumor prognosis. J Natl Cancer Inst 87:1603–1612
Bond JA, Blaydes JP, Rowson J, Haughton MF, Smith JR, Thomas DW, Wyllie FS (1995) Mutant p53 rescues human dip-
  loid cells from senescence without inhibiting the induction
  of SDI1/WAF1. Cancer Res 55:2404–2409
Borg A, Baldetorp B, Ferno M, Killander D, Olsson H,
  Sigurdsson H (1991) *erb*B-2 amplification in breast cancer
  with a high rate of proliferation. Oncogene 6:137–143
Brawer MK, Deering RE, Brown M, Preston SD, Bigler SA
  (1994) Predictors of pathologic stage in prostatic carcinoma. The role of neovascularity. Cancer 73:678–687
Bretton P, Cordon-Cardo C, Wartinger D, Kimmel M, Fair
  WR, Melamed MR, Fradet Y (1990) Expression of the T-138
  antigen and survival of patients with bladder cancer. Proc
  Am Assoc Cancer Res 31:186 (abstract 1105)
Bringuier PP, Umbas R, Schaafsma HE, Karthaus HFM,
  Debruyne FMJ, Schalken JA (1993) Decreased E-cadherin
  immunoreactivity correlates with poor survival in patients
  with bladder tumors. Cancer Res 53:3241–3245
Brown DC, Gatter KC (1990) Monoclonal antibody Ki-67: its
  use in histopathology. Histopathology 17:489–503
Bush C, Price P, Norten J, et al. (1991) Proliferation in human
  bladder carcinoma measured by Ki-67 antibody labelling:
  its potential clinical importance. Br J Cancer 64:357–360
Cairns P, Proctor AJ, Knowles MA (1991) Loss of heterozygosity at the Rb locus is frequent and correlates with
  muscle invasion in bladder carcinoma. Oncogene 6:2305–
  2309
Cambell SC, Bouck N (1996) Harnessing the tumor-fighting
  power of angiogenesis. Contemp Urol June:27–40
Chodak GW, Scheiner CJ, Zetter BR (1981) Urine from
  patients with transitional-cell carcinoma stimulates
  migration of capillary endothelial cells. N Engl J Med
  305:869–874
Chopin DK, Caruelle J-P, Colombel M, et al. (1993) Increased
  immunodetection of acidic fibroblast growth factor
  in bladder cancer, detectable in urine. J Urol 150:1126–
  1130
Cohen MB, Waldman FM, Carroll PR, Kerschmann R, Chew K,
  Mayall BH (1993) Comparison of five histopathologic
  methods to assess cellular proliferation in transitional
  cell carcinoma of the urinary bladder. Hum Pathol 24:772–
  778
Cordon-Cardo C (1995) Mutation of cell cycle regulators. Biological and clinical implications of human neoplasia. Am J
  Pathol 147:545–560
Cordon-Cardo C, Lloyd KO, Finstad CL, et al. (1986)
  Immunoanatomic distribution of blood group antigens in
  the human urinary tract: influence of secretor status. Lab
  Invest 55:444–454

Cordon-Cardo C, Reuter VE, Lloyd KO, Sheinfeld J, Fair WR, Old LJ, Melamed MR (1988) Blood group-related antigens in human urothelium: enhanced expression of precursors, Le^x, and Le^y determinants in urothelial carcinoma. Cancer Res 48:4113–4120

Cordon-Cardo C, Wartinger D, Petrylak D, Dalbagni G, Fair WF, Fuks Z, Reuter VE (1992) Altered expression of the retinoblastoma gene product: prognostic indicator in bladder cancer. J Natl Cancer Inst 84:1251–1256

Cordon-Cardo C, Dalbagni G, Saez GT, et al. (1994) p53 mutations in human bladder cancer: genotypic versus phenotypic patterns. Int J Cancer 56:347–353

Crawford ED, Davis MA (1987) Nontransitional cell carcinomas of the bladder. In: deKernian JB, Paulson DF (eds) Genitourinary cancer management. Lea & Febiger, Philadelphia, chapter 4, pp 95–105

Dalbagni G, Reuter VE, Sheinfeld J, Fradet Y, Fair WR, Cardon-Cardo C (1992) Cell surface differentiation antigens of normal urothelium and bladder tumors. Semin Surg Oncol 8:293–307

Dalbagni G, Cordon-Cardo C, Reuter V, Fair W (1995) Tumor suppressor alterations in bladder cancer. Surg Oncol Clin North Am 4:231–240

Dameron KM, Volpert OV, Tainsky MA, Bouck N (1994) Control of angiogenesis in fibroblasts by p53 regulation of thrombospondin-1. Science 265:1582–1584

Decenzo JM, Howard P, Irish CE (1975) Antigenic deletion and prognosis of patients with stage A transitional cell carcinoma. J Uro 114:874–878

D'Elia FL, Cooper HS, Mulholland SG (1982) ABH isoantigens in stage O papillary transitional cell carcinoma of the bladder: correlation with biological behavior. J Urol 127:665–667

Dickinson AJ, Fox SB, Persad RA, Hollyer J, Sibley GN, Harris AL (1994) Quantification of angiogenesis as an independent predictor of prognosis in invasive bladder carcinomas. Br J Urol 74:762–766

Droller MJ (1990) Individualizing the approach to invasive bladder cancer. Contemp Urol July/August:54–61

Esrig D, Spruch CH III, Nichols PW, et al. (1993) p53 nuclear protein accumulation correlates with mutations in the p53 gene, tumor grade, and stage in bladder cancer. Am J Pathol 143:1389–1397

Esrig D, Elmajian D, Groshen S, et al. (1994) Accumulation of nuclear p53 and tumor progression in bladder cancer. N Engl J Med 331:1259–1264

Esrig D, Shi S-R, Bochner B, et al. (1995) Prognostic importance of p53 and Rb alterations in transitional cell carcinoma of the bladder. J Urol 153:362A (abstract 536)

Folkman J, Klagsbrun M (1987) Angiogenic factors. Science 235:442–447

Folkman J, Cole P, Zimmerman S (1966) Tumor behavior in isolated perfused organs: in vitro growth and metastases of biopsy material in rabbit thyroid and canine intestinal segment. Ann Surg 164:491–502

Fontana D, Bellina M, Gubetta L, et al. (1992) Monoclonal antibody Ki-67 in the study of the proliferative activity of bladder carcinoma. J Urol 148:1149–1151

Fradet Y, Cordon-Cardo C (1993) Critical appraisal of tumor markers in bladder cancer. Semin Urol 11:145–153

Fradet Y, Tardif M, Bourget L, Robert J and the Laval University Urology Group. (1990) Clinical cancer progression in urinary bladder tumors evaluated by multiparameter flow cytometry with monoclonal antibodies. Cancer Res 50:432–437

Fradet Y, Gauthier J, Bedard G, Charrois R, Naua A (1991) Monitoring and prognostic determination of bladder tumors by flow cytometry with monoclonal antibodies on bladder irrigations. J Urol 145:250A (abstract 149)

Fradet Y, Lafleur L, La Rue H (1992) Strategies of chemoprevention based on antigenic and molecular markers of early and premalignant lesions of the bladder. J Cell Biochem 161:85–92

Frixen UH, Behrens J, Sachs M, et al. (1991) E-cadherin-mediated cell-cell adhesion prevents invasiveness of human carcinoma cells. J Cell Biol 113:173–185

Fung Y-KT, Murphree AL, T'Ang A, Qian J, Hinrichs SH, Benedict WF (1987) Structural evidence for the authenticity of the human retinoblastoma gene. Science 236:1657–1661

Geradts J, Hu S-X, Lincoln C, Benedict WF, Xu H-J (1994) Aberrant Rb gene expression in routinely processed, archival tumor tissues determined by three different anti-Rb antibodies. Int J Cancer 58:161–167

Gerdes J, Schwab U, Lemke H, Stein H (1983) Production of a mouse monoclonal antibody reactive with a human nuclear antigen associated with cell proliferation. Int J Cancer 31:13–20

Gimbrone MA Jr, Leapman SB, Coltran RS, Folkman J (1972) Tumor dormancy in vivo by prevention of neovascularization. J Exp Med 136:261–276

Gimbrone MA Jr, Cotran RS, Leapman SB, Folkman J (1974) Tumor growth neovascularization: an experimental model using the rabbit cornea. J Natl Cancer Inst 52:413–417

Golijanin D, Sherman Y, Shapiro A, Pode D (1995) Detection of bladder tumors by immunostaining of Lewis X antigen in cells from voided urine. Urology 46:173–177

Good DJ, Polverini PJ, Rastinejad F, LeBeau MM, Lemons RS, Frazier WA, Bouck NP (1990) A tumor suppressor-dependent inhibitor of angiogenesis is immunologically and functionally indistinguishable from a fragment of thrombospondin. Proc Natl Acad Sci 87:6624–6628

Gorgoulis VG, Barbatis C, Poulias I, Karameris AM (1995) Molecular and immunohistochemical evaluation of epidermal growth factor receptor and c-erbB-2 gene product in transitional cell carcinomas of the urinary bladder. A study in Greek patients. Mod Pathol 8:758–764

Grossfeld GD, Ginsberg D, Stein JP, et al. (1996a) Thrombospondin-1 expression in bladder cancer: association with p53 alterations, tumor angiogenesis and tumor progression. J Natl Cancer Inst (in press)

Grossfeld GD, Shi SR, Ginsberg DA, Rich KA, Skinner DG, Taylor CR, Cote RJ (1996b) Immunohistochemical detection of thrombospondin-1 in formalin-fixed, paraffin-embedded tissue. J Histochem Cytochem 44:761–766

Hakomori SI (1985) Aberrant glycosylation in cancer cell membranes as focused on glycolipids: overview and perspectives. Cancer Res 45:2405–2414

Hollstein M, Sidransky D, Volgelstein B, Harris CC (1991) p53 mutations in human cancers. Science 253:49–53

Horak ER, Leek R, Klenk N, et al. (1992) Angiogenesis, assessed by platelet/endothelial cell adhesion molecule antibodies, as indicator of node metastases and survival in breast cancer. Lancet 340:1120–1124

Ishikawa J, Xu H-J, Hu S-X, et al. (1991) Inactivation of the retinoblastoma gene in human bladder and renal cell carcinomas. Cancer Res 51:5736–5743

Jaeger TM, Weidner N, Chew K, Moore DH, Kerschmann RL, Waldman FM, Carroll PR (1995) Tumor angiogenesis correlates with lymph node metastases in invasive bladder cancer. J Urol 154:69–71

Jouanneau J, Gavrilovic J, Caruelle D, Jaye M, Moens G, Caruelle J-P, Thiery JP (1991) Secreted or nonsecreted forms of acidic fibroblast growth factor produced by transfected epithelial cells influence cell morphology, motility, and invasive potential. Proc Natl Acad Sci 88:2893–2897

King ED, Matteson J, Jacobs SC, Kyprianou N (1996) Incidence of apoptosis, cell proliferation and bcl-2 expression in transitional cell carcinoma of the bladder: association with tumor progression. J Urol 155:316–320

Kohler G, Milstein C (1975) Continuous cultures of fused cells secreting antibody of predefined specificity. Nature 256:495–497

Lane DP (1992) Cancer: p53, guardian of the genome. Nature 358:15–16

Lange PH, Limas C, Fraley EE (1978) Tissue blood-group antigens and prognosis in low stage transitional cell carcinoma of the bladder. J Urol 119:52–55

Larjava H, Peltonen J, Akiyama SK, Yamada SS, Gralnick HR, Uitto J, Yamada KM (1990) Novel function of *B1* integrins in keratinocyte cell-cell interactions. J Cell Biol 110:803–815

Lawler J, Derick LH, Connolly JE, Chen J-H, Chao FC (1985) The structure of human platelet thrombospondin. J Biol Chem 260:3762–3772

Lee J, Dull TJ, Lax I, Schlessinger J, Ullrich A (1989) HER2 cytoplasmic domain generates normal mitogenic and transforming signals in a chimeric receptor. EMBO J 8:167–173

Lerner S, Linn D, Chakraborty S, et al. (1995) Correlation of p53 and retinoblastoma protein expression with established pathologic prognostic features in radical cystoprostatectomy specimens. J Urol 153:363A (abstract 537)

Liebert M (1995) Growth factors in bladder cancer World J Urol 13:349–355

Liebert M, Wedemeyer G, Stein J, Washington RW Jr, Van Waes C, Carey TE, Grossman HB (1993) The monoclonal antibody BQ16 identifies the alpha-6*B4* integrin on bladder cancer. Hybridoma 12:67–80

Liebert M, Washington R, Stein J, Wedemeyer G, Grossman B (1994a) Expression of the VLA *B1* integrin family in bladder cancer. Am J Pathol 144:1016–1022

Liebert M, Washington R, Wedemeyer G, Carey TE, Grossman BH (1994b) Loss of co-localization of alpha-6*B4* integrin and collagen VII in bladder cancer. Am J Pathol 144:787–795

Limas C, Lange P, Fraley EE, Vessella RL (1979) A, B, H antigens in transitional cell tumors of the urinary bladder: correlation with the clinical course. Cancer 44:2099–2107

Lipponen PK (1993a) Expression of c-*erb*B-2 oncoprotein in transitional cell bladder cancer. Eur J Cancer 29A:749–753

Lipponen PK (1993b) Over-expression of the p53 nuclear oncoprotein in transitional cell carcinoma of the bladder and its prognostic value. Int J Cancer 53:365–370

Lipponen PK, Eskelinen MJ (1994) Expression of epidermal growth factor receptor in bladder cancer as related to established prognostic factors, oncoprotein (c-*erb*B-2, p53) expression and long-term prognosis. Br J Cancer 69:1120–1125

Lipponen PK, Eskelinen MJ (1995) Reduced expression of E-cadherin is related to invasive disease and frequent recurrence in bladder cancer. J Cancer Res Clin Oncol 121:303–308

Lloyd KO (1987) Blood group antigens as markers for normal differentiation and malignant change in human tissues. Am J Clin Pathol 87:129–139

Logothetis CJ, Xu H-J, Ro JY, Hu S-X, Sahin A, Ordonez N, Benedict WF (1992) Altered expression of retinoblastoma protein and known prognostic variables in locally advanced bladder cancer. J Natl Cancer Inst 84:1256–1261

Loke SL, Jaffe ES, Neckers LM (1987) Inhibition of in vitro DNA synthesis by the monoclonal antibody Ki-67. Blood Suppl 70:1579–1583

Mellon JK, Lunec J, Wright C, Horne CHW, Kelly P, Neal DE (1996) C-*erb*B-2 in bladder cancer: molecular biology, correlation with epidermal growth factor receptors and prognostic value. J Urol 155:321–326

Messing EM (1990) Clinical implications of the expression of epidermal growth factor receptors in human transitional cell carcinoma. Cancer Res 50:2530–2537

Messing EM, Hanson P, Ulrich P, Erturk E (1987) Epidermal growth factor – interactions with normal and malignant urothelium: in vivo and in situ studies. J Urol 138:1329–1335

Michieli P, Chedid M, Lin D, Pierce JH, Mercer EW, Givol D (1994) Induction of WAF1/CIP1 by a p53–independent pathway. Cancer Res 54:3391–3395

Moch H, Sauter G, Moore D, Mihatsch MJ, Gudat F, Waldman F (1993) p53 and *erb*B-2 protein overexpression are associated with early invasion and metastasis in bladder cancer. Virchows Arch [A] 423:329–334

Moriyama M, Akiyama T, Yamamoto T, et al. (1991) Expression of c-*erb*B-2 gene product in urinary bladder cancer. J Urol 145:423–427

Mulder AH, Van Hootegem JCSP, Sylvester R, Ten Kate FJW, Kurth KH, Ooms ECM, Van Der Kwast TH (1992) Prognostic factors in bladder carcinoma: histologic parameters and expression of a cell cycle-related nuclear antigen (Ki-67). J Pathol 166:37–43

Neal DE, Marsh C, Bennett MK, Abel PD, Hall RR, Sainsbury JRC, Harris AL (1985) Epidermal-growth-factor receptors in human bladder cancer: comparison of invasive and superficial tumors. Lancet I:366–368

Neal DE, Sharples L, Smith K, Frennelly J, Hall RR, Harris AL (1990) The epidermal growth factor receptor and the prognosis of bladder cancer. Cancer 65:1619–1625

Newman AJ Jr, Carlton CE Jr, Johnson S (1980) Cell surface A, B, or O(H) blood group antigens as an indicator of malignant potential in stage A bladder carcinoma. J Urol 124:27–29

Nguyen M, Watanabe H, Budson AE, Richie JP, Folkman J (1993) Elevated levels of the angiogenic peptide basic fibroblast growth factor in urine of bladder cancer patients. J Natl Cancer Inst 85:241–242

O'Brien T, Cranston D, Fuggle S, Dicknell R, Harris AL (1995) Different angiogenic pathways characterize superficial and invasive bladder cancer. Cancer Res 55:510–513

Ogata K, Celis JE, Tan EM (1987) Proliferating cell nuclear antigen: cyclin. Methods Enzymol 150:147–159

Okamura K, Miyake K, Koshikawa T, Asai J (1990) Growth fractions of transitional cell carcinomas of the bladder defined by the monoclonal antibody Ki-67. J Urol 144:875–878

Otto T, Birchmeier W, Schmidt U, Hinke A, Schipper J, Rubben H, Raz A (1994) Inverse relation of E-cadherin and autocrine motility factor receptor expression as a prognostic factor in patients with bladder cancer. Cancer Res 54:3120–3123

Parker SB, Eichele G, Zhang P, et al. (1995) p53-independent expression of p21 in muscle and other terminal differentiating cells. Science 267:1024–1027

Parker SL, Tong T, Bolden S, Wing PA (1996) Cancer statistics, 1996. CA Cancer J Clin 46:8–9

Partanen AM (1990) Epidermal growth factor and transforming growth factor-A in the development of epithelial-mesenchymal organs of the mouse. Curr Top Dev Biol 24:31–55

Polverini PJ, Leibovich SJ (1984) Induction of neovascularization in vivo and endothelial proliferation in vitro by tumor-associated macrophages. Lab Invest 51:635–642

Presti JC Jr, Reuter VE, Galan T, Fair WR, Cordon-Cardo C (1991) Molecular genetic alterations in superficial and locally advanced human bladder cancer. Cancer Res 51:5405–5409

Robbins BA, de la Vega D, Ogata K, Tan EM, Nakamura RN (1987) Immunohistochemical detection of proliferating cell nuclear antigen in solid human malignancies. Arch Pathol Lab Med 111:841–845

Sarkis AS, Dalbagni G, Cordon-Cardo C, et al. (1993) Nuclear over-expression of p53 protein in transitional cell bladder carcinoma: a marker for disease progression. J Natl Cancer Inst 85:53–59

Sarkis AS, Charytonowicz E, Cordon-Cardo C (1994) Blood group antigen expression in bladder tumors: an immunohistochemical study of superficial bladder lesions. J Exp Clin Cancer Res 13:139–144

Sarosdy MF, de Vere White RW, Soloway MS, et al. (1995) Results of a multicenter trial using the BTA test to monitor for and diagnose recurrent bladder cancer. J Urol 154:379–384

Sato K, Moriyama M, Mori S, et al. (1992) An immunohistologic evaluation of c-erbB-2 gene product in patients with urinary bladder carcinoma. Cancer 70:2493–2498

Sauter G, Haley J, Chew K, et al. (1994) Epidermal growth factor receptor expression is associated with rapid tumor proliferation in bladder cancer. Int J Cancer 57:508–514

Sheinfeld J, Reuter VE, Melamed MR, et al. (1990) Enhanced bladder cancer detection with the Lewis X antigen as a marker of neoplastic transformation. J Urol 143:285–288

Sheinfeld J, Sarkis AS, Reuter VE, Fair WR, Cordon-Cardo C (1992) The Lewis X antigen as a predictor of tumor recurrence in high risk disease-free bladder cancer patients. J Urol 147:423A (abstract 841)

Shiozaki H, Tahara H, Oka H, et al. (1991) Expression of immunoreactive E-cadherin adhesion molecules in human cancers. Am J Pathol 139:17–23

Skinner DG, Lieskovsky G (1988) Management of invasive and high-grade bladder cancer. In: Skinner DG, Lieskovsky G (eds) Diagnosis and management of genitourinary cancer, vol 1. Saunders, Philadelphia, pp 295–312

Slamon DJ, Godolphin W, Jones LA, et al. (1989) Studies of the HER-2/neu proto-oncogene in human breast and ovarian cancer. Science 244:707–712

Srivastava A, Laidler P, Davies RP, Horgan K, Hughes LE (1988) The prognostic significance of tumor vascularity in intermediate-thickness (0.76–4.0 mm thick) skin melanoma. Am J Pathol 33:419–423

Stein JP, Ginsberg DA, Grossfeld GD, et al. (1996) The effect of p21 expression on tumor progression in p53 altered bladder cancer. J Urol 155:628A (abstract 1270)

Stern DF, Heffernan PA, Weinberg RA (1986) p185, a product of the neu proto-oncogene, is a receptor like protein associated with tyrosine kinase activity. Mol Cell Biol 6:1729–1740

Sutherland RM, McCredie JA, Inch WR (1971) Growth of multicell spheroids in tissue culture as a model of nodular carcinomas. J Natl Cancer Inst 46:113–120

Symington BE, Takada Y, Carter WG (1993) Interaction of intergrins alpha 3 beta 1 and alpha 2 beta 1: potential role in keratinocyte intercellular adhesion. J Cell Biol 120:523–535

Tsujihashi H, Nakanishi A, Matsuda H, Uejima S, Kurita T (1991) Cell proliferation of human bladder tumors determined by BRDURD and Ki-67 immunostaining. J Urol 145:846–849

Underwood M, Bartlett J, Reeves J, Gardiner S, Scott R, Cooke T (1995) C-erbB-2 gene amplification: a molecular marker in recurrent bladder tumors? Cancer Res 55:2422–2430

Valles AM, Boyer B, Badet J, Tucker GC, Barritault D, Thiery JP (1990) Acidic fibroblast growth factor is a modulator of epithelial plasticity in a rat bladder carcinoma cell line. Proc Natl Acad Sci USA 87:1124–1128

Walz DA (1992) Thrombospondin as a mediator of cancer cell adhesion in metastasis. Cancer Metastasis Rev 11:313–324

Wang JY, Knudsen ES, Welch PJ (1994) The retinoblastoma tumor suppressor protein. Adv Cancer Res 64:25–87

Weidner N, Folkman J, Pozza F, et al. (1992) Tumor angiogenesis: a new significant and independent prognostic indicator in early-stage breast carcinoma. J Natl Cancer Inst 84:1875–1887

Weidner N, Carrol PR, Flax J, Blumenfeld W, Folkman J (1993) Tumor angiogenesis correlates with metastasis in invasive prostate carcinoma. Am J Pathol 143:401–409

Weinstein RS, Alroy J, Farrow GM, Miller AW, Davidsohn I (1979) Blood group isoantigen deletion in carcinoma in situ of the urinary bladder. Cancer 43:661–668

Wiley EL, Mendelsohn G, Droller MJ, Eggleston JC (1982) Immunoperoxidase detection of carcinoembryonic antigen and blood group substances in papillary transitional cell carcinoma of the bladder. J Urol 128:276–280

Xu H-J, Cairns P, Hu S-X, Knowles MA, Benedict WF (1993) Loss of Rb protein expression in primary bladder cancer correlates with loss of heterozygosity at the Rb locus and tumor progression. Int J Cancer 53:781–784

Yamamoto T, Ikawa S, Akiyama T, et al. (1986) Similarity of protein encoded by the human c-erbB-2 gene to epidermal growth factor receptor. Nature 319:230

Young AK, Hammond E, Middleton AW Jr (1979) The prognostic value of cell surface antigens in low grade, noninvasive, transitional cell carcinoma of the bladder. J Urol 122:462–464

4 Molecular Genetics in Carcinoma of the Bladder

C.M. Bender and P.A. Jones

CONTENTS

4.1 Introduction

Bladder cancer represents the fifth most common cancer in the United States (Silverberg et al. 1989). Epidemiological investigations suggest that cigarette smoking and occupational exposure to arylamines are the two leading risk factors contributing to this disease (Augustine et al. 1988). Carcinomas of the bladder arise from the neoplastic transformation of uroepithelial cells into the several morphologically and genetically distinct subsets of bladder cancer. For example, approximately 90% of bladder cancer malignancies in the United States are transitional cell carcinomas (TCCs), and the remaining 10% are classified as either squamous cell carcinomas (SCCs),

C.M. Bender, PhD, Department of Biochemistry and Molecular Biology, Urologic Cancer Research Laboratory, University of Southern California, USC/Norris Comprehensive Cancer Center, 1441 Eastlake Avenue, Los Angeles, CA 90033, USA
P.A. Jones, PhD, Professor of Biochemistry and Molecular Biology, Urologic Cancer Research Laboratory, University of Southern California, USC/Norris Comprehensive Cancer Center, 1441 Eastlake Avenue, Los Angeles, CA 90033, USA

undifferentiated adenocarcinomas, or undifferentiated cancers of the bladder. In contrast, SCCs predominate in Middle Eastern countries, Egypt, and Africa, representing the leading cancer in men and accounting for 80% of all bladder cancer cases. The prevalence of SCC in these regions is associated with the endemic occurrence of infections by the *Schistosoma haematobium* trematode (Mostofi et al. 1988).

Bladder cancer varies both histologically and clinically, ranging from a benign, superficial papillary disease to a metastatic, muscle-invasive disease. Approximately 80% of transitional cell carcinomas are low-grade, superficial Ta and T1 papillary tumors, and the remaining 20% include both the noninvasive carcinomas in situ and high-grade, invasive tumors. Although most superficial papillary tumors recur after local resection, only 10%–30% of these recurrences progress to invasive disease. Carcinomas in situ, however, exhibit a greater tendency to progress despite their noninvasive character. Once a tumor invades the underlying stroma of the bladder, this cancer usually progresses into a more invasive disease.

Recent molecular investigations suggest that specific genetic alterations determine whether a particular cancer will progress. Various molecular and genetic events may be responsible for the histologically and clinically distinct subsets of bladder cancer, and the order in which these events occur may determine whether a transformed cell forms a benign papillary tumor which can be easily resected, or an aggressive metastatic tumor which invades the underlying stroma of the bladder. The existence of diverse morphologies and histopathologies in bladder cancer supports the hypothesis that multiple molecular and genetic pathways during the developmental course of the disease are responsible for its initiation and progression. Identifying specific genetic alterations associated with the different stages of bladder cancer will prove useful. In addition, understanding the molecular biological phenomena underlying carcinogenesis in order to develop new cancer therapies and improve clinical prognoses (via genetic intervention) will have both scientific and clinical significance.

4.2
Analytical Methods to Study Bladder Cancer

4.2.1
Cytogenetic Studies

Established cytogenetic methodologies, together with more recent molecular biological innovations, have facilitated the advancement of genetic investigations in bladder cancer. Methods in molecular biology are useful because they often complement cytogenetic studies by revealing chromosomal changes not visible through a microscope. The analytical methodologies of both technical areas will be described.

Cytogenetic studies include karyotyping, flow cytometry, and fluorescence in situ hybridization (FISH). These methods are all designed to detect gross chromosomal anomalies which include chromosomal duplications, translocations, amplifications, and deletions (SANDBERG and BRIDGE 1992). Although karyotyping is still popular, the cell culturing procedures involved in this method have potential drawbacks. In particular, karyotyping requires that tumor cells be incubated until their mitotic activity peaks; however, this may confer a selective growth advantage for smaller cell subpopulations which acquire chromosomal aberrations during culturing. As a result, karyotypic results from these cell subpopulations may not reveal chromosomal aberrations which actually occurred in vivo. Alternatively, flow cytometric analyses offer a much more rapid and reliable method to determine the ploidy status of cell populations in which cells are fixed, stained, and analyzed according to their relative DNA content (SANDBERG and BRIDGE 1992). This method is useful for the identification of aneuploidy, which is known to be associated with tumor cell progression; however, a major limitation of flow cytometric analysis resides in the fact that subsets of cells with different chromosomal anomalies may not be deciphered. FISH, therefore, represents the most convenient cytogenetic method to date because both individual and nondividing cells can be analyzed (HOPMAN et al. 1991).

4.2.2
In Vitro Studies

An interesting experimental model for the analysis of nonrandom chromosomal losses in bladder cancer has been designed by WU et al. (1991) in which an in vivo and in vitro transformation system was used to identify specific chromosomal losses associated with the stepwise neoplastic transformation and progression of uroepithelial cells. In this procedure, the propensity for ten transformed cell lines with variable phenotypes (representing low- and high-grade TCCs, SCCs, and undifferentiated bladder cancers) to progress was analyzed. Next, nonrandom allelic chromosomal losses associated with both transformation and progression were documented. Their results implicate that losses on 3p, 6q, and 18q are nonrandom. In another in vitro study utilizing human bladder carcinoma cell lines, RIEGER et al. (1995) searched for genetic changes in the p53, MDM2, RB1, E-cadherin, and APC genes which have been previously implicated in urothelial neoplastic progression. Interestingly, the genetic alterations reported in bladder tumor cell lines were consistent with molecular events previously demonstrated in primary bladder cancers. The artifacts of cell culture must be observed with caution because genetic alterations found in cell lines may not always reflect what occurs in vivo. Nevertheless, molecular changes associated with the H-ras, RB1, and c-src genes initially discovered in bladder tumor cell lines were subsequently confirmed to be altered in primary bladder tumor tissue (DER et al. 1982; HOROWITZ et al. 1990; FANNING et al. 1992). The implementation of similar in vitro systems will facilitate the rapid and convenient analyses of chromosomal losses and genetic mutations during the stepwise progression of urothelial tumors. In addition, assessing the susceptibilities of particular cell lines to DNA damage upon exposure to particular carcinogens will prove useful (SOUTHGATE et al. 1995).

4.2.3
Molecular Studies

The recent advancements of molecular techniques complement the previously established cytogenetic studies by expanding beyond the identification of gross chromosomal anomalies to the detection of alterations at specific genetic loci. The two primary methods to identify either chromosomal deletions or allelic losses of tumor suppressor genes are Southern

Blot analyses which utilize recombinant DNA markers to detect restriction fragment length polymorphisms (RFLPs), and polymorphic microsatellite analyses in which polymorphisms are detected via the polymerase chain reaction (PCR). In RFLP analysis, genomic DNA is digested with restriction endonucleases specific for DNA sequences whose locations frequently vary in position within polymorphic loci. Heterozygosity at a particular locus is represented when restriction enzyme digestions yield two different electrophoretic DNA fragment patterns. Loss of heterozygosity (LOH), therefore, is confirmed by performing Southern Blot analyses in which the absence of an allele-specific DNA electrophoretic pattern is demonstrated. Alternatively, polymorphic microsatellite analyses have implemented PCR technology which utilizes the presence of repetitive microsatellite sequences in the genome whose variabilities in repeat number render them polymorphic. Once PCR is performed, a particular allele is identified via polyacrylamide gel electrophoresis. The integration of this procedure allows the rapid analysis of limited DNA samples (Ovita et al. 1989). In addition, microsatellite analysis has become particularly popular because the sensitivity of PCR has facilitated the analysis of limited quantities of DNA from archival tissues (Litt and Luty 1989).

Mutations in either oncogenes or tumor suppressor genes are rapidly screened during single-stranded conformational polymorphism (SSCP) analysis. With this method, amplification of a gene sequence with a single point mutation can generate a PCR product which forms a different 3D conformation than its wild-type counterpart (which is detected during nondenaturing polyacrylamide gel electrophoresis). SSCP represents a rapid and sensitive preliminary screening step preceding the identification of a specific point mutation by direct DNA sequencing (Sambrook et al. 1989).

Immunohistochemistry (IHC) analysis is performed to identify structurally abnormal proteins which can arise from a single point mutation. Monoclonal antibodies are specifically designed to detect the overabundance of proteins with abnormal structural features which prohibit their normal cellular regulation, resulting in an increased half-life. IHC can be used to screen proteins on histological sections, and it also provides an alternative approach to identify molecular changes beyond the DNA level. RFLP analysis, polymorphic microsatellite analysis, SSCP, and IHC have all contributed to a more precise and detailed analysis of bladder cancer genetics.

4.3
Cancer as a Genetic Disease

Carcinogenesis is a multistep process in which multiple genetic alterations accumulate in rapidly dividing tumor cells which acquire a selective growth advantage over their neighboring normal cells. Neoplastic transformation arises from the loss or inactivation of tumor suppressor genes, the activation of proto-oncogenes, or the abnormal expression of growth factors or their corresponding receptors (Bishop 1987; Fearon and Jones 1992). Proto-oncogenes are activated into oncogenes by amplification, point mutation, translocation, or the random insertion of viral sequences (Solomon et al. 1991). Tumor suppressor genes are inactivated to establish the same tumorigenic phenotype through the silencing or inactivation of one allele coupled to the loss of the other allele (Bishop 1987). Alterations of oncogenes and tumor suppressor genes usually occur together in the establishment of a variety of different human malignancies. Interestingly, bladder cancer is a heterogeneous disease in which familial studies have not definitively revealed a pattern of Mendelian inheritance. Nevertheless, inherited genetic traits (like N-acetyltransferase activity) may affect the incidence of bladder cancer in certain high-risk populations. Hopefully, molecular analyses will determine whether the specific genotype of a tumor can be phenotypically manifested through clinical features including tumor stage, histopathology, and grade. Cytogenetic and molecular studies to date implicate that multiple cumulative genetic events govern the genesis of bladder carcinomas and predispose a given tumor to a particular disease phenotype.

4.4
The Monoclonality of Bladder Cancer

The monoclonal origin of neoplasia explains how tumorigenesis begins with a single transformed cell which itself gives rise to progenitor cells. These cells then continue to accumulate more genetic alterations which provide them with a selective growth advantage over neighboring cells. Nevertheless, some aspects of bladder carcinogenesis are apparently not concordant with this concept of monoclonality in neoplasia. For example, patients with bladder cancer often develop numerous spatially distinct tumors in the urothelial lining at different times, and this phenomenon is not suggestive of a single precursor cell in the genesis of these independent tumors. Therefore, the idea of a "field defect" in bladder carcinogenesis has been established which proposes that numerous uroepithelial cells can transform simultaneously and independently via the same causative agent, resulting in multiple tumors in different regions of the bladder. In contrast, an alternative theory proposes that the existence of a single transforming event in one cell can possibly explain the presence of metachronous urothelial tumors if the progeny of this cell were to migrate and eventually generate spatially distinct tumors.

SIDRANSKY et al. (1992) investigated the conflicting concepts of either a "field defect" or a "monoclonal origin" in bladder carcinogenesis to understand the multifocal nature of bladder TCC. X chromosome inactivation patterns in female patients with multiple bladder tumors were analyzed to determine whether individual tumors of one patient were derived from the same precursor cell. Their results provide evidence for the monoclonal origin of bladder cancer because every tumor of a given patient was shown to possess the same pattern of X chromosome inactivation, supporting the hypothesis that several bladder tumors can arise from the dispersion of a single transformed cell. HABUCHI et al. (1993c) also investigated the monoclonal origin of urothelial cells by analyzing mutation patterns in the p53 tumor suppressor gene of both primary and recurrent bladder tumors from one patient. The independent occurrence of identical p53 mutations in the cells of each tumor is unlikely, especially since the p53 gene is so large and a broad spectrum of mutations have already been characterized for this gene (SHIBATA et al. 1994). Likewise, their results suggest that multifocal urothelial tumors can arise from the initial dispersion of a single transformed cell (LANE and BENCHIMOL 1990).

A challenge to the widely accepted concept of monoclonality in bladder neoplasia has been presented by TSAI et al. (1994), who have demonstrated that large, macroscopic patches of urothelial cells harbor the same inactivated X chromosome. The pre-existence of large patches of genetically similar urothelial cells suggests that they arise from a single urothelial cell precursor. Such a patch of cells may be equally predisposed to tumorigenesis, explaining why bladder tumors can appear multifocally, thus demonstrating a field defect in the bladder. Although the monoclonal origin of multifocal bladder tumors is probable, the concept of a field defect represents another explanation for the multifocal nature of bladder tumors.

4.5
Oncogenes in Bladder Cancer

The role of oncogene activation in bladder cancer was initially suggested upon discovery of the first isolated human oncogene, H-ras, in the T24 bladder tumor-derived cell line. The H-ras oncogene is known to be activated in many human cancers, and this gene encodes a 21-kDa membrane-associated signal transduction molecule. Specific activating H-ras mutations have been identified (ANDERSON et al. 1992), and increased H-ras expression has been demonstrated in high-grade bladder tumors, carcinomas in situ, and dysplasia of the bladder (VIOLA et al. 1985). Overexpression and ectopic expression of the c-erbB-1 proto-oncogene, which encodes the epidermal growth factor receptor (EGFr), has also been demonstrated in bladder cancers (WRIGHT et al. 1991). Investigations have revealed the increased expression of other oncogenes in bladder cancer which include c-erbB-2 (ASAMOTO et al. 1990), c-myc (KOTAKE et al. 1990), and c-src (FANNING et al. 1992), however, their precise roles in bladder cancer have not been well defined (SANDBERG 1992). In general, immunohistochemical analyses have confirmed overexpression of several oncogenes in bladder tumors, but only the H-ras oncogene appears to be susceptible to activating mutations. Because oncogenic alterations do not appear to play a primary role in bladder carcinoma, molecular studies currently emphasize the role of tumor suppressor genes in the etiology of bladder carcinogenesis.

4.6
Tumor Suppressor Genes
in Bladder Cancer

The concept of the tumor suppressor gene was established following the discovery of specific chromosomal deletions characteristic of particular tumor types. Tumor suppressor gene inactivation is also believed to play a primary role in the initiation and progression of bladder cancer. Unlike activated proto-oncogenes, which influence tumor progression in a dominant fashion, tumor suppressor genes are susceptible to inactivating recessive mutations. Both copies of these genes are usually altered to effectively impair their abilities to regulate cell proliferation. This usually occurs via the mutation or silencing of one allele combined with a deletion of the other allele. Occasionally, a mutated tumor suppressor gene can also behave in a dominant-negative fashion. For example, a mutant tumor suppressor protein product-subunit can inactivate a functional protein by interacting with its wild-type subunits (HERSKOWITZ 1991). Nonrandom chromosomal losses associated with tumor formation have been discovered using cytogenetic and molecular approaches, and such studies have enabled the mapping of genetic loci whose alterations correlate with a phenotypic predisposition to specific cancer syndromes. A multitude of chromosomal deletions are associated with bladder cancer, suggesting that important tumor suppressor genes reside in these deleted regions. Current investigations in bladder cancer research have focused on the search for candidate tumor suppressor genes.

4.6.1
Allelic Losses in Bladder Cancer

Molecular and cytogenetic studies have revealed a frequent loss of heterozygosity on chromosomes 8, 9, 11, 13, and 17 in bladder TCC. Although such deletions have been identified on all 22 autosomes including the Y chromosome at a high frequency (SANDBERG and BERGER 1994), only those chromosomal regions with frequent deletion will be described in the context of their associated tumor suppressor loci (Fig. 4.1).

The LOH findings in Fig. 4.1 demonstrate that loss of all or part of chromosome 9 is the most frequent chromosomal abnormality in bladder cancer, confirming earlier cytogenetic evidence for the importance of chromosome 9 in this disease (GIBAS et al. 1984; VANNI and SCARPA 1986). Identifying the putative tumor suppressor gene (or genes) on chromosome 9q has been more challenging than for 9p, because results from positional cloning strategies seldom reveal smaller partial deletions of this chromosomal arm without the entire loss of chromosome 9 (Fig. 4.2). It has been recently suggested that at least two tumor suppressor genes reside on chromosome 9 (RUPPERT et al. 1993; SIMONEAU et al. 1996). The role of chromosome 9 in bladder TCC will be described more thoroughly in the following section.

Allelic loss of chromosome 17p, the location of the *p53* gene, represents the second most common site of allelic loss in bladder cancer. The high frequency of 17p loss correlates with the evidence of *p53* mutations in approximately half of all human cancers (HARRIS 1993; HOLLSTEIN et al. 1991). The *p53* tumor suppressor gene encodes a 53-kDa nuclear phosphoprotein which functions as a transcription factor to regulate the cell cycle in response to DNA damage. Although *p53* alterations (including mutation, deletion, and abnormal expression) are

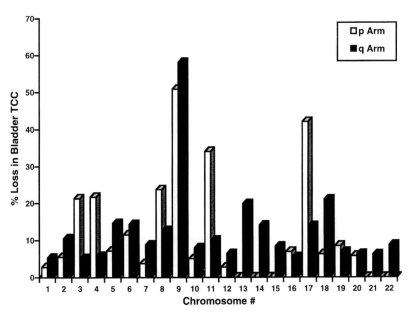

Fig. 4.1. Allelotype demonstrating the frequency of allelic loss for each human chromosome in bladder cancer. This allelotype has been expanded from the original data published by KNOWLES et al. (1994) to include combined studies by TSAI et al. (1990), OLUMI et al. (1990), PRESTI et al. (1991), DALBAGNI et al. (1993b), BREWSTER et al. (1994), HABUCHI et al. (1993a, 1995), CHANG et al. (1995), and SIMONEAU et al. (1996)

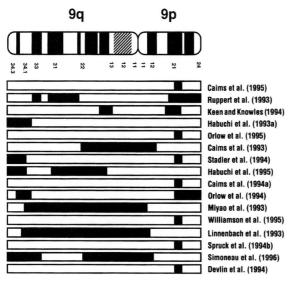

Fig. 4.2. Chromosome 9 regions frequently deleted in bladder cancer. The *black areas* represent regions of deletion confirmed during independent studies

associated with the progression of bladder TCC, alterations in this gene are not unique to bladder cancer.

In contrast, the high frequency of 11p loss in bladder TCC does not appear to be associated with the progression of bladder cancer. The two Wilms' tumor loci have been mapped to 11p13 and 11p15 respectively, but no evidence for their inactivation in

bladder TCC has been demonstrated (CALL et al. 1990; KOUFOS et al. 1989).

LOH of 13q, the location of the *RB1* gene, is also associated with bladder cancer. The *RB1* gene encodes a nuclear phosphoprotein which negatively regulates the transition of cells from the G_1 into the S phase of the cell cycle. This protein participates in the same regulatory pathway as p16, and an inverse correlation between alterations in either gene has been observed in numerous cancers. YEAGER et al. (1995) demonstrated that increased p16 levels correlate with alterations of the RB protein in cultured urothelial cells. Both LOH of the *RB1* genetic locus (CAIRNS et al. 1991) and decreased protein expression levels (XU et al. 1993) have been identified in a proportion of bladder cancers. Since *RB1* alterations are more frequent in higher bladder tumor stages, they may play a pivotal role in disease progression.

Approximately 23% of bladder TCCs demonstrate 8p allelic loss (KNOWLES et al. 1993). The polymorphic *N*-acetyltransferase gene (*PNA2*) represents a likely candidate tumor suppressor gene in this region because *PNA2* encodes an enzyme already demonstrated to be associated with bladder cancer (CARTWRIGHT et al. 1982). The roles of the DNA polymerase β (POLβ) and the β catalytic subunit of protein phosphatase 2A (PPP2CB) in bladder cancer are unknown and must be considered too because these putative tumor suppressor loci also map to chromosome 8p.

Table 4.1. Alterations affecting tumor suppressor genes in bladder cancer

Gene (region)	Type of alteration	Method of detection	Clinical correlates	References	
p16 (9p)	LOH (9p)	RFLP analysis Microsatellite polymorphism	High and low stages	TSAI et al. (1990) KEEN and KNOWLES (1994)	KNOWLES et al. (1994) DEVLIN et al. (1994)
	LOH (p16)	RFLP analysis Microsatellite polymorphism	High and low stages	SPRUCK et al. (1994b) CAIRNS et al. (1995) WILLIAMSON et al. (1995)	ORLOW et al. (1995) ROSIN et al. (1995)
p53 (17p)	Point mutation	DNA sequencing	Progression	SHIBATA et al. (1994) SPRUCK et al. (1994a) HABUCHI et al. (1993b)	SIDRANSKY et al. (1991) FUJIMOTO et al. (1992)
	Abnormal expression	Immunohistochemistry	Progression	WRIGHT et al. (1991) JAHNSON et al. (1995) DALBAGNI et al. (1993a)	SARKIS et al. (1993) ESRIG et al. (1993) SERTH et al. (1995)
RB1 (13q)	LOH	RFLP analysis	Progression	MIYAMOTO et al. (1994) XU et al. (1993)	CAIRNS et al. (1991) ISHIKAWA et al. (1991)
	Abnormal expression	Immunohistochemistry	Progression	LOGOTHETIS et al. (1992) PRESTI et al. (1991) JAHNSON et al. (1995)	XU et al. (1993) LIPPONEN (1993)
	No protein	Immunohistochemistry	Progression	ISHIKAWA et al. (1991)	
	Point mutation	DNA sequencing	High and low stages	MIYAMOTO et al. (1994)	

Linkage analysis and positional cloning techniques can be performed to identify candidate tumor suppressors associated with familial cancers; however, preliminary LOH studies must be applied to identify general regions of loss relevant to sporadic cancer syndromes. Table 4.1 describes the alterations affecting the three major candidate tumor suppressor genes (*p16*, *p53*, and *RB1*) in many human malignancies, which also reside in the described chromosomal regions frequently deleted in bladder cancer. The specific role of each tumor suppressor gene in carcinoma of the bladder will be described in following sections.

4.6.2
The Role of Chromosome 9 in Bladder Cancer

Cytogenetic and molecular analyses have demonstrated a high frequency of chromosome 9 alterations associated with all grades and stages of bladder tumor progression. In fact, the deletion of all or part of chromosome 9 was identified in 319 of 580 (55%) bladder tumors analyzed during independent studies. Such a high frequency of loss implicates the presence of at least one tumor suppressor locus on chromosome 9 (DALBAGNI et al. 1993b; HABUCHI et al. 1993a). Figure 4.2 illustrates the regions of frequent chromosome 9 deletion defined during numerous investigations.

In 1990, TSAI et al. initially observed 9q loss in 17 out of 25 (68%) of advanced stage bladder tumors. Subsequently, OLUMI et al. (1990) discovered that 9q loss is common in all stages of bladder tumor progression. The significance of this finding resides in the fact that the remaining chromosomal losses frequently found in bladder cancer are usually confined to high-stage tumors; therefore, the specific loss of 9q may be a hallmark of bladder cancer. Figure 4.3 illustrates the relative frequencies of chromosome 9q and 9p loss categorized according to bladder tumor stage, and although loss of genetic information on both chromosomal arms has been reported for all stages of bladder cancer, the common occurrence of 9q loss in low-grade, low-stage tumors is important. Recent evidence implicates the coexistence of more than one tumor suppressor locus on chromosome 9q (SIMONEAU et al. 1996). Unfortunately, positional cloning strategies are often not sensitive enough to define smaller regions of 9q deletion associated with bladder TCC.

Although a putative tumor suppressor gene on 9q may be unique to bladder cancer, alterations of spe-

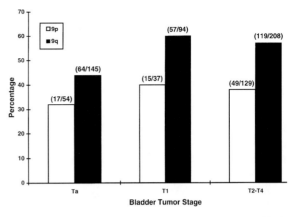

Fig. 4.3. Stratification of 9p loss and 9q loss according to bladder tumor stage. Data for 9p represent compiled results obtained by SPRUCK et al. (1994b), ORLOW et al. (1994, 1995), and SIMONEAU et al. (1996). Data for 9q represent compiled results obtained by SPRUCK et al. (1994a; 1994b), DALBAGNI et al. (1993b), HABUCHI et al. (1993a), LINNENBACH et al. (1993), ORLOW et al. (1994), and SIMONEAU et al. (1996)

cific genes on 9p may predispose individuals to a variety of other cancer syndromes. For example, a defined region localized to 9p21–22 is frequently deleted in leukemias (DIAZ et al. 1990), gliomas (OLOPADE et al. 1992), and melanomas (FOUNTAIN et al. 1992) in addition to bladder cancer (CAIRNS et al. 1994a; WILLIAMSON et al. 1995; ORLOW et al. 1995). The *p16* cell cycle regulatory gene located in this region represents the most attractive 9p tumor suppressor gene candidate to date; however, its precise role in bladder cancer has been difficult to determine because the observance of its frequent deletion in bladder tumor cell lines does not directly coincide with deletion analysis results for uncultured tumors (SPRUCK et al. 1994b). A significant frequency of 9p LOH is demonstrated in both low-stage and high-stage bladder tumors (Fig. 4.3), but it does not appear to occur at the frequency of 9q LOH. Recently, investigations of LOH in bladder TCC have focused on the 9p21–22 region because the *p16* cell cycle regulatory gene mapping to this region exhibits frequent homozygous loss in numerous tumor types, contributing to the genesis of many different cancers (NOBORI et al. 1994; KAMB et al. 1994).

NOBORI et al. (1994) initially demonstrated *p16* homozygous deletion in 133 out of 290 tumor cell lines (including bladder, breast, lung, renal carcinoma, melanoma, astrocytoma, and osteosarcoma). The *p16* gene encodes a 16-kDa polypeptide that directly inactivates cyclin-dependent kinases 4 and 6, which phosphorylate the retinoblastoma gene product, thus inhibiting the transcription of S phase-specific genes and resulting in G_1 arrest. Consequently, *p16* functions as a negative cell cycle regulator (SERRANO et al. 1993), and inactivation of *p16* may confer a selective growth advantage to a rapidly dividing subpopulation of bladder tumor cells.

A conflicting body of evidence from independent studies has been generated regarding the frequency of *p16* homozygous deletion in bladder cancer and its precise role in this disease. Although homozygous deletions of 9p21 (which include *p16*) occur frequently in cultured TCCs of the bladder (SPRUCK et al. 1994b), *p16* homozygous deletions and intragenic mutations occur at somewhat lower frequencies in uncultured TCCs. Evidence from two independent investigations of the *p16* gene in bladder TCC suggests that its frequent homozygous deletion could represent a cell line phenomenon (CAIRNS et al. 1994a; SPRUCK et al. 1994b). For example, when SPRUCK et al. (1994b) examined a panel of primary bladder tumors and bladder TCC-derived cell lines for mutation and homozygous deletion of the *p16* gene, 54% of the bladder tumor cell lines displayed *p16* alterations, but only 19% of the primary bladder tumors exhibited such alterations. Table 4.2 demonstrates an average frequency of *p16* homozygous deletion and mutation established from several studies of *p16* in bladder cancer. The compiled results show that an estimated 3% of primary bladder tumors contain a *p16* point mutation, and another 27% harbor a *p16* homozygous deletion, implicating a significant 30% frequency of *p16* alterations in bladder tumors. Moreover, the observed frequencies of *p16* homozygous deletions determined from these studies are most likely underrepresentations because identifying lost genetic material in DNA obtained from bladder tumor specimens (which is often contaminated with surrounding normal tissue) will be masked by the amplification of retained alleles from surrounding normal cells.

The described studies of *p16* homozygous deletion in carcinomas of the bladder have been complemented by additional mutation analyses performed by CAIRNS et al. (1994b), SPRUCK et al. (1994b), and KAI et al. (1995), all of which demonstrated a low frequency of *p16* mutation, in 2/75, 0/31, and 2/39 bladder tumors respectively (Table 4.2). Point mutations, therefore, appear to be a minor mechanism for *p16* inactivation in the genesis of bladder cancer.

One explanation for the lower frequency of *p16* alterations, namely point mutations, observed in bladder cancer may be the existence of an alternative mechanism for *p16* inactivation. More specifically, hypermethylation of the 5′ CpG island of *p16* has been shown to be associated with its transcriptional repression in a variety of human cancers (MERLO et al. 1995; GONZALEZ-ZULUETA et al. 1995b; HERMAN et al. 1995). Evidence for the hypermethylation of *p16* in tumor cell lines and uncultured tumors not expressing *p16*, in addition to the demonstration of *p16* reactivation in tumor cell lines exposed to 5-aza-CdR, suggests that de novo methylation is associated with *p16* inactivation both in vitro and in vivo (MERLO et al. 1995; HERMAN et al. 1995). Cell growth inhibition has also been shown to directly correlate with 5-aza-CdR-mediated *p16* induction in cultured bladder tumor cells (unpublished data). This observation implicates a possible role for *p16* de novo methylation during successive cell passages which may confer a selective growth advantage to bladder tumor cells in vitro. Our laboratory is currently analyzing specific patterns of CpG demethylation in the 5′ upstream CpG island of *p16* in bladder tumor cell lines treated with 5-aza-CdR to elucidate the precise relationship between CpG demethylation and trans-criptional activation, and between de novo methylation and gene silencing. Understanding the mechanism by which cytidine analogs induce a dormant, hypermethylated tumor suppressor gene will also prove useful as a possible alternative for cancer therapy. More specifically, reactivating a dormant growth regulatory gene in the tumors of patients will bypass the technical challenges attributed to targeting a vector containing an exogenous gene into specific tumor cells.

Although most studies focus on the role of this candidate tumor suppressor gene in bladder TCCs, more recent evaluation of bladder SCCs suggests that *p16* alterations are very common in this other sub-

Table 4.2. Frequency of *p16* mutation and homozygous deletion in primary bladder tumors

Reference	Homozygous deletion	Mutation
SPRUCK et al. (1994b)	6/31	0/31
KAI et al. (1995)	–	2/39
ORLOW et al. (1995)	11/110	–
WILLIAMSON et al. (1995)	31/140	–
CAIRNS et al. (1994a)	10/112	–
CAIRNS et al. (1994b)	–	2/75
CAIRNS et al. (1995)	126/285	–
Totals	184/678 (27%)	4/145 (3%)

type of bladder cancer (GONZALEZ-ZULUETA et al. 1995a). The search for the *9p21* tumor suppressor gene in bladder cancer is currently ongoing, and although *p16* represents a promising candidate gene, the existence of different tumor suppressor loci within this chromosomal region should be acknowledged.

4.6.3
The Role of the *p53* Gene in Bladder Cancer

The *p53* tumor suppressor gene located on chromosome 17p represents the most frequently altered tumor suppressor gene in many human cancers. Evidence for *p53* mutations in colon cancer (BAKER et al. 1989; FEARON and JONES 1992) and the detection of frequent 17p loss associated with later stages of many human malignancies (FEARON and VOGELSTEIN 1990) introduced the concept that *p53* loss may be associated with tumor progression in general. Alterations in this gene, therefore, are not unique to bladder cancer. The *p53* gene encodes a 393 amino acid nucleo-phosphoprotein which associates with the alpha subunit of DNA polymerase to regulate transcription (GANNON and LANE 1987). *p53* functions as a G_1 cell cycle check point molecule in response to DNA damage (DILLER et al. 1990; YIN et al. 1992). Alterations in the *p53* gene, therefore, may cause genomic instability, which is known to be a hallmark of many cancers. The complete inactivation of *p53* can proceed in a recessive fashion (characteristic of a typical tumor suppressor gene) in which mutation of one allele is accompanied by deletion of the other allele. Alternatively, mutant forms of *p53* can behave in a *trans*-dominant manner by complexing with wild-type *p53* to form inactive hetero-oligomers which exhibit a longer than normal half-life (SARKIS et al. 1993; WRIGHT et al. 1991).

An abnormal increase in cellular *p53* levels can be detected via immunohistochemical analysis, and the immunohistochemical detection of mutations in *p53* offers a technique for the investigation of fresh, frozen, or paraffin-embedded tumor specimens. Preliminary studies using this method have demonstrated that in patients with TCC confined to the bladder, nuclear *p53* accumulation predicts a significantly increased risk of disease progression, recurrence, and death (SOINI et al. 1993; DALBAGNI et al. 1993a; LIPPONEN 1993; ESRIG et al. 1993). ESRIG (1993) continued to investigate the prognostic value of *p53* mutations in bladder cancer for two reasons.

Table 4.3. Stratification of *p53* mutations according to bladder tumor stage (modified from YANG and JONES 1996)

Reference	Ta	CIS and Dysplasia	T1	T2–T4
SPRUCK et al. (1994a)	1/36	15/23	9/28	25/49
FUJIMOTO et al. (1992)	0/7	1/1	0/5	6/12
HABUCHI et al. (1993b)	0/11	–	5/17	12/18
SHIBATA et al. (1994)	–	–	1/3	6/9
SPRUCK et al. (1994b)	0/12	–	3/6	7/16
Totals	1/66 (1.5%)	16/24 (67%)	18/59 (30%)	56/104 (54%)

CIS, Carcinoma in situ.

First, earlier work focused on *p53* alterations and the propensity for progression in superficial disease (SARKIS et al. 1993), and second, a subsequent study reported that the prognostic value of *p53* accumulation was not independent of stage (LIPPONEN et al. 1993). Interestingly, ESRIG and colleagues confirmed that nuclear accumulation of abnormal *p53* correlates with an increased propensity for disease progression, independent of tumor stage and grade.

p53 mutations are associated with TCCs of the bladder in general; however, the specific timing of mutation occurrence in relation to clinical stages and grades must be considered. Table 4.3 stratifies *p53* mutations according to bladder tumor stage and grade. The increased frequency of mutations in carcinomas in situ and the more invasive high-grade bladder tumors (detected by direct DNA sequencing) further confirms that *p53* alterations are associated with disease progression. Such a dramatic trend for *p53* mutation and chromosome 17p allelic loss during later stages of bladder cancer (Table 4.3) is not observed for loci on chromosomal regions 9p and 9q (Fig. 4.3).

Understanding the mutational spectrum of *p53* from a molecular epidemiological perspective provides additional information regarding the mechanism of carcinogenesis in bladder TCC (GREENBLATT et al. 1994). For example, transition mutations (purine → purine or pyrimidine → pyrimidine) usually arise from endogenous carcinogens, whereas transversion mutations (purine → pyrimidine or pyrimidine → purine) are likely to arise from exogenous carcinogens, including cigarette smoke. SHIBATA et al. (1994) established a distinct pattern of *p53* mutations in bladder TCC in the endemic area of black foot disease Taiwan. Their results revealed a *p53* mutational spectrum quite different from previously reported *p53* mutations in bladder neoplasms, implicating a different endogenous agent in the etiology of bladder cancer in this geographical location. Therefore, the nature of *p53* alterations, in addition to the frequencies of their occurrence, may provide insight regarding the etiology of bladder carcinomas.

4.6.4
The Role of the *RB1* Gene in Bladder Cancer

Functional inactivation of the retinoblastoma susceptibility gene (*RB1*) on chromosome 13q14 is known to contribute to the development of several types of human cancers. The *RB1* gene encodes a nucleophosphoprotein which forms complexes with the adenovirus (E1A) and SV40 large T antigen oncoproteins to regulate progression through the G_1 phase of the cell cycle (GOODRICH et al. 1991). Frequent *RB1* alterations have been identified in retinoblastoma (FRIEND et al. 1986), osteosarcoma (FRIEND et al. 1986), lung cancer (HARBOUR et al. 1988), breast cancer (T'ANG et al. 1988), and prostate cancer (BOOKSTEIN et al. 1990). In addition, results from immunohistochemical analyses and LOH analyses have also implicated a role for the *RB1* gene in bladder cancer. Interestingly, GOODRICH et al. (1991) demonstrated that transfecting the *RB1* gene into bladder cancer cells suppressed tumorigenicity, suggesting a role for this gene in tumor progression. Alterations in *RB1* occur more frequently in high-grade, high-stage tumors (PRESTI et al. 1991; XU et al. 1993). CAIRNS et al. (1991) demonstrated LOH at the *RB1* locus in 28 tumors from 126 patients, and only two of these tumors were observed to be low-stage, low-grade tumors. This observation again confirms that RB loss of function does not represent an initiating event in bladder TCC, but is associated with the onset of progressive disease. The *RB1* gene is too large (with 27 exons spanning 190kb) to be rapidly screened for inactivating point mutations; therefore, the implementation of immunocytochemistry to detect RB protein expression will be more convenient in a clinical setting. Studies by CORDON-CARDO et al. (1992) and LOGOTHETIS et al. (1992) independently reported significant alterations in RB protein expression levels in muscle-invasive TCCs. The assessment of RB protein expression levels by immunocytochemical techniques could be a valuable prognostic indicator for tumor progression in bladder cancer.

4.7
Divergent Molecular Pathways in Bladder Cancer

The multistep accumulation of genetic alterations in a precise combination may govern the development of specific subsets of tumors. Comparison of these genetic changes in large groups of tumors at each clinical stage of bladder tumor progression, therefore, should allow a detailed sequence of molecular progression to be defined. The variable histopathological subsets of bladder cancer and the identification of distinct molecular defects present in superficial papillary TCCs, carcinomas in situ, and invasive bladder TCCs support the hypothesis that bladder carcinogenesis possibly occurs via two molecular pathways (SPRUCK et al. 1994a). More recent investigations of SCC of the bladder suggest the existence of yet a third pathway for bladder carcinogenesis (GONZALEZ-ZULUETA et al. 1995a,b). *p16* homozygous deletions were reported in 6 out of 12 SCCs analyzed, which is a significantly higher

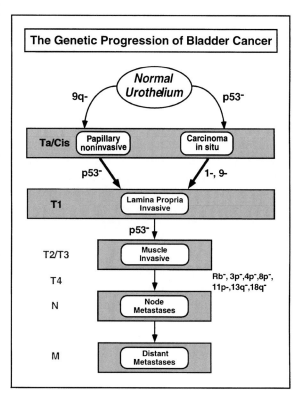

Fig 4.4. Model for the divergent pathways of genetic events associated with bladder tumor progression. (Modified from YANG and JONES 1996)

frequency than observed for TCCs of the bladder. Nevertheless, conflicting evidence reported by ROSIN et al. (1995) suggests that *p16* alterations are actually more common in TCCs of the bladder, particularly in carcinomas in situ. More extensive analyses must be performed on a larger number of TCCs and SCCs to clarify the specific role of 9p (and more precisely, *p16*) deletion in different kinds of bladder cancer during tumor progression. Figure 4.4 represents a model for the genetic progression of bladder cancer derived from numerous cytogenetic and molecular genetic analyses (BABU et al. 1987; JONES and DROLLER 1993; SPRUCK et al. 1994a).

This model illustrates specific genetic losses in both early and late stages of bladder TCC and SCC. Loss of at least one tumor suppressor gene on chromosome 9q may be an initiating event in the onset of papillary, noninvasive bladder tumors. In addition, increased *p53* mutations correlate with the progression to muscle-invasive bladder cancer. In contrast, *p53* mutations are believed to occur early in the establishment of dysplasias and carcinomas in situ of the bladder with chromosome 9 defects following to facilitate the progression of these tumors. Since *p53* mutations are known to destabilize the genome, the observation of *p53* mutations in carcinomas in situ may explain their propensity to progress to invasive disease. A possible third pathway involves the development of SCC, which is associated with frequent *p53* mutations and chromosome 9p alterations believed to be at the *p16* locus. These observations indicate that that there may be two independent pathways in TCC tumorigenesis which differ in their initiating event, represented by either a 9q deletion or a *p53* genetic alteration. Following transformation, however, subsequent molecular changes determine the onset of invasive disease, which usually involve deletions within chromosomes 3p, 4p, 8p, 11p, 13q, or 18q.

4.8
Microsatellite Instability in Bladder Cancer

The human genome contains regions of highly polymorphic microsatellite sequences comprising mono-, di-, tri-, or tetranucleotide repeats (WEBER 1990; KWIATKOWSKI et al. 1992). Microsatellite DNA markers provide a useful tool for both the detection of genomic instability and the loss of heterozygosity in primary tumors. Initially, these short tandem repeats were reported to be genetically unstable in sporadic and familial cases of colon cancer (IONOV et al. 1993). Such instability is characterized by variations in the repeat number within specific microsatellites in tumor DNA when compared to the DNA of normal cells, resulting from a combination of replication errors and defective DNA repair activity. Alterations in the *hMSH2* gene on chromosome 2 have been linked to microsatellite instability in colon cancer (LEACH et al. 1993). The *hMSH2* gene represents a human homolog of the yeast *Mut S* gene, which encodes a DNA repair enzyme. GONZALEZ-ZULUETA et al. (1993) identified microsatellite instabilities in one or more loci on chromosome 9 in 3% of the TCCs examined, and ORLOW and colleagues (1994) subsequently reported a higher frequency of genomic instability in 41% of bladder cancers, indicative of a nonrandom event.

MAO et al. (1996) suggest that microsatellite markers may prove useful as specific clonal markers for the detection of human cancer. PCR technology can be utilized to rapidly detect alterations in microsatellite sequences. In a blinded study, urine samples from 25 patients with bladder lesions were examined first by this proposed molecular method, and second by conventional cytology. Interestingly, microsatellite alterations were detected in DNA from the urine samples of 19 out of 20 patients diagnosed with bladder cancer. In contrast, cytological techniques detected cancer cells in only 9 out of 18 of the same urine samples. Microsatellite analysis represents another alternative screening method for the early detection of bladder cancer.

4.9
Conclusions

Understanding the molecular genetic changes responsible for the progression of bladder cancer will facilitate the clinical management of this disease. Recent innovations in molecular biology and immunohistochemistry have already contributed much to the genetic dissection of bladder carcinogenesis. Activating mutations in the H-*ras* oncogene (among other proto-oncogenes) have been demonstrated in some bladder tumors, but activated oncogenes appear to play a minor role in this disease. In contrast, the inactivation of tumor suppressor genes occurs quite frequently in bladder cancer. Likewise, current investigations have focused on the identification of putative tumor suppressor loci residing in chromosomal regions whose losses are associated with bladder cancer. The specific genes on chromosome 9 which contribute to bladder cancer still remain unidentified, and the role of *p16* inactivation in bladder cancer appears to be significant. While chromosome 9 alterations are believed to be a primary event in the genesis of papillary TCCs, *p53* inactivation represents the initiating event in carcinoma in situ lesions, this being followed by alterations on chromosome 9. Two independent genes on either arm of chromosome 9 could be responsible for the distinct pathways of bladder cancer development. Alterations in the *RB1* gene are also associated with high-grade, high-stage tumors. In addition, numerous other genetic alterations in bladder cancer include alterations in chromosomes 3p, 4p, 8p, 11p, and trisomy 7 to generate a more invasive phenotype. Characterizing the specific molecular and genetic changes which lead to bladder tumorigenesis will elucidate the natural history of bladder TCC and provide insight for the improvement of diagnoses and therapies which may involve genetic intervention.

Acknowledgment. This work was supported by grant R35 CA49758 from the National Cancer Institute.

References

Anderson JA, Irish JC, Ngen BY (1992) Prevalence of *ras* oncogene mutations in head and neck carcinomas. J Otolaryngol 21:321–326

Asamoto C, Mellon K, Neal DE, Johnston P, Corbett IP, Harris AL, Horne CHW (1990) Expression of the c-*erb*B-2 protein product in bladder cancer. Br J Cancer 62:764–765

Augustine A, Herbert JR, Kabat GC, Wynder EL (1988) Bladder cancer in relation to cigarette smoking. Cancer Res 48:4405–4408

Babu VR, Lutz MD, Miles BJ, Farah RN, Weiss L, Van DD (1987) Tumor behavior in transitional cell carcinoma of the bladder in relation to chromosome markers and histopathology. Cancer Res 47:6800–6805

Baker SJ, Fearon ER, Nigro JM, et al. (1989) Chromosome 17 deletions and *p53* gene mutations in colorectal carcinomas. Science 244:217–221

Bishop JM (1987) The molecular genetics of cancer. Science 235:305–311

Bookstein R, Shew J-Y, Chen P-L, Scully P, Lee W-H (1990) Suppression of tumorigenicity of human prostate carcinoma cells by replacing a mutated *RB* gene. Science 247:712–715

Brewster SF, Gingell JC, Browne S, Brown KW (1994) Loss of heterozygosity on chromosome 18q is associated with muscle-invasive transitional cell carcinoma of the bladder. Br J Cancer 70:697–700

Cairns P, Proctor AJ, Knowles MA (1991) Loss of heterozygosity at the *RB* locus is frequent and correlates with muscle invasion in bladder carcinoma. Oncogene 6:2305–2309

Cairns P, Shaw ME, Knowles MA (1993) Preliminary mapping of the deleted region of chromosome 9 in bladder cancer. Cancer Res 53:1230–1232

Cairns P, Tokino K, Eby Y, Sidransky D (1994a) Homozygous deletions of 9p21 in primary human bladder tumors detected by multiplex polymerase chain reaction. Cancer Res 54:2060–2063

Cairns P, Mao L, Merlo A, et al. (1994b) Rates of *p16* (*MTS1*) mutations in primary tumors with 9p loss. Science 265:415–416

Cairns P, Polascik TJ, Eby Y, et al. (1995) Frequency of homozygous deletion at p16/CDKN2 in primary human tumors. Nat Genet 11:210–212

Call KM, Glaser T, Ito CY, et al. (1990) Isolation and characterization of a zinc finger polypeptide gene at human chromosome 11 Wilms' tumor locus. Cell 60:509–520

Cartwright RA, Glashan RW, Rogers HJ, Ahmad RA, Barham-Hall D, Higgins E, Kahn MA (1982) The role of *N*-acetyltransferase phenotypes in bladder carcinogenesis: a pharmaco-genetic epidemiological approach to bladder cancer. Lancet:842–846

Chang WY, Cairns P, Schoenberg MP, Polascik TJ, Sidransky D (1995) Novel suppressor loci on chromosome 14q in primary bladder cancer. Cancer Res 55:3246–3249

Cordon-Cardo C, Wartinger D, Petrilak D, Dalbagni G, Fair WR, Fuk SG, Reuter VE (1992) Altered expression of the retinoblastoma gene product is a prognostic indicator in bladder cancer. J Natl Cancer Inst 84:1251–1256

Dalbagni G, Presti JC, Reuter VE, Zhang Z, Sarkis AS, Fair WR, Cordon-Cardo C (1993a) Molecular genetic alterations of chromosome 17 and p53 nuclear overexpression in human bladder cancer. Diagn Mol Pathol 2:4–13

Dalbagni G, Presti J, Reuter V, Fair WR, Cordon-Cardo C (1993b) Genetic alterations in bladder cancer. Lancet 342:469–471

Davidoff AM, Kerns BM, Iglehart JD, Marks JR (1991) Maintenance of *p53* alterations throughout breast cancer progression. Cancer Res 51:2605–2610

Der CJ, Krontiris TG, Cooper EM (1982) Transforming genes of human bladder and lung carcinoma cell lines are homologous to the *ras* genes of Harvey and Kirsten sarcoma viruses. Proc Natl Acad Sci U S A 79:3637–3660

Devlin J, Keen AJ, Knowles MA (1994) Homozygous deletion mapping at 9p21 in bladder carcinoma defines a critical region within 2 cm of IFNA. Oncogene 9:2757–2760

Diaz MO, Rubin CM, Harden A, Larson RA, Le Beau MM, Rowley JD (1990) Deletions of interferon genes in acute lymphoblastic leukemia. N Engl J Med 322:77–82

Diller R, Kassel J, Nelson CE, et al. (1990) p53 functions as a cell cycle control protein in osteosarcomas. Mol Cell Biol 10:5772–5781

Esrig D, Spruck CH III, Nichols PW, et al. (1993) *p53* nuclear accumulation correlates with mutations in the *p53* gene, tumor grade, and stage in bladder cancer. Am J Pathol 143:1389–1397

Fanning P, Bulovas K, Saini KS, Libertino JA, Joyce AD, Summerhayes IC (1992) Elevated expression of pp60c-*src* in low grade human bladder carcinomas. Cancer Res 52:1457–1462

Fearon ER, Jones PA (1992) Progressing toward a molecular description of colorectal cancer development. FASEB J 6:2783–2790

Fearon ER, Vogelstein B (1990) A genetic model for colorectal tumorigenesis. Cell 61:759–767

Fountain JW, Karayiorgou M, Ernstoff MS, et al. (1992) Homozygous deletions within human chromosome band

9p21 in melanoma. Proc Natl Acad Sci U S A 89:10557–10561

Friend SH, Bernards R, Rogeli S, Weinberg RA, Rapaport JM, Albert DM, Dryta TP (1986) A human DNA segment with properties of the gene that predisposes to retinoblastoma and osteosarcoma. Nature 323:643–646

Fujimoto K, Yamada Y, Okajima E, Kakizoe T, Sasaki H, Sugimura T, Terada M (1992) Frequent association of p53 gene mutations in invasive bladder cancer. Cancer Res 52:1393–1398

Gannon JV, Lane DP (1987) p53 and DNA polymerase-alpha compete for binding to SV40 T antigen. Nature 329:456–458

Gibas Z, Prout GR, Connelly JG, Pontis JE, Sandberg AA (1984) Nonrandom chromosomal changes in transitional cell carcinoma of the bladder. Cancer Res 44:1257–1264

Gonzalez-Zulueta M, Ruppert JM, Tokino K, et al. (1993) Microsatellite instability in bladder cancer. Cancer Res 53:5620–5623

Gonzalez-Zulueta M, Shibata A, Ohneseit PF, et al. (1995a) High frequency of chromosome 9p allelic loss and CDKN2 tumor suppressor gene alterations in squamous cell carcinoma of the bladder. J Natl Cancer Inst 87:1383–1393

Gonzalez-Zulueta, Bender CM, Yang AS, Nguyen T, Beart RW, Van Tornout JM, Jones PA (1995b) Methylation of the 5' CpG island of the p16/CDKN2 tumor suppressor gene in normal and transformed human tissues correlates with gene silencing. Cancer Res 55:4531–4535

Goodrich DW, Wang NP, Qian Y-W, Lee EY-HP, Lee W-H (1991) The retinoblastoma gene product regulates progression through the G_1 phase of the cell cycle. Cell 67:293–302

Greenblatt MS, Bennett WP, Hollstein M, Harris CC (1994) Mutations in the p53 tumor suppressor gene: clues to cancer etiology and molecular pathogenesis. cancer Res 54:4855–4878

Habuchi T, Ogawa O, Kakehi Y, et al. (1993a) Accumulated allelic losses in the development of invasive urothelial cancer. Int J Cancer 53:579–584

Habuchi T, Takahashi R, Yamada H, et al. (1993b) Influence of cigarette smoking and schistosomiasis on p53 gene mutation in urothelial cancer. Cancer Res 53:3795–3799

Habuchi T, Takahashi R, Yamada H, Kakehi Y, Sugiyama T, Yoshida O (1993c) Metachronous multifocal development of urothelial cancers by interaluminal seeding. Lancet 342:1087–1088

Habuchi T, Devlin J, Elder PA, Knowles MA (1995) Detailed deletion mapping of chromosome 9q in bladder cancer: evidence for two tumor suppresor loci. Oncogene 11:1671–1674

Harbour JW, Lai S-L, Whang-Peng J, Gazdar AF, Minna JD, Kaye FJ (1988) Abnormalities in structure and expression of the human retinoblastoma gene in SCLC. Science 241:353–357

Harris C (1993) p53: at the crossroads of molecular carcinogenesis and risk assignment. Science 262:1980–1981

Herman JG, Merlo A, Mao L, et al. (1995) Inactivation of the CDKN2/p16/MTS1 gene is frequently associated with aberrant DNA methylation in all common human cancers. Cancer Res 55:4525–4530

Herskowitz I (1991) Functional inactivation of genes by dominant negative mutations. Nature 329:219–222

Hollstein M, Sidransky D, Vogelstein B, Harris CC (1991) p53 mutations in human cancer. Science 253:49–53

Hopman AHN, Moesken O, Smeets AWGB, Pairnels RPF, Vooijs P, Ramaekers FCS (1991) Numerical chromosome 1, 7, 9, and 11 aberrations in bladder cancer detected by in situ hybridization. Cancer Res 51:644–651

Horowitz JM, Park S-H, Bogenmann E, et al. (1990) Frequent inactivation of the retinoblastoma anti-oncogene is restricted to a subset of human tumor cells. Proc Natl Acad Sci U S A 87:2775–2779

Ionov Y, Peinado MA, Malkhosyan S, Shibata D, Perucho M (1993) Ubiquitous somatic mutations in simple repeated sequences reveal a new mechanism for colonic carcinogenesis. Nature 363:558–561

Ishikawa J, Xu HJ, Hu SX, et al. (1991) Inactivation of the human retinoblastoma gene in human bladder and renal cell carcinoma. Cancer Res 51:5736–5743

Jahnson S, Risberg B, Karlsson MG, Westman G, Bergstrom R, Pedersen J (1995) p53 and RB staining in locally advanced bladder cancer: relation to prognostic variables and predictive value for the local response to radical radiotherapy. Eur Urol 28:135–142

Jones PA, Droller MJ (1993) Pathways of development and progression in bladder cancer: new correlations between clinical observations and molecular mechanisms. Semin Urol XI:177–192

Kai M, Arakawa H, Sugimoto Y, Murata Y, Ogawa M, Nakamura Y (1995) Infrequent somatic mutation of the MTS1 gene in primary bladder carcinomas. Jpn J Cancer Res 86:249–251

Kamb A, Gruis N, Weaver-Feldhaus J, et al. (1994) A cell cycle regulator potentially involved in the genesis of many tumor types. Science 264:436–439

Keen AJ, Knowles MA (1994) Definition of two regions of deletion on chromosome 9 in carcinoma of the bladder. Oncogene 9:2083–2088

Knowles MA, Shaw ME, Proctor MA (1993) Deletion mapping of chromosome 8 in cancers of the urinary bladder using restriction fragment length polymorphisms and microsatellite polymorphisms. Oncogene 8:1357–1364

Knowles MA, Elder PA, Williamson M, Cairns JP, Shaw ME, Law MG (1994) Allelotype of human bladder cancer. Cancer Res 54:531–538

Kotake T, Saiki S, Kinouchi T, Shiku H, Nakayama E (1990) Detection of the c-myc gene product in urinary bladder cancer. Jpn J Cancer Res 81:1198–1201

Koufos A, Grundy P, Morgan K, et al. (1989) Familial Wiedemann-Beckwith syndrome and a second Wilms' tumor locus map to 11p15.5. Am Hum Genet 44:711–719

Kwiatkowski DJ, Henske EP, Weimer K, Ozelius L, Gusella JF, Haines J (1992) Construction of a GT polymorphism map of human 9q. Genomics 12:229–240

Lane DP, Benchimol S (1990) p53: oncogene or antioncogene? Genes Dev 4:1–8

Leach FS, Nicolaides NC, Papadopoulus N, Liu B, Vogelstein B (1993) Mutations of a Mut S homolog in hereditary nonpolyposis colorectal cancer. Cell 75:1215–1225

Linnenbach AJ, Pressler LB, Seng BA, Kimmel BS, Tomaszewski JE, Malkowicz SB (1993) Characterization of chromosome 9 deletions in transitional cell carcinoma by microsatellite assay. Hum Mol Genet 2:1407–1411

Lipponen PK (1993) Over-expression of p53 nuclear oncoprotein in transitional-cell bladder cancer and its prognostic value. Int J Cancer 53:368–370

Litt M, Luty JA (1989) A hypervariable microsatellite revealed by in vitro amplification of a dinucleotide repeat within the cardiac muscle actin gene. Am Hum Genet 44:397–401

Logothetis CJ, Xu HJ, Ro JY, Hu SX, Sahin A, Orodonez N, Benedict WF (1992) Altered expression of the retinoblastoma protein and known prognostic variables in locally advanced bladder cancer. J Natl Cancer Inst 84:1256–1261

Mao L, Schoenberg MP, Scicchitano M, Erozan YS, Merlo A, Scwab D, Sidransky D (1996) Molecular detection of primary bladder cancer by microsatellite analysis. Science 271:659–662

Merlo A, Herman JG, Mao L, Lee DJ, Gabrielson E, Burgo PC, Baylin SB, Sidransky D (1995) 5′ CpG island methylation is associated with transcriptional silencing of the tumor suppressor p16/CDKN2/MTS1 in human cancers. Nature Medicine 1:686–692

Miyamoto H, Shuin T, Torigoe S, Iwasaki Y, Kubota Y (1994) Retinoblastoma gene mutations in primary human bladder cancer. Br J Cancer 71:831–835

Miyao N, Tsai YC, Lerner SP, et al. (1993) Role of chromosome 9 in human bladder cancer. Cancer Res 53:4066–4070

Mostofi FK, Davis CJ, Sesterhenn IA (1988) Pathology of tumors of the urinary tract. In: Skinner DG, Lieskovsky G (eds) Diagnosis and management of genitourinary cancer. Saunders, Philadelphia, pp 83–117

Nobori T, Miura K, Wu DJ, Lois A, Takabayashi K, Carson DA (1994) Deletions of the cyclin-dependent-kinase-4 inhibitor gene in multiple human cancers. Nature 368:753–756

Olopade OI, Jenkins RB, Ransom DT, et al. (1992) Molecular analysis of deletions of the short arm of chromosome 9 in human gliomas. Cancer Res 52:2523–2529

Olumi AF, Tsai YC, Nichols PW, Skinner DG, Cain DR, Bender LI, Jones PA (1990) Allelic loss of chromosome 17p distinguishes high-grade from low-grade transitional cell carcinomas of the bladder. Cancer Res 50:7081–7083

Orlow I, Lianes P, Lacombe L, Dalbagni G, Reuter VE, Cardon-Cardo C (1994) Chromosome 9 allelic losses and microsatellite alterations in human bladder tumors. Cancer Res 54:2848–2851

Orlow I, Lacombe L, Hannon GJ, et al. (1995) Deletion of the p16 and p15 genes in human bladder tumors. J Natl Cancer Inst 87:1524–1529

Ovita M, Suzuki MY, Sekiya T, Hayashi K (1989) Rapid and sensitive detection of point mutations and DNA polymorphisms using the polymerase chain reaction. Genomics 5:874–879

Presti JC, Reuter VE, Galan T, Fair WR, Cardon-Cardo C (1991) Molecular genetic alterations in superficially and locally advanced human bladder cancer. Cancer Res 51:5405–5409

Rieger KM, Little AF, Swart JM, et al. (1995) Human bladder carcinoma cell lines as indicators of oncogeneic change relevant to urothelial neoplastic progression. Br J Cancer 72:683–690

Rosin MP, Cairns P, Epstein JI, Schoenberg MP, Sidransky D (1995) Partial allelotype of carcinoma in situ of the human bladder. Cancer Res 55:5213–5216

Ruppert JM, Tokino K, Sidransky D (1993) Evidence for two bladder cancer suppressor gene loci on human chromosome 9. Cancer Res 53:5093–5095

Sambrook J, Fritsch EF, Maniatis T (1989) Molecular cloning: a laboratory manual. Cold Spring Harbor Laboratory, Cold Spring Harbour, New York

Sandberg AA (1992) Chromosome changes in early bladder neoplasms. J Cell Biochem 161:76–79

Sandberg AA, Berger CS (1994) Review of chromosome studies in urological tumors. II. Cytogenetics and molecular genetics of bladder cancer. J Urol 151:545–560

Sandberg AA, Bridge JA (1992) Techniques in cancer cytogenetics: an overview and update. Cancer Invest 10:163–172

Sarkis AS, Dalbagni G, Cordon-Cardo C, et al. (1993) Nuclear overexpression of p53 protein in transitional cell bladder carcinoma: a marker for disease progression. J Natl Cancer Inst 85:53–59

Serrano M, Hannon GJ, Beach D (1993) A new regulatory motif in cell-cycle control causing specific inhibition of cyclin D/CDK4. Nature 370:704–707

Serth J, Kuczyk, Bokemeyer C, Hervatin C, Nafe R, Tan HK, Jonas U (1995) p53 immunohistochemistry as an independent prognostic factor for superficial transitional cell carcinoma of the bladder. Br J Cancer 71:201–205

Shibata A, Ohnset PF, Tsai YC, et al. (1994) Mutational spectrum of the p53 gene in bladder tumors from the endemic area of black foot disease in Taiwan. Carcinogenesis 15:1085–1087

Sidransky D, Von Eschenbach A, Tsai YC, et al. (1991) Identification of p53 mutations in bladder cancers and urine samples. Science 252:706–709

Sidransky D, Frost P, Von Eschenbach A, Oyashu R, Preisinger AC, Vogelstein B (1992) Clonal origin of bladder cancer. N Engl J Med 326:737–740

Silverberg E, Boring CC, Squires TS (1989) Cancer statistics. CA Cancer J Clin 39:1–26

Simoneau AR, Spruck CH, Gonzalez-Zulueta M, et al. (1996) Evidence for two tumor suppressor loci associated with proximal chromosome 9p to 9q and distal chromosome 9q in bladder cancer and the initial screening for GAS1 and PTC mutations. Cancer Res 56:5039–5043

Soini Y, Turpeenniemi-Hujanen T, Kamel D, et al. (1993) p53 immunohistochemistry in transitional cell carcinoma and dysplasia of the urinary bladder correlates with disease progression. J Natl Cancer Inst 85:1029–1035

Solomon E, Borrow J, Goddard A (1991) Chromosome aberrations and cancer. Science 254:1153–1160

Southgate J, Profitt J, Roberts P, Smith B, Selby P (1995) Loss of cyclin-dependent kinase inhibitor genes and chromosome 9 abnormalities in human bladder cancer cell lines. Br J Cancer 72:1214–1218

Spruck CH, Ohnseit P, Gonzalez-Zulueta M, et al. (1994a) Two molecular pathways to transitional cell carcinoma of the bladder. Cancer Res 54:784–788

Spruck CS, Gonzalez-Zulueta M, Shibata A, et al. (1994b) p16 alterations are more common in tumor cell lines than uncultured tumors. Nature 370:183–184

Stadler WM, Sherman J, Bohlander S, Roulston D, Dreyling M, Rukstalis D, Olopade OI (1994) Homozygous deletions within chromosomal bands 9p21–22 in bladder cancer. Cancer Res 54:2060–2063

T'Ang A, Varley JM, Chakraborty S, Murphree AL, Fung Y-KT (1988) Structural rearrangement of the retinoblastoma gene in human breast carcinoma. Science 242:263–266

Tsai YC, Nichols PW, Hiti AL, William Z, Skinner DG, Jones PA (1990) Allelic losses of chromosome 9, 11, and 17 in human bladder cancer. Cancer Res 50:44–47

Tsai YC, Simoneau AR, Spruck CH, Nichols PW, Steven K, Buckley J, Jones PA (1994) Mosaicism in human epithelium: macroscopic monoclonal patches cover the urothelium. J Urol 153:1697–1700

Vanni R, Scarpa RM (1986) Non-random chromosomal changes in transitional cell carcinoma of the bladder. Cancer Res 46:4873

Viola MW, Fromowitz F, Oravez S, Deb S, Schlom J (1985) Ras oncogene-p21 expression is increased in premalignant lesions and high-grade bladder carcinoma. J Exp Med 161:1213–1218

Weber JL (1990) Informativeness of (dC-dA)n (dG-dT)n polymorphisms. Genomics 7:524–530

Williamson MP, Elder PA, Shaw ME, Devlin J, Knowles MA (1995) *p16* (*CDKN2*) is a major deletion target at 9p21 in bladder cancer. Hum Mol Genet 4:1569–1577

Wright C, Mellon K, Johnston P, Lane DP, Harris AL, Horne CHW, Neal DE (1991) Expression of mutant *p53*, c-*erb*B-2 and the epidermal growth factor receptor in transitional cell carcinoma of the human urinary bladder. Br J Cancer 63:967–970

Wu S, Storer BE, Bookland EA, et al. (1991) Nonrandom chromosome losses in stepwise neoplastic transformation in vitro of human uroepithelial cells. Cancer Res 51:3323–3326

Xu H, Cairns P, Hu S, Knowles MA, Benedict WF (1993) Loss of RB protein expression in primary bladder cancer correlates with loss of heterozygosity at the *RB* locus and tumor progression. Int J Cancer 53:781–784

Yang AY, Jones PA (1996) The molecular progression of bladder cancer. In: Liciani L, Debruyne FMJ, Schlaken JA (eds) Basic research in urological oncology. Karger, Basel, pp 97–112

Yeager T, Stadler W, Belair C, Puthenveettil J, Olopade O, Reznikoff C (1995) Increased *p16* levels correlate with alterations in human urothelial cells. Cancer Res 55:493–497

Yin Y, Tainsky MA, Bischoff FZ, Strong LC, Wahl GM (1992) Wild-type *p53* restores cell cycle control and inhibits gene amplification in cells with mutant *p53* alleles. Cell 70:923–935

5 Pathology of Bladder Cancer

E.C.M. Ooms and R.W. Veldhuizen

CONTENTS

5.1 Introduction

The urinary bladder is lined by highly specialized epithelium, so-called urothelium or transitional cell epithelium. One specific characteristic of this urothelium is the ability to protect the human body against reabsorption of toxic elements excreted by the kidney. The constantly changing volume of urine in the bladder requires a high degree of stretching of the covering epithelium, while maintaining an intact barrier function. Unfortunately this highly specialized epithelium shows a strong tendency to develop neoplastic disease. In most industrialized parts of the world, bladder cancer constitutes an important issue in oncological health care (RÜBBEN 1985).

Although the urinary bladder is the site of origin for a large variety of tumors, this chapter deals mainly with neoplastic disease derived from transitional cell epithelium since this group accounts for approximately 98% of all primary bladder tumors in adults in the Western world (YOUNG 1989a). At the end of this chapter a brief overview of remaining tumor types occurring at this location will be given.

Like the epithelium from which the transitional cell tumors are derived, transitional cell carcinoma (TCC) is characterized by specific properties which can have a major influence on the natural history of the disease and consequently on the choice of treatment.

A complicating factor is that cystectomy is a major procedure and the use of an organ-sparing treatment modality would be preferable. The fact that most tumors are sensitive to radiotherapy, immunotherapy, and chemotherapy compounds the complexity of the treatment of TCC and its precursors.

Since TCC is obviously not comparable in all ways to other malignant diseases, the cooperation between the clinician and pathologist demands a high level of expertise on both sides. The same holds true for scientific work related to the development of new diagnostic techniques for TCC.

5.2 Characteristics of Transitional Cell Carcinoma

Since cystectomy in most patients is not the first choice of treatment, the urinary bladder has provided us with a great deal of information concerning the clinical biology of TCC. After treatment of the primary tumor the patient remains at risk for developing new tumors in the bladder since TCC is char-

E.C.M. OOMS, MD, Head of department of Pathology, Westeinde Ziekenhuis, Lijnbaan 32, Postbus 432, NL-2501 CK Den Haag, The Netherlands
R.W. VELDHUIZEN, MD, Departent of Pathology, Westeinde Ziekenhuis, Lijnbaan 32, Postbus 432, NL-2501 CK Den Haag, The Netherlands

acterized by multifocality and recurrences (GILBERT et al. 1976; Koss 1979).

Primary diagnosis of TCC not only indicates that the patient has a tumor but also serves to indicate that the entire urothelium of the patient is abnormal and at risk for developing neoplastic disease. This implies that besides the urinary bladder, the renal pelvis, ureter, and urethra are also at risk. These so-called field changes in the urothelium force the clinician to monitor the entire urothelium of the patient and not only the urinary bladder.

This unique condition in which the organs at risk are generally not initially removed has stimulated many scientists to investigate TCC, its precursors, and related prognostic factors. Not surprisingly, this has led to a large variety of scientific data which may be of importance for individual patient care. Unfortunately the complexity of the disease and the obtained scientific data both give rise to confusion. This confusion is possibly the reason why, in the recent past, no major advances have been made in the contribution of pathology to the treatment of the individual TCC patient.

5.3
Tumor Progression

5.3.1
Introduction

The most important clinical signs of tumor progression arise from local tumor invasion and the development of distant metastases.

Tumor progression in TCC is probably a multistep process in which several mechanisms are involved. Since in most patients the involved organ is initially not removed, tumor recurrence at the primary site is a possible means of progression (local recurrence). Furthermore, as TCC is an expression of dysregulation of the entire urothelium (field change), the development of a new tumor in a different locus is an additional mode of progression (multifocality). As a result of these conditions the tumor may develop local invasive growth in the bladder wall and neighboring structures. The extent to which the tumor shows invasive growth is a major parameter influencing clinical outcome, and is often complicated by the development of distant metastases (BLOMJOUS et al. 1989; REUTER 1990; JEWETT and STRONG 1946; MARSHALL 1962). Progressive disease may be the result of one of

these mechanisms (local recurrence, multifocality, invasive growth, metastases) or a combination of two or more of these pathways.

This complex multistep mode of tumor progression is probably a source of confusion in the scientific approach to the clinical problem. Therefore it seems logical that clinical pathologic studies of TCC progression should take these different pathways into consideration. Following this approach the significance of potential "progression markers" in TCC can be established.

Significant prognostic parameters at the time of primary diagnosis are the local extension of the tumor (the pathologic stage and growth pattern) and the histologic grade of the resected specimen (BERGKVIST et al. 1965; FRIEDELL et al. 1976; JORDAN et al. 1987).

5.3.2
Prognostic Parameters

5.3.2.1
Classical Parameters

In general, clinical decisions are based on classical, standard parameters obtained by routine examination. These parameters include the extent of local invasion (tumor stage), the growth pattern (papillary versus nonpapillary/nodular, flat lesions), and the tumor grade.

5.3.2.1.1 TUMOR STAGE AND GROWTH PATTERN. In the evaluation of patients with bladder cancer the determination of tumor stage has become an essential step. Current methods of staging rely primarily on bimanual palpation, cystoscopy, imaging techniques, and histopathologic examination. A widely accepted staging system is the TNM classification of malignant tumors (HERMANEK and SOBIN 1987; BEAHRS and MEYERS 1983). Several modifications of this system have been developed and are in use. Tumor staging is of paramount importance since tumor behavior is directly related to the depth of tumor invasion in the bladder wall and neighboring structures. (For more detail see Chap. 8.)

In general, tumors showing muscle invasion have a significantly worse clinical outcome than superficially invasive tumors. On the other hand, taking the growth pattern into consideration, the distinction between a papillary and nonpapillary/nodular tumor is of prognostic significance. This means that muscle-invasive and nonpapillary tumors carry an unfavorable outcome, and in such patients additional pathologic techniques and parameters are probably not required.

On the other hand, papillary and superficial tumors in general may have a favorable outcome, and this group of patients may therefore benefit from evaluation of additional prognostic parameters in order to avoid unnecessary treatment or diagnostic procedures. Such evaluation will define those patients in need of more aggressive and often mutilating therapy (Ooms et al. 1981; Lipponen et al. 1990a,b,c; Devere White et al. 1988; Schapers et al. 1990; Vasco et al. 1991; Baak and Oort 1983). Tumors with a flat, noninvasive growth pattern are called carcinoma in situ (CIS) and are described elsewhere in this chapter (Sect. 5.4.2).

5.3.2.1.2 TUMOR GRADE. Grading is one of the basic techniques used in pathology to create order in processes which are characterized by "sliding scales" of severity. This is particularly useful when pathologic changes do not form discrete patterns but rather continuous (or gradual) transitions. A good example of a gradual, nondiscrete transition is the histologic variety of TCC. Since the pathologist is challenged to provide the clinician with useful information concerning the biologic properties of a tumor, many attempts have been made at creating a clinically useful grading system for TCC (Bergkvist et al. 1965; Mostofi et al. 1973; Broders 1922; Friedell et al. 1976; Ooms et al. 1983, 1985; Farrow 1987; Collan 1979). Before going into detail we have to answer the question of how we define grading and subsequently we have to define the characteristics of a good grading system.

Grading is an attempt to correlate histologic images with the biologic properties of a disease and subsequently to subdivide this disease into specific groups in such a way that each defined subgroup is characterized by differences in clinical behavior. This implies that each grading system has to fulfill criteria of clinical relevance and reproducibility.

In 1922 Broders was one of the first to introduce a grading system for TCC. Since then several changes have been made in the grading system, leading to lively discussion among pathologists and other clinicians. One of the more successful grading systems was published by Bergkvist et al. in 1965. The most widely used system was presented by Mostofi et al. in 1973: the World Health Organization (WHO) system, accredited by the American Bladder Tumor Registry.

A major problem in all grading systems is the high inter-and intraobserver variation, leading to concern about the reproducibility of pathologic diagnoses (Ooms et al. 1983, 1985). In most, if not all, grading systems a sharp distinction between different grades cannot be made, probably because of the large number of cytologic and histologic variables which should be taken into consideration. Therefore comparison of the results from different studies using histopathologic grading as a prognostic factor should always be done prudently.

Grading systems which are based on very detailed cytologic and histologic criteria may form a challenge to the experienced pathologist but seem to be of little value in daily routine practice. To facilitate clinical decision making it is advisable to abandon such sophisticated grading systems and replace them with a simple grading system where tumors are divided into only two groups: low grade and high grade. In the WHO system the border between these two groups can be found somewhere in the middle of the grade II carcinomas. Since most pathologists should now be familiar with this WHO system, it is important to learn to divide the grade II carcinoma group into low-grade and high-grade lesions.

Although it may seem attractive to use standard cytologic and histologic criteria of anaplasia for the purpose of grading, it has been proven that this leads to results with a disappointingly low reproducibility (Ooms et al. 1983, 1985). Consequently the application of other techniques, e.g., morphometry and flow cytometry, to solve this problem is unavoidable (Blomjous et al. 1988, 1989).

In the recently published American Air Force Institute of Pathology (AFIP) *Atlas of Tumor Pathology*, Murphy et al. (1993a) support the idea of a two-step grading system for bladder tumors. In this system low-grade TCC is defined as: "a well differentiated malignant neoplasm composed of relatively small, uniform cells covering on a fibrovascular stalk", while high-grade TCC is defined as: "a moderately to poorly differentiated malignant neoplasm composed of pleomorphic cells most often arranged in nodules." The experienced pathologist will understand that this definition is very much akin to the WHO grading system concerning the problems of reproducibility. The big advantage of the AFIP system, however, is that it is composed of two instead of three or four grades.

In summary, it is advised that TCCs be divided into low-grade and high-grade tumors and that additional techniques be used only in those tumors which are classified as WHO grade II carcinoma and superficial tumors.

5.3.2.2
Additional Parameters

Since the "classical" parameters (stage, growth pattern, and grade) are not capable of predicting the prognosis of all tumors, especially the superficial low-grade carcinomas, additional parameters are required for accurate prognostication in the individual patient. This urgent need for additional parameters has resulted in much research in this field. Among the additional parameters and techniques investigated and proposed for use in the diagnosis of TCC are: mitotic index, immunohistochemical investigation of the basement membrane, DNA cytometry, morphometry, p53, Ki-67 Bcl2, cytogenetic analysis, interphase cytogenetics, electron microscopy, polymerase chain reaction (PCR) techniques, in situ hybridization, and ABH blood group deletion (BLOMJOUS et al. 1988, 1989; BORLAND et al. 1993; LIPPONEN et al. 1990a,b,c; LIPPONEN 1993a,b; LIPPONEN and AALTOOMAA 1994; LIPPONEN and ESKELINEN 1994; MALMSTRÖM et al. 1989; NIELSEN et al. 1986; OOMS et al. 1983, 1985; VAN DER POEL et al. 1992; RUSSELL et al. 1990; SARKIS et al. 1993; SHIMAZUI et al. 1990; SOINY et al. 1993; WOOD et al. 1991; WRIGHT et al. 1990; ZING and WALLACE 1985).

It is clear that ongoing developments in the molecular biology of TCC will deepen our understanding of the processes of oncogenesis and tumor progression. New techniques, developed on the basis of fundamental research, will certainly prove to be of clinical importance. The combination of these results must lead to the development of powerful algorithms. The final goal in this process is to find a combination of parameters that is able, in the individual TCC patient, to distinguish aggressive tumors from those with a more benign nature. Until now this aim has not been fully realized because of a lack of integration of scientific results and proper biologic thinking. Although the final goal appears distant, it would seem interesting to look more closely at the different approaches mentioned above (see Chaps. 3, 4, and 10 for more detailed information).

5.4
Flat Lesions

5.4.1
Preneoplastic Conditions and Associated Lesions

The relation between morphologic histologic changes and the development of neoplastic lesions in urothelium is, unfortunately, still not as obvious as in other organs such as the uterine cervix and gastrointestinal tract. The significance of hyperplastic and dysplastic changes in transitional cell epithelium for clinical decision making is therefore not at all clear and not fully understood. Another confusing factor in this regard is that histologic abnormalities such as hyperplasia, dysplasia, and carcinoma in situ are not always clearly defined (COUTS et al. 1985; MURPHY and SOLOWAY 1982; MURPHY et al. 1993b; YOUNG 1989b).

Hyperplastic and metaplastic lesions of the urothelium are common lesions in the urinary tract. Although many studies suggest a certain relation between these lesions and the development of TCC, it is not certain whether these lesions are merely a sign of field change in the entire urothelium or whether they themselves will develop into carcinoma. The presence of these lesions is without doubt a sign of potential neoplastic change in the entire urothelium and it seems attractive to suggest that the severity of these lesions is related to the likelihood of developing true neoplastic disease. This theory implies that the presence of dysplastic lesions should be interpreted as a risk factor since dysplasia and TCC are associated lesions (WOLF and HOJGAARD 1983).

By definition normal urothelium has a maximum of seven cell layers. An increase in the number of cell layers is defined as "simple hyperplasia" in the absence of cellular atypia. Simple hyperplasia is considered to be associated with (but not always caused by) inflammation, lithiasis, and neoplasia. When this hyperplastic condition is complicated by cellular atypia, the lesions are defined as "atypical hyperplasia" or "dysplasia." The presence of dysplasia in random biopsies of the urinary bladder is considered to be a risk factor for the development of TCC (WOLF and HOJGAARD 1983).

The diagnosis of dysplasia is, as indicated above, based only on histologic criteria. The division of dysplasia into three or more grades, as in many other organs, may be an attractive idea but seems to be of little or no clinical importance, not least because of reproducibility problems. The best solution may be to differentiate dysplasia into low- and high-grade lesions, as has been done in respect of the uterine cervix, vulva, bronchus, and prostate with the introduction of terms such as CIN, VIN, BIN, and PIN. This might lead to the definition of transitional cell intraepithelial neoplasia – "TIN" – in three different grades: TIN I, TIN II, and TIN III. According to this proposition, TIN I would include simple hyperplasia and low-grade dysplasia, TIN II would include high-grade dysplasia, and TIN III would include carcinoma in situ.

The definition of the different grades of TIN should be based on separate clinical entities which require a different diagnostic and therapeutic approach: TIN I requires only follow-up since it is a low-risk lesion. TIN II requires a more intense follow-up but no treatment. TIN III is a high-risk lesion and consequently requires treatment and close follow-up.

For reasons of reproducibility and clinical relevance it is probably worthwhile to give more attention to the development of this new nomenclature of TIN in diagnosing flat lesions of the urothelium.

5.4.2
Carcinoma In Situ

Carcinoma in situ (CIS) of the urinary bladder is a specific clinicopathologic entity with certain clinical, endoscopic, cytologic, and histopathologic characteristics. Unlike the situation in other organs, not every noninfiltrating carcinoma is included in the definition of CIS. Noninfiltrating papillary TCC is excluded from the definition of CIS of the urinary bladder (WEINSTEIN and GARDNER 1992).

By definition, CIS of the urinary bladder is a flat (nonpapillary) lesion in which the entire thickness of the urothelium is replaced by malignant cells. The thickness of the epithelium is variable and may be more or less than the normal seven layers. Again, by definition, CIS of the urinary bladder is considered a high-grade malignant lesion. This implies that there is no such thing as "low-grade CIS" and "high-grade CIS." The loss of intercellular cohesion in high-grade TCC (including CIS) is a well-known phenomenon. This diminished cell cohesion in CIS results in the shedding of many individual malignant cells in the urine (see Sect. 5.5 for more detail) and in a histologic picture which may be difficult to interpret (denuding cystitis with atypia). Histologically, CIS may be represented by the classical picture without cell loss or by denuding cystitis. In extreme circumstances of cell loss there may be a total denuded surface of the bladder wall, resulting is in denuding cystitis. This histologic picture is a good explanation for the clinical symptoms of CIS (urge, frequency, pain) since the urine is in direct contact with the stroma of the bladder wall. The combination of clinical symptoms, cytology, endoscopy, and histology is usually sufficient to achieve the diagnosis of CIS in the urinary bladder (BOON et al. 1986).

Unlike noninfiltrating papillary carcinoma, CIS is considered an important precursor lesion of high-grade TCC with a poor clinical outcome. Of great clinical importance is the tendency of CIS to demonstrate pagetoid spread involving neighboring organs and structures such as the prostate, seminal vesicle, and urethra.

5.5
Urinary Cytology

5.5.1
Introduction

Cytologic investigation of the patient with TCC has a role to play in both primary diagnosis and follow-up after treatment for the initial lesion. Since TCC is characterized by recurrences and multifocality, urinary cytology is important in the follow-up of patients after initial treatment. However, reports of the value of urinary cytology as a diagnostic tool for TCC have been contradictory, leading to confusion about the diagnostic accuracy (sensitivity and specificity) of this method (BADALAMENT et al. 1987; KOSS et al. 1985; OOMS and VELDHUIZEN 1993). One of the main reasons for this is, in our eyes, the lack of consensus about the way the slides should be interpreted and the terminology which should be used in the cytology report that is sent to the clinician. If pathologists want to promote urinary cytology as a reliable method for the follow-up of patients with bladder tumors, the terminology and the diagnostic criteria must be standardized and agreed upon.

In order to make urinary cytology a useful diagnostic procedure, we have to consider what information the clinician needs in order to make an optimal therapeutic decision and adapt our cytology report to these needs. Since these decisions are partly based on histologic parameters, the cytology report should provide information which permits correlation with histology: cytohistologic correlation (OOMS and VELDHUIZEN 1993).

5.5.2
Technique

5.5.2.1
Introduction

The basis of any diagnostic laboratory test is a reliable technique which ought to be incorporated in a standard operating procedure as part of an integrated quality system in the laboratory. For urinary cytology the "preanalytical" phase is of paramount importance since specimen collection and preservation play an importance role in the procedure. For the "analytical phase" (the processing of the urinary specimen), several techniques are available which all lead to acceptable results. The "Postanalytical" phase includes the interpretation of the slides, cytologic criteria, and terminology and is described later in Sects. 5.5.3 and 5.5.4.

5.5.2.2
Specimen Collection

There are several ways to obtain a urinary spcimen for cytology. The simplest way is to use urine produced by voiding. If a voiding specimen is used for urinary cytology there are a few guidelines which lead to good results. Morning voidings give suboptimal results and should be avoided because of degenerative cell changes probably caused by the long period the urine has been contained in the urinary bladder. Good results are obtained by collecting random morning voidings, the first voiding excluded! A good practical instruction for a community clinic may be to allow a first morning voiding which is not used. Then the patient has to wait until 11 A.M. From th voiding produced at 11 A.M. at the office of the clinician, good cytologic results can be obtained. Because of preservation problems, 24-h collections and drainage bag specimens should be avoided.

Optimal results can be obtained by bladder washings or by using the "waste fluid" of cystoscopy. Although voidings are in general the easiest to obtain, the rsults of bladder washings are far superior.

5.5.2.3
Preservation

The main reason for preservation is to prevent bacterial overgowth in the urine since this is the major cause of disturbing cell changes. Alcoholic solutinso, salt solutinons, and a large variety of fixatives (all having bacteriostatic effects) have been tested with satisfying results. A very simple method that yields excellent results is to store the urine or bladder washing in a normal refrigerator at 4°C as soon as possible after having obtained the urine specimen. Cooling for up to 48h gives good diagnostic results. Consequently the general advice is not to add any fixative but to place the urine specimen in a normal refrigerator as soon as possible after voiding and to keep it cool until the moment of processing in the laboratory.

5.5.2.4
Processing

Several ways of processing urine samples are available to produce high-quality cytologic slides of urine and/or bladder washings. The local expertise of the laboratory staff and cytotechnicians is a major factor in the choice of a specific technique. In general, direct smears are easy to prepare but there is a risk of significant cell loss. Very good cytologic results are obtained using the membrane filter method. A disadvantage of this method is the complex procdure in the laboratory. Cytocentrifugation results in cytologic slides of average to good quality in the hands of most cytotechnicians. Therefore the first choice of processing is usually cytocentrifugation with an optional second technique for "difficult" samples.

Papanicolaou staining gives good results for urinary cytology and should be the first choice. If, because of local experience, a second staining method is desired (Giemsa, H&E), this should be supplementary to the standard Papanicolaou stain.

5.5.3
Terminology

As mentioned above, reports of the accuracy of urinary cytology are contradictory, resulting in confusion about the value of this technique as a diagnostic tool. A plausible explanation for this is the lack of consensus concerning the interpretation of the cytologic findings and the terminology for reporting.

The cytology report must fulfill the following criteria:

1. The report must give detailed diagnostic information.
2. The terminology should be unambiguous.
3. The terminology must be based on correlation between cytology and histology.
4. The cytologic categories should be the same as the histologic categories.
5. The cytologic categories should be based on detailed cytologic diagnostic criteria.
6. Consensus is needed on the terminology, the cytologic categories, and the cytologic criteria.

If cytopathologists want to promote urinary cytology, all these criteria have to been taken into consideration.

We present here a list of cytologic diagnoses which we believe are unambiguous and appropriate for modern clinical practice. The proposed terminology for urinary cytology is as follows:

- Negative cytology
- Atypical cells, significance uncertain
- Atypical cells, suspicious for malignancy
- Grade I carcinoma, low-grade
- Grade II carcinoma, probably low-grade
- Grade II carcinoma, probably high-grade
- Grade III carcinoma, high-grade
- Carcinoma in situ (CIS)
- Squamous cell carcinoma
- Adenocarcinoma
- Small cell carcinoma
- Others

This terminology corresponds to the international cassification of the WHO for tumors of the bladder and the histologic classification which is described in this chapter (Mostofi et al. 1973).

5.5.4
Cytologic Criteria

In order to achieve the above-mentioned cytologic diagnoses, a detailed description of the cytologic patterns associated with each diagnosis is provided. These cytologic descriptions are based on the pattern of exfoliated cells and the morphologic features of individual cells. The number of cells in the smears is also taken into consideration, although this is to some extent influenced by methods of specimen collection and processing. Proliferative lesions of the urothelium generally result in cellular samples. In cases where there are few urothelial cells, it is very unlikely that the patient is suffering from a urothelial tumor. Cellular patterns are based on the ratio of three-dimensional branching papillary clusters to single cells in the smears. Small clusters of transitional cells and sheets of transitional cells are excluded form the evaluation of the specimen. Cytomorphologic features evaluated include nuclear size, nuclear shape, chromatin texture, chromatin content, nucleolar size, number of nuclei, and nuclear-cytoplasmic ratio. The background is also taken into consideration. The characteristic combination of exfoliation pateern and the cytonuclear features for each diagnostic group of proliferative urothelial lesions is summarized below:

1. Since a papilloma, an inverted papilloma, and a grade I carcinoma give the same pattern, they are grouped together. These lesions result in highly cellular smears with many papillary clusters and few single cells. Because of good cell cohesion in low-grade bladder tumors, the clusters are large and compact. Moderate cytonuclear atypia is not present in this group. The background is clean; hematuria may be present.

2. In grade II carcinoma there is a combination of single cells and papillary clusters. Because cell cohesion in these tumors is only moderate, the clusters are smaller than in grade I tumors and less compact. Cytonuclear atypia is found both in the clusters and in the single cells.

3. In grade III carcinoma single cells outnumber papillary clusters. These clusters, if present, are very small. The cytonuclear atypia is very pronounced. Since most of these grade III tumors are advanced, the background contains necrotic cell material, polymorphonuclear leukocyte fragments, fibrin, and degenerated erythrocytes.

4. One of the characteristics of CIS is the lack of cellular cohesion, rsulting in a high cellularity of the urinary specimen. Papillary clusters are in general not found in CIS. The specimen is dominated by single cells with a pronounced nuclear atypia. In contrast to grade III carcinoma, there is no tumor diathesis (i. e., there is a clean background).

This classification system has been extensively tested in Dutch laboratories. From these data and from the literature it is clear that the cytohistologic correlation is not influenced by any therapeutic agent used for bladder cancer. Although different therapies such as radiotherapy, immunotherapy, and chemotherapy induce specific cytologic changes, they do not alter the basic cytologic pattern as described above (Ooms and Veldhuizen 1993).

5.6
Other Tumors

5.6.1
Introduction

In most parts of the world the majority of bladder tumors in adults are transitional cell neoplasms. Other epithelial and nonepithelial tumors play a minor role and therefore are mentioned here only briefly for the sake of completeness. In the light of this chapter it seems adequate to give a global overview without going into histologic detail, which is probably only of interest to the experienced pathologist. The classification in this chapter is not based on molecular-biological or genetic concepts but purely on histologic light microscopic characteristics. Benign tumors and nonneoplastic tumorous conditions are beyond the scope of this chapter and therefore are not included. For the interested reader the AFIP atlas (MURPHY et al. 1993c) and the book by R. H. Young (YOUNG 1989c) can be recommended.

5.6.2
Variants of Transitional Cell Carcinoma

Transitional cell tumors having unexpected histologic patterns or cellular products are defined as variants of TCC. The unexpected histology may concern the formation of gland-like structures, cell nests, or spindle cells, respectively leading to names such as carcinoma with gland-like lumina, TCC nested type, and sarcomatoid carcinoma. Another choice of nomenclature for these tumors is: TCC with glandular differentiation (or metaplasia), TCC with squamous differentiation, etc.

These aberrant differentiation patterns (metaplasia) may be found in both low-grade and high-grade tumors, but the incidence is higher in the latter.

5.6.3
Squamous Cell Carcinoma

In areas where schistosomiasis is not endemic, squamous cell carcinoma accounts for less than 5% of bladder carcinomas. Chronic irritation is a major etiologic factor for this group of tumors. Squamous cell carcinoma is relatively more common in women than is TCC. In general these tumors have a poor prognosis since they are usually of a high stage at the time of diagnosis.

5.6.4
Mixed Carcinoma

Mixed carcinomas are defined as urothelial carcinomas composed of more than one distinctive histologic component. The differential diagnosis with TCC variants is not well defined and probably not of great clinical significance.

5.6.5
Adenocarcinoma

The etiology and pathogenesis of adenocarcinoma of the urinary bladder are unknown. These tumors account for less than 2% of bladder carcinomas. Adenocarcinoma of urachal origin is a distinct entity with specific characteristics such as localization in the bladder.

In general, adenocarcinoma of the urinary bladder has a poor prognosis. The incidence in males is significantly higher than in females.

5.6.6
Small Cell Carcinoma

Small cell carcinoma of the urinary bladder is a very rare highly malignant tumor most commonly occurring in elderly males. Other histologic types of carcinomas are often associated with small cell carcinoma. As in small cell carcinoma of the lung, the neuroendocrine character of this tumor has been established by transmission electron microscopy and immunohistochemisty.

5.6.7
Rare Tumors

Like most other organs in the human body, the urinary baldder may be the site of origin of rare neoplasms. These may be of epithelial or nonepithelial origin. The group of rare epithelial tumors consists, among others, of carcinosarcoma, carcinoid tumor, melanoma, and several histologic variants of carcinomas with a descriptive nomenclature, e.g., giant cell carcinoma. On the nonepithelial side, pediatric tumors such as sarcomas need to be mentioned.

Pheochromocytoma, lymphoma, and germ cell neoplasms are extremely rare tumors of the bladder.

References

Baak JPA, Oort J (1983) A manual of morphometry in diagnostic pathology. Springer, Berlin Heidelberg New York, pp 18–20

Badalament RA, Hermansen DK, Kimmel M (1987) The sensitivity of bladder wash flowcytometry. Bladder wash cytology and voided cytology in the detection of bladder carcinoma. Cancer 60:1423–1427

Beahrs OH, Meyers MD (1983) Manual for staging of cancer, 2nd edn. Lippincott, Philadelphia, p 173

Bergkvist A, Ljungqvist G, Moberger G (1965) Classification of bladder tumours based on the cellular pattern. Acta Chir Scand 130:371–378

Blomjous CE, Smeulders AWM, Vos W, Baak JPA, van Galen EM, Meyer CJLM (1988) Retrospective study of prognostic importance of DNA flowcytometry of urinary bladder transitional cell carcinoma. J Clin Pathol 41:21–25

Blomjous CE, Schipper NW, Vos W, Baak JPA, de Voort HJ, Meijer CJLM (1989) Comparison of quantitative and classic prognosticators in urinary bladder carcinoma. A multivariate analysis of DNA flowcytometric, nuclear morphometric and clinicopathological features. Virchows Arch [A] 415:421–428

Boon ME, Blomjous CEM, Zwartendijk J, Heinhuis RJ, Ooms ECM (1986) Carcinoma in situ of the urinary bladder. Clinical presentation, cytologic pattern and stromal changes. Acta Cytol 30:360

Borland RN, Partin AW, Epstein JI, Brendler CB (1993) The use of nuclear morphometry in predicting recurrence of transitional cell carcinoma. J Urol 149:272–275

Broders AC (1992) Epithelioma of genito-urinary organs. Ann Surg 75:574–580

Collan Y, Makinen J, Heikkinen A (1979) Histologic grading of transitional cell tumors of the bladder: value of histologic grading (WHO). Eur Urol 5:311

Couts AG, Grigor KM, Fowler JW (1985) Urothelial dysplasia and bladder cancer in cystectemy specimens. Br J Urol 57:535

Devere White RW, Deitch AD, West B, Fitzpatrick JM (1988) The predictive value of flowcytometric information in the clinical management of stage 0 – Ta bladder cancer. J Urol 139:279–285

Farrow G (1987) Histopathology and cytopathology of bladder cancer. In: Javadpour N, Barsky SH (eds) Surgical pathology of urologic diseases. Williams and Wilkins, Baltimore, p 154

Friedell GH, Bell JR, Burney SW, Soto EA, Tiltman AJ (1976) Histopathology and classification of urinary bladder carcinoma. Urol Clin North Am 3:53–70

Gilbert HA, Logan JL, Kagan AR (1976) The natural history of papillary transitional cell carcinoma of the bladder and its treatment in an unselected population on the basis of histologic grading. J Urol 119:488

Hermanek B, Sobin LH (1987) T.N.M. classification of malignant tumors, Union International Contre le Cancer (UICC), 4th edn. Springer, Berlin Heidelberg New York, pp 121–144

Jewett HJ, Strong GH (1946) Infiltrating carcinoma of bladder: relation of depth of penetration of bladder wall to incidence of local extension and metastasis. J Urol 55:366–372

Jordan AM, Weingarten J, Murphy WM (1987) Transitional neoplasms of the urinary bladder. Cancer 60:2766–2770

Klein FA, Herr HW, Sogani PC, Withmore WP, Melamed MR (1982) Detection and follow-up of carcinoma of the urinary bladder by flowcytometry. Cancer 50:389

Koss LG (1979) Mapping of the urinary bladder: its impact on the concepts of bladder cancer. Hum Pathol 10:533–548

Koss LG, Dietch D, Ramanathan R, Sherman AB (1985) Diagnostic value of cytology of voided urine. Acta Cytol 29:810–816

Lipponen PK (1993a) Over-expression of p 53 nuclear oncoprotein in transitional cell bladder cancer and its prognostic value. Int J Cancer 53:365–370

Lipponen PK (1993b) Expression of c-erb B-2 oncoprotein in transitional cell bladder cancer. Eur J Cancer 29A:749–753

Lipponen PK, Aaltomaa S (1994) Apoptosis in bladder cancer as related to standard prognostic factors and prognosis. 173:333–339

Lipponen PK, Eskelinen M (1994) Expression of epidermal growth factor receptor in bladder cancer as related to established prognostic factors, oncoprotein (c-erb B-2, p 53) expression and long-term prognosis. Br J Cancer 69:1120–1125

Lipponen PK, Collan Y, Eskelinen MJ, Pesonen E, Sotarauta M, Nordling S (1990a) Comparison of morphometry and DNA flowcytometry with standard prognostic factors in bladder cancer. Br J Urol 65:589

Lipponen PK, Eskelinen MJ, Sotarauta M (1990b) Prediction of superficial bladder cancer by histoquantitative methods. Eur J Cancer 26:1060–1063

Lipponen PK, Kosma VM, Collan Y, Kulju T, Kosunen E, Eskeli nen M (1990c) Potential of nuclear morphometry and volume-corrected mitotic index in grading transitional cell carcinoma of the urinary bladder. Eur Urol 17:333

Malmström PU, Norlen BJ, Andersson B, Busch C (1989) Combination of bloodgroup ABH antigen status and DNA ploidy as independent prognostic factor in transitional cell carcinomas. Scand J Urol Nephrol 64:49–55

Marshall VF (1962) The relation of the preoperative estimate to the pathologic demonstration of the extent of vesicle neoplasms. J Urol 68:714–723

Mostofi FK, Sobin LH, Torloni H (1973) In: Histological typing of urinary bladder tumours. International histological classification of tumours, no 10. World Health Organisation (WHO), Geneva

Murphy WM, Soloway MS (1982) Urothelial dysplasia. J Urol 127:849

Murphy WM, Beckwith JB, Farrow GM (1993a) Atlas of tumor pathology, tumors of the kidney, bladder and related urinary structures. Armed Forces Institute of Pathology, Washington, pp 210–219

Murphy WM, Beckwith JB, Farrow GM (1993b) In: Atlas of tumor pathology, tumors of the kidney, bladder and related urinary structures. Armed Forces Institute of Pathology, Washington, pp 228–230

Murphy WM, et al. (1993c) pp 193–275

Nielsen K, Colstrup H, Nilsson T, Gundersen HJG (1986) Stereological estimates of nuclear volume correlated with histopathological grading and prognosis of bladder tumours. Virchows Arch [A] 52:41

Ooms ECM, Veldhuizen RW (1993) Cytological criteria and diagnostic terminology in urinary cytology. Cytopathology 4:51–54

Ooms ECM, Essed E, Veldhuizen RW, Alons CL, Kurver PHJ, Boon ME (1981) The prognostic significance of morphometry in T1 bladder tumours. Histopathology 5:311–318

Ooms ECM, Kurver PHJ, Veldhuizen RW, Alons CL, Boon ME (1983) Morphometric grading of bladder tumours in comparison with histologic grading by pathologists. Hum Pathol 14:144–150

Ooms ECM, Blok APR, Veldhuizen RW (1985) The reproducibility of a quantitative grading system of bladder tumours. Histopathology 9:501–509

Reuter VE (1990) Pathology of bladder cancer. Assessment of prognostic variables and response to therapy. Semin Oncol 17:524–532

Rübben H, Lutzeyer W, Wallace DMA (1985) The epidemiology and aetiology of bladder cancer. In: Zingg EJ, Wallace DMA (eds) Bladder Cancer. Springer, Berlin Heidelberg New York, p 1

Russell PJ, Brown JL, Grimmond SM, Ragvahan D (1990) Review molecular biology of urological tumours. Br J Urol 65:121–130

Sarkis AS, Dalbagni G, Cordon-Cardo C, et al. (1993) Nuclear over expression of p 53 protein in transitional cell bladder carcinoma: a marker for disease progression. J Natl Cancer Inst 85:53–59

Schapers RFM, Pauwels RPE, Havenith ME, Smeets AWGB, van den Brandt PA, Bosman FT (1990) Prognostic significance of type IV collagen and laminin immunoreactivity in urothelial carcinomas of the bladder. Cancer 66:2583–2588

Shimazui T, Koiso K, Uchiyama Y (1990) Morphometry of nucleoli as an indicator for grade of malignancy of bladder tumors. Virchows Arch [B] 59:179

Soiny Y, Turpeenniemi-Hujanen T, Kamel D (1993) p 53 Immuno histochemistry in transitional cell carcinoma and dysplasia of the urinary bladder correlates with disease progression. Br J Cancer 68:1029–1035

van der Poel HG, van Cambergh RD, Boon ME, Debruyne FMJ, Schalken JA (1992) Karyometry in recurrent superficial transitional cell tumours in the bladder. Urol Res 20:375–381

Vasco J, Malinström PU, Taube A, Wester K, Busch C (1991) Prognostic value of a systematized method for determination of mitotic frequency in bladder cancer assisted by computerized image analysis. J Urogenital Pathol 1:53–59

Weinstein RS, Gardner WA (1992) Urothelial neoplasia. In: Pathology and pathobiology of the urinary bladder and prostate. Williams and Wilkins, Baltimore, pp 77–111

Wolf H, Hojgaard K (1983) Urothelial dysplasia concomittant with bladder tumours as a determinant factor for further new occurrences. Lancet 2:134

Wood DP, Wartinger DD, Reuter V, Cordon-Cardo C, Faiz WR, Changanti RSK (1991) DNA, RNA and immunohistochemical characterisations of the HER – 2 / neu oncogene in transitional cell carcinoma of the bladder. J Urol 146:1398–1401

Wright C, Mellon K, Neal DE, Johnston P, Corbett LP, Horne CHW (1990) Expression of C-erb B-2 protein product in bladder cancer. Br J Cancer 62:764–765

Young RH (1989a) Pathology of the urinary bladder. Churchill Livingstone, New York, pp 78–82

Young RH (1989b) Pathology of the urinary bladder. Churchill Livingstone, New York, p 89

Young RH (1989c) Pathology of the urinary bladder. Churchill Livingstone, New York, pp 139–212

Zing EJ, Wallace DMA (1985) Clinical practice in urology. Bladder cancer. Springer, Berlin Heidelberg New York

6 Imaging Modalities in the Diagnosis and Staging of Carcinoma of the Bladder

R.H. OYEN

CONTENTS

6.1
Examination Techniques

6.1.1
Intravenous Urography

Intravenous urography (IVU) prior to or following diagnostic cystoscopy is commonly performed early in the evaluation of a bladder neoplasm, and is considered a basic imaging study in patients with a suspected bladder neoplasm. The rationale for the use of IVU is to exclude upper tract disease. A diagnosis of multicentric synchronous neoplasm is of major importance since it will change patient management. Urothelial neoplasms of the upper tract are expected in up to 4% of patients with bladder cancer (YOUSEM et al. 1988). Even in the era of cross-sectional techniques, IVU is the most sensitive method of detecting subtle occult upper urinary tract urothelial lesions (Fig. 6.1).

An early film of the bladder, a film of the distended bladder, a prone film, and a postvoiding film are usually recommended in visualizing small lesions (Fig. 6.2). Occasionally, oblique films can be helpful to differentiate between intestinal air and bladder masses.

Despite the use of meticulous technique, small bladder lesions may not be visible. Published reports have shown that only 60% of known bladder tumors can be detected on IVU (HILLMAN et al. 1981). Therefore, IVU is of only limited use for the detection of bladder neoplasms.

6.1.2
Ultrasonography

The following ultrasonographic techniques are currently in use for diagnosis and staging of bladder neoplasms:

1. Transabdominal
2. Suprapubic
3. Transurethral
4. Transrectal

6.1.2.1
Transabdominal Ultrasonography

The distended fluid-filled bladder provides an excellent window for the evaluation of this organ (Fig. 6.3). The bladder should not be distended too much when performing the examination because of the discomfort which this may cause the patient. Particular attention should be paid to the anterior

R.H. OYEN MD, PhD, Associate Professor, Department of Radiology, UZ Gasthuisberg, University Hospitals of Leuven, Herestraat 49, B-3000 Leuven, Belgium

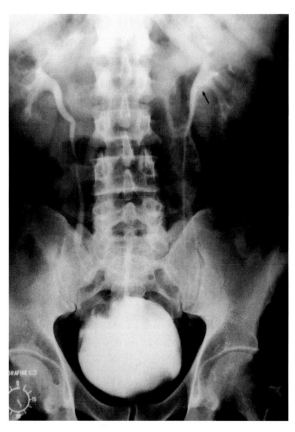

Fig. 6.1. Bladder papillomatosis and urothelial neoplasm in the left renal pelvis. IVU. Multiple filling defects are present at the bladder dome and the bladder base, and a small filling defect is seen at the inferior border of the left renal pelvis (*small arrow*)

neoplasms originating in such bladders can be missed. Flat infiltrating bladder neoplasms can be missed whereas small polypoid tumors are more readily seen. Therefore, in order to evaluate the bladder urothelium adequately cystoscopy is usually required.

The diagnostic accuracy of transabdominal ultrasonography has been reported in several studies (SINGER et al. 1981; ABU-YOUSSEF et al. 1984; ABU-YOUSSEF 1986; DERSHAW and SCHER 1987). As would be expected, diagnostic accuracy depends on the tumor stage, with deep infiltrating tumors being staged more accurately than superficial tumors. In addition, superficial tumors are often overstaged.

6.1.2.2
Transurethral Ultrasonography

Transurethral ultrasonography was introduced a decade ago and has been popularized in Scandinavian countries. Theoretically, it should be the best technique for evaluating the bladder wall. Under optimal conditions, the tumor as well as infiltration of the bladder wall can be visualized. However, use of the technique is now limited to a few centers only, since after the early enthusiasm, certain limitations became obvious. Transurethral ultrasonography is relatively invasive and requires some form of anesthesia – especially in males – for confortable examination. Attenuation of the sound beam by bulky lesions, superficial calcification which produces an acoustic shadow area behind the lesion, blood clots, and air bubbles are important limitations of the technique and may contribute to inaccurate diagnosis and staging (Fig. 6.5). Finally, the routinely used transducers are equipped with crystals that allow only cross-sections of the bladder, i.e., perpendicular to the bladder wall. Complete evaluation of the bladder, including the dome and the base, requires angulated crystals that permit forward view (i.e., towards the bladder dome) and a backward view (i.e., towards the bladder base).

With transurethral ultrasonography, detection rates of greater than 95% have been reported. As with transabdominal ultrasonography, flat infiltrating tumors and tumors of less than 0.5 cm in diameter often cannot be visualized (DERSHAW and SCHER 1987). As with most other imaging techniques, edema, trabeculations, suture material, postoperative status, and postradiotherapy status (external beam or brachytherapy) may

bladder wall. With the use of some transducers the anterior bladder wall is not in the optimal focal area and thus lesions can be missed. On the other hand, reverberation artifacts may also obscure the anterior bladder wall (Fig. 6.3). Changing of the patient's position (i.e., lateral position) may be helpful to differentiate neoplasms from blood clots. Likewise, calcified neoplasms can be differentiated from calculi. Color-Doppler ultrasonography can be used in selected cases to differentiate neoplasms from nonvascularized masses such as blood clots. Color-Doppler ultrasonography, though, is clinically not helpful in the evaluation of transitional cell carcinoma or other tumors as tumor grade, stage, and size are not related to vascularity (HORSTMAN et al. 1995). In some circumstances it can be difficult to detect urothelial neoplasms. Muscular hypertrophy of the bladder wall and formation of trabeculations sometimes mimic multifocal bladder cancer or papillomatosis (Fig. 6.4a). Conversely,

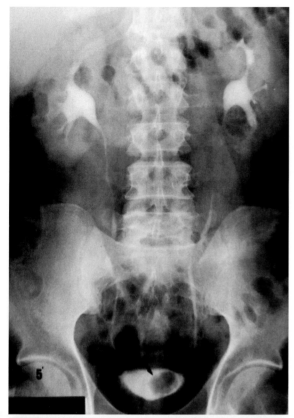

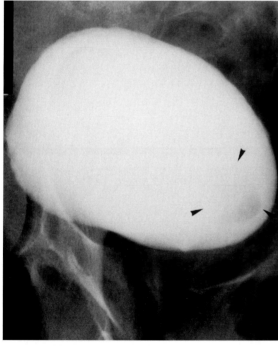

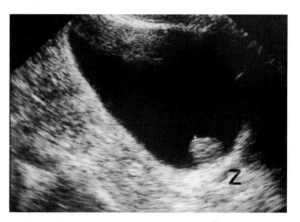

Fig. 6.3. Bladder carcinoma. Transabdominal ultrasonography. A typical polypoid tumor is present at the bladder trigone. Color-Doppler ultrasonography and changing the patient's position may be helpful in distinguishing such lesions from blood clots. *B*, Bladder; *PR*, prostate; *Z*, ••

be mistaken for tumor. This technique is also of some value in detecting tumors in a bladder diverticulum.

6.1.2.3
Transrectal Ultrasonography

Transrectal ultrasonography is not routinely used for the evaluation of bladder neoplasms. Nevertheless, from time to time this route should be considered for evaluation of bladder masses. The bladder should not be distended too much since the limited penetration and focal potential of the transducers employed may prevent accurate evaluation of the anterior bladder wall. The potential advantage of this technique is the detailed evaluation of the area of the bladder neck and of the proximal prostatic urethra. Color-Doppler ultrasonography may be useful to differentiate vascularized (neoplasms) from avascular masses (blood clots). The diagnostic accuracy of transrectal ultrasonography has been investigated in several studies (SINGER et al. 1981; ABU-YOUSSEF et al. 1984; ABU-YOUSSEF 1986; DERSHAW and SCHER 1987). The technique is only used in selected patients.

Fig. 6.2a,b. Bladder carcinoma. IVU. Films at early stages of bladder filling (**a**) or following voiding are essential to evaluate the bladder mucosa. Note the polypoid bladder tumor (*arrow*). Even bulky tumors (*arrowheads*) may be difficult to see when the bladder is distended with contrast medium (**b**)

6.1.3
Cystography

Several techniques, including single contrast, double contrast, and even triple contrast, have been pro-

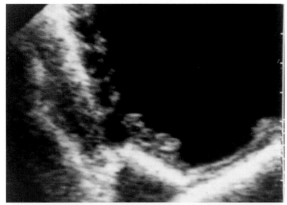

a

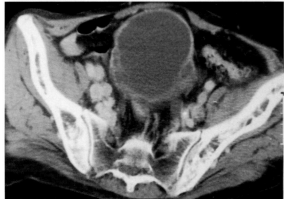

b

Fig. 6.4a,b. Bladder trabeculation. Detail of the bladder wall at transabdominal ultrasonography (**a**) and on CT (**b**). There is irregular thickening of the bladder wall with polypoid-like lesions separated by diverticulum-like outpouchings, representing muscular hypertrophy with small pseudodiverticula because of bladder outlet obstruction. This should not be misinterpreted as bladder neoplasm. It is obvious that if the patient has an associated bladder neoplasm it may be invisible

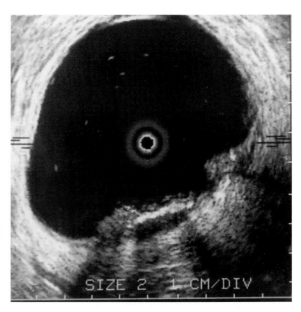

Fig. 6.5. Transurethral ultrasonography. Multiple tumors are present at the bladder base. Because of sound attenuation and superficial calcifications, accurate staging of the neoplasms is impossible

posed (Fig. 6.6). The availability of the cross-sectional techniques, i.e., ultrasonography, CT, and magnetic resonance imaging (MRI) has largely relegated all forms of cystography to history. The technique is no longer useful for the diagnosis of bladder neoplasms.

6.1.4
Computed Tomography

Computed tomography (CT) provides a reliable and effective method of diagnosis and staging of known and invasive bladder cancer. For a period of at least 10 years CT remained unchallenged as the most appropriate technique for staging of these tumors.

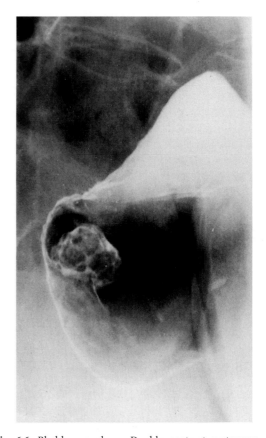

Fig. 6.6. Bladder neoplasm. Double contrast cystogram. A polypoid lesion (TCC) is seen at the right inferolateral bladder wall

6.1.4.1
Technique

The configuration and thickness of the bladder wall largely depend on the degree of filling. For this reason, CT should preferably be performed with a filled bladder, and initially without administration of intravenous contrast medium (Fig. 6.7b). Some patients with bladder cancer may have difficulty in maintaining a full bladder but interpretation of the scans is certainly easier if the bladder is distended as much as possible. Particularly during follow-up

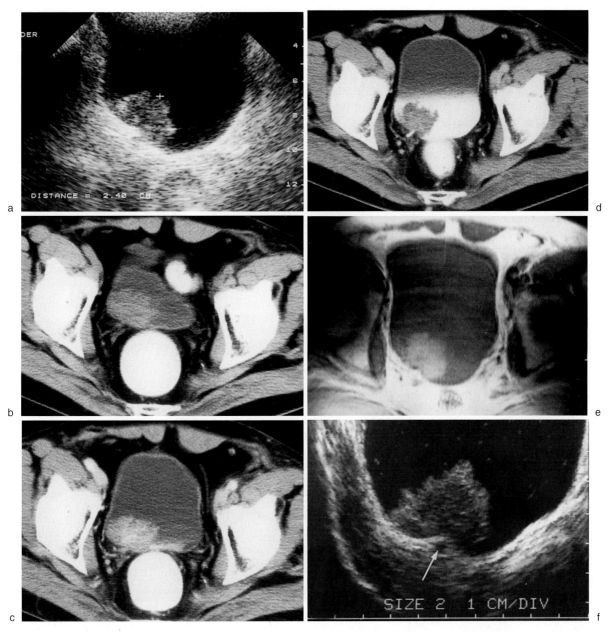

Fig. 6.7a–f. Bladder carcinoma. A polypoid tumor is seen at the right side of the bladder trigone on transabdominal ultrasonography (**a**). On plain CT scan, a mass with attenuation numbers of soft tissue is seen in the posterior part of the bladder (**b**). The mass enhances after IV injection of contrast medium (**c**); a blood clot is ruled out. When the bladder becomes opacified, the mass causes a filling defect (**d**). Note the papillary surface of the tumor. The mass covers the right ureterovesical junction, which is not obstructed. There are some strands in the perivesical fat adjacent to the tumor. The same tumor is clearly visible on the T1-weighted MR image (**e**). **f** Endovesical ultrasonography showing the same tumor. There is no infiltration of the bladder wall. Note the right ureteral orifice (*arrow*) behind the tumor

examination for bladder tumors, the degree of filling should be similar, if visualization of the bladder lesion itself is part of the purpose of the examination. As in the evaluation of other pelvic cancers, all patients should be scanned following the administration of oral and rectal contrast medium. An additional advantage of the ingestion of oral contrast medium is that the bladder will be distended appropriately prior to scanning. In female patients a vaginal tampon to delineate the vaginal vault is helpful but not essential.

Computed tomography should also be carried out following or during a rapid injection of intravenous (IV) contrast medium. This is in order to enhance both the primary tumor and adjacent organs as well as to opacify the pelvic blood vessels (Fig. 6.7c). This technique has the advantage of increasing the contrast between tumor and perivesical fat and also facilitates the diagnosis of enlarged lymph nodes.

With conventional CT techniques, imaging is usually performed using a slice thickness of 7–10 mm, starting at the pelvic floor and continuing up to the pelvic brim. Additional thin sections can be used for improved imaging of suspicious bladder lesions.

When spiral CT is available, usually a pitch of 1.5 is recommended (5/7.5 mm). Scanning starts after IV injection of contrast medium (1.7 ml/s; total amount 120 ml; scan delay 2 min). With both techniques, delayed images after excretion of the contrast through the ureters into the bladder enable improves delineation of the bladder mucosa and the ureters (Fig. 6.7d). In general, no additional information is to be expected from delayed scans when the presence of bladder neoplasm is already known. Occasionally, it may also be possible to identify tumor spread from the bladder into the distal end of the ureter. CT scanning of the abdomen may reveal hydronephrosis and ureteric dilatation in patients with tumors in the region of the trigone.

Films taken in the prone or lateral position sometimes provide a better perspective of certain bladder tumors and permit better differentiation from blood clots (Fig. 6.8). Apart from the obvious advantage of reduction in examination time, spiral CT may be valuable in those patients with tumors of the bladder base or dome. This is because computer reformatting in alternative imaging planes may provide useful additional information. At the present time the diagnostic yield remains doubtful.

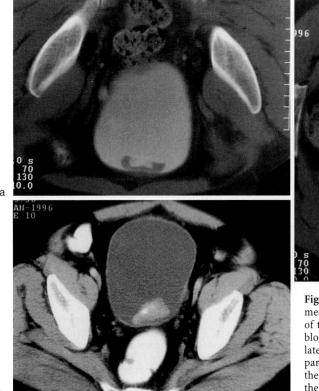

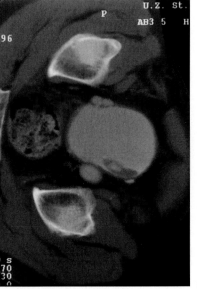

Fig. 6.8a–c. Blood clot. **a** CT scan after IV injection of contrast medium shows a hyperattenuating lesion in the posterior part of the bladder. Because it was suggested that this could be a blood clot, this patient was scanned in the prone (**b**) and lateral (**c**) positions. The mass moved and settled in the lower part of the bladder. Widening of the window and increase of the center permit visualization of small bladder masses when the bladder is opacified with contrast medium

Spiral CT and progress in computer technology have led to the development of a promising new technique for bladder evaluation called CT cystoscopy (VINING et al. 1996). With this technique, a gas-distended bladder is scanned with spiral CT in approximately 10 s. After the routine evaluation of the spiral CT images, the data are transmitted to a graphics workstation for further processing. Real-time three-dimensional (3D) rendering of the CT images is performed to visually simulate a cystoscopic examination. Although this virtual endoscopy does not produce any new information apart from that available in the axial CT slices, it does allow for a rapid and more detailed evaluation of the often complex morphology of this hollow organ. Theoretically, masses of at least 3 mm in diameter should be visible on the CT cystoscopy image. Tumors become readily visible as irregular exophytic masses protrude into the bladder lumen. Experience with CT cystoscopy is still too limited to assess whether there is any advantage in the use of this method in the diagnosis or staging of endophytic bladder neoplasms.

6.1.4.2
Limitations

Despite the excellent CT images of bladder diseases and bladder neoplasms that can be obtained, there are limitations to the technique that should be considered; the major disadvantages of CT are linked to these limitations:

1. Distinct layers of the bladder wall cannot be visualized.
2. The attenuation numbers of the lesion do not allow accurate differentiation of the depth of penetration of the bladder wall.
3. Other conditions such as edema, inflammation, postresection status, status following laser therapy, and status following radiotherapy produce changes in and beyond the bladder wall in the perivesical fat which are completely indiscernible from tumor.
4. Microscopic infiltration in the depth of the bladder wall or in the adjacent fat cannot be seen.

Therefore, the major limitations of CT for staging bladder cancer relate to the following:

1. The inability to stage early tumors
2. Difficulties in identifying minimal deep or extravesical tumor spread

3. Difficulties encountered when attempting to identify adjacent organ invasion

Likewise, problems occur in patients who have previously been investigated by cystoscopy or biopsy or treated with radiotherapy. Thus following endoscopic treatment, edema and inflammation of the bladder wall may be misinterpreted as tumor. For this reason, it is recommended that CT staging be carried out either before cystoscopy or after an interval of at least 2 weeks following this procedure. Sometimes difficulties occur when the bladder wall is hypertrophied due to outlet obstruction or in patients with neuropathic bladder disease. In such conditions, it becomes difficult to differentiate between benign muscular thickening and tumor involvement (Fig. 6.4b).

6.1.5
Magnetic Resonance Imaging

6.1.5.1
Technique

Magnetic resonance imaging has been shown to be well suited for the examination of the pelvic organs and has important general and specific advantages over CT, including superior contrast resolution and the ability to obtain images in multiple planes. Thus, compared with CT, MRI seems to be the more flexible modality for imaging bladder neoplasms and therefore, allows the operator to tailor the examination more appropriately to address a specific clinical question.

As with CT, patients should preferably be examined with a fluid-filled bladder. Axial images are obtained using T1- and T2-weighted sequences. If lymph node staging is required, the images obtained should cover the whole pelvis. Further sequences in alternative planes of imaging are then carried out. The final selection of the spatial orientation depends upon the site of the primary tumor. The use of IV contrast medium can be helpful in selected cases. Oral contrast agents for MRI are just beginning to be used routinely in clinical practice. As in the case of CT, they are promising in differentiating tumor and lymph nodes from the bowel.

Magnetic resonance imaging continues to evolve rapidly and new sequences and new surface coils are continually being introduced into clinical practice. Dedicated surface coils and endorectal coils, together with the use of IV contrast medium, provide images of the bladder wall and of superficial tumors with exquisite anatomic detail. For example, selective fat suppression combined with IV contrast medium may be helpful for evaluating early tumor spread beyond the bladder. Fast imaging sequences combined with the use of IV contrast medium and subtraction techniques may be helpful for demonstrating the pattern of uptake of contrast medium both in the primary neoplasm and in the lymph nodes. Some of these techniques are time consuming, need complex processing, and require highly skilled operators.

6.1.5.2
Limitations

As with the application all imaging techniques, MRI has important limitations with regard to the assessment of bladder cancer. At the present time, it seems unlikely that edema and fibrosis can be reliably distinguished from active tumor within the bladder wall. Additionally, understaging of minimal and microscopic spread beyond the bladder into adjacent organs is likely to remain a problem with MRI just as it is with CT or transurethral ultrasonography. Deep biopsies are still necessary for accurate diagnosis.

An additional problem with MRI and its rapidly evolving techniques is the difficulty in comparing the results of different studies reported in the literature owing to the use of different techniques for imaging of the bladder. Moreover, obtaining optimal MR images with multiplanar reformatting and subtraction requires the use of time-consuming processing techniques. Obtaining and interpreting MR images is becoming more and more operator dependent compared with the reading of CT images.

6.1.6
Angiography

Bladder angiography is only of interest for the embolization of troublesome bleeding or for the local application of chemotherapeutic agents.

6.1.7
Antegrade – Retrograde Ureterography

When, following IVU, the presence of a nonfunctioning kidney is detected due to distal obstruction of the ureter by a bladder neoplasm, a contrast study may be required to evaluate the urothelium of the upper tract. Percutaneous sonographically guided antegrade ureterography and cystoscopic retrograde ureterography at the time of the resection of the bladder tumor are useful alternatives to evaluate the upper tract and to exclude the presence of gross urothelial malignancy.

6.1.8
Positron Emission Tomography

Recently, the use of positron emission tomography (PET) in the diagnosis and staging of bladder cancer was evaluated (AHLSTROM et al. 1996). Employing PET with carbon-11 methionine, it was possible to visualize bladder neoplasms larger than 1 cm in diameter. The value of this method in the staging of bladder lesions is certainly not superior to that of CT or MRI.

6.2
Malignant Bladder Tumors

6.2.1
Transitional Cell Carcinoma

Transitional cell carcinoma (TCC) is the most common malignant tumor of the urinary tract and is responsible for 3% of all cancer deaths. Men are affected 3 times more often than women. The peak incidence of this tumor is between 50 and 80 years of age; TCC is rarely observed in children. Risk factors for tumor development are various chemicals, dyes, and cigarette smoking. In 90% of patients, the tumors are papillary, and in 10% they are solid. One-quarter of the tumors are multifocal at the time of diagnosis. In 3.5% of the upper urinary tract urothelial tumors, bladder tumors develop later in the course of the disease.

The local growth pattern is characterized initially by radial expansion through the bladder wall, and subsequently by circular invasion of the muscle layers. Later in the course of the disease, invasion of the perivesical fat, prostate, seminal vesicle, and internal obturator muscle is known to occur. The involvement of ureteral orifices leads to hydronephrosis. This observation does not necessarily indicate deep tumor invasion. The uterus and cervix are only rarely involved by bladder cancer.

6.2.1.1
Diagnosis

6.2.1.1.1
INTRAVENOUS UROGRAPHY

Bladder neoplasms may have stippled calcification that is either punctate or coarse. Microscopic calcifications are common in bladder neoplasms, but the foci are usually too small to be demonstrated radiographically. The incidence of radiographically demonstrable calcifications has been estimated at about 0.5% (Miller and Pfister 1974). Calcifications are most common in uroepithelial tumors but may also be seen in mesenchymal tumors. Calcium deposits are usually encrusted on the surface of the tumor but may also be present within its substance in the subepithelial layers in degenerating or necrotic foci. From time to time, these calcifications are visible on the KUB film. Punctate calcifications tend to be more often associated with papillary tumors having relatively thin pedicles, characteristic of noninvasive or low-grade invasive neoplasms which have been present for a long time. Calcifications may also be linear or curvilinear. They tend to occur in large papillary or sessile neoplasms and may also develop after radiation therapy. Combinations of these patterns are also known to occur.

On contrast studies, bladder neoplasms generally produce nonspecific intravesical filling defects (Figs. 6.1, 6.2). Urothelial tumors can sometimes be distinguished from mural lesions by some surface characteristics. Primary urothelial neoplasms tend to have an irregular surface while most other diseases have a smooth surface when they are covered by an intact urothelium. Malignant and benign lesions may produce obstruction of one or both ureters, but malig-

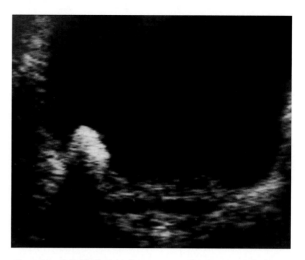

Fig. 6.10. Calcified granuloma. Transabdominal ultrasonography. A calcification is present at the right bladder trigone. A superficially calcified TCC may have exactly the same appearance. In this case the calcification is explained by a granuloma surrounding the sutures after ureter reimplantation for reflux

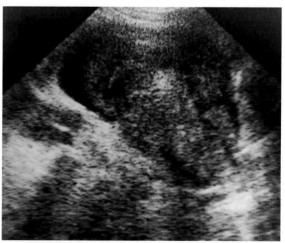

Fig. 6.11. Fresh blood clots in the bladder. Transabdominal ultrasonography. The bladder is filled with blood clots in a patient with massive gross hematuria. In these circumstances a small or even a large intravesical tumor causing the hemorrhage cannot be detected

nant lesions are more likely to do so (HATCH and BARRY 1986). It may be hard to differentiate calcified urothelial neoplasms from other calcified disease processes such as adherent calculi or foreign body granulomas.

6.2.1.1.2
ULTRASONOGRAPHY

Transitional cell carcinomas typically produce soft tissue masses that are flat or pedunculated. These

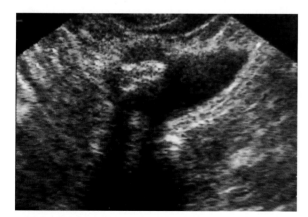

Fig. 6.9. Calcified bladder carcinoma. Transabdominal ultrasonography. Superficial calcifications in a tumor originating at the bladder dome

masses have an irregular surface, whichever imaging approach is used (Figs. 6.3, 6.7a,f). They may be solitary or multifocal. Superficial calcifications produce a typical acoustic shadow (Fig. 6.9). Changing of the patient's position may be helpful to differentiate neoplasms from blood clots. Likewise, calcified neoplasms can be differentiated from calculi or other adherent calcifications (Fig. 6.10). Color-Doppler can be used to differentiate neoplasms from nonvascularized masses such as blood clots (Fig. 6.11). Color-Doppler ultrasonography, however, is not clinically helpful in the evaluation of TCC or other tumors.

Since transrectal ultrasonography is routinely used to evaluate the prostate, bladder masses may be an incidental finding and the operator should be aware of the ultrasonographic characteristics of such neoplasms (HARADA et al. 1977). A prostatic median lobe may erroneously be misinterpreted as a

urothelial neoplasm originating at the bladder trigone behind the bladder neck, or conversely, such a bladder neoplasm may be misinterpreted as a prostatic median lobe (Fig. 6.12a). Two characteristics may assist in the differentiation:

1. The papillary surface of a urothelial tumor causes an irregular outline
2. Cystic areas are frequently seen in a typical prostatic median lobe

6.2.1.1.3
COMPUTED TOMOGRAPHY

CT is usually performed in order to stage bladder cancer in patients in whom the diagnosis has been proven histologically following cystoscopy.

Tumor may be represented as a localized area of thickening of the bladder wall, or by a definite soft tissue mass arising from the bladder wall with or without perivesical extension (Figs. 6.7b, 6.13a). The mass enhances after IV injection of contrast medium (Figs. 6.7c, 6.13b, 6.14). When the bladder becomes filled with excreted contrast medium the tumor produces a filling defect (Figs. 6.7d, 6.13c). If the lesion is small, widening of the window settings and a higher center are recommended for better visualization of the lesion (Figs. 6.8b,c, 6.12b). The surface of the tumor may show calcifications (Fig. 6.15) or be incrusted with fresh hyperattenuating blood clot.

6.2.1.1.4
MAGNETIC RESONANCE IMAGING

On MRI the normal bladder has a completely different appearance on T1-weighted images compared with T2-weighted images. On T1-weighted images the bladder wall has a low signal intensity almost similar to urine within the bladder lumen. The perivesical fat has a high signal intensity. On T2-weighted sequences, the bladder lumen has a high signal intensity whereas the bladder wall has a relatively low signal intensity and appears as a thin line separating the bladder lumen from perivesical fat, which now has an intermediate signal intensity. Bladder tumors appear as relatively low signal intensity lesions on T1-weighted images and as intermediate signal intensity lesions on T2-weighted images (Figs. 6.7e, 6.16). T1-weighted images are therefore the most appropriate ones for detecting perivesical tumor spread, whereas T2-weighted sequences are best for evaluating the bladder wall. In addition the latter are also very helpful for detecting tumor invasion of muscle and adjacent organs such as the prostate, seminal vesicles, and cervix uteri.

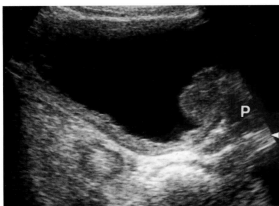

a

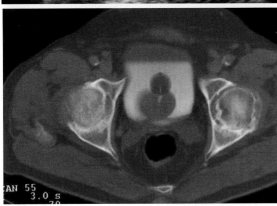

b

Fig. 6.12a,b. Prostatic median lobe. **a** Transabdominal ultrasonography showing diffuse thickening of the bladder wall and an intravesical mass lesion at the bladder neck. Hyperplasia of the prostatic middle lobe causes bladder outlet obstruction and bladder muscle hypertrophy. *P*, Prostate. **b** CT demonstrating an intravesical mass at the midline. The dip in the center of the lesions suggests the prostatic origin of the mass

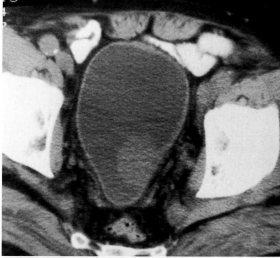

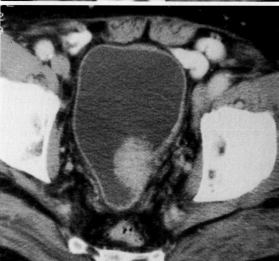

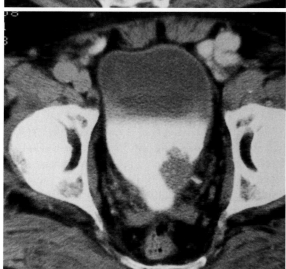

Fig. 6.13a–c. Bladder carcinoma. **a** Unenhanced CT scan revealing a slightly hyperattenuating mass at the left trigone. Note the decreased expansion of the bladder wall compared with the opposite side. The mass enhances after IV injection of contrast medium (**b**) and is seen as a filling defect when the bladder opacifies (**c**). It is impossible to differentiate between transmural infiltration (T3b) or deep infiltration of the bladder wall (T3a) or even only superficial infiltration (<T3)

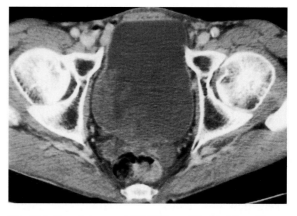

Fig. 6.14. Pseudotumor at CT. Filling of the bladder with excreted contrast medium. The diluted contrast medium causes tumor-like lesions at the posterior and the right bladder wall. These should not be mistaken for tumor

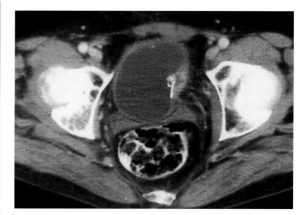

Fig. 6.15. Bladder carcinoma with calcifications. CT shows thickening of the left bladder wall with superficial calcifications. Superficial calcifications are frequently seen in nontreated bladder cancers or after therapy

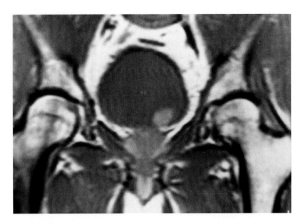

Fig. 6.16. Bladder carcinoma. Coronal T1-weighted MR image showing the polypoid mass at the left bladder base. The infravesical fat has normal signal intensity. Coronal or sagittal images permit better staging of carcinomas at the bladder base or dome

6.2.1.2
Staging

6.2.1.2.1
TUMOR (T-) STAGING

Depth of tumor infiltration through the layers of the bladder wall has a major impact on patient management. Diagnostic workup including cystoscopic evaluation and biopsy demonstrates the tumor growth pattern, the histologic cell type, and its grade. Depth of infiltration through the layers of the bladder wall is determined pathologically by deep biopsy. In patients with advanced disease, when tumor spreads through all the layers of the bladder into the perivesical fat, many urologists are convinced that pathologic staging must be combined with the results of bimanual assessment of tumor bulk. This examination forms the basis of the clinical staging and is accurate for assessing invasive lesions which spread beyond the bladder. For this reason diagnostic imaging plays a key role in the evaluation of bladder tumors, providing information on the following: (a) the depth of infiltration of the primary tumor, and overall assessment of tumor volume, and (b) the presence or absence of lymph node and blood-borne metastases. Once this information has been obtained, the tumor can be classified according to stage and the most appropriate course of management applied.

Ultrasonography. As mentioned in Sect. 6.1.2.1, the diagnostic accuracy of transabdominal ultrasonography has been reported in several studies (McLaughlin et al. 1975; Singer et al. 1981; Abu-

Youssef et al. 1984; Abu-Youssef 1986; Dershaw and Scher 1988) and depends on the stage of the tumor, with deep infiltrating tumors being staged more accurately than superficial ones. In addition, superficial tumors are often overstaged. It is not certain whether ultrasonography is more accurate in staging TCCs than cystoscopic visual assessment by an experienced urologist. Transrectal ultrasonography has been recommended by some authors for the staging of bladder neoplasms (Harada et al. 1977), but its routine use is yet to be established.

It has been mentioned before that transurethral ultrasonography has some advantages in differentiating superficial from deep infiltrating tumors (Naamura and Nijima 1980) (Figs. 6.5, 6.7f). This imaging technique seems to be most valuable in determining the stage of tumor which is confined to the bladder wall (Koraitim et al. 1995). In this recent study, the correlation between transurethral ultrasonography and pathologic staging was 100% in tumors without muscle invasion (stages Ta and T1), 95.7% and 96.8% in muscle-invasive tumors (stages T2 and T3a, respectively) and 70% in tumors with extravesical spread. The diagnostic accuracy in determining perivesical tumor extent in advanced stages, though, is rather limited (Naamura and Nijima 1980; Schuller et al. 1982). Finally, this endoluminal imaging technique also has inherent limitations in evaluating the status of pelvic lymph nodes.

Computed Tomography. On CT, T1 lesions, where there is invasion of the lamina propria, cannot be distinguished from those involving superficial muscle (T2) and deep muscle (T3a) (Koss et al. 1981). Thus CT is impractical for the staging of early lesions; its major advantage lies in the ability to distinguish tumors with extravesical spread from tumors confined to the bladder wall (Sager et al. 1983).

Early extravesical spread is recognized as strands of soft tissue extending into the perivesical fat in direct contiguity with the primary tumor (Figs. 6.17–6.19). Thin sections are often helpful for evaluating doubtful cases but definite histologic staging is impossible.

Early organ invasion can be difficult to detect if the only sign is loss of the fat plane between the bladder wall and an adjacent structure. However, enlargement of the structure or organ as well as contrast enhancement of tissue within the organ in direct contiguity with the primary tumor provides strong evidence of tumor invasion (Fig. 6.20). Inva-

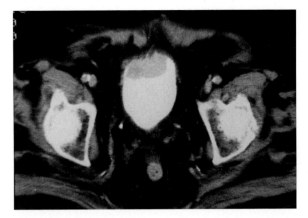

Fig. 6.17. Bladder carcinoma. CT demonstrating a tumor at the anterior bladder wall. The strands into the prevesical fat suggest deep tumor invasion with reactive infiltration of the bladder (T3a) or transmural tumor extension (T3b)

sion of the seminal vesicles is identified relatively easily because of the effacement of the fat angle between the posterior bladder wall and the anterior surface of the seminal vesicles. In more advanced disease, extravesical tumor extension is easily recognized. Spread to the pelvic side wall is diagnosed if tumor extends through the pelvic fat and is contiguous with the pelvic side wall muscles (Fig. 6.20). These muscles may even be enlarged by tumor infiltration or edema. The diagnostic accuracy of CT is reported to be between 88% and 92%, but to a large extent it depends on the stage of the tumor. More "invasive" techniques such as instillation of fat emulsions, air, or CO_2 in the bladder have been proposed but none has been accepted for routine use. These techniques do not significantly improve the staging accuracy (THORNBURY et al. 1983).

The major limitations of the use of CT for staging bladder cancer relate to the following:

1. Its inability to stage early tumors
2. Difficulties in identifying minimal extravesical tumor spread and adjacent organ invasion (HUSBAND et al. 1989)
3. Other problems that occur in patients who have previously been investigated by cystoscopy or treated with radiotherapy

With regard to point 3, following endoscopic treatment, edema and inflammation of the bladder wall may be misinterpreted as tumor and for this reason, CT staging should be carried out either before cystoscopy or after an interval of at least 2 weeks following cystoscopy (Fig. 6.21). Deep infiltrating tumors (T3a) may cause reactive inflammation and

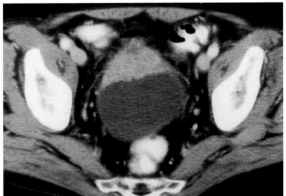

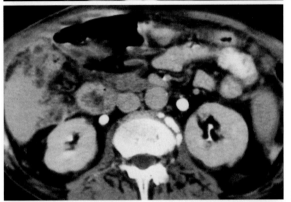

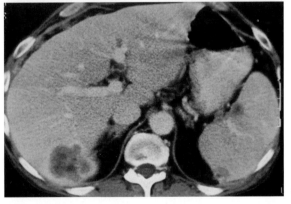

Fig. 6.18a–c. Bladder carcinoma; T3c. **a** CT scan at the time of the diagnosis. A TCC is located at the anterior bladder wall. The prevesical fat is infiltrated, suggestive of transmural tumor extension, which was confirmed at histologic examination after cystectomy (T3cN0). **b** CT 6 months after the cystectomy revealing extensive peritoneal metastases (*arrowheads*) and renal metastasis (*arrow*). **c** There are also metastases in the liver and spleen

infiltration of the adjacent perivesical fat. This reactive phenomenon is indiscernible from true extravesical tumor spread (T3b) (Figs. 6.17, 6.18). For this reason T3a tumors are frequently overstaged at CT. In addition, because of CT's inability to detect microscopic involvement of the perivesical tissues,

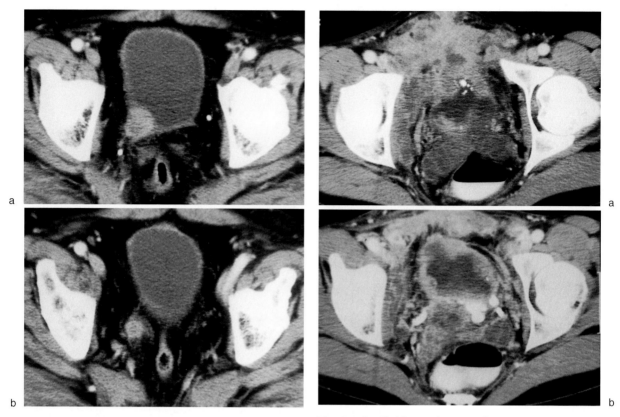

Fig. 6.19a,b. Bladder carcinoma extending into the ureter. **a** CT demonstrating a neoplasm around the right ureterovesical junction. **b** The ureter is dilated and the lumen is enhancing after IV injection of contrast medium. The surrounding fat is infiltrated, suggestive of transmural infiltration

Fig. 6.20a,b. Bladder carcinoma; T4b. CT in a young male a few months after partial cystectomy for TCC. Neoplasm is seen involving the bladder wall, the right seminal vesicle, the right pelvic wall, and the abdominal wall

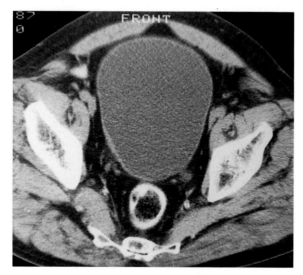

Fig. 6.21. Thickening of the bladder wall after therapy. CT after transurethral resection. The right bladder wall is thickened and rigid. The adjacent perivesical fat is infiltrated by some strands. It is impossible to differentiate local recurrence from sequelae of therapy. CT should be performed at least 2 weeks after therapy to avoid therapy-related infiltration of the perivesical fat

T3b and T4 lesions are frequently understaged. During recent years, several studies have been undertaken comparing the accuracy of MRI with that of CT for staging bladder cancer. The results of these studies have shown that MRI has a similar accuracy to CT, ranging from 72% to 96% (HUSBAND et al. 1989). However, the important advantages of MRI were clearly seen in those studies in which both MRI and CT were performed in the same patients.

Magnetic Resonance Imaging. T1-weighted images are the most appropriate ones for detecting perivesical tumor spread, whereas T2-weighted sequences are best used for evaluating the bladder wall. They are also useful for detecting tumor invasion of muscle and adjacent organs such as the prostate, seminal vesicles and cervix uteri (BUY et al. 1988).

Images in the sagittal or coronal plane may demonstrate tumor spread beyond the bladder wall which cannot readily be appreciated in the transverse plane. This is particularly important for staging tumors of the bladder base and dome. The use of additional planes of imaging frequently increases confidence in diagnosing perivesical disease as well as occasionally upstaging the disease (Figs. 6.7e, 6.16). MRI is also superior to CT in the demonstration of adjacent organ invasion due to the better contrast resolution obtained with the use of this technique (HUSBAND et al. 1989).

Recent studies have suggested that the use of IV contrast medium may be useful for staging early tumors because they enhance to a greater degree than the normal bladder wall. Small tumors down to the size of 7 mm can be detected on contrast-enhanced scans (HAWNAUR et al. 1993). However, in more advanced disease the value of IV contrast medium is not substantiated, because unlike in the case of CT, contrast enhancement of extravesical tissue reduces the contrast between tumor and perivesical fat, which has a high signal intensity on T1-weighted images (NEUERBERG et al. 1991). Contrast enhancement may be useful for detecting organ invasion, but at present insufficient information is available to determine whether the use of IV contrast medium upstages the disease (SPARENBERG et al. 1991). Enhancement after gadolinium enables distinction between necrotic and viable tumor and blood clot. This technique, though, seems to be of only slight advantage for tumors infiltrating perivesical fat or in those patients with lymph node or bone metastases. Selective use in patients with T3a tumors is recommended where the depth of bladder wall invasion is inadequately shown on precontrast sequences (HAWNAUR et al. 1993; KIM et al. 1994).

Studies using IV contrast medium to assess early tumors have revealed a diagnostic accuracy of 69%–89%. Several authors have reported that additional information can be obtained on contrast-enhanced images in more than 10% of patients. However, a recently reported comparison of contrast-enhanced CT, MRI and contrast MRI showed disappointing results. Although all imaging techniques performed moderately well in distinguishing tumors confined to the bladder from tumors extending into the perivesical fat, the depth of infiltration of the bladder wall was poorly demonstrated by all techniques (TACHIBANA et al. 1991). Thus in published reports no technique or sequence has reliably separated the mucosal layer from the muscular layer. Moreover, at present it seems unlikely that edema and fibrosis can be reliably distinguished from active tumor within the bladder wall. Understaging of minimal and microscopic tumor spread beyond the bladder into adjacent organs is likely to remain a problem with MRI just as it is with CT.

Magnetic resonance imaging continues to evolve rapidly and new sequences and new surface coils are continually being introduced. Submillimeter MR images have a higher resolution than the conventional images and are beneficial for the staging of bladder carcinoma (MAEDA et al. 1995). With this technique an accuracy of 96.2%, a sensitivity of 100%, and a specificity of 91.7% have been reported (BARENTSZ et al. 1993). BARENTSZ et al. (1995, 1996) have evaluated a magnetization prepared–rapid gradient-echo (MP-RAGE) sequence as a three-dimensional T1-weighted MR imaging technique for the staging of bladder cancer. The staging accuracy for the combination of three-dimensional techniques, T2-weighted, and dynamic sequences was 93%, compared with 78% for the commonly used two-dimensional T1-weighted spin-echo sequences, T2-weighted sequences, and dynamic sequences. Selective fat suppression combined with IV contrast medium may be helpful for evaluating early tumor spread beyond the bladder and fast imaging sequences combined with the administration of IV contrast medium and the use of subtraction techniques may be helpful for demonstrating the pattern of uptake of contrast medium (BARENTSZ et al. 1993). Dedicated surface coils and endorectal coils, together with the use of IV contrast medium, provide images with exquisite anatomic detail of the bladder wall and of superficial tumors.

6.2.1.2.2
LYMPH NODE (N-) STAGING

A statement on the presence or absence of lymph node and blood-borne metastases is the second major task for the imaging techniques. This information is essential to accurately assess the tumor stage and to consider the most appropriate course of management.

Lymphatic drainage of the bladder is to the external iliac and hypogastric lymph nodes. The posterior bladder wall also partially drains into the hypogastric lymph nodes. Lymph node metastases are found in 3% of T1 tumors, 25% of T2 tumors, and 60% of T3/4 tumors.

Carcinoma of the bladder spreads initially to the regional pelvic lymph nodes. The first involved lymph nodes include the anterior and lateral perivesical, the hypogastric, the obturator, the external iliac, and the lateral sacral nodes. In more advanced disease, lymph nodes in the common iliac, para-aortic, and inguinal chains are involved. The incidence of lymph node metastases increases with advancing disease, rising to approximately 60% in patients with extravesical tumor extension.

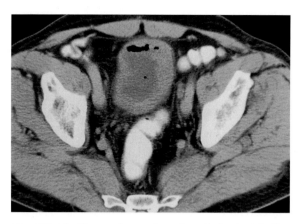

Fig. 6.22. Bladder carcinoma. Lymph node in the left iliac chain in a patient with TCC of the bladder. The size is the only criterion that can be used. This was a reactive enlarged lymph node in a patient with diffuse bladder cancer

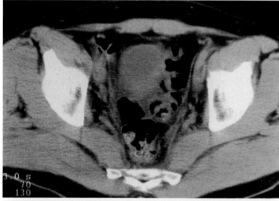

a

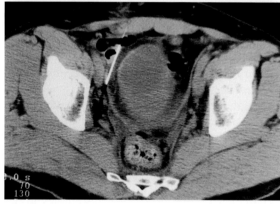

b

Fig. 6.23a,b. Bladder carcinoma. a Lymph node in the right iliac chain in a patient with TCC of the bladder **b** Transperitoneal CT-guided fine-needle aspiration cytology proved metastases of TCC. In patients with TCC of the bladder, only 50%–60% of the enlarged lymph nodes are metastatically involved

Computed Tomography and Magnetic Resonance Imaging. CT and MRI can identify enlarged lymph nodes in the external obturator and internal iliac groups within the pelvis, but unlike lymphangiography, cannot provide any information on the internal architecture of the enlarged nodes. Thus, tumor cannot be distinguished from benign causes of nodal enlargement.

On CT, enlarged lymph nodes appear as an area of soft tissue density (Figs. 6.22, 6.23a). These enlarged lymph nodes may show uniform or heterogeneous enhancement following injection of IV contrast medium, and occasionally may opacify to such an extent that they are difficult to distinguish from opacified blood vessels. On MRI, enlarged lymph nodes show a low signal on T1-weighted images and a relatively high signal on T2-weighted sequences. If there is doubt regarding the presence of an enlarged lymph node on conventional sequences, then fat suppression techniques can be particularly helpful. Three-dimensional techniques for lymph node imaging have also been used (BARENTSZ et al. 1995). For lymph node staging, an accuracy of 93% was reported, compared to 86% for T1-weighted spin-echo sequences. Coronal images may also be helpful in confirming the presence of enlarged lymph nodes suspected on initial axial images.

Since enlargement is the only criterion for detecting metastases in lymph nodes with CT and MRI, the size taken as the upper limit of normal is of critical importance. Guidelines are as follows:

1. Lymph nodes greater than 10 mm in the external iliac group should be considered as suspicious.

2. The upper limit of normal for the internal iliac group and obturator groups should be taken as 7 and 8 mm respectively.

3. If more than one lymph node is enlarged, the likelihood that these nodes contain metastases increases, but if there is doubt, percutaneous fine-needle aspiration under CT control can be readily undertaken (Fig. 6.23b). In our experience approximately 60% of enlarged lymph nodes proved to be metastatically involved at fine-needle aspiration biopsy, while 40% were reactive benign large lymph nodes (OYEN, unpublished data). MRI scanners with easy patient access are now becoming routinely available, opening the way to interventional MRI procedures, so lymph node sampling under MRI control will also be feasible.

In patients with involved pelvic lymph nodes, the likelihood of para-aortic lymph node involvement and liver metastases increases. These patients should undergo both pelvic and abdominal CT or MRI at the time of staging, not only to detect early hematogenous and lymphatic spread, but also to look for hydronephrosis and dilatation of the ureters. In addition, examination of the abdomen provides a baseline for future examinations, so that incidental lesions such as hemangiomas of the liver or benign cysts can be documented and do not cause confusion in interpretation at a later date.

Computed tomography and MRI are considered to be as effective as lymphangiography in the identification of lymph node metastases. For CT, the reported staging accuracy rates range from 70%–96%, and in the few studies reported for MRI similar results have also been obtained (WEINERMAN et al. 1983; WALSH et al. 1980). Other studies have reported on the failure of CT to detect positive lymph nodes in more than 50% of cases (SEE and FULLER 1992). Such observations indeed question the practical utility of CT scanning to stage locally advanced bladder cancer. According to recent work by HERR and HILTON (1996), routine CT scan is not helpful in the management of operable T2 tumors but might change therapy in selected patients with T3–T4 tumors who are considered for cystectomy.

Lymphangiography. A significant disadvantage of lymphography is the inability to demonstrate internal iliac nodes and to reliably demonstrate obturator lymph nodes. Since the obturator lymph nodes are frequently the first nodal stations of involvement to be detected on imaging, they are of particular importance. It seems that with the availability of CT and MRI, lymphangiography no longer to be recommended in the staging of patients with bladder neoplasms.

6.2.1.2.3
DISTANT METASTASES (M-STAGING)
Distant metastases are most commonly located in the liver, lung and bones, and their presence is associated with a poor prognosis (Fig. 6.18b,c). Since hematogenous spread usually occurs late in bladder cancer, the search for metastatic disease is usually carried out when symptoms and signs develop in a particular site. However, occasionally bone metastases may be detected at the time of presentation. These metastases frequently occut in the pelvic bones; therefore, it is of importance that the CT or MRI study covers the entire pelvis, including the pubic rami.

Lung metastases in bladder cancer are usually diagnosed on plain chest radiographs and CT is not indicated as part of the initial staging procedure unless cystectomy is being considered as a primary treatment option. Lung metastases are the most common site of parenchymal distant tumor spread. In the series of GOLDMAN et al. (1979) 6% of the patients with bladder cancer had intrathoracic metastases.

6.2.2
Other Malignant Bladder Neoplasms

6.2.2.1
Neoplasm in a Bladder Diverticulum

It has been reported that from 1% to 5% of bladder cancers develop in bladder diverticula (Figs. 6.24, 6.25). Bladder neoplasms originating in bladder diverticula can be diagnosed with every cross-sectional imaging modality. Accurate staging, however, is at present impossible. Aggressive treatment for patients with carcinoma in a diverticulum is recommended (DAS and AMAR 1986).

6.2.2.2
Adenocarcinoma of the Bladder

Adenocarcinoma of the bladder is an uncommon neoplasm, reported to account for 0.5%–2% of urothelial neoplasms with their origin in the bladder. Adenocarcinoma can exist in a pure form or as part of a mixed tumor with other epithelial elements such as transitional or squamous carcinoma or as part of a carcinosarcoma (KAMAT et al. 1991). It is the most common malignant tumor occurring in an extrophied bladder and is more frequently seen in schistosomiasis-infested bladders. This tumor occurs most frequently from the fifth to the seventh decade of life. It is more prevalent in males, with a reported male to female ratio of 2:1. The symptoms caused by the tumor are usually nonspecific, although urinary mucus may suggest the presence of glandular epithelium. Adenocarcinomas are seen most commonly in the bladder dome, the trigone, and the bladder neck. Primary adenocarcinomas of the bladder also present in advanced stages, irrespective of their site of origin in the bladder, and therefore have a poorer prognosis than other urothelial malignancies.

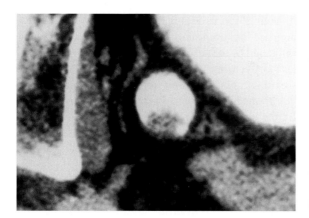

Fig. 6.24. Bladder carcinoma in a diverticulum. CT demonstrates a small soft tissue mass in a bladder diverticulum at the right posterolateral wall

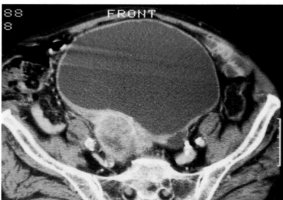

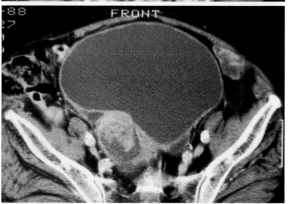

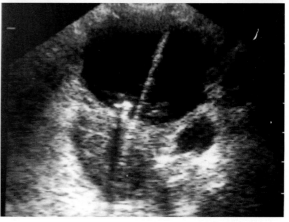

Fig. 6.25a–c. Bladder carcinoma in a bladder diverticulum. **a,b** CT showed a tumor in a bladder diverticulum originating at the right posterior wall. This diverticulum could not be found at cystoscopy. Therefore, sonographically guided percutaneous transvesical puncture was performed (**c**). The needle (*arrowheads*) was inserted in the tumor (*T*); then the tumor was resected (*arrow*: cystoscope)

Urachal carcinomas, mostly mucin-producing adenocarcinomas, have a predilection for calcification and local invasion. Cephalad extension of the tumor toward the anterior abdominal wall and umbilicus is suggestive of urachal carcinoma (BRICK et al. 1988; KOROBKIN et al. 1988; NARUMI et al. 1988). Most of the urachal adenocarcinomas at the time of diagnosis are advanced tumors. Their location and predominantly extramucosal nature explains why they cause symptoms late in the course of disease. Approximately two-thirds of tumors are deeply invasive at the time of presentation (ANDERSTROM et al. 1983).

The distinction between primary bladder adenocarcinoma and urachal adenocarcinoma is important in deciding on the optimal form of management. Primary bladder adenocarcinomas merit radical cystectomy, as compared with partial cystectomy for urachal carcinomas.

6.2.2.3
Melanoma

Melanoma has been reported throughout the genitourinary tract, including the bladder (STEIN and KENDALL 1984). These tumors do not differ histologically from similar lesions arising in the skin. An extravesical primary tumor site must be excluded before the diagnosis of a primary bladder melanoma can be confirmed. The pathogenesis is obscure. It is possible that rare individuals have bladders that contain melanocytes or that melanocytic differentiation infrequently occurs in other-

wise normal bladders. Lesions are not localized to the bladder base and not all lesions are pigmented. This disease process has been uniformly fatal in reported patients.

6.2.2.4
Malignant Lymphoma

Isolated involvement of the bladder by lymphoma is a rarity. The bladder is involved with other organs in 0.3% of patients with generalized lymphoma (WEIMAR et al. 1981). Radiologic manifestations (CT, MRI, ultrasonography) consist in irregular non-specific thickening of the bladder wall, and solitary or multiple nodules may also be observed (YEOMAN et al. 1991).

6.2.2.5
Rare Malignant Tumors

Squamous cell carcinoma is usually caused by chronic irritation such as the chronic infection seen

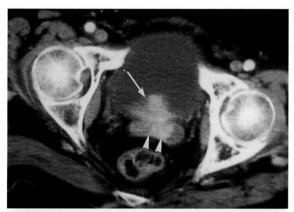

a

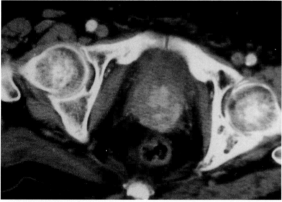

b

Fig. 6.26a,b. Prostatic carcinoma. **a** CT reveals a soft tissue nodule protruding into the bladder on the midline (*arrow*) at the level of the bladder neck. Note the hypervascular aspect of the medial portion of the left seminal vesicle (*arrowheads*). **b** Heterogeneous contrast enhancement and irregular borders of the prostate. Prostatic carcinoma is infiltrating the bladder trigone and the seminal vesicles (T4a). At times it can be difficult to differentiate primary prostatic carcinomas infiltrating the bladder from bladder carcinomas infiltrating the prostate

in patients with neurogenic bladder or in patients with schistosomiasis. These tumors usually present as unifocal solitary lesions (NARUMI et al. 1989). Characteristically they appear as sessile masses, or with predominantly intravesical extension. Papillary tumors or predominantly intravesical growth patterns are not typical.

Signet-ring carcinomas (BLUTE et al. 1989), leiomysarcomas, and fibrosarcomas are very rare malignant bladder lesions.

6.2.2.6
Metastases to Urinary Bladder

Metastases to the bladder from distant sites are rare and almost always associated with widely disseminated disease. The most frequent recorded metastatic lesions have been melanomas and lymphomas, but a wide variety of malignancies have been observed. These include cancers of the stomach, breast, lung, kidney, pancreas, testis, appendix, ovary, uterus, gallbladder, and even tongue (YOUNG 1989). The urothelium is usually spared in metastatic bladder cancer. Metastases to the bladder such as melanoma or other rare tumors such as pheochromocytoma, leiomyosarcoma, or primary bladder lymphoma have similar appearances to those of primary bladder cancer.

6.2.2.7
Involvement by Disease of Other Pelvic Organs

Occasionally a diagnostic problem exists in the distinction of a primary prostatic cancer from a primary bladder tumor. In this situation, CT is usually unhelpful in determining the origin of the tumor, because a large prostate cancer invading the bladder may have identical appearances to a bladder cancer invading the prostate (Figs. 6.12b, 6.26).

The bladder may be invaded directly by primary malignancies from adjacent pelvic organs including rectosigmoid colon, prostate, seminal vesicle, uterine cervix, uterine corpus, and ovary (KIM et al. 1992). Tumors which invade the bladder directly, such as carcinoma of the colon or cervix, can be readily distinguished from a primary bladder tumor because the main bulk of the mass lies outside of the bladder wall. Carcinoma of the uterine cervix or uterine corpus is the most common cause of direct bladder invasion in women, whereas carcinoma of the rectosigmoid colon is the most common cause in men (THOENI 1989) (Fig. 6.27). Differentiation between invasion of the urinary

bladder by tumors originating in the sigmoid colon and primary bladder carcinoma is of major importance since the management of these tumors is very different.

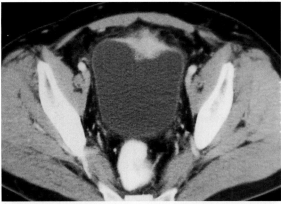

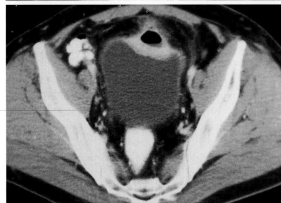

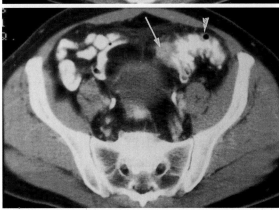

Fig. 6.27a–c. Colonic diverticulitis with extension to the bladder. CT. There is focal hypervascular thickening of the anterior bladder wall near the bladder dome (**a**). Note the air in the lesion and the infiltration of the fat anterior and superior to the bladder (**b**). The wall of the sigmoid colon is thickened (*arrow*) and diverticula (*arrowheads*) are present (**c**). Lower urinary tract infection-like symptoms may be the first indication of inflammatory bowel disease. CT is well suited to differentiate between primary bladder disease and diseases originating in adjacent organs and involving the bladder

6.2.2.8
Recurrence After Local Therapy

Patients who have previously been treated with radiotherapy present a particular diagnostic problem. This is because radiation-induced fibrosis produces thickening and irregularity of the bladder wall. In addition, edema and fibrosis within the perivesical fat lead to a generalized increase in perivesical density. These features frequently make the diagnosis of persistent or recurrent tumor within the bladder wall impossible. This is true even in patients with known tumor recurrence, in whom it may be difficult to accurately define the extent of tumor spread (Fig. 6.21). Changes in the bladder wall due to radiotherapy are often observed and are not specific on CT and ultrasonography. On MRI, mucosal hyperintensity, thickening, and abnormal signal intensity of the muscular layers of the bladder wall, with enhancement after contrast injection, are frequently demonstrated (HAWNAUR et al. 1993). Such changes, however, obscure a small volume or superficial recurrence of tumor after therapy. Therefore, even gadolinium-enhanced MRI imaging does not reliably distinguish between recurrent tumor and radiotherapy changes. Sometimes aggressive tumor appears only a short time after partial cystectomy (Fig. 6.20).

6.2.2.9
Recurrence After Cystectomy

After partial cystectomy it is frequently difficult to differentiate postsurgical scarring from tumor recurrence (Fig. 6.28). If the patient has had a bladder substitution, any of the cross-sectional techniques are indicated to evaluate the new bladder. Sometimes it can be difficult to distinguish intestinal folds from tumor recurrence. One of the more frequent complications is stone formation. Stone formation can be attached to sutures in the bladder wall (Fig. 6.29). CT scans have been recommended for examination of patients at risk for recurrent TCC after cystectomy (Fig. 6.18). Thorough technique requires excellent opacification of bowel (particularly small-bowel loops in the pelvis), IV

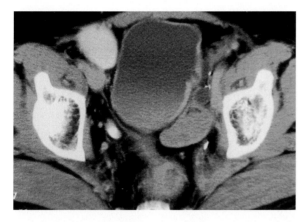

Fig. 6.28. Local recurrence after partial cystectomy and reimplantation of the left ureter. Irregular thickening of the left bladder wall at CT. Note the dilated left ureter (*arrow*). The lesion was histologically proven to be TCC after partial cystectomy. In fact it is not possible to differentiate between scarring and tumor recurrence by any imaging modality

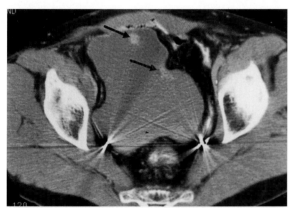

a

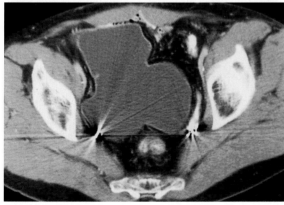

b

Fig. 6.29a,b. Cystectomy and Hartmann pouch. CT of the fluid-filled pouch after IV injection of contrast medium. Heterogeneity of the wall or the content of the pouch may cause tumor-like conditions in the bladder (*arrows*)

contrast material to opacify urinary diversions, and a scanning range that includes the abdomen and perineum.

The pelvis is the most common site of tumor recurrence. Cystectomy site or retroperitoneal nodal recurrences are usually accompanied by pelvic adenopathy, but the converse is not as common. Local recurrence may appear as an asymmetric soft tissue mass within the pelvis or as focal masses. Patients with recurrence at the cystectomy site tend to have associated pelvic adenopathy. Hepatic metastases are usually associated with widespread involvement of multiple sites. CT follow-up of the postcystectomy patient should include abdominal scans and scans through the perineum because of the possibility of deep perineal and isolated abdominal recurrences. According to the study of ELLIS et al. (1991) more than 10% of patients would not have had recurrent disease detected if scans through the perineum and abdomen had been excluded

6.3
Benign Bladder Tumors

6.3.1
Leiomyoma

Leiomyoma is a rare tumor, though the most common benign nonepithelial bladder tumor, with an incidence of less than 1%. These tumors are characterized by slow and noninvasive growth and typically do not show destruction of the mucosa. In the majority of patients the tumor growth is endophytic; one-third show extravesical tumor extension and less than 10% of patients have purely intramural lesions. Malignant degeneration is unlikely. The rate of recurrence after resection is low.

At ultrasonography a soft tissue mass can be seen, usually with preservation of the echogenic bladder urothelium (ILLESCAS et al. 1986).

Solid tumors of the bladder wall with soft tissue densities and bladder displacement are the typical findings. Areas of necrosis are not uncommon in large tumors. To determine the organ of origin for tumors predominantly located at the bladder neck and dome, coronal or sagittal reformatting may be useful (ILLESCAS et al. 1986).

Leiomyomas are hypointense on T1- and T2-weighted images whereas primary urothelial neoplasms tend to have higher signal intensities. The presence of tumor necrosis causes heterogeneity.

6.3.2
Pheochromocytoma

Approximately 1.2% of extra-adrenal pheochrom-ocytomas are located in the bladder trigone or the bladder dome (SCHÜTZ and VOGEL 1984). A discrete solid lesion in the bladder wall isodense to the sur-rounding tissues on noncontrast images but with strong enhancement is the typical finding. T1-weighted and gadolinium-enhanced MRI scans seem to be specific to establish the diagnosis.

6.3.3
Nephrogenic Adenoma

Nephrogenic adenomas are rare benign tumors of the bladder caused by metaplasia of the urothelium. Chronic irritation, injuries and altered immune sta-tus are thought to be predisposing causes (NAVARRE et al. 1982).

Discrete bladder wall thickening and mass lesions, occasionally with calcifications, are typically seen, but unfortunately are not pathognomonic for the presence of nephrogenic adenomas (ZINGAS et al. 1986).

6.3.4
Hemangioma

Hemangiomas of the bladder are generally consid-ered congenital anomalies, although almost 50% of cases are detected in adult patients. The preferred locations of bladder hemangiomas are the bladder dome and the trigone. Bladder hemangiomas may be solitary or may occur in association with hem-angiomas at one or more extravesical loca-tions. There is an increased frequency of hem-angiomas in patients with Klippel-Trenaunay-Feil syndrome.

While a distinct tumor mass is usually seen, dif-fuse bladder wall thickening with calcifications has also been described (GUPTA and BHARGAVA 1987; PAKTER et al. 1988).

6.3.5
Endometriosis

Endometriosis is found in up to 20% of women of childbearing age. Involvement of the urinary bladder is an exception. Discrete solid lesions in the bladder

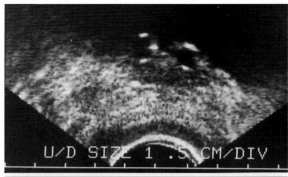
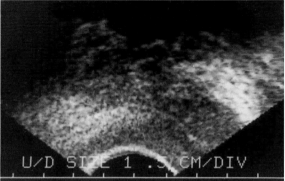

Fig. 6.30a,b. Bullous cystitis. Endovaginal ultrasonography shows the focal thickening of the bladder wall with multiple clearly cystic areas (*arrowheads*) surrounding the bladder neck

wall, with an exophytic growth pattern, are typical but not pathognomonic (ALDRIDGE et al. 1985).

There is nothing specific about the diagnosis of benign bladder tumors. The differential diagnosis always includes all bladder malignancies and other causes of bladder wall thickening.

6.4
Tumor-like Conditions (Inflammatory)

Nonspecific inflammatory diseases of the urinary bladder causes generalized wall thickening. If the eti-ology is unclear, or if an extravesical cause for the inflammation is suspected, CT may be indicated to help to make a diagnosis.

6.4.1
Cystitis Cystica and Glandularis

Cystitis cystica and cystitis glandularis are prolifera-tive inflammatory diseases developing as a result of chronic irritation and may be associated with pelvic lipomatosis. Diffuse or focal wall thickening and prominent trabeculations are characteristic findings (Fig. 6.30) (KAUZLARIC et al. 1987).

6.4.2
Condyloma Acuminatum

Condyloma acuminatum typically affects the muco-cutaneous surfaces of the external genitalia or perianal region. Bladder involvement is rare and almost always occurs in patients with cutaneous condyloma. Ultrasonography of the bladder frequently shows a large mass with lobular contours at the trigone with the ureteral orifice within it (LEVINE et al. 1995).

6.4.3
Amyloidosis

The CT findings of primary amyloidosis of the bladder are nonspecific and include wall thickening and mobile masses (BUTTERWORTH and HART 1990).

6.4.4
Inflammatory Pseudotumor (Pseudosarcoma)

Inflammatory pseudosarcoma is a rare entity indistinguishable from a malignant mesenchymal bladder tumor. Recurrent cystitis and prior bladder surgery may be predisposing factors (GUGLIADA et al. 1991; STARK et al. 1989) (Fig. 6.31).

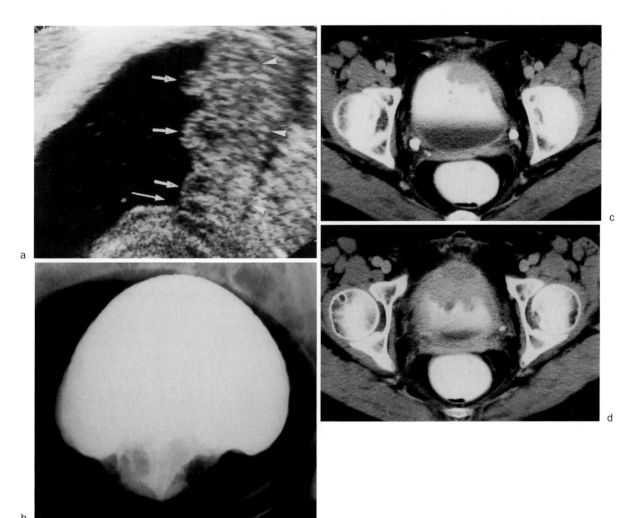

Fig. 6.31a–d. Inflammatory pseudotumor. **a** Endovaginal ultrasonography demonstrates thickening of the bladder wall (*arrowheads*) with cyst-like endophytic outpouchings (*small arrows*) anterior to the bladder neck (*large arrow*). **b** Edematous thickened urothelium is present at the bladder base on this AP film of the cystogram. **c,d** CT, patient in prone position. Note the pronounced thickening of the anterior bladder wall indiscernible from neoplasm

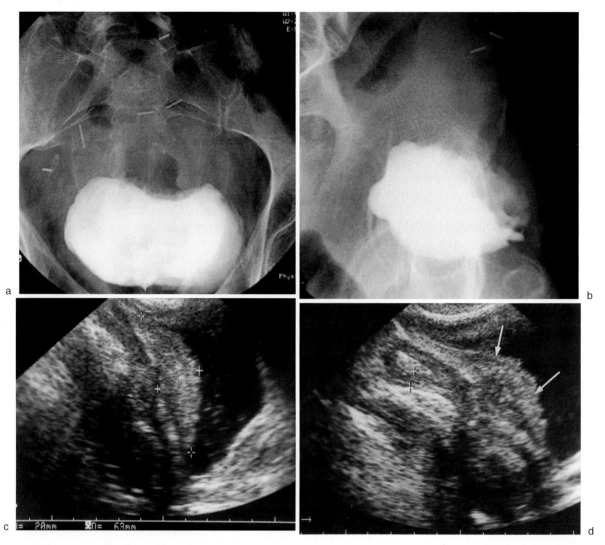

Fig. 6.32a–d. Crohn's disease. **a,b** Contrast study showing irregular thickening of the anterior bladder wall and dome suggestive of extravesical disease. Note that the lesions are easily visible on the lateral film (**a**); this is in contrast with the AP film (**b**), where the heterogeneous opacification might suggest bladder disease. **c,d** Transabdominal ultrasonography. **c** Diffuse thickening of the bladder dome (between the cursors) is seen in a young male. Isolated thickening of the bladder dome warrants thorough investigation of the adjacent bowel structures. **d** Thickening of the bowel wall (between the cursors), disappearance of the fat between the bowel, and the thickened bladder dome (*arrows*) represent inflammatory bowel disease involving the bladder wall

6.4.5
Involvement by Inflammatory Disease of Other Organs

Inflammatory disease of pelvic structures and organs can involve the bladder wall. When intestines are involved in the inflammatory process, fistula between the intestines and the bladder may exist. In patients with intestinal fistula, air bubbles and intestinal discharge may be present in the bladder. The bladder wall is usually thickened and hypervascular when contrast medium is injected intravenously (Figs. 6.27, 6.32). The most frequent inflammatory diseases involving the bladder wall are Crohn's disease and diverticulitis of the sigmoid colon.

6.5
Conclusion

In summary, the diagnosis of bladder neoplasm may be suggested by the following:

1. Detection of stippled calcification on the plain abdominal radiograph
2. Filling defects on IVU
3. The presence of intraluminal masses on ultrasonography, CT, or MRI

Cystoscopy and transurethral biopsy are still the basis of final diagnosis.

As imaging techniques continue to develop and become more sophisticated, their relative roles change. Currently CT is the most widely use technique for evaluating bladder cancer. MRI, however, also provides important information, and in larger medical centers MRI is rapidly becoming the technique of choice. It will be interesting to monitor the impact of spiral CT on radiologic practice. In relation to pelvic cancers, its major advantage will be the ability to carry out 3D volume scanning and to obtain multiplanar reformatted images following extremely rapid image acquisition. These features are likely to have important implications not only for diagnosis, but also for radiotherapy planning.

References

Abu-Youssef MM (1986) Ultrasound of bladder tumors. Semin Ultrasound CT MR 7:275

Abu-Youssef MM, Narayana AS, Brown RC, Franen EA (1984) Urinary bladder tumors studied by cystosonography. II. Staging. Radiology 153:227–231

Ahlstrom H, Malmstrom PU, Letocha H, Andersson J, Langstrom B, Nilsson S (1996) Positron emission tomography in the diagnosis and staging of urinary bladder cancer. Acta Radiol 37:180–185

Aldridge KW, Burns JR, Singh B (1985) Vesical endometriosis: a review and 2 case reports. J Urol 134:539–541

Anderstrom C, Johansson SL, Von Schultz L (1983) Primary adenocarcinoma of the urinary bladder: a clinicopathologic and prognostic study. Cancer 52:1272–1280

Barentsz JO, Ruijs SH, Strijk SP (1993) The role of MR imaging in carcinoma of the urinary bladder. AJR 160:937–947

Barentsz JO, Jager G, Mugler JP, Oosterhog G, Peters H, van Erning LT, Ruijs H (1995) Staging urinary bladder cancer: value of T1-weighted three-dimensional magnetization prepared-rapid gradient-echo and two-dimensional spin-echo sequences. AJR 164:109–115

Barentsz JO, Jager GJ, Witjes JA, Ruijs JHJ (1996) Primary staging of urinary bladder carcinoma: the role of MRI and a comparison with CT. Eur Radiol 6:129–133

Blute ML, Engen DE, Travis WD, Kvols LK (1989) Primary signet ring cell adenocarcinoma of the bladder. J Urol 141:17–21

Brick SH, Frieman AC, Pollack HM, et al. (1988) Urachal carcinoma: CT-findings. Radiology 169:377–381

Butterworth RJ, Hart AJL (1990) Primary amyloidosis of the bladder. Br J Urol 66:434

Buy JN, Moss AA, Guinet C, et al. (1988) MR staging of bladder carcinoma: correlation with pathologic findings. Radiology 169:695–700

Das S, Amar AD (1986) Vesical diverticulum associated with bladder carcinoma: therapeutic implications. J Urol 136:1013–1014

Dershaw DD, Scher HI (1987) Sonography in evaluation of carcinoma of the bladder. Urology 29:454–457

Dershaw DD, Scher HI (1988) Serial transabdominal sonography of bladder cancer. AJR 150:1055–1059

Ellis JH, McCullough NB, Francis IR, Grossman HB, Platt JF (1991) Transitional cell carcinoma of the bladder: patterns of recurrence after cystectomy as determined by CT. AJR 157:999–1002

Goldman SM, Fajardo AA, Naraval RC, Madewell JE (1979) Metastatic transitional cell carcinoma from the bladder: radiographic manifestations. AJR 132:419

Gugliada K, Nardi PM, Borenstein MS, Torno RB (1991) Inflammatory pseudosarcoma (pseudotumor) of the bladder. Radiology 179:66

Gupta AK, Bhargava S (1987) Bladder hemangioma: ultrasonographic demonstration. Urol Radiol 9:181

Harada K, Igari D, Tanathashi Y, et al. (1977) Staging of bladder tumors by means of transrectal ultrasonography. J Clin Ultrasound 5:388

Hatch TR, Barry JM (1986) The value of excretory urography in staging bladder cancer. J Urol 135:49

Hawnaur JM, Hohnson RJ, Read G, et al. (1993) Magnetic resonance imaging with gadolinium-DTPA for assessment of bladder carcinoma and its response to treatment. Clin Radiol 47:302–310

Herr HW, Hilton S (1996) Routine CT scan in cystectomy patients: does it change management? Urology 47:324–325

Hillman BJ, Silvert M, Cook G, et al. (1981) Recognition of bladder tumors by excretory urography. Radiology 138:319–323

Horstman WG, McFarland RM, Gorman D (1995) Color Doppler sonographic findings in patients with transitional cell carcinoma of the bladder and renal pelvis. J Ultrasound Med 14:129–133

Husband JE, Olliff JF, Williams MP, et al. (1989) Bladder cancer: staging with CT and MR. Radiology 173:435–440

Illescas FF, Baker ME, Weinerth JL (1986) Bladder leiomyoma: advantages of sonography over computed tomography. Urol Radiol 8:216–218

Kamat MR, Kulkarni JN, Tongaonakar HB (1991) Adeno-carcinoma of the bladder: study of 14 cases and review of the literature. Br J Urol 68:254–257

Kauzlaric C, Barmeir E, Campana A (1987) Diagnosis of cystitis glandularis. Urol Radiol 9:50–52

Kim B, Semelka RC, Ascher SM, Chalpin DB, Carroll PR, Hricak H (1994) Bladder tumour staging: comparison of contrast-enhanced CT, T1- and T2-weighted MR imaging, dynamic gadolinium-enhanced imaging. Radiology 193:239–245

Kim HS, Na DG, Choi BI, Han JK, Han MC (1992) Direct invasion of urinary bladder from sigmoid colon cancer: CT findings. J Comput Assist Tomogr 16:709–712

Koraitim M, Kamal B, Metwalli N, Zaky Y (1995) Transurethral ultrasonographic assessment of bladder carcinoma: its value and limitation. J Urol 154:375–378

Korobkin M, Cambier L, Drake J (1988) Computed tomography of urachal carcinoma. J Comput Assist Tomogr 12:981–987

Koss JC, Aarger PH, Coleman BG, et al. (1981) CT staging of bladder carcinoma. 137:359

Levine CD, Pramanik BK, Chow SH, Spiegal N, Simmons MZ (1995) Condyloma acuminatum of the bladder: radiologic findings. AJR 165:1467–1468

Maeda H, Kinukawa T, Hattori R, Toyooka N, Furukawa T, Kuhara H (1995) Detection of muscle layer invasion with submillimeter pixel MR images: staging of bladder carcinoma. Magn Reson Imaging 13:9–19

McLaughlin IS, Morley P, Deane RF, et al. (1975) Ultrasound in the staging of bladder tumors. Br J Urol 47:51

Miller SW, Dfister RC (1974) Calcification in uroepithelial tumors of the bladder. Report of 5 cases and survey of the literature. Am J Roentgenol Radium Ther Nucl Med 121:827–831

Naamura S, Nijima T (1980) Staging of bladder cancer by ultrasonography: a new technique by transurethral intravesical scanning. J Urol 124:341–344

Narumi Y, Sato T, Kuriyama K, et al. (1988) Vesical dome tumors: significance of extravesical extension on CT. Radiology 169:383–385

Narumi Y, Sato T, Kuriyama K, et al. (1989) Squamous cell carcinoma of the uroepithelium: CT evaluation. Radiology 173:853

Navarre RJ, Leoning SA, Platz C, Narayana A, Culp DA (1982) Nephrogenic adenoma: a report of 9 cases and review of the literature. J Urol 127:775–779

Neuerberg JM, Bohndorf K, Sohn M, et al. (1991) Staging of urinary bladder neoplasms with MR imaging: is Gd-DTPA helpful? J Comput Assist Tomogr 15:780–786

Pakter R, Nusbaum A, Fishman EK (1988) Hemangioma of the bladder: sonographic and computerized tomography findings. J Urol 140:601–602

Sager EM, Talle K, Fossa S, et al. (1983) The role of CT in demonstrating perivesical tumour growth in the preoperative staging of carcinoma of the urinary bladder. 146:443

Schuller J, Walther V, Schmiedth E, et al. (1982) Intravesical ultrasound tomography in staging bladder carcinoma. J Urol 128:264–266

Schütz W, Vogel E (1984) Pheochromocytoma of the urinary bladder: a case report and review of the literature. Urol Int 39:250–255

See WA, Fuller JR (1992) Staging of advanced bladder cancer. Urol Clin North Am 19:663–683

Singer D, Itzchak Y, Fischelovitch Y (1981) Ultrasonographic assessment of bladder tumors. II. Clinical staging. J Urol 126:34–36

Sparenberg A, Hamm B, Hammerer P, Samberger V, Wolf KJ (1991) The diagnosis of bladder carcinomas by NMR-tomography: an improvement with Gd-DTPA? ROFO 155:117–122

Stark GL, Fedderson R, Lowe BA, Benson CT, Black W, Borden TA (1989) Inflammatory pseudotumor (pseudosarcoma) of the bladder. J Urol 141:610

Stein BS, Kendall AR (1984) Malignant melanoma of the genitourinary tract. J Urol 132:859–868

Tachibana M, Baba S, Deguchi N, et al. (1991) Efficacy of gadolinium-diethyl-enetriaminepentaacetic acid enhanced magnetic resonance imaging for differentiation between superficial and muscle-invasive tumour of the bladder: a comparative study with computer tomography and transurethral ultrasonography. Radiology 181:910

Thoeni RF (1989) CT evaluation of carcinomas of the colon and rectum. Radiol Clin North Am 141:135–138

Thornbury JR, Wicks JD, Eckel CG (1983) Imaging methods for evaluating the adult bladder and urethra: an overview. Semin Roentgenol 18:250–254

Vining DJ, Zagoria RJ, Liu K, Stelts D (1996) CT cystoscopy: an innovation in bladder imaging. AJR 166:409–410

Walsh JW, Amendola MA, Konerding KF, et al. (1980) Computed tomographic detection of pelvic and inguinal lymph-node metastases from primary and recurrent pelvic malignant disease. Radiology 137:157–166

Weimar G, Culp DA, Leoning S, Narayana A (1981) Urogenital involvement by malignant lymphomas. J Urol 125:230–231

Weinerman PM, Arger PH, Coleman BG, et al. (1983) Pelvic adenopathy from bladder and prostate carcinoma: detection by rapid-sequence computed tomography. AJR 140:95–99

Yeoman LJ, Mason MD, Olliff JF (1991) Non Hodgkin's lymphoma of the bladder – CT and MRI appearances. Clin Radiol 44:389–392

Young RH (1989) Unusual variants of primary bladder carcinoma and secondary tumors of the bladder. In: Young RD (ed) Pathology of the urinary bladder. Churchill Livingstone, New York, pp 128–130

Yousem DM, Gatewood OMB, Goldman SM, Marshall FF (1988) Synchronous and metachronous transitional cell carcinoma of the urinary tract: prevalence, incidence, and radiographic detection. Radiology 167:613

Zingas AP, Kling GA, Crotte E, Shumaker E, Vazquez PM (1986) Computed tomography of nephrogenic adenoma of the urinary bladder. J Comput Assist Tomogr 10:979–982

7 Contemporary Nonimaging Methods in the Diagnosis and Prognosis of Carcinoma of the Bladder

M.-A. D'Hallewin, N. De Graeve, and L. Baert

CONTENTS

7.1 Introduction

The standard surveillance technique to detect recurrent bladder cancer or to diagnose primary bladder cancer is cystoscopy. Flexible cystoscopes have made cystoscopy more acceptable to patients but this method still remains invasive. Techniques used in attempts to replace cystoscopy by urine examinations have included cytopathology and flow cytometry. Cytologic examination requires the presence of a pathologist and is always dependent on a personal interpretation. Results of cytologic exami-

M.D'Hallewin, MD, Consultant, Department of Urology, UZ Gasthuisberg, University Hospitals of Leuven, Herestraat 49, B-3000 Leven, Belgium
N. De Graeve, MD, Department of Urology, UZ Gasthuisberg, University Hospitals of Leuven, Herestraat 49, B-3000 Leuven, Belgium
L. Baert, MD, Professor and Chairman, Department of Urology, UZ Gasthuisberg, University Hospitals of Leuven, Herestraat 49, B-3000 Leuven, Belgium and Clinical Professor, Department of Urology and Radiation Oncology, University of Southern California, USC/Norris Comprehensive Cancer Center, 1441 Eastlake Avenue, Los Angeles, CA 90033, USA

nation typically can only be obtained after several hours. Furthermore, the sensitivities of these tests are not high enough to detect the majority of tumor recurrences, particularly those that are well or moderately well differentiated (Badalament et al. 1987; Murphy 1990). A distinction should be made between surveillance and screening for bladder cancer due to the presence of suggestive symptoms. Follow-up algorithms vary from country to country within the European Community and are different from those in U.S. protocols. When routine cystoscopies are not performed every 3 months, especially in low-grade superficial disease, noninvasive diagnostic tests might represent a great benefit to patients. In the screening for bladder cancer, however, such tests might be of less interest since diagnostic endoscopy will be performed in any case.

For the past 20 years, researchers have been investigating and attempting to develop a number of potential markers for bladder cancer. While some have been very promising, most have not proven useful. A distinction has to be made between diagnostic and prognostic markers, though some markers can be used for both purposes. We have chosen to focus on some of the markers currently being investigated that have potential for clinical applicability in the near future.

7.2 Prognostic Markers

7.2.1 Tumor Suppressor Genes

Chromosomal alterations may result in the inactivation of tumor suppressor genes. Of several candidate tumor suppresssor genes that have been identified in recent years, the most extensively studied have been the *p53* and retinoblastoma (*RB*) genes.

The *RB* gene located on chromosome 13q, encodes a phosphoprotein that plays a central role in the control of cell cycle (Cordon-Cardo et al. 1992).

The RB protein can be studied with an antibody that will detect loss of expression. Loss of RB expression will usually be observed in patients with invasive disease and with a low expected survival rate (LOGOTHETIS et al. 1992).

The *p53* gene is also involved in cell cycle regulation. Stressed cells seem to produce a higher amount of p53 protein, which causes cell cycle arrest and gives the damaged DNA time to repair itself (Bos 1989). Altered *p53* can be detected by antibody-directed staining methods. Altered *p53* can be found in approximately 50% of invasive bladder cancers but in only 10% of patients with Ta and T1 disease (SARKIS et al. 1993). Over expression of p53 protein in T1 disease is also associated with a higher probability of tumor progression.

7.2.2
Oncogenes and Growth Factor Receptors

A member of the *ras* family of oncogenes, the Harvey (H-*ras*) oncogene was first identified in bladder cancer (Bos 1989). Point mutations of the proto-oncogene can result in a potent oncogene that can induce cancer. Because the H-*ras* oncogene is found in only 10% of bladder tumors, its clinical usefulness is very limited.

The c-erythoblastosis (*erb*) B-2 can be found in 10%–70% of bladder tumors (DALBAGNI et al. 1995). The prognostic value of c-*erb* B-2 has not yet been determined.

Oncogene products are involved in signal transduction and growth control. One important signal receptor is the epidermal growth factor receptor (EGFR). Increased expression of EGFR in bladder tumors may provide them with a growth advantage. It is also a good predictor of those superficial tumors prone to progress to invasive disease (NEAL et al. 1990).

7.2.3
Blood Group Antigens

All of the blood group antigens are differentiation antigens found on the surface of normal epithelium. Loss of these blood group antigens was described in 1975 by DECENZO et al. and correlated with a higher likelihood of tumor recurrence and progression. This, however, could not be duplicated in larger trials.

Related Lewis antigens have also been extensively tested. The only one which holds some promise is the Le^x antigen. Le^x antigen can be found in 70%–90% of bladder cancers and it may correlate well with tumor progression and recurrence (KONETY et al. 1996).

7.2.4
Tumor-Associated Antigens

Among a large group of monoclonal antibodies studied by FRADET et al. (1990), M344 and 19A211 appeared to have prognostic potential. Of the patients with a positive test, 75% had recurrences within 6 months as compared to 20% of those with a negative test. These bladder mucinous antigens have the advantage of being detectable on voided exfoliated cells.

7.2.5
Markers of Proliferative Activity

Increased expression of Ki-67 and proliferating cell nuclear antigen indicates a high level of proliferative activity and can be associated with tumors that are more aggressive (FRADET and CORDON-CARDO 1993). Their prognostic value, however, needs to be studied more extensively.

7.2.6
Nuclear Matrix Proteins

Nuclear matrix proteins make up the nonchromatin structure that confers nuclear shape, organizes the chromatin, and regulates critical aspects of mitosis. Nuclear matrix protein 22 (NMP 22) appears to be a promising marker. Elevated levels of NMP 22 in urine samples 1 week after transurethral resection can be correlated well with recurrence within 9 months of treatment. The sensitivity of this test is 70% and its specificity, 79% (SOLOWAY et al. 1996).

7.2.7
Markers of Therapeutic Responsiveness

Eleveted serum levels of beta-human chorionic gonadotropin (β-HCG) are mainly detectable in patients with advanced disease, and were found in 76% of patients with metastases by ILES and CHARD

(1991). β-HCG expression may suggest resistance to radiotherapy and higher sensitivity to chemotherapy.

Fibronectin, an extracellular matrix component, can be found in a higher concentration in the urine of patients with bladder cancer (MALMSTROM et al. 1993). Increased levels of urinary fibronectin may prevent bacille Calmette-Guérin (BCG) from binding to the bladder mucosa and thus limit the effects of intravesical BCG instillations.

Resistance to cisplatin may be suggested by overexpression of metallothioneins (BAHNSON et al. 1994). Metallothioneins are involved in the processing of metals such as cadmium, copper, and zinc. Tumors that do not express metallothioneins are more likely to respond to cisplatin and associated chemotherapy.

7.3
Diagnostic Markers

7.3.1
Tumor Suppressor Genes

Chromosomal alterations in the *p53* gene have incidentally been reported in urine cytology specimens, several years prior to the actual diagnosis of bladder cancer (HRUBAN et al. 1994).

7.3.2
Blood Group Antigens

The use of p12 monoclonal antibody against the Le^x antigen on cytocentrifuged preparations from voided urine specimens has proven effective in the diagnosis of bladder cancer. The sensitivity is 80% when this method is performed on a single urine sample, and increases to 97% when it is performed on two separate occasions (GOLIJANIN et al. 1995).

7.3.3
Tumor-Associated Antigens

The antigen recognized as M344 is known to be expressed in 70% of low-grade bladder tumors, in 25% of cases of carcinoma in situ, and in 15% of invasive cancers (FRADET and CORDON-CARDO 1993). The antigen 19A211 is detected in 70% of low-grade tumors, in 60% of cases of carcinoma in situ, and in 50% of invasive cancers. Overall, either one or both antigens can be detected in voided urine specimens in 90% of low-grade tumors and in 80% of carcinomas in situ.

The bladder tumor antigen (BTA) test is a latex agglutination test that qualitatively detects the presence of basement membrane complexes in the urine. It is a quick strip test that can be performed in 5 min. Recent multicenter trials conducted in the United States (SAROSDY et al. 1995) and European trials (D'HALLEWIN and BAERT 1996; LEYH et al. 1996) have shown an overall sensitivity of 65% and an overall specificity of 80%. This compares with the 30% sensitivity expected with the use of urinary cytology.

7.3.4
Markers of Proliferative Activity

Serum tissue polypeptide antigen (TPA) is a differentiation and proliferation marker of nonsquamous epithelium and derived neoplasms. Since too many superficial bladder cancers present with a normal TPA level (MAULARD et al. 1994), it is of little value in screening for cancer detection. It appears to be useful, however, in detecting tumor recurrences in patients previously treated for invasive or metastatic bladder cancer (VAN POPPEL et al. 1996).

7.3.5
Nuclear Matrix Proteins

Recently, GETZENBERG et al. (1996) have described six nuclear matrix proteins (BLCA 1–BLCA 6) that can be detected in all bladder cancers, independent of tumor grade or stage. BLCA 1–BLCA 6 have never been detected in normal bladder tissue. Three other important proteins (BLNL 1–BLNL 3) were found to be specific for normal tissue and have never been found in bladder cancer.

7.4
Conclusion

Most of the tumor markers discussed previously have not been sufficiently tested in clinical settings to draw absolute conclusions as to their usefulness. The exceptions are the following tests: the BTA, the Le^x antigen, and the NMP 22 tests. From the available data, it appears that the sensitivity (ca. 90%) and specificity (ca. 60%) of these tests are more or less comparable to those of cytology, irrespective of grade and stage of the disease. A combination of all available tests would probably make it possible to obtain diagnostic sensitivity and specificity of almost 100%. This approach, however, cannot be supported from an economic point of view. When, however, a noninvasive test is needed in order to avoid cystoscopy, practical and financial considerations should direct the choice towards one of the three tests mentioned above. All three tests can be performed on voided urine specimens. The cost of a BTA test or cytology in Belgium is comparable to that of the NMP 22 test, while the cost of the Le^x antigen test is much higher. A BTA result can be obtained in 5 min, a cytology result and an Le^x test result in 1 day and an NMP 22 test result in a few days.

Diagnostic and prognostic tests based on biomarkers will undoubtedly influence the management of bladder cancer in the near future. Today, however, no single noninvasive test is ready to replace cystoscopy and cytology. When there is a demand for noninvasive testing, financial and practical considerations together with the scientific value of the test should direct the physician's choice.

References

Badalament RA, Hermansen DK, Kimmel M, et al. (1987) The sensitivity of flow cytometry, bladder wash cytology and voided cytology in the detection of bladder carcinoma. Cancer 60:1423–1427

Bahnson RR, Becich M, Ernstoff MS, et al. (1994) Absence of immunohistochemical metallothionein staining in bladder tumor specimens predicts response to neoadjuvant cisplatin, methotrexate and vinblastine chemotherapy. J Urol 152:2272–2275

Bos JL (1989) ras oncogenes in human cancer: a review. Cancer Res 49:4682–4689

Cordon-Cardo C, Dalbagni G, Richon VM (1992) Significance of the retinoblastoma gene in human cancer. Princ Pract Oncol 6:1–9

Dalbagni G, Cordon-Cardo C, Reuter V, et al. (1995) Tumor suppressor gene alterations in bladder carcinoma: translational correlates to clinical practice. Surg Oncol Clin North Am 4:231–240

Decenzo JM, Howard P, Irish CE (1975) Antigenic deletion and prognosis of patients with stage A transitional cell carcinoma. J Urol 114:874–878

D'Hallewin MA, Baert L (1996) Initial evaluation of the bladder tumor antigen test in superficial bladder cancer. J Urol 155:475–476

Fradet Y, Cordon-Cardo C (1993) Critical appraisal of tumor markers in bladder cancer. Semin Urol 11:145–153

Fradet Y, Tardif M, Bourget L, et al. (1990) Clinical cancer progression in urinary bladder tumors: evaluated by multiparameter flow cytometry with monoclonal antibodies. Cancer Res 50:432–437

Getzenberg RH, Konety BR, Oeler TA, et al. (1996) Bladder cancer associated nuclear matrix proteins. Cancer Res 56:1690–1694

Golijanin D, Sherman Y, Shapiro A, et al. (1995) Detection of bladder tumors by immunostaining of the Lewis X antigen in cells from voided urine. Urology 46:173–177

Hruban RH, Van der Riet P, Erozan YS, et al. (1994) Brief report: molecular biology and the early detection of carcinoma of the bladder. The case of Hubert H Humphrey. N Engl J Med 330:1276–1278

Iles RK, Chard T (1991) Human chorionic gonadotropin expression by bladder cancers: biology and clinical potential. J Urol 145:453–458

Konety BR, Ballou B, Jaffe R, et al. (1996) Expression of SSEA-1 (Lewis^x) on transitional cell carcinoma of the bladder. Urol Int (in press)

Leyh H, Mazeman E, Hall RR, et al. (1996) Results of a European multicenter trial comparing the Bard BTA test to urinary cytology in patients suspected of having bladder cancer. J Urol 155:492A

Logothetis CJ, Xu HJ, Ro JY, et al. (1992) Altered expression of retinoblastoma protein and known prognostic variables in locally advanced bladder cancer. J Natl Cancer Inst 84:1256–1261

Malmstrom PU, Larsson A, Johansson S (1993) Urinary fibronectin in diagnosis and follow up of patients with urinary bladder cancer. Br J Urol 72:307–310

Maulard C, Toubert ME, Chretien Y, et al. (1994) Serum tissue polypeptide antigen (S-TPA) in bladder cancer as a tumor marker. A prospective study. Cancer 73:394–398

Murphy WM (1990) Current status of urinary cytology in the evaluation of bladder neoplasma. Hum Pathol 21:429

Neal DE, Sharples L, Smith K, et al. (1990) The epidermal growth factor receptor and the prognosis of bladder cancer. Cancer 65:1619–1625

Sarkis SS, Dalbagni G, Cordon-Cardo C, et al. (1993) Nuclear expression of p53 protein in transitional cell bladder carcinoma. A marker for disease progression. J Natl Cancer Inst 85:53–59

Sarosdy MF, de Vere White RW, Soloway MS, et al. (1995) Results of a multicenter trial using the BTA test to monitor for and diagnose recurrent bladder cancer. J Urol 154:379–384

Soloway MS, Brigmann JV, Carpinito GA, et al. (1996) Use of a new tumor marker, NMP 22, in the detection of occult rapidly recurring transitional cell carcinoma of the urinary tract following surgical treatment. J Urol 156:363–367

Van Poppel H, Billen J, Goethuys H, et al. (1996) Serum tissue polypeptide antigen (STPA) as tumor marker for bladder cancer. Anticancer Res 16:2205–2207

8 Staging of Bladder Cancer

W. IJZERMAN, P. JUNG, and G. JAKSE

CONTENTS

8.1
Introduction

In the Western world about 70% of patients with bladder cancer will have a superficial tumor (Tis, Ta, or T1) at first diagnosis, while only 30% will present with muscle-invasive cancer (T2, T3–4, N+, M+) (STEINBERG et al. 1992). History, physical examination, urine cytology, intravenous pyelography, and endoscopy, together with adequate tissue sampling by transurethral resection (TUR), are considered to be the cornerstones of the diagnostic armamentarium. Procedures such as bimanual examination,

random biopsy, ultrasonography, computer tomography, and bone scintigraphy are considered a routine part of the staging process. The invasive and metastatic behavior of bladder cancer depends on the depth of tumor invasion. We can grossly differentiate superficial tumors, which are only occasionally disseminated at first presentation, from muscle-invasive tumors, which in a significant percentage of cases are accompanied by regional or distant metastases. Both the diagnostic workup and the therapy differ significantly for these two groups, as will be discussed below.

Only distinct staging procedures will enable us to develop statistically valid prognostic parameters, which in turn will help us to compare groups of patients treated at different institutions or with different therapeutic measures. This means that the use of the TNM-oriented classification is essential. However, patient comfort, the prevalence of possible pathologic findings, and financial resources should also be considered. Finally, the value of new investigational methods should be proven in a sample of adequate size, and precise conclusions must be drawn for or against such a staging procedure. Failure to do so would cause unnecessary and costly investigations to be performed as part of the routine staging process.

8.2
TNM Staging System

Staging is currently defined as identification of the type of tumor and the anatomic distribution of the tumor at a microsopic level in the organ of origin, and at a macroscopic level within the host (KOTAKE et al. 1995). The TNM staging system is used on the basis of the consensus reached by Americans, Japanese, and Europeans at the 4th International Consensus Meeting on Bladder Cancer (Table 8.1). The minimum requirements for the assessment of T, N, and M are listed in Table 8.2.

W. IJZERMAN, MD, Urological University Clinic, Aachen Technical University of Rheinisch-Westfalen (RWTH), Pauwelstraße 30, D-52055 Aachen, Germany
P. JUNG, MD, Urological University Clinic, Aachen Technical University of Rheinisch-Westfalen (RWTH), Pauwelstraße 30, D-52055 Aachen, Germany
G. JAKSE, MD, PhD, Professor and Chairman, Urological University Clinic, Aachen Technical University of Rheinisch-Westfalen (RWTH), Pauwelstraße 30, D-52055 Aachen, Germany

Table 8.1. TNM staging system for bladder cancer

Primary tumor (T)

TX	Primary tumor cannot be assessed
T0	No evidence of primary tumor
Ta	Noninvasive papillary carcinoma
Tis	Carcinoma in situ: "flat tumor"
T1	Tumor invading subepithelial connective tissue
T2	Tumor invading superficial muscle (inner half)
T3	Tumor invading deep muscle or perivesical fat

    T3a   Tumor invading deep muscle (outer half)
    T3b   Tumor invading perivesical fat
        i) microscopically
        ii) macroscopically (extravesical mass)

T4	Tumor invading any of the following: prostate, uterus, vagina, pelvic wall, or abdominal wall

    T4a   Tumor invades the prostate, uterus, or vagina
    T4b   Tumor invades the pelvic wall or abdominal wall

Regional lymph nodes (N)
Regional lymph nodes are those within the true pelvis; all others are distant nodes.

NX	Regional lymph nodes cannot be assessed
N0	No regional lymph node metastasis
N1	Metastasis in a single lymph node, 2 cm or less in greatest dimension
N2	Metastasis in a single lymph node, more than 2 cm but not more than 5 cm in greatest dimension, or multiple lymph nodes, none more than 5 cm in greatest dimension
N3	Metastasis in a lymph node more than 5 cm in greatest dimension

Distant metastasis (M)

MX	Presence of distant metastasis cannot assessed
M0	No distant metastasis
M1	Distant metastasis

Histopathologic types
Transitional cell carcinoma (urothelial)
  In situ
    Papillary
    Flat
  With squamous metaplasia
  With glandular metaplasia
  With squamous and glandular metaplasia
Squamous cell carcinoma
Adenocarcinoma
Undifferentiated carcinoma

Histopathologic grade (G)

GX	Grade cannot be assessed
G1	Well differentiated
G2	Moderately differentiated
G3–4	Poorly differentiated or undifferentiated

Table 8.2. Minimum requirements for TNM assessment (from PROUT et al. 1993)

T	Clinical examination, urography, cystoscopy, bimanual examination (under anesthesia), and biopsy or transurethral resection of tumor (if indicated) prior to definitive treatment
N	Clinical examination and imaging studies as indicated (urography, lymphography, ultrasonography, CT)
M	Clinical examination, blood profiles, biochemical studies, and imaging studies as indicated (usually chest film, ultrasonography of the liver, CT of the abdomen, and bone scan)

tumor. Urine cytology, intravenous pyelography, and endoscopy with TUR are considered basic and essential investigations for all patients with bladder cancer and will be discussed in detail.

8.3.1
Urine Cytology

Urine cytology is a sensitive and specific investigation for the noninvasive diagnosis of transitional cell carcinoma. The sensitivity of this examination clearly depends on tumor grade (LEWIS et al. 1976). Specificity is hampered by macrohematuria and infection, leading to both false-positive and false-negative results (Ro et al. 1992). Therefore, urine cytology should not replace endoscopy in patients in whom bladder cancer is suspected. The situation is clearly different for patients with suspected carcinoma in situ or patients undergoing regular follow-up after a bladder preservation procedure. Patients with positive urine cytology but an otherwise normal appearing bladder will show dysplasia or carcinoma in situ on random biopsy. Carcinoma in situ is diagnosed by positive cytology and biopsy result. In addition, the separate collection of urine from both ureters is recommended to exclude the presence of carcinoma in situ or to determine its extension to the ureter (KURTH et al. 1995).

8.3.2
Ultrasonography

Transabdominal or transurethral ultrasonography is used for the diagnosis and staging of bladder cancer (SEE and FULLER 1992). Depending on tumor size, bladder cancer can be diagnosed in about 90% of patients (ITZCHAK et al. 1981). Intravesical ultrasonography initially seemed attractive for

8.3
Basic Staging Procedures

Clinical evaluation and radiographs of the chest are routinely performed as elements of the preoperative evaluation rather than the metastatic workup; however, they are rarely helpful in staging the underlying urologists since endoscopy, ultrasonography, and tumor resection may be performed in one session. Results in the late 1970s looked promising, but there was no real breakthrough. The question has always remained as to what important information can be provided by this investigation that is not necessarily obtained by the urologist performing an adequate TUR (SCHULZE et al. 1991).

8.3.3
Intravenous Pyelography

Although intravenous pyelography (IVP) is not a true staging procedure, and the evidence of a filling defect on the cystogram is of minor diagnostic importance, demonstration of dilatation of the upper urinary tract on this study is considered to represent a sign of invasive growth (GOLDING et al. 1987; HATCH and BARRY 1986). Hydronephrosis on IVP is an independent prognostic parameter for patients undergoing radiotherapy and, therefore, IVP should be included as a staging procedure at least in this group of patients (SHIPLEY et al. 1985). Furthermore, pretherapeutic knowledge of the presence of tumor in the upper urinary tract, although rare (2%–5%), is also essential (MALKOWICZ and SKINNER 1990; PALOU et al. 1992).

8.3.4
Endoscopy and Transurethral Resection

Endoscopy and TUR form the cornerstone of the assessment of the local tumor. Although endoscopy in itself is not a staging procedure, it provides essential information if additional evaluation by imaging techniques such as computed tomography is needed (see below). It is important to know that superficial tumors can be distinguished from infiltrating ones by endoscopy alone in almost 90% of patients (OOSTERLINCK et al. 1993).

Since the information which is gained by TUR is essential for further treatment decisions, exact technique is warranted. The questions which need to be answered are:

1. Tumor type and differentiation
2. Extension of the tumor into or through the bladder wall
3. Completeness of tumor excision

Textbooks illustrate quite well the technique of adequate tumor sampling, considering various points such as resection with low energy, thereby avoiding excessive thermal damage to the tissue. When considering carcinoma in situ or very small tumors, "cold cup" biopsies are preferable to resection. To answer the second question, separate biopsies of the tumor base are needed. In patients with larger tumors, this means that TUR should sometimes be performed in two operative sessions. Finally, the borders of the resection area should be biopsied to locate lateral extensions of the tumor. ALTHAUSEN et al. (1976) showed that biopsies in the immediate surrounding area are positive for dysplasia or carcinoma in situ in 46% of patients. Approximately 53% of patients will develop local recurrence within 6 months when not adequately managed. Furthermore, it has been shown that more than 30% will have residual tumors, detected only by a second TUR (KÖHRMANN et al. 1994).

Although significant time in our professional education is devoted to TUR technique in bladder cancer, a surprisingly high percentage of patients will have residual tumor after the first resection of a Ta, T1 tumor (Table 8.3). The percentage of residual tumors locally or at other sites depends on tumor grade, size, and multifocality. In accordance with these findings, it is our policy not only to adhere strictly to the above-mentioned points of technique but also to perform a second resection in all patients with T1 tumors. The same policy applies to multifocal high-grade tumors irrespective of stage (Ta and T1), and we recommend early cytoscopy in patients with multifocal well-differentiated tumors.

Patients with muscle-invasive tumors who are not candidates for cystectomy, but will receive irradiation with or without concomitant chemotherapy, will have a full-thickness bladder wall resection. The reason for this is, first, to establish the presence of transmural growth by means of histopathologic evaluation and, second, to remove all visible tumor, which favorably influences the result of radiotherapy. SHIPLEY et al. (1985) clearly showed that the complete resection of all visible growths is an inde-

Table 8.3. The frequency of residual disease before and after resection

Authors	Patients	T1 (%)	Positive after resection (%)
FLAMM and STEINER (1991)	60	52	18
KLÄN and HULAND (1990)	33	76	45
KLÄN et al. (1991)	46	100	43
VÖGELI et al. (1992)	71	Only Ta	63
VÖGELI et al. (1992)	91	100	57
KÖHRMANN et al. (1994)	159	48	32

pendent favorable prognostic parameter (see also GOSPODAROWICZ et al. 1995).

8.3.5
Systematic Biopsy of Bladder Mucosa

Transitional bladder cancer may be multifocal as a result of field change disease or implantation (OOSTERLINCK et al. 1993). Numerous investigations have demonstrated that, in patients with visible bladder cancer, normal-looking mucosa may already harbor preneoplastic lesions (ALTHAUSEN et al. 1976; PAULSON et al. 1995). These changes can be detected by systematically taking biopsies at predetermined locations, such as on both sides of the ureter, the trigone, the posterior and anterior wall, and the bladder vault. There is a clear association between the type of preneoplastic lesion (i.e., mild to severe dysplasia and carcinoma in situ) and tumor differentiation (Table 8.4; JAKSE et al. 1980).

However, in the last few years, the necessity for systematic bladder mucosa biopsies has been questioned. In a recent article, KIEMENEY et al. (1994) demonstrated that systematic biopsies provided no additional information regarding the prognosis for recurrence and progression over and above that gained by knowledge of tumor grade, tumor stage, and multiplicity. Therefore, it seems that systematic biopsies should not be taken routinely, but should be restricted to the following patients:

1. Those suspected of having carcinoma in situ
2. Patients with positive cytology after first resection
3. Those with T1 G3 tumors.

Furthermore, cold cup biopsies should be replaced by the TUR-resection biopsy for the assessment of the prostatic urethra. With regard to both disease progression and therapy it is essential to dif-

ferentiate the various types of involvement of the prostatic urethra (PAGANO et al. 1996; MATZKIN et al. 1991).

8.3.6
Bimanual Examination

The TNM classification system demands the bimanual palpation of the tumor for adequate definition of the local extent (Table 8.2). This examination is very subjective and certainly not helpful in obese patients, patients with previous operations in the lower abdomen, and those with tumors behind the symphysis. The tumor extent will be understaged or overstaged in a considerable proportion of patients. Nevertheless, there is also a consensus that the fixation of the bladder and gross residual tumor can be determined with high accuracy (>90%). Therefore, bimanual examination should still be performed and also taught to our residents (FOSSA et al. 1991; MARSHALL 1952).

8.4
Histopathology

Adequate histopathologic evaluation is the most important aspect in the diagnostic workup of a bladder cancer patient. OOMS et al. (1983) demonstrated quite clearly the importance of grading bladder cancer. Moreover, the reports from PARMAR et al. (1989) and KURTH et al. (1995) indicated that the diagnosis of infiltration into the lamina propria is not always easy to make. Review by independent pathologists clearly demonstrated that the initial diagnosis of stage Ta or T1 could be confirmed in only about 50% of cases. In a recent prospective study by GRIGOR and BOLLINA (1996), six experienced uropathologists evaluated 259 newly diagnosed T1, G3 bladder cancer specimens. In 38% of the tumors, lack of agreement in respect of both stage and grade was noted. Furthermore, in 109 cases (42%) there was agreement with regard to either grade (25%) or stage (17%), but not both. Similar results were reported by the pathologists of the French Association of Urology Cancer Committee (BELLOT et al. 1993). More importantly, the initial classification remained unchanged after three assessments in only 78% of Ta and 44% of T1 tumors. Even after open discussion on controversial diagnoses, 12% of cases remained doubtful or controversial. Furthermore, it should

Table 8.4. Correlation between primary lesion stage and grade obtained by biopsy (from JAKSE et al. 1980)

Tumor	Normal	DI	DII	DIII	Tis	Tumor	Total
G1	9	2	–	–	–	–	11
G2	25	8	3	1	–	–	37
G3	12	–	2	8	6	2	30
G4	–	–	–	1	1	2	4
Total	46	10	5	10	7	4	82

D, Dysplasia.

also be admitted that in some cases, due to sampling problems or thermal artifacts, the distinction between Ta and T1 cannot be made. Surprisingly, few reports present a TaT1 category, meaning that a certain number of tumors could not be staged adequately. This misinterpretation of tumors has a significant impact on the individual therapy and creates a problem in the comparison of reported treatment results.

An additional staging parameter of prognostic value for the T1 stage which should be assessed routinely is penetration of the muscularis mucosae, which separates the lamina propria into two compartments (Ro et al. 1987). If the muscularis mucosae is penetrated by T1 tumors, the survival rate has been found to be significantly reduced by comparison with the rate in respect of T1 tumors without such involvement (YOUNES et al. 1990; ANGULO et al. 1995). However, these data have to be confirmed by prospective studies. Moreover, the muscularis mucosae can be demontrated in only about 70% of T1 tumors (Ro et al. 1987; ANGULO et al. 1995).

8.5
Superficial Tumors (Ta, T1, Nx, Mx)

The basic staging procedures indicated above are sufficient for almost all patients with Ta, T1 tumors. However, two tumor presentations need additional and specific staging procedures: carcinoma in situ (CIS) and T1, G3 lesions.

Carcinoma in situ is a multifocal intraepithelial neoplastic lesion with a high rate of extravesical tumor growth at the time of diagnosis (UTZ and FARROW 1984). Tumors of the ureter, renal pelvis, and prostatic urethra have to be identified to permit appropriate treatment decisions. During the 4th International Bladder Cancer Consensus Conference (1992), agreement was reached that resection biopsies of the prostatic urethra are needed to exclude or to diagnose transitional cell carcinoma. The use of cold cup forceps biopsies is inferior to that of TUR biopsies. No consensus has been reached on whether selective urine cytology of the upper urinary tract is sufficient to rule out involvement of the upper urinary tract or whether the use of endoscopy is more appropriate. Both procedures should be evaluated prospectively.

T1, G3 tumors are similar to carcinoma in situ in that there is a high recurrence rate (80%) and a pronouced invasive potential, a 50% progression rate being seen within 5 years (JAKSE et al. 1987). Early cystectomy and TUR with intravesical BCG therapy are the available therapeutic options. In order to base the treatment decision on objective parameters, additional indicators for tumor progression are needed. In a retrospective study, VINCENTE et al. (1991) demonstrated that associated carcinoma in situ may be such an indicator. Seventy-five percent of patients with carcinoma in situ developed invasive cancer despite the use of adjuvant chemotherapy and/or immunotherapy, whereas only 10% of patients without carcinoma in situ did so. Therefore, it is of importance to take two additional staging measures:

1. A second TUR to confirm the tumor stage and completeness of tumor eradication
2. Exfoliative urinary cytology and systematic cold cup biopsies to confirm the presence of carcinoma in situ

8.6
Invasive Bladder Cancer
(T2–4, N0/+, M0/+)

Lymph node metastases are rarely observed in superficial tumors at initial diagnosis; therefore, diagnostic workup to detect regional and distant metastases is restricted to tumors that have invaded bladder muscle or beyond. Lymph node metastases are present in 20%–60% of these patients, and distant metastases are present in 30% (KISHI et al. 1981).

The value of computed tomography, magnetic resonance imaging, bone scintigraphy, and other diagnostic modalities will be discussed subsequently. These investigations should not only demonstrate the presence of metastases but also differentiate tumors confined locally to the bladder from those which already extend into the perivesical fat or other pelvic organs. Although this distinction is not of major importance in the planning of a regular radical cystectomy, it may be significant if the use of nerve-sparing cystectomy or bladder substitution is considered in a female. Furthermore, the above distinction is essential in all those patients in whom radiotherapy, with or without concomitant chemotherapy, is considered, since planning and results of therapy are based on clinical staging only.

8.7
Computed Tomography and Magnetic Resonance Imaging

The techniques of computed tomography (CT) and magnetic resonance imaging (MRI), as well as the results of relevant clinical investigations, are discussed in Chap. 6. For this reason we shall restrict our considerations here to other essential questions. It is of importance to realize that CT and MRI studies should be performed before any manipulation (biopsy, TUR) of the tumor is carried out. Furthermore, the reported sensitivity, specificity, and accuracy of imaging studies should be considered valid only when histopathologic confirmation is obtained by cystectomy (total or partial). The exact T category, that is T2, T3a, or T3b, is of no importance if a straightforward cystectomy is planned: In this situation only the presence of muscle-invasive tumor in the TUR specimens and mobile bladder on bimanual palpation needs to be known. Prognosis depends on histopathologic features. However, the use of imaging studies is of importance if consideration is given to the preservation of neurovascular bundles in men or the anterior vaginal wall in females undergoing bladder substitution. Moreover, exact definition of the clinical T category is of importance for patients undergoing neoadjuvant treatment or any kind of bladder-preserving therapy, such as radiotherapy or radio-chemotherapy. The results obtained with these two treatment modalities can only be compared with cystectomy series if the clinical staging error is significantly reduced. In this respect, it is important to remember that at present the error of clinical staging is 30%–50% for both under- and overstaging (Table 8.5). Therefore, modern imaging techniques are needed to define local tumor extent more acurately. Furthermore, modern imaging techniques such as gadolinium-enhanced MRI may also improve the accuracy of radiotherapeutic planning and thus, theoretically, lead to better treatment results (NEUERBURG et al. 1991). Finally, aside from efforts to improve staging accuracy, advantage should be taken of imaging studies to objectively measure tumor size, which certainly has an impact on the results of chemotherapy or radiotherapy (JAKSE et al. 1985).

Lymph node metastases are present in up to 43% of patients with muscle-invasive tumors and in up to 60% when the prostatic stroma is infiltrated (MATZKIN et al. 1991). Several cystectomy series have shown that about 30% of patients with N1 disease will be long-term survivors depending on the associated pT stage (LERNER et al. 1993). Adjuvant chemotherapy may improve these results (HERR et al. 1990). However, patients with N2 or N3 disease rarely survive 5 years. Inductive chemotherapy is an alternative therapeutic approach in patients with positive lymph nodes. Recent publications indicate that a significant remission rate may be achieved by the use of MVAC or MCV polychemotherapy (see Chap. 20). Patients undergoing surgery after successful chemotherapy remain in complete remission for a considerable time (Table 8.6). Finally, patients with lymph node metastases are not candidates for radiotherapy or chemo-radiotherapy. Therefore, there are several good reasons for the accurate preoperative assessment of lymph node status.

A summary of five published series addressing the diagnosis of lymph node metastases by CT scanning indicates a low specificity of 48%, but a high sensitivity of 94.5% (Table 8.7) (SEE and FULLER 1992). Using CT, VOGES et al. (1989) evaluated 164 patients with bladder cancer prior to cystectomy. Out of 19 cases of histologically proven lymph node metastases, CT correctly recognized only two; on the other hand, there was an 80% rate of false-positive diagnoses. At the other end of the spectrum are the

Table 8.5. Clinical T stage versus pathologic T stage (from PAULSON et al. 1995)

Clinical T stage	No.	No residual tumor pTO (%)	T stage better of final pathology (%)	T stage worse on final pathology (%)
Tis	23	8 (34.8)	7 (30.4)	8 (34.8)
Ta	31	3 (9.7)	11 (35.5)	17 (54.8)
T1	166	32 (19.3)	76 (45.8)	58 (34.9)
T2	213	23 (10.8)	75 (35.2)	115 (54.0)
T3a	33	3 (9.1)	13 (39.4)	17 (51.5)
T3b	4	0	2 (50)	2 (50)
T4	61	6 (9.8)	55 (90.2)	0
Total	531	75 (14.1)	239 (45)	217 (40.9)

Table 8.6. Results of inductive chemotherapy in 31 N+ patients documented by surgery and pathology

Investigator(s)	Patients	Chemotherapy	pCR	sCR	Duration of CR (months)
Sternberg et al. (1989)	11	M-VAC	4	7	33 (12–47+)
Miller et al. (1993)	14	MCV	5	9	23–98+
Jakse et al. (1996)	6	MCV	3	3	22 (10–42+)

pCR, Pathologically documented complete remission; sCR, complete surgical resection of residual tumor; M-VAC, methotrexate, vinblastine, adriamycun, and cisplatin; MCV, methotrexate, cisplatin, and vinblastine.

Table 8.7. Sensitivity and specificity (%) of CT for determining nodal status in cases of bladder cancer (from See and Fuller 1992)

Series	No.	Sensitivity (%)	Specificity (%)
Voges et al. (1989)	164	10	95
Koss et al. (1981)	25	60	100
Vock et al. (1982)	44	94	85
Weinerman et al. (1982)	36	57	100
Sawczuk et al. (1983)	8	0	83
Giri et al. (1984)	17	37	89
Total	294	48	94

results of van Poppel et al. (1994), who used CT to evaluate patients with prostate cancer for the presence of lymph node metastases. The reported sensitivity was 78% and the specificity was 100%. Although both groups of investigators used the same CT scanning techniques, the results are rather contradictory. The difference can be explained by the fact that, in van Poppel's group, any enlarged lymph node was assessed by fine-needle aspiration cytology. In this way, the rate of false-positive and false-negative results was significantly reduced. According to these results, CT scanning is certainly indicated in the following situations:

1. When preoperative chemotherapy is considered as a therapeutic option in the presence of lymph node metastases
2. When cystectomy is not considered in the presence of grossly involved lymph nodes
3. In T4a patients with a significant risk of metastases
4. In all patients undergoing organ-preserving therapy

Aside from the assessment of lymph node metastases, detection of metastases to the liver is of importance for adequate staging and the application of appropriate therapy. According to autopsy studies, liver metastases may occur in 30% of patients with locally advanced tumors (Kishi et al. 1981). Therefore, intravenous contrast should be routinely employed whenever CT is used for the staging of the local tumor and lymph nodes. Otherwise, ultrasonography can be used, which has a sensitivity of 100% and specificity of 75% (Vlachos et al. 1990).

8.8
Laparoscopic Lymphadenectomy

The incidence of metastases to the regional lymph nodes increases in accordance with tumor stage. Herr (1988) observed a 5% incidence of lymph node metastases in patients with pT1 tumors. Guiliani et al. (1988) demonstrated that, when meticulous and extended lymphadenectomy was performed, the incidence of positive lymph nodes increased. They found a 60% incidence of positive lymph nodes in patients with pT4 tumors. Furthermore, Lerner et al. (1993) clearly showed that deeply invasive but still organ-confined tumors have lymph node metastases less often than tumors which have already infiltrated perivesical fat (24% vs 42%, respectively).

In patients who undergo cystectomy in the presence of lymph node metastases, survival rates are expected to depend on the following factors:

1. The extent of the primary tumor
2. The number of involved lymph nodes
3. Possibly the administration of adjuvant chemotherapy (Herr 1993; Lerner et al. 1993; Stöckle et al. 1992).

The 5-year survival rate is approximately 50% in patients with minimal lymphatic disease (Herr et al. 1990; Wishnow and Tenney 1991). Therefore, at present, cystectomy is performed in the presence of lymph node metastases except when there is gross and extensive lymph node involvement. When it is desired to spare the latter group an open surgical approach, laparoscopic lymphadenectomy can be contemplated.

Radiotherapy is essential to treatment of the localized tumor, a complete remission rate of about 40% being achieved in patients with T3 tumors. The impact of lymph node metastases on the therapeutic outcome is unknown. Moreover, the effect of radiotherapy on regional lymph node metastases can only be speculated upon. Therefore, it seems reasonable to perform laparoscopic lymphadenectomy routinely before initiating radiotherapy. In this way, patients with positive lymph nodes could receive adequate systemic chemotherapy. The benefit of such an approach would be twofold. First, the value of radiotherapy in bladder cancer therapy could be evaluated on more scientific grounds and, second, patients without lymph node metastases would need smaller radiation fields, thus lowering the incidence of side-effects seen with the use of this treatment modality.

8.9
Bone Scintigraphy

Bone metastases will be detected in 6% of patients with locally advanced tumors (DAVEY et al. 1985). Conventional radiography, bone scintigraphy, and alkaline phosphatase determination are the techniques used for the detection of bone metastases. The sensitivity of alkaline phosphatase determination is low, and this is unlikely to be useful as a screening test. Only 50% of patients with bone metastases will have an increased serum alkaline phosphatase level, whereas 30% of patients without bone metastases will show increased serum levels (GORIS and BRETILLE 1984; McNEIL 1984). In contrast, bone scintigraphy has a sensitivity of more than 95% and a specificity of 85%–95% (PEDRAZZINI et al. 1986). Considering the data generated by DAVEY et al. (1985), indicating that 12% of patients with T3 tumors will have bone metastases, it is evident that bone scintigraphy is an adequate diagnostic tool for this group of patients. On the other hand, BERGER et al. (1981) detected only one case of bone metastases in 58 patients with bladder tumors scheduled for cystectomy. This indicates that patient selection may play a significant role in the detected incidence of positive studies obtained with the use of this technique. Similar results have been obtained in a recent study (BRAENDENGEN et al. 1996).

However, there are three major reasons to perform bone scintigraphy:

1. The likelihood of achieving cure by means of cystectomy or radiotherapy in patients with bone metastases is certainly less than 5%.

2. The published data consider only patients who had already been referred to institutions for specific therapy and therefore, do not provide the true prevalence of bone metastases.

3. If cost is considered a factor of major importance, we should reflect not only on the cost of bone scintigraphy but also on that of cystectomy when performed without proper indications (LINDNER and DEKERNION 1982).

8.10
Conclusions

Our daily clinical practice should entail the application of stage-oriented therapy. Therefore, improvements in the staging of the local tumor and adequate assessment of lymph node metastases by noninvasive methods are to be greatly desired. Especially treatment strategies aimed at bladder preservation rely on adequate clinical staging. Posttherapeutic staging is a special problem in this context, which has not yet been resolved. The diagnostic possibilities of the use of the classical imaging techniques such as CT and MRI certainly have not been exhausted. But the use of newer techniques for the staging of patients with carcinoma of the bladder, such as positron emission tomography and single-photon emission tomography, should be evaluated.

Critical prospective evaluation of the TNM classification in terms of accuracy and reproducibility (T2 vs T3a) as well as prognosis (T4a mucosa versus stroma) will certainly lead to changes in the present staging system, which has already been revised several times. Defining tumor stage more accurately will enable us to compare more accurately patients who are treated by the same techniques at different institutions or are treated with different treatment techniques. Molecular biological evaluation of the primary tumor will, in addition, provide important prognostic and staging information.

References

Althausen AF, Prout GR, Dalye JJ (1976) Non-invasive papillary carcinoma of the bladder associated with carcinoma in situ. J Urol 116:575–580
Angulo JC, Lopez JI, Gignon DJ, Sanchez-Chapado M (1995) Muscularis mucosa differentiates two populations with different prognosis in stage T1 bladder cancer. Urol 45:47–53
Bellot J, et al. Pathologists of the French Association of Urology Cancer Committee (1993) Lamina propria

microinvasion of bladder tumors, incidence on stage allocation (pTa vs pT1): recommended approach. World J Urol 11:161–164

Berger GL, Sadlowski RW, Sharpe JR, Finney RP (1981) Lack of value of routine preoperative bone and liver scans in cystectomy candidates. J Urol 125:637–639

Braendengen M, Winderen M, Fossa SD (1996) Clinical significance of routine pre-cystectomy bone scans in patients with muscle-invasive bladder cancer. Br J Urol 77:36–40

Davey P, Merrick MV, Duncan W, Redpath T (1985) Bladder cancer: the value of routine bone scintigraphy. Clin Radiol 36:77–79

Flamm J, Steiner R (1991) Stellenwert der differenzierten transurethralen Resektion beim primären oberflächichen Harnblasenkarizinem. Urologe A 30:111–113

Fossa SD, Ous S, Berner A (1991) Clinical significance of the "palpable mass" in patients with muscle infiltrating bladder cancer undergoing cystectomy after pre-operative radiotherapy. Br J Urol 67:54–60

Giri PG, Walsh JW, Hara TA (1984) Computed tomography in the management of bladder carcinoma. Int J Radiat Oncol Biol Phys 10:1121

Golding RP, van Zanten TEG, Tierie AH, Batterman JJ, Hart G (1987) Intravenous urography as a prognostic indicator in vesical carcinoma. Cancer 60:883–886

Goris ML, Bretille J (1984) Skeletal scintigraphy for the diagnosis of malignant metastatic disease to the bones. Radiother Oncol 3:319–329

Gospodarowicz MK, Quilty PM, Scalliet P, et al. (1995) The place of radiation therapy as definitive treatment of bladder cancer. Int J Urol 2(Suppl 2):41–48

Grigor KM, Bollina PR (1996) Interpathologist variation in the assessment of G3T1 bladder carcinoma. Eur Urol 30(Suppl 2):850

Guiliani L, Giberti C, Martorana G, Pizzorno R (1988) Lymphadenectomy during radical cystectomy for bladder cancer. In: Smith PH, Pavone-Macaluso M (eds) Management of advanced cancer of prostate and bladder. Liss, New York, pp 329–339

Hatch TR, Barry JM (1986) The value of excretory urography in staging bladder cancer. J Urol 135:49

Herr HW (1988) Bladder cancer: pelvic lymphadenectomy revisted. J Surg Oncol 37:242

Herr HW (1993) Impact of T and N stage on the prognosis of invasive bladder cancer. In: Breul J, Hartung R (eds) Prognostic factors in urological cancers. Zuckschwerdt, München, pp 104–109

Herr HW, Withmore WF, Morse MJ, Sogani PC, Russo P, Fair WR (1990) Neoadjuvant chemotherapy in invasive bladder cancer: the evolving role of surgery. J Urol 144:1083–1088

Itzchak Y, Singer D, Fischelowitsch Y (1981) Ultrasonographic assessment of bladder tumors. I. Tumor detection. J Urol 126:31–33

Jakse G, Hofstadter F, Marberger H (1980) Wert der Harnzytologie und Quadrantbiopsie bei oberflächichen Blasenkarzinom. Akt Urol 11:309–315

Jakse G, Frommhold H, zur Nedden D (1985) Combined radiation and chemotherapy for locally advanced transitional cell carcinoma of the urinary bladder. Cancer 55:1659–1664

Jakse G, Loidl W, Seeber G, Hofstädter F (1987) Stage T1, grade 3 transitional cell carcinoma of the bladder: an unfavorable tumor. J Urol 137:39–43

Jakse G (1996) Personal communication

Kiemeney LA, Witjes JA, Heijbroek RP, Koper NP, Verbeek ALM, Dubruyne •• (1994) Should at random urothelial biopsies be taken from patients with primary superficial bladder cancer. Br J Urol 73:164–170

Kishi K, Hirota T, Matsumoto K, Kalazoe T, Murase T, Fujita J (1981) Carcinoma of the bladder: a clinical and pathological analysis of 87 autopsy cases. J Urol 123:36–39

Klän R, Huland H (1990) Residualtumor nath Resektion oberflächicher Blasentumsren – eine wesentliche Ursache für "Frührezidivë". Urologe A 29:A18 (Suppl)

Klän R, Loy V, Huland H (1991) Residual tumor discovered in routine second transurethral resection in patients with T1 transitional cell carcinoma of the bladder. J Urol 146:316–318

Köhrmann KU, Woeste M, Kappes J, Rassweiler J, Alken P (1994) Der Wert der transurethralen Nachresektion beim oberflächlichen Harnblasenkarzinom. Akt Urol 25:208–213

Koss JC, Arger PH, Coleman BG, et al. (1981) CT staging of bladder carcinoma. J Urol 137:359

Kotake T, Flamigan RC, Kirkels WJ, et al. (1995) The current TNM-classification of bladder carcinoma – is it as good as we need it to be? Int J Urol 2(Suppl 2):36–40

Kurth KH, Schellhammer PF, Okajima E, et al. (1992) Current methods of assessing and treating carcinoma in situ of the bladder with or without involvement of the prostatic urethra. Int J Urol 2(Suppl 2):8–22

Kurth KH, Denis L, Bouffioux C, Sylvester R, Debruyne FMJ, Pavone-Macaluso M, Oosterlinck W (1995) Factors affecting recurrence and progression in superficial bladder tumours. Eur J Cancer 31A:1840–1846

Lerner SP, Skinner DG, Lieskovsky G, et al. (1993) The rationale for en bloc pelvic lymph node dissection for bladder cancer patients with nodal metastases: long-term results. J Urol 149:758–765

Lewis RW, Jackson AC, Murphy WM, Leblane GA, Meehan WL (1976) Cytology in the diagnosis and follow-up of transitional cell carcinoma of the urothelium. A review with a case series. J Urol 116:43–47

Lindner A, DeKernion JB (1982) Cost-effective analysis of pre-cystectomy radioisotope scans. J Urol 128:1181–1182

Malkowicz SB, Skinner DG (1990) Development of upper urinary tract carcinoma after cystectomy for bladder carcinoma. Urology 36:20

Marshall VF (1952) The relation of the pre-operative estimate to the pathologic demonstration of the extent of vesical neoplasms. J Urol 68:714–723

Matzkin H, Soloway MA, Hardeman S (1991) Transitional cell carcinoma of the prostate. J Urol 146:1207-1212

McNeil BJ (1984) Value of bone scanning in neoplastic disease. Semin Nucl Med XIV: 277–286

Miller RS, Freiha FS, Reese JH, Ozen H, Torti FM (1993) Cisplatin, methotrexate and vinblastine plus surgical restaging for patients with advanced transitional cell carcinoma of the urothelium. J Urol 150:65–69

Neuerburg JM, Bohndorf K, Sohn M, Feul F, Günther RW (1991) Staging of urinary bladder neoplasms with MR imaging. Is Gd. PTPA helpful? J Comput Assist Tomogr 15:780–786

Ooms ECM, Anderson WAD, Alons CL, Boon M, Veldhuizen RW (1983) Analysis of the performance of pathologist in the grading of bladder tumors. Hum Pathol 14:140–143

Oosterlinck W, Kurth KH, Schröder F, Bultinck J, Hammond B, Sylvester R and members of the European Organization for Research and Treatment of Cancer Genitourinary Group (1993) A prospective European organization for research and treatment of cancer genitourinary group randomized trial comparing transurethral resection followed by a single intravesical instillation of epirubicin or water in single stage Ta, T1 papillary carcinoma of the bladder. J Urol 149:749–752

Pagano F, Bassi P, Drago Ferrante LD, Piazza N, Abatangelo G, Pappagallo GL, Garbeglio A (1996) Is stage pT4a (D) reliable in assessing transitional cell carcinoma involvement of the prostate in patients with a concurrent bladder cancer? A necessary distinction for contiguous or noncontiguous involvement. J Urol 155:244–247

Palou J, Farina LA, Villavicencio H, Vicente J (1992) Upper tract urothelial tumor after transurethral resection of bladder tumor. Eur Urol 21:110–114

Parmar MKB, Freedman LS, Hargreave TB, Tolley DA (1989) Prognostic factors for recurrence and follow-up policies in the treatment of superficial bladder cancer: report from the British Medical Research Council subgroup on superficial bladder cancer (urological cancer working party). J Urol 142:284–288

Paulson D, Denis L, Orikasa S, et al. (1995) Optimal staging procedures, including imaging, to define prognosis of bladder cancer. Int J Urol 2(suppl 2):1–7

Pedrazzini A, Gelber R, Isley M, Castiglione M, Goldhirsch A (1996) First repeated bone scan in the observation of patients with operable breast cancer. J Clin Oncol 4:389–394

Prout GR Jr, Kotake T, Pavone-Maculaso M, et al. (1993) TNM classification of bladder carcinoma. In: Consensus development in clinical bladder cancer research. Proceedings of the second and third international consensus development conferences. 1:259–265

Ro JY, Ayala AG, El-Naggar A (1987) Muscularis mucosa of urinary bladder: importance of staging and treatment. Am J Surg Pathol 11:668–673

Ro JY, Staerkel GA, Ayala AG (1992) Cytologic and histologic features of superficial bladder cancer. Urol Clin North Am 19:435–455

Sawczuk IS, deVere White R, Gole RP, et al. (1983) Sensitivity of computed tomography in evaluation of pelvic lymph node metastases from carcinoma of the bladder and prostate. Urology 21:81

Schulze S, Holm-Mielsen A, Mogensen P (1991) Transurethral ultrasound scanning in the evaluation of invasive bladder cancer. Scand J Urol Nephrol 25:215–217

See WA, Fuller JR (1992) Staging of advanced bladder cancer. Urol Clin North Am 19:455

Shipley WU, Rose MA, Perrone TL, Mannix CM, Heney NM, Prout GR (1985) Full-dose irradiation for patients with invasive bladder carcinoma: clinical and histological factors prognostic of improved survival. J Urol 134:679–683

Steinberg GD, Trump DL, Cummings KB (1992) Staging advanced bladder cancer. Urol Clin North Am 19:735–746

Sternberg CN, Yagoda A, Scher HI, et al. (1989) MVAC for advanced transitional cell carcinoma of the urothelium: efficacy and pattern of response. Cancer 64:2448–2458

Stöckle M, Meyenburg W, Wellek S, et al. (1992) Advanced bladder carcinoma. Improved survival rates after radical cystectomy and 3 cycles of adjuvant chemotherapy. Results of a controlled prospective study. J Urol 302–307

Utz CC, Farrow GM (1984) Carcinoma in situ of the urinary tract. Urol Clin North Am 11:735

van Poppel H, Ameye F, Oyen R, van de Voorde W, Baert L (1994) Accuracy of combined computerized tomography and fine needle aspiration cytology in lymph node staging of localized prostatic carcinoma. J Urol 151:1310–1314

Vincente J, Laguna MP, Duarte D, Algaba F, Chechile G (1991) Carcinoma in situ as a prognostic factor in G3$_p$T1 bladder tumors. Br J Urol 68:380–382

Vlachos L, Trakadas S, Gouliamos A, et al. (1990) Comparative study between ultrasound, computed tomography intra-arterial digital subtraction angiography and magnetic resonance imaging the differentiation of tumors of the liver. Gastrointest Radiology 15:102–106

Vock P, Haeertel M, Fuchs WA, et al. (1982) Computed tomography in staging of carcinoma of the urinary bladder. Br J Urol 54:158

Vögeli TA, Marx G, Ackermann R (1992) Zur Notwendigkeit der Nachresektion beim urothelialen Blasenkarzinom als Kontrolle der Erstresektion. Urologe A:A59 (Suppl)

Voges GE, Tauschke E, Söckle M, Alken M, Hohenfellner R (1989) Computerized tomography: an unreliable method for accurate staging of bladder tumors in patients who are candidates for radical cystectomy. J Urol 142:972–974

Weinerman PM, Arger PH, Polloch HM (1982) CT evaluation of bladder and prostate neoplasms. Urol Radiol 4:105

Wishnow KI, Tenney DM (1991) Radical cystectomy for invasive bladder cancer. Urol Clin North Am 18:529–537

Younes M, Sussmann J, True LD (1990) The usefulness of the level of the muscularis mucosa in the staging of invasive transitional cell carcinoma of the urinary bladder. Cancer 66:543–548

9 Photodynamic Therapy of Bladder Cancer

M.-A. D'Hallewin and L. Baert

9.1 Introduction

Photodynamic therapy (PDT) is based on interactions between light and a photosensitizer in the presence of oxygen. Photosensitizer-tagged cells are selectively destroyed. Medical interest in the cytotoxic responses of photosensitizers was recorded as long ago as 1900 by Raab (1900), who showed that a nonpigmented protozoan could be sensitized to visible light by the introduction of an appropriate dye (acridine). The protozoans that took up the dye were killed when exposed to sunlight. Neither the dye nor the light alone could achieve this. The use of porphyrins as photosensitizers has quite a long history. The first observation of porphyrin accumulation was made by Policrd (1924). In 1961, a new porphyrin composition, referred to as hematoporphyrin de-

rivative (HPD), was introduced by Lipson et al. (1961). Pioneering efforts in clinical HPD photosensitization were made by Dougherty, who published reports on a series of PDT-treated patients from 1978 onward. (Dougherty et al. 1978; Dougherty 1984). Urologic use of PDT was first reported by Kelly et al. (1975), with the successful destruction of human transitional cell carcinoma in mice.

9.2 Photosensitizers

The two-step process of PDT requires the delivery of a sensitizer to the target tissue followed by its activation by light. Once in the circulation, the sensitizer concentrates in normal as well as in neoplastic tissue, but with a predilection for accumulation within tissues containing significant reticuloendothelial components (Henderson and Dougherty 1992). Organ retention of photosensitizers is most persistent in the liver, spleen, and kidney (Gomer and Ferraio 1990). The lowest concentration of sensitizer can be detected in skin, muscle, and brain in decreasing order (Bellnier et al. 1989). Sensitizer uptake is thus not restricted to neoplastic tissue but there is some selectivity that is enhanced in certain human malignancies. With regard to the different human organs, the ratio of tumor to nontumor sensitizer concentration varies from 2:1 (bladder) to 10:1 (brain) (Henderson and Dougherty 1992). The maximum ratio between tumor and normal tissue concentration occurs from 4–6 h for benzoporphyrin derivative mono-acid ring A (BPD MA) (Richter et al. 1992) to 24–96 h for dihematoporphyrin ethers and esters (DHE) (Brown and Vernon 1990). The mechanism for selective retention of the photosensitizer in tumor is poorly understood.

The increased concentration of HPD in traumatized or embryonic tissue suggests that the retention may preferentially occur in rapidly proliferating tissues. It has been suggested that leakage of the

M.-A. D' Hallewin, MD, Consultant, Department of Urology, UZ Gasthuisberg, University Hospitals of Leuven, Herestraat 49, B 3000, Belgium
L. Baert, MD, PhD, Professor and Chairman, Department of Urology, UZ Gasthuisberg, University Hospitals of Leuven, Herestraat 49, B-3000 Leuven, Belgium and Clinical Professor, Department of Urology and Radiation Oncology, University of Southern California, USC/Norris Comprehensive Cancer Center, 1441 Eastlake Ave., Los Angeles, CA 90033, USA

sensitizer through the tumoral neovascular network leads to molecular aggregation and that the clearance of these macromolecules is retarded by poorly functioning lymphatics (HENDERSON and DOUGHERTY 1992).

The largest clinical PDT experience has been obtained using the porphyrin variants HPD and porphimer sodium, commercially known as Photofrin II. Photofrin contains less than 20% of inactive monomers and more than 80% of active dimers and oligomers. Photofrin has a weak light absorption at wavelengths above 600 nm and causes prolonged cutaneous photosensitivity. A growing number of second-generation photosensitizers are being synthesized to overcome these problems such as chlorines (PANDEY et al. 1991), purpurins (MORGAN 1992), benzoporphyrins (RICHTER et al. 1990) and phtalocyanines (VAN LIER 1990). Second-generation photosensitizers undergoing clinical investigation include BPD MA, mono-asparty chlorine e6 (NPe6), mesotetrahydroxyphenyl chlorine (mTHPC), and tin etiopurpurin (SnET2). BPD MA has the advantage of reaching a maximal concentration ratio after 4–6 h, thus minimizing cutaneous toxicity to a few hours. mTHPC is a very selective and also very effective sensitizer which makes it possible to use low drug and light doses. Aminolevulinic acid (ALA) is another promising new drug for PDT. Protoporphyrin IX (pPIX) is a precursor in the biosynthetic pathway of heme. As heme-containing enzymes are required by cells for energy metabolism, all nucleated cells should theoretically have the capacity to synthesize pPIX. In many types of cells, heme biosynthesis is regulated by negative feedback on the rate-limiting step of the pathway, the synthesis of ALA. This step may be bypassed by the addition of exogenous ALA, allowing cells to produce heme at a rate governed by their individual enzyme profiles (DIVARIS et al. 1990). Following exposure to light, a clinical PDT effect can be achieved. Systemic administration of ALA (orally or intravenously) produces a rapid rise in the pPIX content of the bladder, followed by a reduction to control values after 24 h (POTTIER et al. 1986). pPIX appears to localize preferentially in the mucosa rather than the muscle (JORI and REDDI 1993), which makes it an interesting prospect for PDT. Another approach to improve photosensitizer selectivity in tumors consists in binding the dye to targeting molecules. The incorporation of photosensitizers in liposomes produces increased delivery into lipoproteins and a higher tumor uptake, as compared to saline administration of the same dye (JORI and REDDI 1993). This is due to the higher amount of LDL receptors in highly mitotic

cells (JORI 1992). This, however, has only been demonstrated in mouse or rat models and cannot be directly extrapolated to humans. Photoimmunotherapy is another targeting technique in which anti-tumor monoclonal antibodies are used as carriers for the photosensitizer. Clinical limitations to this technique are mostly due to the fact that few specific tumor antibodies are known today. A preliminary report, however, has been documented in three patients with advanced ovarian cancer (SCHMIDT et al. 1992).

9.3
Cytotoxic Mechanisms

Upon absorption of a photon, the photosensitizer will be excited to a higher energy level. When excited from the ground state to a singlet excited state, decay back to the ground state will result in fluorescence; this will be discussed in the next chapter. Decay to a triplet excited state with subsequent decay to the singlet ground state will result in energy transfer to oxygen and the production of singlet oxygen ($^1O_2$), hydroxyl radicals and superoxide anions (O_2-) (WEISHAUPT et al. 1976; BUETTNER and NEED 1985). Multiple subcellular sites and types of cellular photooxidation result from PDT since none of the photosensitizers are site specific (GOMER et al. 1989). Damage to mitochondria and endoplasmic reticulum membranes is observed with inactivation of various enzymes (cytochrome C oxidase, succinate dehydrogenase, and acyl coenzyme A) and inhibition of cellular respiration (GOMER et al. 1989). Plasma membrane depolarization and inactivation of transmembrane pumps (Ca^{2+}/ATPase, Na^+/K^+ ATPase) is another cytotoxic mechanism (Specht and RODGERS 1990). DNA damage, such as single strand breaks and sister chromatid exchanges, has also been demonstrated (MOAN et al. 1980), but does not appear to be a critical determinant of cytotoxicity since cell sensitivity to photosensitization was found to be identical in cells proficient or deficient in DNA damage repair (GOMER et al. 1988). Animal models stress the major role played by vascular damage since vascular stasis and hemorrhage are first observed, followed by tumor cell death secondary to oxygen and nutrient deprivation (STAR et al. 1986). Irradiation of sensitized mast cells and macrophages results in the release of vasoactive inflammatory agents and cytokines (prostaglandins, lymphokines, and thromboxanes) and the administration of cyclooxygenase inhibitors decreases vascular damage and tumor destruction (REED et al. 1989). Vascular effects, however, might not be predominant in clinical settings since the amount of tumor necrosis is more related to the light penetration depth and is independent of the sites of vascular occlusion (HENDERSON and DOUGHERTY 1992).

9.4
Light Delivery and Dosimetry

Photodynamic therapy is initiated when the sensitizer is excited by the absorbed light. Nonlaser sources of light were used in the early clinical PDT studies and will probably continue to play a useful role. Lasers, however, have become the standard light source because the light beam can be efficiently coupled to optical fibers, inserted in rigid or flexible endoscopes used in clinical practice.

The wavelength used will depend on the absorption spectrum of the sensitizer. Gold vapor lasers, with a pulsed output at 628 nm, copper vapor lasers (578 nm), and solid state lasers [frequency doubled Nd-YAG laser (532 nm)] have been used. Optically pumped dye lasers, however, such as the argon ion pumped dye laser, copper vapor pumped dye laser, or excimer pumped dye laser, remain the most popular light source since single dyes can cover a significant range of wavelength and different dyes allow for the alteration of the wavelength to suit different drugs with varying absorption properties. A certain minimum of light energy is required to activate the photosensitizer; lower energy levels will only result in photodestruction of the dye or photobleaching. It is believed that normal irradiated tissue will be relatively spared from photodynamic destruction (POTTER et al. 1987). The penetration depth of the light and the depth of the PDT effect will depend on the wavelength used, the power density of the light source, and the tissue characteristics of the target. Tissue characteristics can be evaluated in vitro (PREUSS et al. 1983), but are difficult to predict in vivo since the final light delivery will be affected by various changes within the tissue such as vascularization, cell composition, oxygenation, and photosensitizer concentration (WILSON 1989). This might account for the different tumor responses observed in clinical practice. Techniques to noninvasively monitor those variables are currently under investigation. The local fluence rate can be measured using optical fiber light detectors (MARIJNISSEN and STAR 1987). Photosensitizer concentration in tissue can be evaluated by quantitative fluorometry (BERNSTEIN et al. 1991) or reflectance spectrophotometry (PATTERSON et al. 1989). Local oxygen concentration

can be measured during treatment (TROMBERG et al. 1990). Attempts have also been made to determine in vivo the singlet oxygen production (GORMAN and RODGERS 1992). Optimization and clinical use of these techniques in the future will improve control of clinical photodynamic treatments.

9.5
Clinical Photodynamic Therapy of Superficial Bladder Cancer

9.5.1
Light Delivery and Dosimetry

9.5.1.1
Light Delivery

Intralipid is a fat emulsion that acts as a light-scattering medium and makes it possible to use a flat cut fiber for laser treatment (JOCHAM et al. 1984). A computer-aided motor-driven irradiation system with a circular radiation pattern has been designed (HISAZUMI et al. 1984). The light beam is moved at various speeds depending on the distance between the light source and the bladder wall. Most investigators use a spherical diffuser tip at the end of a bare cut fiber.

9.5.1.2
Dosimetry

Light dosimetry is essential in bladder PDT due to the low drug concentration ratio between tumor and normal tissue (HENDERSON and DOUGHERTY 1992). Excessive power delivery will result in overtreatment and greater tissue damage than desired. Underestimation of the true treatment area and delivery of a lesser energy density than desired will lead to treatment failure. The spherical diffuser tips do not always emit light in a perfect isotropic way. It has been demonstrated that at least twice as much light is directed along the long axis of the fiber toward the posterior bladder wall as is reflected back toward the anterior wall (MANYAK 1993). Because light irradiance varies with the square of the distance, this discrepancy is magnified when comparing actual light dose in various parts of the bladder wall. Tissue reflectance is also an important factor for dosimetric error. The true light dose that strikes the urothelial surface is 2–7 times higher than calculated from the laser output (MARIJNISSEN et al. 1989; STAR et al. 1987; MARIJNISSEN et al. 1993). The manner in which the optical fiber is placed is another source of dosimetric error. A deviation of approximately 1 cm of the fiber tip may provoke changes in the energy fluence rate at the bladder wall of approximately 100% (MARIJNISSEN et al. 1989).

Since 1984, various methods have been devised to obtain homogeneous illumination. Balloons coated with a special light scattering material, exhibiting 90% reflectivity, have been designed (UNSOELD et al. 1990). Once inserted into the bladder, the balloon is filled with water to unfold it spherically. A different kind of balloon system has also been developed, the intravesical laser catheter delivery and monitoring system (NSEYO et al. 1990). Inflation of the catheter's balloon transforms an asymmetrical bladder into a sphere of known diameter with the fiber tip automatically positioned in its center. A light sensor is incorporated in the balloon wall to monitor light fluence and dose. Another dosimetry system, without a balloon, consists of a modified cystoscope to introduce a fiber with a diffusing tip into the bladder and three nylon catheters that are expanded in the bladder, in close contact with the bladder wall (MARIJNISSEN et al. 1989; STAR et al. 1987; MARIJNISSEN et al. 1993). Each catheter incorporates an isotropic light detector, providing a measure of integrated light dose throughout the treatment. This system will be discussed more extensively in the next paragraph. Integrated light dose measurement is essential since a large variation in ratio between nonscattered and total light dose was observed between patients (2.5–7) and also within the

same patient during treatment (−13% to +21%) (MARIJNISSEN et al. 1993).

9.5.2
Results

Bladder tumors were among the first malignancies investigated for photodynamic destruction (KELLY et al. 1975). Papillary tumors as well as flat carcinoma in situ have been treated. It is very difficult to compare the results obtained owing to the use of different drugs, drug doses, light doses, light delivery systems, and time intervals between injection of the drug and light illumination.

9.5.2.1
Papillary Tumors

BENSON (1986) reported on four patients with Ta/T1 disease who received 2–5 mg/kg body weight HPD at 3 and 48 h prior to combined focal and whole bladder wall illumination to 150 J/cm². Only partial responses were achieved after 3 months (Table 9.1) PROUT et al. (1987) described 19 patients with papillary Ta/T1 disease, treated with 2.5 mg/kg Photofrin II, injected 48 h prior to focal illumination up to a light dose of 200 J/cm². Nine (47%) complete responses and ten (53%) partial responses were observed after 3 months. NSEYO et al. (1987) reported on 20 patients with papillary Ta (8), T1 (8), T2 (3), and T3 (1) tumors who received either whole bladder wall, focal,

Table 9.1 PDT for papillary bladder cancer: review of the literature

Author	Drug	Drug dose (mg/kg)	Time interval (h)	Illumination	Light does (J/cm²)	No. of patients	Response	Follow-up (months)
BENSON (1986)	HPD	2–5	3, 48	F + WBW	150	4	PR	3
PROUT et al. (1987)	PF II	2.5	48	F	200	19	CR: 47% PR: 53%	3
NSEYO et al. (1987)	PF II	2	72	F, WBW F + WBW	15–200	20	CR T1: 25% CR Ta: 37%	3
HARTY et al. (1989)	PF II	2	72	F + WBW	100	5	CR 3 mo Ta rec. 1 yr T1 rec. 3 mo	12
NAITO et al. (1991)	HPD DHE	2	72	WBW	10–50	24	CR: 62%	3
WINDHAL and LOFGREN (1993)	HPD PF II	2.5 2	48	WBW	30–50	4	CR 3 mo 2 rec. 3 mo	12
KRIEGMAIR et al. (1995)	PF II Photosan	2	48	WBW	15–30	17	CR 3 mo: 53% CR 2 yr: 17%	24
KRIEGMAIR et al. (1996)	ALA (intravsical)	5 mg	5	WBW	60	10	CR 3 mo: 40% 9 mo: 75% rec. CR 3 mo: 50/103 (49%)	18

HPD, Hematoporphyrin derivative; PF II, Photofrin II; DHE, Dihematoporphyrin ethers and esters; ALA, aminolevulinic acid; F, focal; WBW, whole bladder wall; PR, partial response; CR, complete response; mo, months; yr, years; rec., recurrence(s).

or combined PDT ($15–200\,J/cm^2$) 72 h after systemic administration of $2\,mg/kg$ Photofrin II. Complete response was obtained in two T1 tumors (25%) and three Ta tumors (37%). HARTY et al. (1989) presented a report on five patients with Ta/T1 disease who received $2\,mg/kg$ Photofrin II, 72 h prior to combined illumination ($100\,J/cm^2$). All Ta tumors had disappeared after 3 months, but one recurred after 1 year. One of the T1 tumors showed a complete response after 3 months but recurred 3 months later. NAITO et al. (1991) reviewed 24 patients with superficial papillary tumors treated with whole bladder wall PDT ($10–50\,J/cm^2$) 72 h after injection of $2\,mg/kg$ DHE or HPD. A complete response was obtained in 15 patients (62%). WINDHAL and LOFGREN (1993) reported on four patients with Ta, T1, and T3 disease. who received either $2.5\,mg/kg$ HPD or $2\,mg/kg$ Photofrin II, followed 48 h later by integral illumination up to $30–50\,J/cm^2$. A 100% complete response rate was reported after 3 months, but two recurrences were noted 3 months later.

KRIEGMAIR et al. (1995) reported on 17 patients with Ta and T1 tumors who received $2\,mg/kg$ Photosan or Photofrin II 48 h prior to integral illumination ($15–30\,J/cm^2$). Fifty-three percent (9/17) showed a complete response after 3 months, but only three (17%) were still disease-free after 2 years. KRIEGMAIR et al. (1996) have also reported more recently on a series of ten patients treated with ALA. Five milligrams of ALA was administered intravesically for about 5 h and whole bladder wall illumination was performed to $60\,J/cm^2$. Complete response was obtained in four patients (40%) after 3 months, but recurrences were noted after 6–18

months. The overall success rate after 3 months for the different patient series is 49% (50/103). In view of the poor cure rate, and given the effectiveness of current treatments such as transurethral resection or laser coagulation, these results clearly show that papillary tumors are not a good indication for PDT treatments.

9.5.2.2
Carcinoma In Situ

Since carcinoma in situ cannot be fully resected because of its flat appearance, PDT seems to be an interesting approach from a theoretical point of view. The same authors as were cited above have reported on the results of PDT for carcinoma in situ (Table 9.2). BENSON (1986) observed a complete response rate of 100% after 3 months, but described three recurrences after 6, 6, and 9 months (success rate 73%). NSEYO et al. (1987) and NSEYO (1992) mentioned three complete remissions out of four patients at 3 months (75%). HARTY et al. (1989) obtained a complete response rate of 50% (1/2) at 3 months. After 1 year of follow up, the patient was still free of disease. NAITO et al. (1991) reported a complete response rate of 82% (9/11) after 3 months. WINDHAL and LOFGREN (1993) reported a success rate of 100% at 3 months, which had reduced to 66% 3 months later. KRIEGMAIR et al. (1995) observed a success rate of 75% (3/4) after 3 months. Two patients were still disease-free after nearly 2 years. JOCHAM et al. (1989) reported a complete response rate of 86% (13/15) after 3 months. The two patients

Table 9.2. PDT for carcinoma in situ: a review of the literature

Author	Drug	Drug dose (mg/kg)	Time interval	Light dose (J/cm^2)	No. of patients	Follow-up (months)	Response
BENSON (1986)	HPD	4–5	3, 48	25–45	11	9	CR 3 mo: 100% CR 9 mo: 73%
NSEYO et al. (1987) NSEYO (1992)	DHE	2	72	5–60	3	6	CR 3 mo: 3/4 CR 6 mo: 1/3
HARTY et al. (1989)	DHE	2	72	25	2	12	CR 3 mo: 1/2 CR 12 mo: 1/2
NAITO et al. (1991)	PF II	2	72	10–30	11	3	CR: 82%
WINDHAL and LOFGREN (1993)	HPD PF II	2.5 2	48	15–50	7	14	CR 3 mo: 100% CR 14 mo: 66%
KRIEGMAIR et al. (1995)	PF II Photosan	2	48	15–30	4	23	CR 3 mo: 3/4 CR 23 mo: 2/4
JOCHAM et al. (1989)	DHE HPD	2.3	72 48	15–70	15	54	CR 3 mo: 13/15 CR 54 mo: 11/13
D'HALLEWIN	PF II	2	48	75–100	15	66	CR 3 mo: 100%

Abbreviations as in Table 9.1.

who failed to respond to the first PDT session were retreated and obtained a complete response.

9.5.3
Side-effects

Skin phototoxicity is always mentioned. It lasts for approximately 2–4 weeks and is usually moderate. Severe frequency, urgency, and irritative symptoms are mentioned by most authors and are proportional to the light doses, but are reversible in most of the cases after 3 months. HARTY et al. (1989), nevertheless, described severe side-effects consisting of extensive muscular fibrosis and bladder shrinking associated with vesicoureteral reflux in five out of eight patients. Four patients had received combined whole bladder wall ($25 \, J/cm^2$) and focal treatment ($100 \, J/cm^2$) and one patient had received only integral bladder treatment. WINDHAL and LOFGREN (1993) described the same shrinking (bladder capacity <50 ml at cystoscopy) and fibrosis in five out of 11 patients. These patients were treated with whole bladder wall treatment ($30–40 \, J/cm^2$) and four had received previous external beam radiation therapy.

9.6
The Leuven Experience

9.6.1
Dosimetric Considerations

Light dosimetry is essential in bladder PDT owing to the poor therapeutic ratio between tumor and normal tissue. However, the surface configuration of the urinary bladder poses several problems for PDT as several factors may contribute to dosimetry inaccuracies when large bladder surface areas have to be treated simultaneously. Accurate surface area calculation depends on accurate measurements of the urothelial surface. Excessive power delivery will result in overtreatment and create greater tissue damage than desired. Underestimation of the true treatment area and delivery of a lesser energy density than desired will lead to treatment failure.

9.6.1.1
The Isotropic Light Source

The commercially available spherical tip optical fiber that can emit light isotropically is most frequently used. This tip is placed in the center of a saline-filled bladder before laser activation. It is assumed that the light is distributed equally from the fiber tip to all points on the bladder mucosa. It has been demonstrated, however, that at least twice as much light is directed along the long axis of the fiber toward the posterior bladder wall than is reflected back toward the anterior wall (MANYAK 1993). Because light irradiance varies with the square of the distance, this discrepancy is magnified when comparing actual light doses in various parts of the bladder wall.

9.6.1.2
The Positioning of the Fiber

The manner in which the optical fiber is placed is another source of dosimetric error. The fiber is usually placed in two different ways: under direct vision of what is presumed to be the center of the bladder or at the midpoint of the ureteral catheter placed against the posterior bladder wall. Transabdominal ultrasonography, however, provides a more accurate assessment of the true bladder contour for more accurate fiber positioning. It is to be noted that a deviation of approximately 1 cm of the fiber tip creates changes in energy fluence rate at the bladder wall of approximately 100% (MARIJNISSEN et al. 1989).

9.6.1.3
Calculation of Bladder Surface Area

Before the recent use of ultrasonography, bladder surface was calculated by extrapolation from volume measurements, assuming the bladder to be a perfect sphere. Variances in bladder compliance, however, are not easily detected and overdistention was seen rather frequently, causing too deep penetration of the light and undesired damage to the deeper muscle layers. Compensation for this problem by partially filling the bladder will not allow full distention of the total urothelium and will create a shadowing effect which will induce treatment failure.

9.6.1.4
Tissue Reflectance

Since the bladder is a hollow organ, tissue light reflectance will enhance the light energy dose that reaches the target tissue. As mentioned above, it has been estimated that the true light dose that strikes the urothelial surface is 2–7 times greater than is calculated from the laser output alone (STAR et al. 1987; MARIJNISSEN et al. 1989, 1993).

9.6.2
Dosimetry System

Presently, the factors determining success or failure and recurrence of carcinoma in situ or bladder shrinking are not well known. As described above, one important factor is the light dosimetry. The total light dose, including scattered light, is not known and neither is the uniformity of the light dose distribution across the bladder wall. A treatment system for in vivo monitoring and control of light dose rate and total light dose (scattered and nonscattered), during whole bladder wall PDT has been developed in Rotterdam by MARIJNISSEN et al. (1989) and tested in vivo on dogs. Once the system was proven safe and the light dosimetry was sufficiently understood, the first patient treatments in vivo were started in Leuven in 1989.

9.6.2.1
Description of the Treatment System

The system consists of a modified cystoscope, a preamplifier, and an amplifier with gauges displaying light fluence rate and integrated light fluence at three points of the bladder wall. The modified cystoscope consists of the following parts: (1) a 21-French cystoscope shaft that has been shortened by 3.5 cm so that the telescope protrudes from the shaft; (2) a light dosimetry unit including three translucent nylon catheters and three light detectors with isotropic response; (3) a light irradiation unit. The bridge within the cystoscope has been modified so that the telescope can be rotated independently from the shaft and the whole bladder wall can be observed. The light dosimetry unit, incorporated in the bridge, admits three nylon catheters with a diameter of 1 mm. These are hinged at the tip with a semirigid stainless steel rod. A miniature isotropic light dosimetry detector can be inserted into each of the capillaries. The light irradiation unit admits an isotropic light source, which consists of another sphere of light-scattering material, 3.2 mm in diameter, mounted on a quartz fiber and connected to an argon-pumped DCM dye laser. The isotropic light source can be radially displaced by an Albarran lever and can also be rotated and moved back and forth along the axis. By these movements the light source can be placed in an optimal position, resulting in a uniform light distribution across the bladder wall.

9.6.2.2
Treatment Procedure

Since 1989, 15 patients with carcinoma in situ of the bladder with or without a previous history of superficial transitional cell carcinoma have been treated with PDT (Table 9.3). PDT was performed at least 6 weeks after transurethral resection or biopsy in order to avoid excessive photosensitizer retention in reactive inflammatory tissue. The patients were injected with 2 mg/kg Photofrin II, 48 h before illumination. Once the patient is under general anesthesia, the bladder is inspected and the maximal bladder capacity is measured. The bladder is then filled with saline to an average volume of 100 ml, which is generally sufficient to smooth out mucosal folds and to yield the most spherical bladder shape possible without overdistention of the bladder wall. Then, the shaft of the cystoscope is retracted until the tip just protrudes from the urethra but does not reach beyond the bladder neck. The joint of the nylon catheters, guided by the steel rod, is pushed under cystoscopic vision to the bladder fundus. This is to determine the distance from the neck to the dome. The nylon catheters are then pushed further through the metal capillaries and unfolded in three directions approximately 120° apart, in contact with the bladder mucosa. The telescope is then removed and replaced by the irradiation unit. Into each of the catheters, an isotropic light dosimetry detector is inserted and connected to an electronic amplifier. The fiber of the isotropic light source is connected to the laser. The detectors are moved back and forth in the nylon catheters and using a low light level, the position of the light source is changed until all meters indicate nearly the same energy fluence rate. After optimizing the position of the light source, therapeutic irradiation can start.

9.6.2.3
Dosimetry Data

The first four patients received a total light dose of 100 J/cm^2 (Table 9.3) This dose was based on 15 J/cm^2 non-scattered light as prescribed in whole bladder wall PDT protocols, without in situ light measurements, taking into account a mean ratio of up to 7 between total and nonscattered light dose as measured in a previous series of dogs (MARIJNISSEN et

Table 9.3. Details regarding the use of PDT in Leuven

Case no.	History	Dose (J/cm^2)	Bladder capacity (volume change, %)^a	BCG shrinking	Recurrence (months)	Follow-up (months)
1	Ta	100	+50			84
2	Ta	100	−60	++		
3	Ta	100	−50	++		
4		100	+66		29	
5	Ta, CIS	75	+100	+		74
6		75	+150			71
7	Ta, CIS	75	+43	+	9	
8		75	+100		32	
9	Ta	75	+28		25	
10	Ta	75	−14			65
11	CIS	75	+50	+		65
12	Ta	75	+100			65
13		75	−80	++	54	
14		75	0		9	
15		75	−20			50
					6/15	67^b

^{a} Change in bladder capacity, comparing measurements under general anesthesia before and 3 months after PDT.
^{b} Mean follow-up.

al. 1989). After six patients had been treated, this ratio between total and nonscattered light in humans appeared to be close to 5. Therefore, the following patients were treated with a total light dose of 15 × 5 = 75 J/cm^2 (D'HALLEWIN et al. 1992; MARIJNISSEN et al. 1993). A very large variation in the ratio between nonscattered and total light dose was observed between patients (from 2.5 to 7) (D'HALLEWIN et al. 1992). This ratio is related to the diffused reflection factor of the bladder wall and its optical properties. Differences in optical properties of bladder tissue from patient to patient have not previously been reported (CHEONG et al. 1990) in normal bladders. The differences in our patient series can be explained by the fact that the bladders were diseased (carcinoma in situ) and had previously been heavily pretreated (transurethral resection, Nd-YAG laser irradiation, instillations). We also reported a variation in ratio between total and nonscattered light within the same patient, throughout the treatment (−13% to +21%).

9.6.2.4
Clinical Results

9.6.2.4.1
PHOTOTOXICITY

Strict avoidance of contact with sunlight was advised for the first 3 weeks after photosensitizer injection. Progressive exposure was allowed in the following weeks, and no severe (grade 2 or 3) sunburns were noted.

9.6.2.4.2
BLADDER SYMPTOMS

Urgency symptoms occurred in all patients after PDT and remained for up to 4 weeks. These symptoms were less pronounced in the patients who received a reduced light dose of 75 J/cm^2. Irreversible bladder shrinking and fibrosis occurred in two patients (50%) treated with the high light dose of 100 J/cm^2 and only in one patient (7%) with a light dose of 75 J/cm^2.

9.6.2.4.3
TUMOR RESPONSE

A complete response rate of 100% was noted after 3 months, but recurrences occurred in six patients after 9 months to 4$^1/_2$ years (D'Hallewin and Baert 1995). Two patients developed recurrences only in the prostatic urethra, without evidence of disease in the bladder. The response rate after a mean follow-up of 5 years is 60%.

9.7
Conclusions

Although the concept of PDT has existed for almost 100 years, its full working mechanism is unknown and it still has to be considered as an experimental treatment modality. In the urologic field, its use should be limited to the treatment of carcinoma in situ. With regard to the nature of this disease and superficial bladder cancer in general, 'recurrences' after complete response should not be considered as treatment failures but rather as new occurrences. From this point of view, PDT (with Photofrin II) appears to be extremely effective. However, side-effects, mostly bladder irritative symptoms, are a major drawback. The poor selective retention of Photofrin II and the complex physical properties of the bladder necessitate the use of time-consuming and expensive dosimetry systems. Future prospects are twofold: new sensitizers and, connected with this, new light sources. ALA is probably one of the most promising drugs for various reasons. The first concerns the administration of ALA, which can be given intravesically as well as by the intravenous route. The former option allows for a reduction in the amount of ALA needed, thus reducing the cost of treatment and avoiding the problem of phototoxicity. Even when intravenous administration is chosen, phototoxicity is very low since the skin is completely cleared of ALA after 24h. ALA also has the advantage of being localized in the mucosa only, without muscle deposition; this reduces bladder symptoms, though it might constitute a drawback to its use for carcinoma in situ when microinvasive lesions can be expected. Another interesting new drug is mTHPC. Since it is extremely effective, the drug as well as the light dose can be reduced, thus lowering costs and phototoxicity. No clinical trials with mTHPC for bladder cancer have been performed as of today, however. With the advent of new drugs and new excitation wavelengths, new and less expensive light sources will be available, such as light-emitting diodes. These future prospects can be expected to significantly change the clinical outcome of PDT. PDT is a truly dynamic process.

References

Bellnier DA, Ho YK, Panday RK, Missert JR, Dougherty TJ (1989) Distribution and elimination of Photofrin II in mice. Photochem Photobiol 50:221–228

Benson RC (1986) Integral photoradiation therapy of multifocal bladder tumors. Eur Urol 12(Suppl 1):47–53

Bernstein EF, Friayf WS, Smith PD, et al. (1991) Transcutaneous determination of tissue dihematoporphyrin ether content: a device to optimize photodynamic therapy. Arch Dermatol 127:1794–1798

Brown SB, Vernon DI (1990) The quantitative determination of porphyrins in tissues and body fluids: applications in studies of photodynamic therapy. In: Kessel D (ed) Photodynamic therapy of neoplastic disease, vol. 1. CRC Press, Boca Raton, Fl., pp 109–208

Buettner GR, Need MJ (1985) Hydrogen peroxide and hydroxyl free radical production by hematoporphyrin derivative, ascorbate and light. Cancer Lett 25:297–304

Cheong WF, Pral SA, Welch AJ (1990) Review of the optical properties of biological tissues. IEEE J Quant Electr 26:2166-2172

D'Hallewin MA, Baert L (1995) Long term results of whole bladder wall photodynamic therapy for carcinoma in situ of the bladder. Urol 45:763–767

D'Hallewin MA, Baert L, Marijnissen JP, Star WM (1992) Whole bladder wall photodynamic therapy with in situ light dosimetry for carcinoma in situ of the bladder. J Urol 148:1152–1155

Divaris DX, Kennedy JC, Pottier RH (1990) Phototoxic damage to sebaceous glands and hair follicles of mice after systemic administration of 5-aminolevulinic acid correlates with localized protoporphyrin production. Am J Pathol 136:891–896

Dougherty TJ (1984) Photodynamic therapy of malignant tumors. CRC Crit Rev Biochem 2:83–116

Dougherty TJ, Kaufman JE, Goldfarb A, Weishaupt KR, Boyle D, Mittleman A (1978) Photoradiation therapy for the treatment of malignant tumors. Cancer Res 38:2628–2635

Dougherty TJ, Henderson BW, Schwartz S, Winkelman JW, Lipson RL (1992) Historical perspective. In: Henderson BW, Dougherty TJ (eds) Photodynamic therapy. Basic principles and clinical applications. Dekker, New York, p 1

Gomer CJ, Ferrario A (1990) Tissue distribution and photosensitizing properties of mono-L-aspartyl chlorine 6 in a mouse tumor model. Cancer Res 50:3985-3990

Gomer CJ, Rucker N, Murphree AL (1988) Differential cell photosensitivity following porphyrin photodynamic therapy. Cancer Res 48:4539–4542

Gomer CJ, Rucker N, Ferario A, Wong S (1989) Properties and applications of photodynamic therapy. Radiat Res 120:1–18

Gorman AA, Rodgers MA (1992) Current perspectives of singlet oxygen detection in biological environments. J Photochem Photobiol B 14:159–176

Harty JI, Amin M, Wieman TJ, Tseng MT, Ackerman D, Broghamer W (1989) Complications of whole bladder dihematoporphyrin ether photodynamic therapy. J Urol 141:1341–1346

Henderson BA, Dougherty TJ (1992) How does photodynamic therapy work? Photochem Photobiol 55:145–157

Hisazumi H, Miyoshi N, Naito K and Misaki T (1984) Whole bladder wall photoradiation therapy for carcinoma in situ of the bladder. A preliminary report J Urol 131:884–887

Jocham D, Staehler G, Chaussy C (1984) Integral dye laser irradiation of photosensitized bladder tumors with the aid of a light scattering medium In: Doiron DR, Gomer CJ (eds) Porphyrin localization and treatment of tumors. Liss, New York, pp 249–257

Jocham D, Beer M, Baumgartner R, Staehler G, Unsold E (1989) Long-term experience with integral photodynamic therapy of Tis bladder carcinoma. Ciba Found Symp 146:199–205

Jori G (1992) Low density lipoproteins – liposome delivery systems for tumor photosensitizers in vitro. In: Henderson BW, Dougherty TJ (eds) Photodynamic therapy. Basic principles and clinical applications. Dekker, New York, pp 173–186

Jori G, Reddi E (1993) The role of lipoproteins in the delivery of tumor-targettin photosensitizers. Int J Biochem 25:-1369–1375

Kelly JF, Snell ME, Berenbaum MC (1975) Photodynamic destruction of human bladder carcinoma. Br J Cancer 31:237–244

Kriegmair M, Waidelich R, Ehsan A, Baumgartner R, Hofstetter A (1995) Integral photodynamic therapy of refractory superficial bladder cancer. J Urol 154:1339–1341

Kriegmair M, Baumgartner R, Lumper W, Waidelich R, Hofstter A (1996) Early clinical experience with 5-aminolevulinic acid for the photodynamic therapy of superficial bladder cancer. Br J Urol 77:667–671

Lipson RL, Baldes EJ, Olsen AM (1961) The use of a derivative of hematoporphyrin in tumor detection. J Natl Cancer Inst 26:1–15

Manyak MJ (1993) Photodynamic therapy for superficial bladder carcinoma. Curr Opin Urol 3:220–233

Marijnissen JP, Star WM (1987) Quantitative light dosimetry in vitro and in vivo. Lasers Med Sci 2:235–242

Marijnissen JP, Jansen H, Star WM (1989) Treatment system for whole bladder wall photodynamic therapy with in vivo monitoring and control of light dose rate and dose. J Urol 142:1351–1355

Marijnissen JP, Star WM, in 't Zandt HJ, D'Hallewin MA, Baert L (1993) In situ light dosimetry during whole bladder wall photodynamic therapy: clinical results and experimental verifications. Phys Med Biol 38:567–582

Moan J, Waksvik H, Christensen T (1980) DNA single-strand and sister chromatid exchanges induced by treatment with hematoporphyrin and light or by X-rays in human NHIK 3025 cells. Cancer Res 40:2915–2918

Morgan AR (1992) Reduced porphyrins as photosensitizers: synthesis and biological effects. In: Henderson BW, Dougherty TJ (eds) Photodynamic therapy, basic principles and clinical applications. Dekker, New York, pp 157–172

Naito K, Hisazumi H, Uchibayashi T, et al. (1991) Integral laser photodynamic treatment of refractory multifocal bladder tumors. J Urol 146:1541–1545

Nseyo UO (1992) Photodynamic therapy. Urol Clin North Am 19:591–599

Nseyo UO, Dougherty TJ, Sullivan L (1987) Photodynamic therapy in the management of resistant lower urinary tract carcinoma. Cancer 60:3113–3119

Nseyo UO, Lundhal SL, Merrill DC (1990) Whole bladder photodynamic therapy: critical review of present day technology and rationale for development of intravesical laser catheter and monitoring system. Urology 36:398–402

Pandey RK, Bellnier DA, Smith KM, Dougherty TJ (1991) Chlorine and porphyrin derivatives as potential photosensitizers in photodynamic therapy. Photochem Photobiol 53:65–72

Patterson MS, Chance B, Wilson BC (1989) Quantitative reflectance spectrophotometry for the noninvasive measurement of photosensitizer concentration in tissue during photodynamic therapy. Proc International Society for Optical Engineering (SPIE) 1065:115–122

Policard A (1924) Etude sur les aspects offerts par des tumeurs expérimentales examinées à la lumier de Wood. Compterendus Soc Biol 91:1423–1424

Potter WR, Mang TS, Dougherty TJ (1987) The theory of PDT dosimetry: consequences of photodestruction of sensitizer. Photochem Photobiol 46:97–101

Pottier RH, Chow YF, LaPlant JP, Truscott TG, Kennedy JC, Beiner LA (1986) Non-invasive technique for obtaining fluorescence excitation and emission spectra in vivo. Photochem Photobiol 44:679–683

Preuss LE, Bolin FP, Cain BW (1983) A comment on spectral transmittance in mammalian skeletal muscle. Photochem Photobiol 37:113–116

Prout GR, Lin CW, Benson RC, et al. (1987) Photodynamic therapy with hematoporphyrin derivative in the treatment of superficial transitional-cell carcinoma of the bladder. N Engl J Med 12:1251–1255

Raab O (1900) Über die Wirkung fluoreszierenden Stoffen. Infusuria Z Biol 39:524–546

Reed MWR, Wieman J, Doak KW, Pietsch CG, Schuschke G (1989) The microvascular effects of photody-namic therapy: evidence for a possible role of cyclooxygenase products. Photochem Photobiol 50:419–423

Richter AM, Waterfield E, Jain AK, Sternberg ED, Dolphin D, Levy JG (1990) In vitro evaluation of phototoxic properties of four structurally related benzoporphyrin derivatives. Photochem Photobiol 52:495–500

Richter AM, Jain AK, Canaan AJ, Waterfield E, Sternberg ED, Levy JG (1992) Photosensitisation efficiency of two regioisomers of the benzoporphyrin derivative mono acid ring A. Biochem Pharmacol 43:2349–2358

Schmidt S, Wagner U, Popat S, et al. (1992) Photodynamic therapy in gynecological oncology. In: Spinelli P, Dal Fante M, Marchesini R (eds) Photodynamic therapy and biomedical lasers. Excerpta Medica, Internation Congress Series 1011, pp 327–332

Specht K, Rodgers M (1990) Depolarization of mouse myeloma cell membranes during photodynamic action. Photochem Photobiol 51:319–324

Star WM, Marijnissen HP, van den Berg-Blok AE, Versteeg JA, Franken KA, Reinhold HS (1986) Destruction of rat mammary tumor and normal tissue microcirculation by hematoporphyrin derivative photoradiation observed in in vivo sandwich observation chambers. Cancer Res 46:2532–2540

Star WM, Marijnissen JP, Jansen H, Keijzer M, Van Gemert MJ (1987) Light dosimetry for photodynamic therapy by whole bladder wall irradiation. Photochem Photobiol 46:619–624

Tromberg BJ, Orenstein A, Kimel S, Barker SJ, Hyatt J, Nelson JS, Berns MW (1990) In vivo tumor oxygen tension measurements for the evaluation of the efficiency of photodynamic therapy. Photochem Photobiol 52:375–385.

Unsoeld E, Baumgartner R, Beyer W, Jocham D, Stepp H (1990) Fluorescence detection and photodynamic treatment of photosensitized tumors in special considerations of urology. Lasers Med Sci 5:207–212

Van Lier JE (1990) Phtalocyanines as sensitizers for PDT of cancer. In: Kessel D (ed) Photodynamic therapy of neoplastic disease, vol 1. CRC Press, Boca Raton, FL., pp 279–291

Weishaupt K, Gomer CJ, Dougherty TJ (1976) Identification of singlet oxygen as the cytotoxic agent in photoinactivation of a murine tumor. Cancer Res 36:2326–2329

Wilson BC (1989) Photodynamic therapy: light delivery and dosage for second-generation sensitizers. Ciba Found Symp 146:60–73

Windhal T, Lofgren A (1993) Two years' experience with photodynamic therapy of bladder carcinoma. Br J Urol 71:187–191

10 Fluorescence Detection of Bladder Cancer

M.-A. D'Hallewin, H. Vanherzeele, and L. Baert

CONTENTS

10.1 Introduction

Visual differentiation of normal tissue from transitional cell carcinoma (TCC) is relatively easy, but carcinoma in situ (CIS) or nonmalignant diseases, such as cystitis (bacterial, chemical, or due to radiotherapy), are often invisible to the naked eye. Therefore, biopsies have to be taken for determination of histopathology. Unfortunately, a biopsy represents only a small sample area, and the final pathology results are available only after several days. Hence there is a need for a more practical diagnostic technique, which would provide an in vivo classification of the tissue type in real time.

In recent years, there has been growing interest in the use of lasers and other light sources to "optically diagnose" pathology in human tissues. Although a

M.-A. D'Hallewin, MD, Consultant, Department of Urology, UZ Gasthuisberg, University Hospitals of Leuven, Herestraat 49, B-3000 Leuven, Belgium
H. Vanherzeele, PhD Department of Applied Sciences, Vrije Universiteit Brussel, Pleinlaan 2, B-1050 Brussels, Belgium
L. Baert, MD, PhD, Professor and Chairman, Department of Urology, UZ Gasthuisberg, University Hospitals of Leuven, Herestraat 49, B-3000 Leuven, Belgium and Clinical Professor, Department of Urology and Radiation Oncology, University of Southern California, USC/Norris Comprehensive Cancer Center, 1441 Eastlake Ave., Los Angeles, CA 90033, USA

wide variety of optical techniques have been suggested as potentially useful tools, the methods explored to date have mostly been based on diffuse reflectance spectroscopy and fluorescence spectroscopy. The latter has generated the most interest. Upon excitation by (linear) absorption of light, molecules quickly return to their ground state, thereby emitting photons at longer wavelengths than the excitation wavelength. This phenomenon is called fluorescence. The fluorescence of large biologic molecules exhibits a rather broad and featureless spectrum, reflecting the distribution of the substates in the ground electronic level. Nevertheless, by properly choosing the excitation wavelength and accurately analyzing the fluorescence spectrum, it is frequently possible to obtain information about the tissue molecules. Many different chromophores may contribute to the fluorescence signal: endogenous molecules such as NADH, collagen, and elastin, as well as exogenous added tumor-seeking agents (called photosensitizers), such as those described in Chap. 9.

In this chapter, we will review commonly explored light-induced fluorescence (LIF) methods and their ability to identify bladder malignancies. Exogenous fluorescence will be addressed first (Sect. 10.2), followed by a discussion of endogenous fluorescence (Sect. 10.3). Concluding remarks about the usefulness of the presently known techniques for detecting bladder malignancies will be presented in Sect. 10.4. Although we have included many important published results, even from other disciplines, no attempt has been made to give a complete review of the existing literature. Instead, attention has been focused on our practical experience with LIF.

10.2 Exogenous Fluorescence Spectroscopy

Currently, two photosensitizers are commonly used in clinical practice: Photofrin II (P II) and aminolevulinic acid (ALA).

10.2.1
Fluorescence with Photofrin II

Fluorescence of porphyrins has been exploited in vivo since 1924 (POLICARD 1924). To some extent, P II is preferentially retained by tumor tissue and, as a result, a larger fluorescence signal will be obtained from malignant tissue than from the surrounding normal tissue (upon equal excitation): hence, the basic idea of exploiting the relative fluorescence yield as a tumor demarcation function.

Photofrin II is composed of different fractions of hematoporphyrin derivatives such as monomers, dimers, oligomers, and larger aggregates of porphyrin (KESSEL 1982; KESSEL and CHOU 1983). The absorption band occurs at different wavelengths for the various compounds dissolved in saline: 390 nm for the monomers, 370 nm for the dimers, and 365 nm for the larger aggregates (PROFIO et al. 1984). Other parameters which affect absorption and fluorescence are temperature and pH (POTTIER et al. 1985). The fluorescence properties of P II are altered when bound to serum proteins. In this case, the spectra are red shifted to 405 nm (MOAN and SOMMER 1981). Therefore, 405 nm is the best wavelength to excite P II in vivo. The resulting emission spectrum exhibits two typical (red) peaks at 630 and 690 nm, which are superimposed on the tissue autofluorescence resulting from native chromophores (PROFIO et al. 1984).

Several phenomena may adversely affect the tumor demarcation capabilities of the technique. The observed fluorescence signal depends on the amount of scattering and absorption in the tissue. Both these effects are wavelength and tissue dependent. Generally, shorter wavelengths will be more scattered and, therefore, also be more attenuated. Nonlinear effects, such as saturation and photo-bleaching, also may occur and cause a decrease in the fluorescence signal, particularly from tumor areas. Equally important, the stronger exogenous fluorescence from malignant tissue is counteracted by a decrease in the endogenous fluorescence (PROFIO and BALCHUM 1985). Endogenous fluorescence, or autofluorescence, will be discussed in Sect. 10.3 for various types of tissue.

Hematoporphyrin fluorescence to detect cancer in various organs was first described by LIPSON et al. (1961). KELLY and SNELL (1976), followed by JOCHAM et al. (1981), BENSON et al. (1982), and LIN et al. (1984), later used it to detect bladder cancer. They used high doses of hematoporphyrin (2–4 mg/kg) in order to obtain a visually observable red

fluorescence from tumor areas. The rather poor tumor demarcation contrast ratio they obtained accounts for their large number of false-positive results.

To avoid false-positive results, BAERT et al. (1993) have used a spectroscopic detection system. Such a system can be made at orders of magnitude more sensitive than the human eye, thus permitting lowering of the sensitizer dose and reduction of the P II uptake by normal tissue. A crucial advantage of a spectroscopic system is its capability to separately evaluate the exogenous and endogenous contributions to the overall tissue fluorescence spectrum. This leads to a further significant reduction of false-positive results (see hereinafter). The system, based on the fluorosensor as described by ANDERSSON-ENGELS et al. (1991), uses a nitrogen laser (337 nm) to pump a DPS dye laser which emits short excitation pulses at 405 nm. A dichroic beam splitter reflects the excitation light into a 600-nm single fiber. The fiber is introduced into a 21-French cystoscope and carefully placed in contact with the tissue to be examined. The induced fluorescent light propagates back through the fiber, travels through the dichroic mirror, and is focused onto the entrance slit of a grating monochromator. An intensified diode array, linked to an optical multichannel analyzer (OMA) and a PC computer, allows the fluorescence spectra to be captured and stored. Finally, a programmed spectroscopic algorithm is executed to calculate a specific tumor demarcation index.

Twenty-one patients with suspicious bladder areas and/or exophytic tumors were examined in vivo. Fluorescence measurements were performed on various apparently normal, suspicious, or manifest malignant areas. Cold cup biopsies were taken from the same areas and later diagnosed by a pathologist. In this way, more than 800 fluorescence spectra were recorded and correlated with almost 300 biopsies. Some 48 h prior to investigation, the patients were injected with 0.5 or 0.35 mg/kg body weight P II. The patients were advised to avoid direct sunlight for 48 h. After 48 h, no signs of skin porphyrin fluorescence could be detected, either with the high P II dose of 0.5 mg/kg or with the lower dose of 0.35 mg/kg.

All the fluorescence spectra show the characteristic P II peaks at 630 nm and 690 nm, superimposed on the tissue autofluorescence (Fig. 10.1). As explained earlier, these peaks are stronger in malignant tissue than in normal tissue, but the autofluorescence from malignant tissue is about a factor of 2 weaker compared with normal tissue.

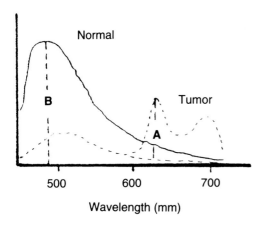

Fig. 10.1. Fluorescence spectra of normal bladder and TCC following P II injection (0.35 mg/kg) upon 405-nm excitation. *A*, P II-related fluorescence; *B*, endogenous fluorescence

Table 10.1. Demarcation index (DI) for TCC after Photofrin II injection (0.35 mg/kg) upon 405-nm excitation

Patient	Tumor type		DI	
	Papillary	Flat	Papillary	Flat
1	Ta GI		10.2	
2	Ta GI	Dys	14.0	1.5
3	Ta GII		1.3	
4	Ta GII		68.4	
5	Ta GII		133.0	
6	Ta GII	CIS	13.4	8.2
7	Ta GII		10.0	
8	Ta GII		8.7	
9	Ta GII		55.8	
10	Ta GIII		17.5	
11	Ta GIII	CIS	3.3	1.2
12	Ta GIII	CIS	91.4	3.3
13	Ta GIII		68.8	
14	Ta GIII	CIS	3.9	2.1
15	T1 GII		11.3	
16	T1 GIII		14.5	
17	T2 GIII	CIS	42.6	22.3
Mean			33.4	6.4
St. dev.			37.7	8.2

Dys, Dysplasia.

Consequently, the demarcation contrast can be digitally enhanced by taking the ratio of the background-free P II fluorescence peak at 630 nm (denoted A) to the endogenous fluorescence intensity at 470 nm (denoted B). A large A/B ratio, thus, is indicative of malignant tissue. Since this ratio is without dimensions, it is also independent of the various experimental parameters which determine both the excitation and the detection efficiency. In particular, the distance between the excitation source (i.e., the tip of the fiber) and the tissue does not affect the A/B ratio.

The results are summarized in Table 10.1. For each patient who showed some malignancy, this table lists the ratio of the average A/B value for cancerous (dysplastic) to normal tissue versus the type of malignancy. This ratio of average A/B values is our demarcation index (DI). Clearly, DI was greater than 1 for all cases, albeit only marginally so for a few of them where one might suspect inaccurate optical sampling and/or insufficient photosensitizer retention. However, the vast majority of the data show a clear distinction between TCC, CIS, and normal tissue (DI = 1). On average, the DI for TCC is about a factor of 4.5 larger than for CIS. Unfortunately, the individual A/B values in each category vary substantially among patients. Therefore, standardized threshold values for A/B cannot be defined and, as a result, only TCC can be unambiguously distinguished from normal mucosa with a diagnosis solely based on this ratio. Moreover, it should be noted that the ratio of mean A values of TCC (or CIS) to normal tissue for an individual patient is quite low: on average 1.88 for TCC and 1.65 for CIS. While these values cannot be directly translated into ratios of P II molecule concentrations, because of possibly different absorption and scattering properties of normal and malignant tissue, they nevertheless suggest that the selective low-dose P II uptake in malignancies is less than has usually been assumed.

10.2.2
Fluorescence with Aminolevulinic Acid

Protoporphyrin IX (pPIX) is a precursor in the biosynthetic pathway of heme. As heme-containing enzymes are required by cells for energy metabolism, all nucleated cells theoretically should have the capability to synthesize pPIX. In many types of cells, heme biosynthesis is regulated by negative feedback on the rate-limiting step of the pathway (for the synthesis of ALA, see Fig. 10.2) (Konig et al. 1994). This step can be bypassed by the addition of exogenous ALA, allowing cells to produce heme at a rate governed by their individual enzyme profiles (Kappas et al. 1992). Systemic administration of ALA (orally or intravenously) produces a rapid rise in pPIX content of the bladder, followed by a reduction to control values after 24 h (Leveckis et al. 1994). pPIX appears to localize preferentially in the mucosa rather than the muscle (Bedwell et al. 1992). Intravesical administration of ALA to normal bladders, on the other

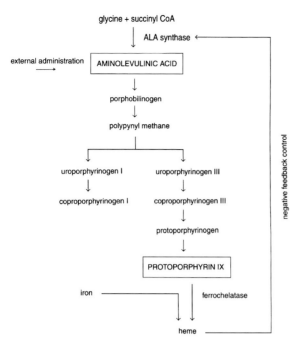

glycine + succinyl CoA

ALA synthase

external administration → AMINOLEVULINIC ACID

porphobilinogen

polypynyl methane

uroporphyrinogen I   uroporphyrinogen III

coproporphyrinogen I   coproporphyrinogen III

protoporphyrinogen

PROTOPORPHYRIN IX

iron ——— ferrochelatase

heme

negative feedback control

Fig. 10.2. Schematic representation of the pathway of heme synthesis

hand, does not provoke any increase in pPIX amount (BEDWELL et al. 1992). This is comparable with the behavior of ALA in the skin, where fluorescence can be observed after topical administration to abnormal areas but not to normal skin (KENNEDY et al. 1990). In principle, intravesical administration of ALA has many advantages compared with systemic porphyrin sensitization, such as the absence of skin sensitization and a fast tumor retention (3 vs 48 h). Intravesical administration of a 3% solution of ALA has been successfully used to visualize bladder cancer upon excitation with a krypton ion laser at 406 nm (KRIEGMAIR et al. 1996). The laser-induced fluorescence was imaged with an integrating color video camera. KRIEGMAIR et al. observed 3% false-negative results, and 80% false-positive results.

In our department, we investigated ALA-induced bladder fluorescence with an excitation source developed by the Storz company (D Light System). It consists of a 300 W Xenon arc lamp, coupled to a fiber bundle. By activating a foot switch, a 380–450 nm bandpass filter can be inserted between the lamp and the fiber bundle, so that either blue or white excitation light is available. A conventional cystoscope is used for endoscopic examination, but the telescopes (0° and 30°) are equipped with a 520-nm cutoff filter, which absorbs the reflected blue excitation light

without blocking the red fluorescence light. The bladders were first inspected under conventional white light, before being exposed to the blue excitation beam. After excitation with the blue beam, all red fluorescent areas were once more inspected with white light, and their macroscopic appearances were noted (nonspecific inflammatory appearance was generally considered to be normal, but if CIS was suspected, it was considered pathologic). Biopsies were taken from every red fluorescent area, from every macroscopically suspicious nonfluorescent area, and from at least two apparently normal and nonfluorescent zones. All biopsies were interpreted by the same pathologist, who was unaware of fluorescence results and macroscopic appearances. The ALA solution was prepared on ice by dissolving the ALA (Merck) in sterile distilled water, with a 5 ml phosphate buffer solution (Merck) for adjusting the pH to 5–5.5 in a 50 ml volume. The first two patients with TCC received a 3% solution (1.5 g), the next two a 2% solution (1 g), and the remaining patients a 1% solution (0.5 g). Three hours prior to investigation, an indwelling catheter was placed, the bladder content evacuated, and the ALA solution instilled. The patients were asked to change their position regularly to bring the ALA solution into mucosal contact for the entire bladder wall. The catheter was removed in the operating room, immediately before fluorescence inspection. A total of 15 patients were included in this study. Initially, dose-related effects were examined in five patients with superficial papillary bladder carcinoma. Neither CIS nor dysplasia was diagnosed for these patients. Four more patients suffered from papillary TCC and associated CIS. One patient had dysplasia associated with TCC. Pure CIS was found in two patients and three more had CIS associated with dysplasia but without papillary TCC. Three of these patients had previously been treated with Calmette-Guérin becillus (BCG) for CIS. Two patients among them had had positive urinary cytology for a few months, but previous biopsies (without fluorescence detection) failed to show any signs of recurrence.

The first group of five patients who were examined with LIF had multifocal superficial papillary TCC GI, II, and III. All of the lesions showed a bright red fluorescence, regardless of the dose of ALA (Fig. 10.3). However, these lesions were also readily identified after careful inspection with white light. The remaining ten patients were suspected of having CIS, either associated with macroscopically invasive and poorly differentiated TCC, or pure CIS, because of

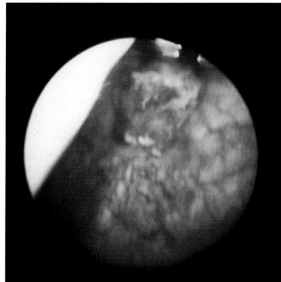

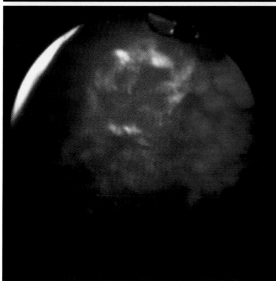

Fig. 10.3. White (**a**) and blue light (**b**) examination of a bladder after 3 h of sensitization with 0.5 g ALA. White light examination shows a sessile tumor with apparently normal surroundings. Blue light illumination shows bright red fluorescence of the tumor, but also surrounding red fluorescence that proved to be CIS

Table 10.2. Comparison between macroscopic appearance, fluorescence, and pathology of 96 biopsies of flat mucosal areas

Pathology	Fl+ WL+	Fl+ WL−	Fl− WL+	Fl− WL−
CIS	9	18	0	1
Dysplasia	4	12	0	2
Normal	12	16	4	28

Fl, Fluorescence; WL, white light observation.

was correctly diagnosed with fluorescence emission in 27 (96%) patients, but with conventional cystoscopy in only nine (32%) patients. Mild or moderate dysplasia was found in 18 biopsies. Of these, 16 (89%) were fluorescence-positive, while only four (22%) could be detected with white light illumination. False-positive fluorescence was observed in 28 (46%) biopsies.

Fluorescence detection after ALA sensitization appears to be very helpful in detecting CIS, although there is a relatively high proportion of false-positive results. This might be lessened in the future by reducing the ALA dose even further, and detecting the fluorescence with more sensitive devices than visual detection.

10.3
Endogenous Fluorescence Spectroscopy

10.3.1
Introduction

Although tissue is a complex heterogeneous mixture of a large number of molecular species containing numerous fluorophores, the observed autofluorescence spectra are broad and relatively featureless. It is generally accepted that they originate from contributions of only a few fluorophores. Nevertheless, the sensitivity of fluorescence to tissue composition makes it reasonable to hypothesize that light-induced autofluorescence might be a valuable tool for determining tissue types. The absence of photosensitizers has the advantage that no expensive drugs are needed, thereby eliminating skin sensitization and false-positive results due to poor tissue selectivity. Endogenous fluorescence diagnosis was first suggested and described by ALFANO et al. (1984). They used blue light (488 nm) from an argon ion laser to excite urinary tract tissue in vitro, and demonstrated that spectral features not evident in

positive urinary cytology without papillary lesions on cystoscopy or intravenous urography. They were instilled with a low dose of 0.5 g ALA. Five patients had concomitant invasive papillary TCC. The macroscopic appearance agreed with a positive fluorescence for all the lesions. Next, 106 biopsies were taken from flat mucosal areas and a comparison was made between pathology, macroscopic aspect, and fluorescence (Table 10.2). Of these 106 biopsies, 28 (29%) showed the presence of CIS. This normal tissues were present in subcutaneously implanted rodent bladder and prostate cancers.

10.3.2
Clinical Experience in Different Disciplines

The aforementioned decrease in the autofluorescence yield in malignant tissue has been observed in the green region of the spectrum for the bronchial tree (HUNG et al. 1991). PALCIC et al. (1991) developed a lung imaging fluorescence endoscope (LIFE system). The excitation source is a helium cadmium laser (442 nm) and the induced fluorescence is amplified and digitized to give a composite pseudo image of the excited tissue on a color television screen. Similar tissue characteristics have been found by imaging of the larynx (HARRIES et al. 1995).

The autofluorescence from cervical neoplasms has been extensively studied by RAMANUJAM et al. (1994), who excited with a pulsed nitrogen laser (337 nm) and developed a two-stage algorithm which differentiates colposcopically normal from histologically abnormal tissue with a sensitivity of 92%, a specificity of 90%, and a positive predictive value of 88%. The second stage differentiates preneoplastic and neoplastic tissue from nonneoplastic abnormal tissue with a sensitivity of 87%, a specificity of 73%, and a positive predictive value of 74%. These algorithms can also be used to differentiate normal cervix from inflammatory lesions, human papilloma virus-infected lesions, and CIS grades I, II, and III.

The most extensively studied organ is the colon. In contrast to the lungs and cervix, where the aim is to detect intraepithelial lesions, the key issue here is to distinguish polyp types (adenoma or adenocarcinoma). KAPADIA et al. (1990) excited with a helium cadmium laser (325 nm) and developed an algorithm to differentiate neoplastic from normal colonic tissue. They were able to identify adenomatous polyps with a sensitivity and a specificity of 100% and 99%, respectively. However, with a similar system, YASHKE et al. (1989) were unable to differentiate normal from abnormal tissue. RICHARDS-KORTUM et al. (1991) used a laboratory spectrofluorometer to examine the excitation-emission properties of surgically excised colons from patients with familial adenomatous polyposis. This group identified several promising excitation bands for differentiating normal from adenomatous tissue, and achieved an accuracy of better than 95%.

MARCHESINI et al. (1992) examined biopsy specimens of colonic mucosa with blue light excitation (410 nm). They achieved a sensitivity of 81% and a selectivity of 90% for discriminating neoplastic from nonneoplastic mucosa. These in vitro studies have subsequently led to in vivo studies. SCHOMACKER et al. (1992) used a pulsed nitrogen laser (337 nm) to examine patients with polyps discovered during routine diagnostic colonoscopy. A spectroscopic algorithm allowed correct classification of 80% of the hyperplastic polyps and 86% of adenomatous polyps. COTHREN et al. (1990) excited with a dye laser (370 nm) pumped by a nitrogen laser, and correctly distinguished adenomatous polyps from normal mucosa in 97% of the cases.

10.3.3
Biologic Considerations

As tissue progresses from normal to abnormal, all the aforementioned organs show a corresponding decrease in autofluorescence yield from the ultraviolet (UV) through the entire visible (VIS) spectrum (approximately 350–650 nm). There is, however, no unique spectroscopic explanation for this general observation.

SCHOMACKER et al. (1992) pointed out that, in their setup, roughly 90% of the collected fluorescence originates from the upper 0.5 mm of the tissue. These values are orders of magnitude only; depth-related effects obviously depend on various experimental parameters and the type of tissue examined. Fluorescence in the 360–420 nm region can be attributed to collagen (NEUMAN and LOGAN 1950). Since neoplasia is associated with mucosal thickening, the decrease in fluorescence yield in this spectral band might be due to a screening of collagen by the thickened epithelium. A decrease near 420 nm undoubtedly stems from an increase in oxyhemoglobin absorption due to the neovascularization of tumors. Thus, in the 360–420 nm part of the spectrum, a reduced fluorescence yield in malignant tissue is likely caused by morphologic changes rather than changes to specific fluorophores.

In addition to morphology, other effects might be involved. Fluorescence in the 430–520 nm band mainly stems from NADH (reduced form of nicotine amide adenine dinucleotide). Lesser NADH fluorescence in normal than in transformed cells has been observed in relation to the absolute co-enzyme concentration (SCHWARTZ et al. 1974). Moreover, a reduction of binding sites for NADH in cancerous tissue has been observed (GALEOTTI et al. 1970). This reduction results in a higher amount of free NADH, which has a smaller fluorescence yield (SALMON et al. 1982). Finally, in the green and red parts of the spectrum (520–650 nm), differences in the amount of oxidized and reduced forms of flavins in tumor and normal tissues may account for the decreased fluorescence yield (POLLACK et al. 1942).

10.3.4
Experimental Studies and Clinical Results

We have extensively studied autofluorescence spectroscopy as a technique to identify bladder malignancies. Several experimental parameters should be optimized before the potential of the technique can be evaluated. These include a determination of the best excitation and emission wavelengths, the identification of appropriate spectroscopic algorithms, and a proper engineering of the hardware. Our program first consisted in recording autofluorescence spectra at several excitation wavelengths both in vitro and in vivo for various types of bladder tissue. Next, these spectra were fitted with the observed emission spectra (obtained at the same excitation wavelengths) from a variety of important fluorophores. In this way, relevant fluorophores were identified for each excitation wavelength. Detailed knowledge of the absorption spectra of these fluorophores, in turn, allowed us to select suitable excitation and corresponding emission bands. With these insights, we engineered a compact fiber-optic instrument, which was tested on a large group of patients.

10.3.4.1
Spectroscopic Results

For spectroscopic studies, we mainly used our OMA detection system described in Sect. 10.2.1. Three pulsed lasers were used as the excitation source: a nitrogen laser (337 nm), a frequency-tripled and Q-switched Nd:YAG laser (355 nm), and a DPS dye laser (405 nm), pumped by a nitrogen laser. We also used the UV-VIS spectral lines of a mercury arc lamp for excitation to obtain additional information. All spectral data presented hereafter, are corrected for reflection and transmission losses in the various optical components of the setup, as well as for the quantum efficiency of the detector, and will be plotted in arbitrary units with peak intensity set equal to 1.

10.3.4.2
Excitation at 405 nm

The autofluorescence spectra for normal tissue and TCC upon 405-nm excitation are identical to that shown in Fig. 10.1 if the characteristic P II peaks are subtracted. There are no spectral differences between normal tissue and TCC, but the fluorescence yield for TCC is about a factor of 2 lower than for normal tissue, as already noted in Sect. 10.2.1. Obviously, 405-nm-excited autofluorescence yields less information about malignancies than does P II fluorescence at this wavelength. Therefore, a discussion of our results at this excitation wavelength is not relevant, and will be omitted.

10.3.4.3
Excitation in the Range 355–365 nm

The autofluorescence spectrum of normal bladder tissue upon excitation in the range 355–365 nm is shown by the solid line in Fig. 10.4. It was obtained by averaging out the data from more than 10 patients. The spectrum shows a relatively broad peak centered at 455 nm, accompanied by a long tail extending into the red. Spectral differences between individual patients show up either as small shifts (± 5 nm) of the peak of the spectrum, or larger shifts (± 20 nm) of the position of the 50% intensity point of the leading edge of the spectrum. This suggests that several components contribute to the spectrum, and

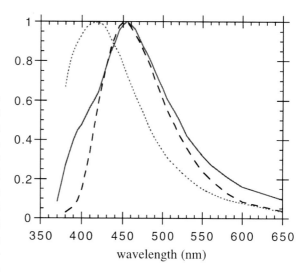

Fig. 10.4. Fluorescence spectra (in arbitrary units) of human bladder tissue (*solid line*), NADH (*dashed line*), and collagen I and III (*dotted line*) upon excitation in the range 355–365 nm

that the absorption and fluorescence yield of each of them differs somewhat from patient to patient. To identify these fluorophores, we collected the spectra of biologically selected important molecules upon excitation in the range 355–365 nm. The fluorescence spectra of powders of both NADH and a mixture of collagen I and III (the spectrum of the latter is red shifted) are shown in Fig. 10.4 by the dashed and dotted lines, respectively. The spectrum of NADH clearly corresponds well with the central part of the bladder spectrum. On the other hand, the fluorescence spectrum of collagen peaks at 415 nm, with a tail extending to 650 nm. The combined spectrum of these fluorophores agrees reasonably well with the observed bladder spectrum if absorption by oxyhemoglobin is taken into account. In this excitation range, the spectra for both CIS and TCC are nearly identical to that for normal bladder tissue. However, compared with normal tissue, the fluorescence yield is about a factor of 2.5 lower for CIS, and about a factor of 3 lower for TCC. This decrease in fluorescence yield is caused by a corresponding decrease in NADH levels, and in particular for TCC, by an additional decrease in excited collagen and/or an increase in hemoglobin absorption.

10.3.4.4
Excitation in the Range 330–340 nm

Figure 10.5 shows an average autofluorescence spectrum of both normal human bladder tissue (solid line) and TCC (dashed line) upon 334 nm excitation in the range 330–340 nm. Both spectra have a different line shape. We first discuss the spectrum of normal tissue. It shows two distinct peaks (385 nm and 455 nm), again accompanied by a long tail extending into the red. A pronounced valley at 420 nm is caused by hemoglobin absorption. Spectral differences among patients are marked by differences in the ratio of the (relative) intensity of the 455-nm peak to the 385-nm peak. Occasionally, the 385-nm peak was found to be stronger than the 455-nm one. This indicates that at least two different fluorophores are excited in normal tissue (each corresponding to one peak), and that the relative fluorescence yield of these fluorophores varies substantially among patients. In contrast, the average autofluorescence spectrum of TCC has a single broad peak centered at 455 nm. Within the experimental errors, this spectrum is identical to the one obtained for the 355–365 nm excitation range. Compared with normal

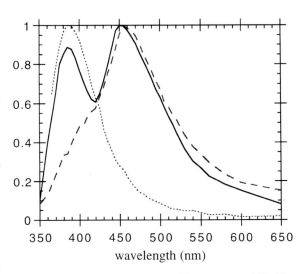

Fig. 10.5. Fluorescence spectrum of human normal bladder tissue (*solid line*), TCC (*dashed line*), and collagen I (*dotted line*) upon 334-nm excitation

tissue, the average fluorescence yield of the 455-nm peak is again approximately a factor of 3 lower for TCC. The spectrum of collagen I in this excitation range is also shown in Fig. 10.5. It peaks at 385 nm. The spectrum of NADH is identical to that shown in Fig. 10.4. Again, a combination of these spectra represents the observed normal bladder spectrum fairly well, if absorption around 420 nm is taken into account. It thus seems reasonable to assume that the two main fluorophores which contribute to the bladder spectrum in the UV and blue part of the spectrum are indeed collagen and NADH. This conclusion is supported by other more direct experimental evidence. To probe the presence of NADH (in vitro), we have incubated malignant tissue in a 2% SDS (sodium dodecyl sulfate) solution (for 15 min at 58°C) to remove the NADH from the tissue, while leaving the collagen unaffected. After incubation, the fluorescence yield from TCC almost completely vanished, thereby confirming that NADH is indeed the main excited fluorophore.

In summary, we feel safe to say that our experimental spectroscopic results corroborate the basic statements in Sect. 10.3.3. Hence, suitable excitation/detection wavelengths for optically diagnosing bladder malignancies are located in about 20-nm-wide bands, centered around the absorption/emission maxima of collagen (330/390 nm), NADH (350/460 nm), flavins (410/550 nm), and oxyhemoglobin (absorption peak at 420 nm). Additional spectroscopic information at intermittent wavelengths is redundant.

10.4
Design of a Compact Fluorometer

With these insights, we have developed a versatile instrument which samples the autofluorescence spectrum of bladder tissue at up to three different wavelengths simultaneously, and displays in real time specific functions of these spectral intensities. The layout is schematically represented in Fig. 10.6. The instrument consists of a small mercury (Hg) arc lamp, the radiation of which is selected by interference filters (IF), depending on the desired excitation wavelength. The excitation beam is modulated by a chopper wheel, and focused into one leg of a bifurcated fiber bundle. The common section of this fiber bundle is inserted into the bladder through one of the biopsy channels of a standard 21-French cystoscope, and brought into contact with the bladder wall during in vivo measurements. The induced autofluorescence propagates back through the fiber bundle and is collected at the other leg by a phase-sensitive detection system, which allows a regular bladder illumination with a quartz tungsten halogen (QTH) lamp for visual inspection with a CCD camera connected to a television monitor. The detection system consists of three channels. In each channel, a specific part of the spectrum is recorded by a photomultiplier tube, the signal of which is processed by a current-to-voltage amplifier followed by a locking amplifier. Analog ratiometers normalize the data in any one of the channels to those in another channel. This normalization is essential to make the data independent of varying experimental parameters such as lamp power, coupling efficiency into the fiber bundle, distance between the end of this bundle and the examined tissue, and gain of the photomultiplier tubes. Fluctuations in the outputs of the radiometers

are effectively eliminated in this way, since the integration times in all channels are identical. Finally, the outputs of the radiometers are processed by another analog device to execute in real time a programmed spectroscopic algorithm.

The advantages of this instrument are manifold. First, the use of an Hg lamp instead of a laser simplifies both the design and the maintenance of the apparatus, thus making it cost-effective, compact, and portable. Second, in contrast to a laser, the Hg lamp offers a wide wavelength tunability and, therefore, makes it possible to select different excitation wavelengths. Third, the use of a weak excitation source prevents optical damage to the fibers and eliminates tissue bleaching, two problems which we experienced with our high peak power pulsed laser systems. On the other hand, the use of a bifurcated fiber bundle instead of a single fiber, also adds to the versatility of the instrument. First, the need for expensive dichroic mirrors to separate excitation and fluorescence beams (one dichroic per excitation wavelength) is avoided. Second, and equally important, parasitic signals arising from the fiber input, which obviously have the same modulation frequency as the fluorescence signal from the tissue, are eliminated. Moreover, the larger cross-section of the fiber bundle (compared with a single fiber) eliminates a previously encountered risk of penetration of the fiber tip into the bladder tissue. Finally, the use of photomultiplier tubes instead of an OMA eliminates nonlinearities and cross-talk between adjacent channels, and yields a significantly better signal to noise ratio. Several surgeons who were asked to evaluate the apparatus found it easy to operate and particularly appreciated the lack of functional switches and control buttons.

10.4.1
Evaluation upon 365-nm Excitation

Upon 365-nm excitation, the autofluorescence spectra of normal tissue, CIS, and TCC are identical but the fluorescence yield is lower for CIS, and still lower for TCC. As a result, normalization of one part of the spectrum to another is impossible and one has to make absolute measurements. As pointed out previously, the best detection wavelength is centered around 460 nm (we actually used an interference filter at 450 nm). To eliminate errors due to fluctuations in both excitation power and gain of the photomultiplier, we slightly modified our instrument and used a ratiometer to normalize the data at

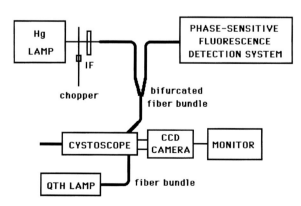

Fig. 10.6 Schematic representation of the experimental apparatus as used at the Catholic University of Leuven

450 nm to a fraction of the excitation beam. More-over, the end of the fiber bundle was always carefully brought into close contact with the bladder wall without pushing it into the tissue in order to enhance the repeatability of the measurements.

We examined 16 patients with papillary TCC and/ or flat CIS with the system. Table 10.3 lists, for each patient, the DI for both TCC and CIS. Here, we define DI as the ratio of the average (normalized) 450-nm signal for cancerous to normal tissue. As expected, DI was less than 1 for all malignancies. Conse-quently, no false-negative results were obtained. On average, the DIs for TCC and for CIS are, respec-tively, factors of 2.6 and 2.1 lower than for normal tissue (DI = 1). Unfortunately, the individual data vary by about a factor of 2 from patient to patient and they also depend somewhat on the way the op-erator brings the fiber bundle into contact with the bladder wall. Therefore, threshold values cannot be defined without referring to the response of normal tissue on a patient to patient basis. In practice, any signal below 70% of the average signal for normal tissue should be considered indicative of a cancerous state. Improved results can be expected from a spe-cific modification of the end of the fiber bundle to ensure a constant illumination and collection geom-etry during measurements (QU et al. 1994). We con-clude that while absolute intensities may provide a way to detect malignancies, they also require some modifications of our instrument. This will be ex-plored in the near future.

10.4.2
Evaluation upon 334-nm Excitation

The pronounced difference in line shape between the autofluorescence spectra of normal tissue and TCC upon 334-nm excitation suggests a simple spectro-scopic algorithm for differentiating normal from malignant tissue. From a study of the data presented in Fig. 10.5, it will be clear that the main features of the spectra can be characterized by the fluorescence at only three wavelengths: 390 nm, 450 nm (the loca-tion of both peaks), and 420 nm (the location of the valley). Our instrument simultaneously measures the spectral intensity $I(1)$ at each of these wave-lengths and the analog ratiometers calculate the two quantities without dimensions $R_1 = I(390\,nm)/I(420\,nm)$ and $R_2 = I(390\,nm)/I(450\,nm)$. An analog multiplier then calculates the product $P = R_1R_2$, which is our algorithm for differentiating normal from malignant tissue. Both R_1 and R_2 and, conse-quently, also their product P are smaller for malig-nancies than for normal tissue.

With this set up, we examined 71 patients both in vitro and in vivo. We took more than 500 biopsies and correlated them to fluorescence data. For each patient, we calculated the DI, defined as the ratio of the average P value for malignant to normal tissue. Any DI of less than 1 indicates a malignancy. The results for TCC obtained in vivo are summarized in Table 10.4. Table 10.5 shows the results for both TCC and CIS obtained in vitro. Measurements in vivo are slightly more repeatable than those made in vitro. On average, the DIs for TCC in vivo and in vitro are, respectively, factors of 4.5 and 3.7 lower than for normal tissue (DI = 1). Tables 10.4 and 10.5 show no false-negative results for TCC. From the data in Table 10.5, it is obvious that our algorithm does not work equally well for CIS. Although for this type of malignancy we obtained only one false-negative result, the DI for CIS is on average only a factor of 1.7 lower than for normal tissue. This result is in fact slightly worse than that obtained upon 365-nm excitation. There is a simple explanation for this deficiency. Our algorithm essentially probes the presence (or absence) of fluorescence at 390 nm from submucosal collagen fibers versus the NADH fluorescence at 450 nm. This works quite well for TCC, where a noticeable thickening of the epithelial layer prevents excitation of the submu-cosa. Apparently, this effect is strongly reduced (or in some cases even absent) for CIS, where a (smaller) decrease in collagen fluorescence is some-what masked in our algorithm by the decrease in

Table 10.3. Demarcation index (DI) for TCC and CIS upon 355-nm excitation (autofluorescence)

Patient	DI (TCC)	DI (CIS)
1	0.27	0.45
2	0.52	
3	0.39	
4		0.62
5	0.34	0.32
6		0.52
7	0.3	
8	0.32	
9	0.5	
10	0.51	
11	0.29	
12	0.51	
13	0.36	
14	0.33	
15	0.43	
16	0.33	
Mean	0.39	0.48
St. dev.	0.09	0.12

Table 10.4. Demarcation index (DI) for TCC upon 334-nm excitation (in vivo autofluorescence)

Patient	DI (TCC)
1	0.45
2	0.17
3	0.11
4	0.36
5	0.28
6	0.23
7	0.52
8	0.3
9	0.43
10	0.12
11	0.34
12	0.08
13	0.08
14	0.15
15	0.11
16	0.15
17	0.27
18	0.34
19	0.35
20	0.08
21	0.08
22	0.18
23	0.06
24	0.03
25	0.14
26	0.27
Mean	0.22
St. dev.	0.14

Table 10.5. Demarcation index (DI) for TCC and CIS upon 334-nm excitation (in vitro autofluorescence)

Patient	DI (TCC)	DI (CIS)
1	0.17	
2	0.13	
3	0.12	
4	0.14	
5	0.53	
6	0.65	
7	0.25	
8		0.51
9	0.23	
10	0.17	
11	0.08	
12	0.05	
13	0.25	
14		0.76
15	0.40	
16		0.54
17		0.82
18	0.34	0.40
19	0.23	
20	0.14	
21	0.07	
22		1.10
23	0.97	0.44
24	0.093	
25	0.46	
26	0.14	0.36
27	0.47	
Mean	0.27	0.60
St. dev.	0.23	0.24

NADH fluorescence and the increased oxyhemoglobin absorption. In addition, it should be noted that, particularly for CIS, individual data for both R_1 and R_2 (and therefore also their product) vary substantially among patients, again making threshold values difficult to define.

10.5
Conclusions

We have reviewed several light-induced fluorescence methods, so-called optical biopsies, all of which are intended to differentiate normal from malignant bladder tissue. Since papillary TCC most often can be observed visually, optical biopsies provide only complementary, and not always strictly needed, information. On the other hand, detection of CIS and other flat diseases currently requires histopathology. The key question, therefore, is whether an optical biopsy can identify flat malignancies with sufficient reliability to provide a simple screening technique for high-risk patients. We believe that the answer is

positive, albeit marginally so with the techniques presently at our disposition.

Basically, two options can be selected: endogenous or exogenous fluorescence spectroscopy. Both have inherent advantages and disadvantages. In principle, endogenous fluorescence is most desirable since no drugs are needed and the results are obtained in real time. Although we (and others) have shown that endogenous fluorescence spectroscopy does indeed identify papillary tumors with a high specificity, particularly upon excitation at 334 nm, the technique seems far less adequate for detecting flat malignancies. Different spectroscopic algorithms and perhaps also different excitation wavelengths are needed to evaluate the true potential of the technique. This work is currently in progress in our laboratories.

For exogenous spectroscopy, on the other hand, ALA presently seems to give the best results. In contrast to the point monitoring detection inherent to endogenous inspection with a fiber bundle, ALA-induced fluorescence allows a visual inspection of the whole bladder at once. False-negative results are extremely rare and, therefore, the sensitivity of the technique is very good. However, many false-positive results occur with the currently used doses, which results in a low specificity. Additional disadvantages are the high cost of the drug and the still rather long incubation period during which patients have to move around.

In conclusion, in our opinion much more research is needed to improve the capabilities of optical biopsies and to make them generally acceptable as a substitute for traditional biopsies.

References

Alfano RR, Tata DB, Cordero J, Tomashefsky P, Longo FW, Alfano MA (1984) Laser induced fluorescence spectroscopy from native cancerous and normal tissue. IEEE J Quantum Electron 20:1507–1511

Andersson-Engels S, Elner A, Johansson J, et al. (1991) Clinical recordings of laser induced fluorescence spectra for evaluation of tumor demarcation feasibility in selected clinical specialties. Lasers Med Sci 6:415–421

Baert L, Berg R, D'Hallewin MA, Van Damme B, Johansson J, Svanberg S, Svanberg K (1991) Clinical fluorescence diagnosis of human bladder carcinoma following low dose Photofrin injection. SPIE Proc 1525:385–390

Baert L, Berg R, Van Damme B, D'Hallewin MA, Johansson J, Svanberg K, Svanberg S (1993) Clinical fluorescence diagnosis of human bladder carcinoma following low-dose Photofrin infection. Urol 41:322–330

Bedwell J, MacRobert A, Philips D, Bown SG (1992) Fluorescence distribution and photodynamic effect of ALA induced pPLX in the DMH rat colonic tumor model. Br J Cancer 65:818–824

Benson RC, Farrow GM, Kinsey JH, Cortese DA, Zincke H, Utz DC (1982) Detection and localization of in situ carcinoma of the bladder with hematoporphyrin derivative. Mayo Clin Proc 57:548–555

Cothren RM, Richards-Kortum R, Sivak MV, Fitzmaurice M, Rava RP (1990) Gastrointestinal tissue diagnosis by laser induced fluorescence spectroscopy at endoscopy. Endoscopy 36:105–111

D'Hallewin MA, Baert L (1996) Fluorescence detection of flat transitional cell carcinoma after intravesical instillation of aminolevulinic acid. (submitted to J Urol)

D'Hallewin MA, Baert L, Vanherzeele H (1993) Cystoscopic photodetection of human bladder carcinoma without sensitizing agents. LEOS '93 Conference. Proc IEEE Lasers and Electro Optics Soc 245

D'Hallewin MA, Baert L, Vanherzeele H (1994a) In vivo fluorescence detection of human bladder carcinoma without sensitizing agents. J Am paraplegia Soc 17:161–164

D'Hallewin MA, Baert L, Vanherzeele H (1994b) Fluorescence imaging of bladder cancer. Acta Urol Belg 62:59–63

D'Hallewin MA, Baert L, Vanherzeele H (1995) In vivo detection of human bladder carcinoma without sensitizing agents. SPIE Proc 2395:110–114

Galeotti T, Van Rossum GD, Mayer DH, Chance B (1970) On the fluorescence of NAD(P)H in whole cell preparations of tumours and normal tissues. Eur J Biochem 17:485–496

Harries ML, Lam S, MacAulay C, Qu J, Palcic B (1995) Diagnostic imaging of the larynx: autofluorescence of laryngeal tumours using the helium cadmium laser. Laryng Otol 109:108–110

Hung J, Lam S, LeRiche JC (1991) Autofluorescence of normal and malignant bronchial tissue. Lasers Surg Med 11:1035–1040

Jichlinski P, Forrer M, Mizeret J, et al. (1995) Comparison of two detection methods for screening superficial bladder transitional cell carcinoma: conventional white light cystoscopy versus fluorescence imaging of protoporphyrin IX induced by a topical application of aminolevulinic acid. Abstract Bios Europe 95

Jocham D, Staehler G, Chaussy C, Hammer C, Lohrs U (1981) Laserbehandlung von Blasertumoren nach Photosensibilisierung mit Hematoporphyrin-derivat. Urologe [A] 20:340–343

Kapadia CR, Cutruzzola FW, O'Brial KM, Stetz ML, Enriquez R, Deckelbaum L (1990) Laser induced fluorescence spectroscopy on human colonic mucosa. Gastroenterology 99:150–157

Kappas A, Sassa S, Galbraith RA, Nordman Y (1992) The Porphyrias. In: Scriver CR, Baudet AL, Sly WS, Valle D (eds) The metabolic basis of inherited disease 6th edn. McGraw Hill, New York, pp 1305–1365

Kelly JF, Snell ME (1976) Hematoporphyrin derivative: a possible aid in the diagnosis and treatment of carcinoma of the bladder. J Urol 155:150–153

Kennedy JC, Pottier RH, Pross DC (1990) Photodynamic therapy with endogenous protoporphyrin IX: basic principles and present clinical experience. J Photochem Photobiol B 6:143–148

Kessel DF (1982) Components of hematoporphyrin derivatives and their tumor localizing capacity. Cancer Res 42:1703–1708

Kessel DF, Chou TH (1983) Tumor localizing components of the porphyrin preparation hematoporphyrin derivative. Cancer Res 43:1994–1999

König K, Kienle A, Boehncke WH, Kaufmann R, Rück A, Meier, T, Steiner R (1994) Photodynamic tumor therapy and on-line fluorescence spectroscopy after ALA administration using 633-nm light as therapeutic and fluorescence excitation radiation. Opt Engineer 33:2945–2952

Kriegmair M, Baumgartner R, Knuechel R, Stepp H, Hofstetter F, Hofstetter A (1996) Detection of early bladder cancer by 5-aminolevulinic acid induced porphyrin fluorescence. J Urol 155:105–110

Leveckis J, Burn JL, Brown NJ, Reed MW (1994) Kinetics of endogenous protoporphyrin IX induction by aminolevulinic acid: preliminary studies in the bladder. J Urol 152:550–553

Lin CW, Bellnier DA, Prout GR, Andrus WS, Prescott R (1984) Cystoscopic fluorescence detector for photodetection of bladder carcinoma with hematoporphyrin derivative. J Urol 131:587–590

Lipson RL, Baldes EJ, Olsen AM (1961) The use of a derivative of hematoporphyrin in tumour detection. J Natl Cancer Inst 26:1–11

Marchesini R, Brambilla M, Pignoli E, et al. (1992) Light induced fluorescence spectroscopy of adenomas, adenocarcinomas and non neoplastic mucosa in human colon: in vitro measurements. J Photochem Photobiol B 14:219–230

Moan J, Sommer S (1981) Fluorescence and absorption properties of the components of hematoporphyrin derivative. Photobiochem Photobiophys 3:93–102

Neuman RE, Logan MA (1950) The determination of collagen and elastin in tissues. J Biol Chem 186:549–556

Palcic B, Lam S, Hung J, MacAulay C (1991) Detection and localization of early lung cancer by imaging techniques. Chest 99:742–743

Policard A (1924) Etude sur les aspects offerts par des tumeurs expérimentales axaminées à la lumière de Wood. Compte Rendus Soc Biol 91:1423–1424

Pollack MA, Taylor A, Williams RJ (1942) B vitamins in cancerous tissues. I. Riboflavin. Cancer Res 2:739–743

Pottier R, Laplante JP, Chow YF (1985) Photofrins; a spectral study. Can J Chem 63:1463–1469

Profio AE, Balchum OJ (1985) Fluorescence diagnosis of cancer. In: Kessel D (ed) Methods in porphyrin sensitization. Plenum Press, New York pp 43–52

Profio AE, Carvin MJ, Sarnaik J, Wudl LR (1984) Fluorescence of hematoporphyrin derivative for detection and characterization of tumors. In: Andreoni A, Cubeddu R (eds) Porphyrins in tumor phototherapy. Plenum Press, New York, pp 321–337

Qu J, MacAulay C, Lam S, Palcic B (1994) Laser-induced fluorescence spectroscopy at endoscopy. SPIE Proc 2133:162–169

Ramanujam N, Mitchell M, Mahadevan A, et al. (1994) In vivo diagnosis of cervical intraepithelial neoplasia using 337 nm excited laser induced fluorescence. Proc Natl Acad Sci USA 91:10193–10197

Richards-Kortum R, Rava RP, Petras RE, Fitzmaurice M, Sivak M, Feld M (1991) Spectroscopic diagnosis of colonic dysplasia. Photochem Photobiol 53:777–786

Salmon JM, Kohen E, Viallet P, Hirschberg JG, Wouters AW, Kohen C, Thorell B (1982) Microspectrofluorometric approach to the study of free/bound NAD(P)H ratio as metabolic indicator in various cell types. Photochem Photobiol 36:585–593

Schomacker KT, Frisoli JK, Compton CC, Flotte TJ, Richter JM, Deutsch TF, Nishioka NS (1992) Ultraviolet laser induced fluorescence of colonic polyps. Gastroenterol 104:1155–1160

Schwartz IP, Possoneau JV, Johnson S, Pasta I (1974) The effect of growth conditions on NAD^+ and NADH concentration and the NAD^+/NADH ratio on normal and transformed fibroblasts. J Biol Chem 249:4138–4143

Yashke PN, Bonner RF, Cohen P, Leon MB, Fleisher DE (1989) Laser induced fluorescence spectroscopy may distinguish colon cancer from normal human colon. Gastrointest Endosc 35:184–189

11 Treatment of Ta, T1 Bladder Tumors: Recent Results of the EORTC-GU Group

A.P.M. van der Meijden, R. Sylvester, and Members of the Superficial Bladder Committee[1]

CONTENTS

11.1 Introduction

Superficial bladder cancer is one of the most frequently encountered tumors in urologic practice. The best management at present is a matter of controversy. Transurethral resection (TUR) remains the treatment of choice, but there is a considerable risk of recurrence of tumors thus treated (50%–70%), as well as a lower risk (10%–15%) of progression to muscle-invasive disease (Kurth et al. 1995). Adjuvant treatment has been advocated for 30 years in order to reduce the number of locally recurrent tumors, the incidence of metastatic disease, and the risk of progression to muscle-invasive disease. Numerous randomized trials have been reported in which the effectiveness of multiple intravesically instilled chemo- and immunotherapeutic agents has been investigated. These adjuvant therapies have been investigated for more than 20 years by the

A.P.M. van der Meijden, MD, PhD, Department of Urology, Bosch Medical Center, P.O. Box 90153 5200 ME 's-Hertogenbosch, The Netherlands
R. Sylvester, Data Center EORTC, Brussels, Belgium
1. Members of the Superficial Bladder Committee:
A.P.M. van der Meijden, Bosch Medical Center, 's-Hertogenbosch, The Netherlands
C. Bouffioux, University Hospital Sart Tilman, Liege, Belgium
R. van Velthoven, Institut Bordet, Brussels, Belgium
K.-H. Kurth, Academic Medical Center, Amsterdam, The Netherlands
W. Höltl, Krankenanstalt Rudolfstiftung, Wien, Austria
M. Brausi, B. Ramazzini Hospital, Capri, Italy
D. Mack, Landeskrankenanstalten, Salzburg, Austria

European Organization for Research and Treatment of Cancer (EORTC) Genito-Urinary (GU) Group (Bouffioux 1995). The conclusions drawn from these studies have been:

1. Primary, solitary, low-stage, low-grade tumors should be resected and should not be treated by adjuvant intravesical therapies. One instillation of a chemotherapeutic agent soon after TUR may favorably influence the recurrence rate.
2. TUR alone results in a higher recurrence rate than TUR followed by instillation therapy, whatever drug is used.
3. There are no hard data to demonstrate that a superior drug exists, although bacille Calmette-Guérin (BCG) might be superior for high-risk tumors.
4. It is not possible to conclude from individual trials whether intravesical chemotherapy is able to prevent the occurrence of muscle-invasive disease and metastases.

11.2 Indications

Most of the studies performed so far indicate that a lower recurrence rate is achieved with TUR plus instillation than with TUR alone. However, this does not mean that every patient should be treated with adjuvant therapy or that every patient needs the same treatment schedule or the same chemotherapeutic agent. In several studies performed since the late 1970s, prognostic factors have been used by the EORTC GU Group to calculate the risk of recurrence or invasion in subgroups of patients.

A multivariate analysis (Kurth et al. 1995) revealed that the three most important factors for recurrence are:

1. G grade
2. Prior recurrence rate
3. Number of tumors at diagnosis (multiplicity)

For progression to muscle-invasive disease the three most important factors were found to be:

1. G grade
2. Prior recurrence rate
3. Tumor size

The fact that T category does not appear in these lists does not mean that T category is not an important factor for recurrence or progression to muscle-invasive disease, but simply that it is not among the three most important prognostic factors.

Based on the prognostic factors it is possible to calculate an index reflecting the risk of invasion and/or recurrence. This results in the identification of three prognostic groups: low-risk, intermediate-risk, and high-risk patients. Classification of patients into one of these three categories provides insight into the prognosis of their bladder tumors and enables a drug and a treatment schedule to be chosen in accordance with the needs of the individual patient. It also enables an alternative therapy to be selected at an earlier time, helping to avoid invasion or metastases of bladder cancer.

11.3
Treatment Modalities

Considering the prognostic factors it seems logical from an oncologic point of view to treat low-risk tumors with less aggressive therapy and high-risk tumors with more aggressive high-dose, intensive, or long-term adjuvant intravesical therapy. Before prognostic factors were taken into account, a number of patients were overtreated. The most favorable group certainly does not need 6 months or more of instillation therapy. On the other hand, patients with carcinoma in situ (CIS) or high-risk papillary tumors might need more intensive schedules, higher doses, or long-term adjuvant treatment (Lamm et al. 1995).

About 50% of all patients with superficial tumors belong to the low-risk group, while 30% have an intermediate risk and 20% have a high risk for recurrence and/or progression. In EORTC protocol 30863, patients with relatively low-risk disease were investigated. Patients presenting with a solitary papillary superficial tumor, primary or recurrent, were randomized between one single instillation of 80 mg epirubicin in one arm and a single instillation of sterile water in the other arm after TUR (Oosterlinck et al. 1993). Instillations were administered within 6 h of TUR (early instillation). Analy-sis of 386 patients with a mean follow-up of 16 months showed a recurrence rate for the epirubicin arm of 0.20 while in the sterile water arm a recurrence rate of 0.39 was noted ($P = 0.0001$). In this low-risk population it can be concluded that adjuvant treatment is better than no treatment, and that one early instillation is capable of considerably reducing the recurrence rate.

The next question was whether or not it would be possible to lower the recurrence rate of 0.20 in the epirubicin arm by increasing the number of instillations. The answer was provided by the EORTC Data Center without embarking upon such a study, by looking at the recurrence rates of low-risk patients treated in previous protocols with more than one instillation. Calculations revealed that the patients categorized in the low-risk group showed a recurrence rate of 0.16 after 6 months or 1 year of instillation therapy. This value does not differ significantly from the recurrence rate of 0.20 obtained in protocol 30863. In practice, this means that at least half of our patients, namely those who are at low risk, may benefit from a single early instillation of a chemotherapeutic agent.

At least in this protocol, this new treatment scheme was shown to be the optimal one with regard to efficacy and toxicity, as well as cost. However, more studies are needed to confirm the above results.

11.4
Limitations

Not all patients benefit from intravesical chemo- or immunotherapy. The biologic behavior of certain tumors is not always predictable. More objective studies such as flow cytometry, chromosomal analysis, and nuclear imaging should be included in the analysis of prognostic factors for the individual patient. However, for the present most of the advanced laboratory techniques are not available for use in an average clinical practice. This means that tumor histology, grade, and cytology are the three studies available in most cases.

The use of intravesical therapy is limited by its failure rate. Not every patient benefits from this therapy. A meticulous and frequent follow-up is warranted to estimate the patient benefit. If cytology does not become negative, if CIS does not disappear, or if tumor recurrence is rapid, one may question the efficacy of the therapy. Change to another agent may be considered but aggressive therapy such as cystectomy also remains an option for those patients who do not respond adequately to chemotherapeutic agents or biologic response modifiers such as BCG. Although at present BCG is considered one of the most potent drugs for CIS and papillary tumors, it is clear that BCG is not a panacea for all tumors.

11.5
Endpoints in Ta and T1 Trials

The most important objective in the treatment of malignant disease is to improve survival. Thus survival is the endpoint of most cancer trials. However, Ta and T1 bladder cancer patients may easily survive 10 years or longer because only a small proportion of them will develop muscle-invasive disease. To achieve statistically reliable conclusions based on this endpoint, very large numbers of patients and a very long period of follow-up are needed. Therefore substitute endpoints have been proposed which ultimately may correlate with survival. Such surrogate endpoints are recurrence rate and invasion into the bladder wall (muscle invasion).

After 30 years of intravesical adjuvant therapy a number of questions remain relevant. Does intravesical chemotherapy prevent recurrent tumors in the long run? Does it prevent progression to muscle-invasive disease? Can it prolong survival? These issues are addressed in this chapter. Recent investigations by the EORTC GU Group and the British Medical Research Council (MRC) subgroup on superficial bladder cancer have provided important answers and conclusions.

Over the past 15 years the EORTC Genito-Urinary Tract Cancer Cooperative Group and the Working Party on Superficial Bladder Cancer have carried out a series of randomized phase III studies investigating the prophylactic treatment of Ta, T1 bladder cancer. Many of these trials have demonstrated the advantage of adjuvant prophylactic treatment after TUR as compared to TUR alone in decreasing the recurrence rate or in prolonging the disease-free interval of Ta, T1 bladder cancer patients (OOSTERLINCK et al. 1993; HERR et al. 1987; SCHULMAN et al. 1982; SOLOWAY 1989; KURTH et al. 1984; NEWLING et al. 1995; MRC Working Party on Urological Cancer 1985; 1994; TOLLEY et al. 1988). These trials have failed, however, to demonstrate the definitive superiority of one agent over another (BOUFFIOUX et al. 1992; 1995; DEBRUYNE et al. 1988). There is also no evidence that adjuvant prophylactic treatment is of

long-term benefit as compared to TUR alone in terms of the time to muscle-invasive disease and the duration of survival. These two crucial endpoints cannot generally be assessed in individual trials because only 10%–15% of the patients entered in such trials can be expected to show disease progression. Despite long-term follow-up, individual trials have only a very low statistical power to detect medically plausible differences with respect to muscle invasion and death.

One possible way to overcome this problem is to carry out a combined analysis of completed trials using meta-analysis techniques: a formal statistical methodology used to combine the results of separate but similar studies in a quantitative manner (GELBER and GOLDHIRSCH 1991). The statistical power of the tests used to compare treatments is increased by using all the evidence from a number of randomized trials. These statistical techniques may be used in an attempt to draw conclusions concerning both the short- and the long-term benefits of different therapeutic options in the treatment of Ta, T1 bladder cancer.

Such a combined analysis was performed on EORTC and MRC trials in order to compare (a) the use of adjuvant prophylactic treatment after TUR and (b) TUR alone, with respect to the disease-free interval, time to progression to muscle-invasive disease, and duration of survival (for both all causes of death and death due to malignant disease).

Patients were randomized to receive either adjuvant prophylactic treatment or no adjuvant prophylactic treatment. Upon recurrence the treatment that the patient was initially randomized to receive was generally restarted after TUR, and patients were followed up for further recurrence. However, patients were eventually taken off the original treatment at subsequent recurrences and further treatment was at the investigator's discretion. Hence, for long-term endpoints such as invasion and death, it should be noted that patients in the no adjuvant treatment group are often likely to have received delayed adjuvant treatment. It is not known exactly how many patients never received intravesical treatment. No trials with BCG were included in the analysis because neither the EORTC nor the MRC conducted any trials in which TUR alone was compared with TUR plus BCG. Six randomized controlled trials (four EORTC and two MRC, 2535 patients in total) met the trial selection criteria. The trials included in this analysis are specified in Table 11.1.

For all patients the baseline data collected included the date of randomization, the treatment allo-

Table 11.1. EORTC and MRC trials included in the combined analysis

Trial number	Reference	Drugs used	Total no. of patients	No. of patients in control arm
EORTC trials				
30751	SCHULMAN et al. (1982)	Thiotepa, VM-26	370	124
30791	KURTH et al. (1984)	Adriamycin, Epodyl	443	73
80863	OOSTERLINCK et al. (1993)	Epirubicin	512	255
30781	NEWLING et al. (1995)	Pyridoxine (oral)	291	144
MRC trials				
BSO1	MRC Working Party on Urological Cancer (1985, 1994)	Thiotepa	417	139
BSO3	TOLLEY et al. (1988)	Mitomycin C	502	171
Total			2535	906

Table 11.2. Patient characteristics

	No.	%
Total no. of patients	2535	100
T category		
T0	53	2
Ta	1244	49
Ta or T1	370	15
T1	668	26
>T1	76	3
Unknown	124	5
G grade		
0	53	2
1	1183	47
2	871	34
3	316	12
Unknown	112	4
No. of tumors		
0	14	1
1	1686	67
2–5	590	23
>5	139	5
Unknown	106	4
Size of tumor (cm)		
0	15	1
<2	1155	46
<4	905	36
<6	261	10
≥6	71	3
Unknown	128	5

The criteria of evaluation and definitions of endpoints were:

1. Time to first recurrence (disease-free interval): time from randomization to the date of the first bladder recurrence. Patients without recurrence were censored at the date of the last available follow-up cystoscopy.
2. Time of progression to muscle-invasive disease: time from randomization until progression to stage T2 or higher within the bladder. Patients without muscle invasion were censored at the date of the last available follow-up cystoscopy.
3. Duration of survival (all causes of death): time from randomization until death. Patients still alive or lost to follow-up were censored at the last date they were known to be alive.

The incidence of recurrence and muscle invasion, as well as survival status as of January 1995 and the cause of death, are presented by treatment arm in Table 11.3. These tables are purely descriptive in nature and should not be used for comparative purposes since they do not take into account the duration of follow-up.

11.6
Effect of Prophylactic Treatment

The treatment efficacy comparisons were based on all 2535 patients randomized; however, for 135 patients no follow-up data were available. The median duration of follow-up for the disease-free interval was 4.6 years, for invasion 5.5 years, and for survival 7.8 years, with a maximum of 18.2 years of follow-up. A comparison of disease-free survival in patients who received adjuvant therapy versus

cated, age, sex, tumor status (primary or recurrent), prior recurrence rate, prior intravesical treatment, T category and G grade (local and review pathology), presence of CIS, and the number and size of tumors (Table 11.2).

Stage and grade of the tumors were assessed in accordance with the 1974 TNM Classification, confirmed in 1978 (International Union Against Cancer 1978).

Table 11.3. Treatment results

	Adjuvant treatment		No adjuvant treatment		All patients	
	No.	%	No.	%	No.	%
Total no. of patients	1629	100	906	100	2535	100
Recurrence						
Yes	766	47	477	53	1243	49
No	863	53	429	47	1292	51
Muscle invasion						
Yes	189	12	80	9	269	11
No	1440	88	826	91	2266	89
Survival						
Alive	1001	61	625	69	1626	64
Death	628	39	281	31	909	36
Cause of death						
Malignant disease	229	36	93	33	322	35
Infection	55	9	20	7	75	8
Cardiovascular disease	209	33	101	36	310	34
Other chronic disease	16	3	4	2	20	2
Other	41	7	26	9	67	7
Unknown	78	12	37	13	115	13

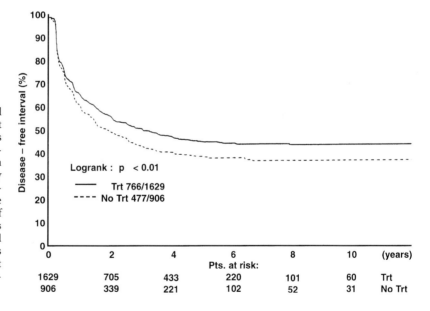

Fig. 11.1. Disease-free interval curves according to the treatment group (adjuvant treatment versus no adjuvant treatment). The difference in the disease-free interval in favor of treatment is statistically significant ($P < 0.01$). It was estimated that the average absolute benefit in terms of the percentage of patients free of disease at 8 years was 8.2% for patients randomized to adjuvant treatment (44.9% vs 36.7% in the no adjuvant treatment arm), with a 95% confidence interval of 3.8%–12.5%

those who received no adjuvant treatment is shown in Fig. 11.1.

The time to progression to muscle-invasive disease in the two treatment groups is given in Fig. 11.2. No statistically significant difference in the time to progression to invasive disease was observed between the two treatment groups, though there was a trend in favor of the patients in no treatment group. There were also no statistically significant differences between the groups with regard to

overall survival (Fig. 11.3) and time to death due to malignant disease. The causes of death are shown in Table 11.3.

The results presented confirm the favorable impact of adjuvant treatment on the disease-free interval in patients with Ta and T1 bladder cancer. The analysis has, however, shown no evidence that prophylactic treatment is of long-term benefit as compared to TUR alone in terms of either time to invasive disease or duration of survival. No signifi-

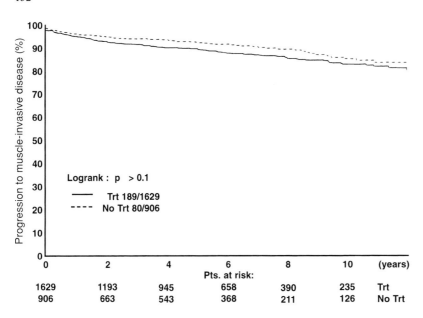

Fig. 11.2. Comparison of time to muscle-invasive disease in patients who received adjuvant therapy versus those who received no adjuvant treatment

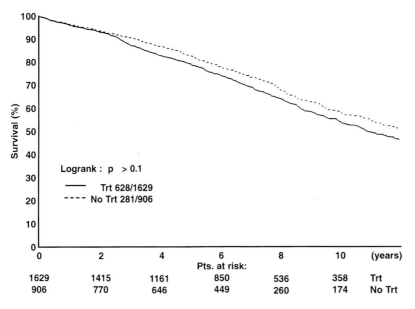

Fig. 11.3. Overall actuarial survival for the group receiving adjuvant therapy as compared to the group of patients who received no adjuvant treatment

cant differences were detected with respect to these endpoints despite the analysis of some 2500 patients and a median follow-up for survival of 7.8 years. The total number of patients with invasion (269) and death due to malignant disease (322) remains relatively small, accounting for only slightly more than 10% of the patients followed up.

The results of this analysis might be criticized from various points of view. First, criticism might be raised as to the heterogeneity of the patients in the trials included in the meta-analysis. These trials

evaluated seven different chemotherapeutic agents and varied according to:

1. Mode of administration (intravesical or oral)
2. Dose
3. Duration of instillations
4. Interval between instillations and duration of treatment

Both patients with primary tumors and patients with recurrences were included, and the trials also varied with regard to the prognosis of the patients included. The use of proper meta-analysis techniques overcomes some of these criticisms by only comparing treatment results within a given trial and then combining the results across all trials to obtain an "average" result.

Second, the long-term results for invasion and survival might be criticized due to the lack of a pure "no treatment arm." As patients taken off the original treatment because of recurrences were then treated at the investigator's discretion, adjuvant prophylactic treatment can only be compared to no treatment or delayed treatment, thus possibly diluting the size of the treatment effect.

11.7
Conclusions

It is concluded that adjuvant prophylactic treatment as given in the studies included in the reported combined analysis has a favorable effect over no (or delayed) prophylactic treatment in terms of the duration of the disease-free interval. Despite a median follow-up of 7.8 years, this short-term effect has not been translated into a long-term benefit. No significant advantage of prophylactic treatment has been shown with respect to the time to progression to muscle-invasive disease or the duration of survival.

Based on this analysis it is clear that while the long-term prognosis of Ta and T1 bladder cancer patients remains good, the use of adjuvant prophylactic treatment has little apparent effect on the long-term results and new modes of treatment should be developed.

References

Bouffioux CH (1995) Intravesical chemoprophylaxis of superficial transitional cell carcinoma of the bladder. When should the drug be given? In: Schroder FH, Richards B (eds) Superficial bladder cancer. Part B. EORTC. Monograph 2. Liss, New York, pp 47–55

Bouffioux CH, Denis L, Oosterlinck W, et al. and members of EORTC-GU Group (1992) Adjuvant chemotherapy of recurrent superficial transitional cell carcinoma: results of EORTC (30782) randomized trial comparing intravesical instillation of thiotepa, doxorubicin and cisplatin. J Urol 148:297–301

Bouffioux CH, Kurth KH, Bono A, Oosterlinck W, Kruger CB, De Pauw M, Sylvester R (1995) Intravesical adjuvant chemotherapy for superficial transitional cell bladder carcinoma: results of 2 European Organization for Research and Treatment of Cancer randomized trials with mitomycin C and doxorubicin comparing early versus delayed instillations and short term versus long term treatment. European Organization for Research and Treatment of Cancer Genito-Urinary Group. J Urol 153:934–941

Debruyne FMJ, Van der Meijden APM, Witjes JA, et al. (1988) BCG versus mitomycin intravesical therapy in superficial bladder cancer (EORTC 30845) Urology 331(Suppl 3):20

Gelber RD, Goldhirsch A (1991) Meta-analysis: the fashion of summing-up evidence. Ann Oncol 2:461–468

Herr HW, Laudone VP, Whitmore WF (1987) An overview of intravesical therapy for superficial bladder tumors. J Urol 138:1363–1368

International Union Against Cancer (1978) TNM classification of malignant tumors, 3rd edn., Geneva

Kurth KH, Tunn A, Ay R, et al. (1984) Adjuvant chemotherapy in superficial transitional cell bladder carcinoma: an EORTC (30791) randomized trial comparing doxorubicin hydrochloride, ethoglucid and TUR alone. J Urol 132:258–262

Kurth KH, Denis L, Bouffioux CH, Sylvester R, Debruijne FMJ, Pavone-Macaluso M, Oosterlinck W (1995) Factors affecting recurrence and progression is superficial bladder tumors. Eur J Cancer 31:1840–1846

Lamm DL, Van der Meijden APM, Akaza H, et al. (1995) Intravesical chemo-and immunotherapy. How do we assess their effectiveness and what are their limitations and uses? Proceedings in the Fourth International Bladder Cancer Consensus Conference. Int J Urol 2(Suppl 2):23–25

MRC Working Party on Urological Cancer (1985) The effect of intravesical thiotepa on the recurrence rate of newly diagnosed superficial bladder cancer: a MRC study. Br J Urol 57:680–685

MRC Working Party on Urological Cancer (1994) The effect of intravesical thiotepa on the tumor recurrence after endoscopic treatment of newly diagnosed superficial bladder cancer. A further report with long term follow-up of a MRC randomized trial. Br J Urol 73:632–638

Newling DWW, Robinson MRG, Smith PH, et al. (1995) Tryptophan metabolites, pyridoxine (vitamin B6) and their influence on the recurrence rate of superficial bladder cancer. Eur Urol 27:110–116

Oosterlinck W, Kurth KH, Schroder F, Bultinck J, Hammond B, Sylvester R and members of EORTC-GU Group (1993) A prospective EORTC-GU Group randomized trial (30863) comparing transurethral resection followed by a single intravesical instillation of epirubicin or water in single stage Ta, T1 papillary carcinoma of the bladder. J Urol 149:749–752

Schulman C, Robinson M, Denis L, et al. (1982) Prophylactic chemotherapy of superficial transitional cell bladder carcinoma: an EORTC (30751) randomized trial comparing thiotepa, an epipodophyllotoxin (VM26) and TUR alone. Eur Urol 8:207–212

Soloway MS (1989) Diagnosis and management of superficial bladder cancer. Semin Surg Oncol 5:247–254

Tolley DA, Hargreave TB, Smith PA, et al. (1988) Effect of intravesical mitomycin C on recurrence of newly diagnosed superficial bladder cancer: interim report from the Medical Research Council subgroup on superficial bladder cancer (Urological Cancer Working Party). BMJ 296:1759–1761

12 Surgical Treatment of Carcinoma of the Bladder: The USC Experience

E.C. Skinner, S. Boyd, G. Lieskovsky, and D.G. Skinner

CONTENTS

12.1
Introduction

Radical cystectomy is currently the treatment of choice for localized high-grade or muscle-invasive carcinoma of the bladder. Over the last 25 years our group has compiled a significant experience in this treatment modality, and we have recently developed a comprehensive database for these patients which has allowed us to study them in more detail.

The indications for radical cystectomy are listed in Table 12.1. Additional indications include patients who have failed definitive radiation therapy (salvage cystectomy) and patients with metastatic carcinoma who require palliative cystectomy because of severe local symptoms. The vast majority of our patients had either documented muscle-invasive transitional cell carcinoma (TCC), high-grade superficially invasive disease (T1), or high-grade superficial disease or carcinoma in situ (CIS) which had not responded to intravesical therapy.

12.2
Patient Population

We reviewed the charts of all patients who underwent radical cysto-prostatectomy or anterior exenteration for cancer between July 1971 and June 1995, and the information was entered into a database. A total of 1131 patients underwent a surgical exploration for bladder cancer during that time. Of those, 242 are excluded from the current discussion, as listed in Table 12.2. This leaves 889 patients with primary TCC, with or without glandular or squamous differentiation, who underwent primary cystectomy with a complete surgical resection.

Of the 889 patients, 80% were male, and 20% female. Their average age was 66 years (range 23–90). Patients were followed up until death or through December, 1995, with a median follow-up for the entire group of 7 years. Prior to 1978 patients routinely received 1600 cGy of external beam radiation therapy in four fractions immediately prior to cystectomy. Since that time patients have generally undergone primary cystectomy with or without adjuvant chemotherapy as indicated. Only 45 of the patients received primary chemotherapy prior to cystectomy.

The type of urinary diversion offered to patients has changed considerably over these 25 years. Prior to 1982 all patients received a standard ileal conduit. From 1982 through 1986 most received a continent Kock ileal reservoir with a cutaneous stoma. From 1986 to the present, the majority of men have opted for an orthotopic ileal reservoir

E.C. Skinner, MD, Assistant Professor, Department of Urology, University of southern California, USC/Norris Comprehensive Cancer Center, 1441 Eastlake Avenue, Los Angeles, CA 90033, USA
S.D. Boyd, MD, Professor, Department of Urology, University of Southern California, USC/Norris Comprehensive Cancer Center, 1441 Eastlake Avenue, Los Angeles, CA 90033, USA
G. Lieskovsky, MD, Department of Urology, University of Southern California, USC/Norris Comprehensive Cancer Center, 1441 Eastlake Avenue, Los Angeles, CA 90033, USA
D.G. Skinner, MD, Professor and Chairman, Department of Urology, University of Southern California, USC/Norris Comprehensive Cancer Center, 1441 Eastlake Avenue, Los Angeles, CA 90033, USA

Table 12.1. Indications for radical cystectomy

1. Muscle-invasive transitional cell carcinoma (stage T2 or above, any grade)
2. High-grade, superficially invasive carcinoma (stage T1, grade 3 or 4)
3. High-grade, superficial disease or carcinoma in situ, failed intravesical therapy (stage Ta, grade 3 or 4, or Tis)
4. Primary adenocarcinoma, squamous cell carcinoma, or sarcoma of the bladder
5. Extensive unresectable low-grade superficial carcinoma (rare)
6. Metastatic disease with severe local symptoms (palliative)

Table 12.2. Patients excluded from analysis

Salvage procedures after failure of definitive radiation	102
Unresectable disease at time of surgery	6
Incomplete resection (gross disease left)	44
Pure adenocarcinoma	25
Pure squamous cell carcinoma	39
Sarcoma or other histology	26
Total	242

Table 12.3. Basic surgical principles of radical cystectomy

Intensive preoperative and postoperative management
Hypotensive anesthesia
Hyperextended supine position – opens the pelvis
Long incision to allow adequate visibility
Extended bilateral pelvic node dissection
Divide lateral and posterior vascular pedicles to bladder first
Careful handling of the urethra if neobladder planned

anastomosed to the urethra. Since 1992 we have also offered orthotopic ileal reservoirs to selected female patients. These changes will be discussed in more detail in Chap. 14.

12.3
Surgical Technique

The details of the surgical technique have been well described and are available elsewhere (SKINNER and LIESKOVSKY, 1988a). Several basic principles have allowed us to improve the safety and efficacy of this surgery. These are listed in Table 12.3. The key is maintaining a standardized, controlled approach, from which we only deviate in unusual cases. This has also allowed us to teach the technique effectively in our training program. The principle of controlling the blood supply prior to manipulating the bladder is a basic concept of cancer surgery, and this is easily followed in the case of radical cystectomy.

Preoperative preparation includes a 1-day bowel preparation with laxatives and oral neomycin and erythromycin base. Any coexisting medical problems, such as cardiac or pulmonary disease, must be optimized prior to surgery. Intravenous hydration is started the night before surgery. Prophylactic antibiotics are generally given on the morning of surgery. If the patient has an indwelling catheter we give sev-

eral preoperative doses of antibiotics beginning on the day of admission.

At surgery we use a hyperextended supine position which effectively opens the pelvis for easier dissection. We also routinely use hypotensive anesthesia, which has allowed us to keep our average blood loss at less than 800 cc. A midline incision is made, extending from the xyphoid to the pubic symphysis.

We begin the surgery with a wide pelvic lymph node dissection, extending from the aortic bifurcation to each genitofemoral nerve laterally, and inferiorly to the femoral canal. A complete dissection of the obturator fossa and the internal and external iliac nodes is included.

We then take down the lateral pedicle to the bladder which includes the anterior branches off the internal iliac artery, including the superior vesicle, uterine, inferior vesicle, and obturator branches. The peritoneum is incised in the cul-de-sac and the space of Denonvillier is developed to the apex of the prostate. The posterior pedicles which extend anteriorly around the rectum to the bladder and prostate are divided. This leaves the specimen attached only by the urethra.

In male patients who are to undergo an orthotopic neobladder we take down the urethra in an identical manner to that used for a radical prostatectomy. We leave eight absorbable sutures circumferentially placed around the urethra to be used in the anastomosis. We do not leave a cuff of apical prostate tissue behind, as up to 40% of patients will be found to have occult prostate cancer.

In female patients the cervix, if present, is circumscribed. The anterior vaginal wall may be excised with the specimen, and this is necessary if the tumor is on the trigone or posterior bladder neck. Otherwise, the plane between the vagina and bladder may be sharply developed down to the urethra. The posterior pedicle is divided along the lateral edge of the vagina rather than along the rectum. If an orthotopic diversion is planned we avoid any dissection over the ventral urethra, and divide the urethra just distal to the bladder neck. In these patients we also place an omental pedicle graft down into the pelvis between the repaired vagina and the neobladder to decrease the risk of fistula formation. If a neobladder is not planned, we excise the entire urethra.

Pelvic drains are placed in all patients, and we have routinely used gastrostomy tube drainage rather than nasogastric tubes, primarily for patient comfort and to decrease any airway compromise. The pelvic drains are left until all catheters are removed, usually at 3 weeks in patients with continent diversion. The gastrostomy tube is removed after 6 or 7 days, or when the patient is tolerating a diet.

We have not routinely performed nerve-sparing cystectomy in our patients, for several reasons. Because of the older age group of the male patients, the expected efficacy of a nerve-sparing approach is less than 50%. We are also concerned about the potential for increasing the risk of local recurrence in a disease in which such a recurrence inevitably leads to an early death. The nerve-sparing approach clearly requires considerable manipulation of the bladder and prostate before division of the posterior vascular pedicles, and limits the surgical margins at the level of the bladder neck and trigone. However, we have occasionally offered nerve-sparing surgery to young men (>50) with high-grade Ta or T1 disease, or CIS only.

12.4
Postoperative Management and Early Complications

Patients are observed in the intensive care unit for the first 24 h. Fluid requirements may be high the first day, but are kept carefully balanced thereafter. Prophylaxis against venous thrombosis is important, since pulmonary embolus is potentially a major cause of postoperative morbidity and mortality. We use oral warfarin therapy beginning in the recovery room, managed to keep the therapeutic ratio between 1.5 and 2.0 times normal. Other alternatives include subcutaneous heparin sulfate and serial pneumatic compression stockings. We also now routinely use H_2 blockers to protect against stomach ulcers, and continued prophylactic antibiotics throughout the hospital stay and for the first 2 weeks at home. Postoperative ileus usually resolves within 3–5 days, but occasionally is prolonged. Laboratory values (complete blood count and electrolytes) are checked daily for the first several days, and then every other day thereafter.

Table 12.4. Most common early complications

Major	Minor
Hemorrhage	Prolonged ileus
Pulmonary embolus	Arrhythmias
Urinary leakage/abscess	Wound infection
Myocardial infarction/severe cardiac problems	Urinary tract infections
Sepsis	
Pneumonia	
Gastrointestinal bleed	

Operative mortality in the entire group was only 2%. The two most frequent causes of death were sepsis and pulmonary embolus. Average hospital stay was 11 days. Early complications, including both major and minor complications, were seen in 27% of the patients, with about half of these having significant major complications requiring reoperation or extension of the postoperative stay. The most common major and minor complications are listed in Table 12.4. We did not observe any difference in early morbidity or mortality when patients received preoperative low-dose radiation therapy, chemotherapy, or combined treatment. In addition, the use of continent forms of urinary diversion has not resulted in any increase in early complication rates or length of stay.

The availability of skilled interventional radiologists has markedly decreased the need for reoperation in these patients over the past 10 years. An undrained urine leak or intra-abdominal abscess can nearly always be managed with percutaneous drainage, with the addition of nephrostomy tube drainage if needed in the former case.

Late complications (after 3 months) do vary with the type of urinary diversion used. The type and incidence of diversion-related late complications are discussed in detail in Chap. 14. Those not related to the diversion include bowel obstruction, incisional hernia, and occasional lower extremity edema. The overall incidence of these late complications in our experience has been under 5%. In general, however, postoperative recovery may be prolonged, with many patients not regaining preoperative strength and vigor for 2–3 months or more.

12.5
USC Studies of Cystectomy Patients

The completion of the database for these patients, along with collaboration with our basic science colleagues, has allowed us to make some important contributions to our understanding of bladder cancer and the role of surgery. These studies will be briefly reviewed here.

12.5.1
Role of Preoperative Radiation

In an early study by SKINNER and LIESKOVSKY, comparison of 81 patients who received 1600 cGy preoperatively (1971–78) with 248 patients who had cystectomy alone with or without postoperative chemotherapy showed no advantage of the preoperative radiation therapy in terms of time to recurrence or overall survival (SKINNER and LIESKOVSKY 1988b). Since then we have abandoned routine preoperative radiation therapy, unless there has been gross tumor spill (e.g., with an open cystotomy or incomplete partial cystectomy).

12.5.2
Cystectomy for Low Pathologic Stage Disease

There is controversy regarding the optimal treatment for patients with low-stage bladder cancer who are at high risk for progression (high-grade stage Ta or T1, or CIS). Many series on conservative treatment of superficial disease combine patients with low-grade and patients with high-grade disease. ZHANG and colleagues looked specifically at 23 patients with grade III, T1 disease treated with transurethral rsection and bacille Calmette-Guérin, and noted a 74% local recurrence rate and 35% progression to muscle invasion or metastatic disease. Only four of the seven patients who underwent delayed cystectomy were salvaged, and a total of 5 of the 23 patients (22%) died of cancer. With longer follow-up these recurrence and progression rates will likely increase (ZHANG et al. 1995).

We reviewed 218 patients in our database who were treated with early cystectomy for high-grade T1 or Ta disease or CIS. The majority had failed an initial trial with intravesical chemotherapy or immunotherapy. As shown in Table 12.5, we found that 36% were clinically understaged, and 9% had positive nodes. Five-year survival for the entire group of patients was 75% (Table 12.5), and for patients with confirmed superficial disease survival increased to more than 80%.

Early cystectomy becomes more attractive with the advances made in the safety of surgery and the

Table 12.5. Results of cystectomy for clinical stage Ta or T1 high-grade TCC or CIS

Pathologic stage	No. of patients	Five-year survival
P0–Pa	13	100%
P1–PIS	126	83%
P2	20	75%
P3A	17	54%
P3B	11	55%
P4A	11	62%
N+, any P stage	20	42%
Total	218	75%

options for urinary tract reconstruction. Based on these results, we continue to recommend early cystectomy for patients with known high-risk tumors, rather than trying multiple courses of intravesical therapy.

12.5.3
Risk of Urethral Recurrence Following Orthotopic Urinary Diversion

Many in the urologic community were initially worried about the long-term risks of urethral recurrence in men undergoing orthotopic urinary diversion after cystectomy for bladder cancer. We and others expected to see up to 10% of our patients develop urethral recurrence, and all patients were advised of this risk. However, as our experience with orthotopic diversion increased, we noted that we were seeing very few urethral recurrences, especially in those men who would have been considered high risk (i.e., those with extensive CIS or prostatic stroma invasion by TCC on the final pathology specimen). Using our database, Tarter and colleagues retrospectively compared 176 men with orthotopic diversion with 262 who underwent diversion to the skin without simultaneous urethrectomy. They found only 4% of the orthotopic patients had evidence of urethral recurrence by 3 years, compared with 10% of the latter group. More importantly, in patients with documented CIS of the prostatic urethra, 24% of 51 patients in the nonorthotopic group developed urethral recurrence, compared to only $1/_{24}$ (<5%) of the Kock to urethra group. This suggests a possible protective effect of urine passing through the intact urethra, or perhaps some effect of the bowel mucosa. Studies are currently underway to try to delineate these findings further (TARTER et al. 1996).

12.5.4
Survival in Patients with Positive Lymph Nodes

There has also been controversy regarding the role of an extended lymph node dissection in invasive bladder cancer, and the appropriateness of proceeding with cystectomy in the face of obvious or microscopic positive nodes. Various investigators have reported 5-year survival rates in node-positive patients ranging from 0% to 29%. Radical cystectomy at USC has always included a wide pelvic node dissection, and we have routinely completed the cystectomy even in the presence of positive nodes whenever possible.

In 1993 LERNER et al. updated our results in 132 patients with positive nodes (22% of the total patients up to 1989), with a median follow-up of 5.5 years. Sixty-seven percent of the patients had developed recurrent disease, most within 3 years of cystectomy. Initial pelvic recurrence was seen in only 11%. The actuarial 5-year survival rate at 5 years was 29%.

Both the number of positive nodes and the pathologic stage of the primary tumor were predictors of survival. Among patients with five or fewer nodes, recurrence-free survival increased to 35%. Patients with primary tumors confined to the bladder had a 50% estimated 5-year survival, with 80% of those with P1 or PIS disease surviving 5 years (Fig 12.1) (LERNER et al, 1993). Therefore, we continue to advocate an aggressive surgical approach for patients with disease localized to the pelvis, even in the presence of nodal metastases.

12.5.5
Role of Adjuvant Chemotherapy

Between 1980 and 1988 a randomized study was completed comparing early adjuvant chemotherapy

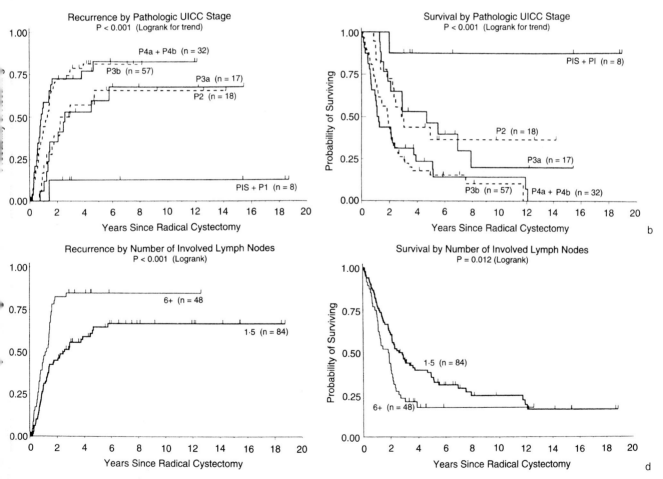

Fig. 12.1a–d. Probability of recurrence and survival in patients with positive lymph nodes, by pathologic stage of primary tumor (**a, b**) and by number of positive lymph nodes (**c, d**). (From LERNER et al. 1993)

with delayed therapy for documented recurrence. Patients eligible for this study all had initial complete resection, and had pathologic stage P3a, P3b, or P4 disease, or positive lymph nodes with any primary tumor stage. Ninety-one patients were randomized to receive four cycles of PAC (cisplatin, doxorubicin, and cyclophosphamide). Forty-four patients were randomized to receive chemotherapy. Eleven patients (25%) subsequently refused any chemotherapy, 21 (48%) received the full four cycles, and 12 (27%) received one to three cycles. All of these were included in the chemotherapy group in an intent-to-treat analysis. Forty-seven were randomized to the observation (delayed treatment) arm.

At 3 years there was a significant delay in time to progression in the adjuvant therapy group, with 70% of the patients in the chemotherapy arm free of recurrence compared to 46% of the observation patients. Median survival was 4.3 years compared to 2.6

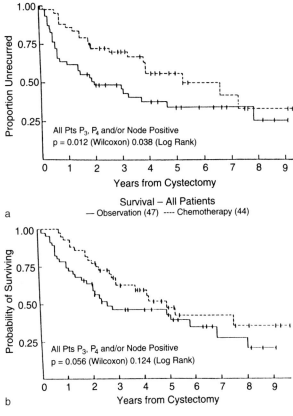

Fig. 12.2. Time to recurrence (**a**) and overall survival (**b**) in 91 patients randomized to receive surgery alone (observation) or surgery plus adjuvant chemotherapy (chemotherapy). (From Skinner et al. 1991)

years, respectively (Fig. 12.2). When stratified for nodal status, patients with negative nodes or only one microscopically positive node seemed to receive the most benefit from adjuvant therapy (Skinner et al. 1991). Although this study has received considerable criticism for methodological problems, the results have been confirmed by at least one other randomized trial (Stockle et al. 1995).

12.5.6
Genetic Studies

For many years the basic scientists studying bladder cancer at USC have had access to tissue and blood samples from patients undergoing cystectomy, and the database has allowed us to put together scientific observations with clinical outcome. The results of these studies are reported in much more detail in Chaps. 3 and 4.

An initial study resulting from this collaboration looking at the loss of chromosomal heterozygosity showed that there were important differences in the genetic alterations seen with superficial tumors compared with invasive tumors and CIS (Tsai et al, 1990). Chromosome 9 alterations were seen commonly in both superficial and invasive tumors, while chromosome 17 alterations were seen only in invasive tumors and CIS. The latter is thought to reflect the impact of the tumor suppressor gene, *p53*, which resides on chromosome 17.

Further studies at USC of *p53* mutations through sequencing and immuno-histochemical techniques have documented a dramatic impact on prognosis of the *p53* status of a particular tumor. The incidence of *p53* alterations increases with higher disease stage. However, at every pathologic stage of disease, the presence of an altered p53 protein correlated with a much higher risk of recurrence and death from bladder cancer. This effect was most dramatically seen with organ-confined disease (Fig. 12.3). Even with deep muscle invasion (stage p3a), patients with normal p53 had a less than 20% rate of progression at 5 years, compared to 71% for those with altered p53 (Esrig et al. 1994).

Recently, focus has been shifted to the p21 protein, a down-stream protein which can "salvage" the repair mechanisms effected by a normal *p53* in the presence of *p53* mutations. The patients with altered *p53* who have intact p21 activity have survival stage-for-stage which is identical to patients with a normal *p53* (Stein et al. 1996).

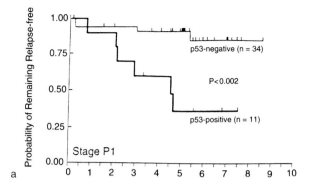

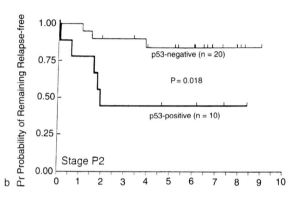

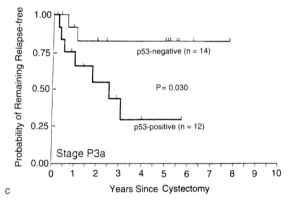

Fig. 12.3a–c. Probability of relapse-free survival in 243 patients with bladder cancer by status of p53 (negative = wild type, positive = altered protein) and pathologic stage. (From ESRIG et al. 1994)

12.6
Future Research

These studies have opened the way for further work to understand the genetics of invasive bladder can-cer, and perhaps to customize current therapy decisions and design gene therapy in the future. Studies are also underway to examine other aspects of tumor biology which might also be amenable to intervention, such as angiogenesis pathways. Finally, it is clear that any future clinical studies of bladder cancer treatment need to take into consideration the genetic status of tumors in individual patients.

References

Esrig D, Elmajian D, Groshen S, et al. (1994) Accumulation of nuclear p53 and tumor progression in bladder cancer. N Engl J Med 331:1259–1264

Esrig D, Groshen S, Freeman JA, et al. (1996) Impact of p53 alterations on the chemosensitivity of bladder cancer: results of a randomized trial of adjuvant chemotherapy. Abstract. J Urol 155:664A

Lerner SP, Skinner DG, Lieskovsky G, et al. (1993) The rationale for en bloc pelvic lymph node dissection for bladder cancer patients with nodal metastases: long-term results. J Urol 149:758–765

Skinner DG, Lieskovsky G (1988a) Technique of radical cystectomy. In: Skinner DG, Lieskovsky G (eds) Diagnosis and management of genitourinary cancer. Saunders, Philadelphia, pp 607–621

Skinner DG, Lieskovsky G (1988b) Contemporary cystectomy with pelvic node dissection compared to peroperative radiation therapy plus cystectomy in management of invasive bladder cancer. J Urol 131:1069–1072

Skinner DG, Daniels JR, Russell CA, et al. (1991) The role of adjuvant chemotherapy following cystectomy for invasive bladder cancer: a prospective comparative trial. J Urol 145:459–467

Stein JP, Ginsberg DA, Grossfeld GD, et al. (1996) The effect of p21 expression on tumor progression in p53 altered bladder cancer. Abstract. J Urol 155:628A

Stockle M, Meyenburg W, Wellek S, et al. (1995) Adjuvant polychemotherapy of nonorgan-confined bladder cancer after radical cystectomy revisited: long-term results of a controlled prospective study and further clinical experience. J Urol 153:47–52

Tarter TH, Freeman JA, Chen S-C, Groshen S, Skinner DG (1996) Urethral recurrence after cystectomy for cancer in the era of orthotopic bladder replacement. Abstract. J Urol 155:691A

Tsai YC, Nichols PW, Hiti AL, et al. (1990) Allelic losses of chromosomes 9, 11, and 17 in human bladder cancer. Cancer Res 50:44–47

Zhang G, Uke E, Sharer W, et al. (1995) Reassessment of conservative management for stage T1N0M0 transitional cell carcinoma of the bladder. Abstract. J Urol 153:232A

13 Prophylactic Urethrectomy: When and How?

H. Van Poppel and L. Baert

13.1 Introduction

Transitional cell carcinoma primarily involves the bladder, but quite frequently it also involves either simultaneously or metachronously the urothelium of the urethra and the upper urinary tract (MELICOW 1945). When urethral involvement is not recognized at the time of cystectomy, or occurs during the follow-up after cystectomy, it leads to urethral tumor recurrence.

It is not very clear why the urethra can be a site of recurrence of transitional cell carcinoma. Transitional cell carcinoma is a multifocal disease and one presumes that the urothelial lining of the pyelocaliceal system, the ureters, and the proximal urethra are at equal risk to the bladder because of a uniform sensitivity of the urothelium to neo-plastic stimuli. However, the penile urethra is not lined by a transitional cell epithelium but by a stratified columnar epithelium. The fossa navicularis and glandular urethra are covered by a stratified squamous epithelium (CARROLL and DIXON 1992). One might speculate that pseudo-columnar or squamous epithelium should not be sensitive to the same carcinogenic stimuli as affect the transitional cell epithelium. Nevertheless, the occurrence of transitional cell carcinoma in the anterior and glandular urethra is well recognized. Therefore, seeding and implantation of exfoliated cells, as well as lymphatic spread, has been proposed to explain urethral recurrence although definitive proof of the existence of this pathway is yet to be presented (STAMS et al. 1974). It is conceivable that the traumatized urothelium is more susceptible to the implantation of malignant cells, with a similar susceptibility to carcinogens.

It is clear that involvement of the upper urinary tract by transitional cell carcinoma after cystectomy is not treated by nephrourethrectomy before its diagnosis is confirmed. Even in the presence of positive cytology without proven transitional cell carcinoma, one will attempt conservative measures (e.g., BCG) or just follow the patient closely. In the urethra the problem is different. Indeed, recently, bladder substitution procedures in male patients have become routine practice and, therefore, the presence of the urethra may be of importance in the overall management of the patient. In females, the urethra is almost always removed during cystectomy and the expertise with bladder substitution in women is still limited to major and highly specialized medical centers. However, when the urethra remains intact without function after cystoprostatectomy, it presents a risk as a likely site for tumor recurrence. So, even when no tumor is obviously present, but no continent reconstruction is contemplated, resection of the urethra seems indicated.

H. Van Poppel, MD, PhD, Professor, Department of Urology, UZ Gasthuisberg, University Hospitals of Leuven, Herestraat 49, B-3000 Leuven, Belgium
L. Baert, MD, PhD, Professor and Chairman, Department of Urology, UZ Gasthuisberg, University Hospitals of Leuven, Herestraat 49, B-3000 Leuven, Belgium and Clinical Professor, Department of Urology and Radiation Oncology, University of Southern California, USC/Norris Comprehensive Cancer Center, 1441 Eastlake Avenue, Los Angeles, CA 90033, USA

13.2
Arguments in Favor of Prophylactic Urethrectomy

Historically, simultaneous removal of the male urethra during cystoprostatectomy was advisable in patients with: (a) diffuse carcinoma in situ, (b) multifocal tumors, and (c) tumors invading the trigone, the bladder neck, and the prostatic urethra (SAROSDY 1992). The main reason why urethrectomy at the time of, or shortly after, exenterative surgery has been advocated is the risk of subsequent urethral recurrence, which is estimated to range from 4% to 19% (Table 13.1).

The large variation in the reported incidence of urethral recurrence is due to several factors. All reported treatment results and the incidence of tumor recurrence have been based on retrospective reviews of patients who were selected for surgical treatment according to different criteria. Some investigators have routinely performed prophylactic urethrectomies, while others have felt that this procedure is rarely indicated. The incidences of carcinoma in situ and of bladder neck or prostatic urethral involvement have not been comparable in the reported studies. Duration of follow-up has also varied widely, and it is obvious that the longer patients survive

Table 13.1. Incidence (%) of urethral involvement after radical cystoprostatectomy

Author	Total number	Percentage with urethral involvement
CORDONNIER and SPJUT (1962)	174	4.02
ASHWORTH (1956)	1307	4.1
LEVINSON et al. (1990)	200	4.8
ZABBO and MONTIE (1984)	119	5.9
SCHELLHAMMER and WHITMORE (1976a)	461	7
STÖCKLE et al. (1990)	273	9.2
RAZ et al. (1978)	17	9.7
HICKEY et al. (1986)	75	10
POOLE-WILSON and BARNARD (1971)	33	12
CLARK (1984)	84	13
FAYSAL (1980)	90	13.5
HARDEMAN and SOLOWAY (1990)	102	15
BEAHRS et al. (1984)	358	17
GOWING (1960)	33	18
HENDRY et al. (1974)	101	19
VAN POPPEL and BAERT (1991a)	114	19

(because their primary tumor is cured), the more chance they have of developing a urethral recurrence (STÖCKLE et al. 1990). This is clearly demonstrated by the findings of BEAHRS et al. (1984) and CLARK (1984), who showed a doubling in the incidence of recurrence at 10 years following surgery (17% and 27%, respectively), as compared to the recurrence rate at 5 years after surgery (9% and 13%, respectively). Some investigators have considered only clinically overt urethral recurrence, while others have also included patients with carcinoma in situ or even those with urothelial dysplasia. In an unselected patient population the incidence of urethral recurrence after cystoprostatectomy is estimated to be about 10%.

A second argument in favor of prophylactic urethrectomy at the time of cystoprostatectomy is the fact that delayed urethrectomy can be a very tedious procedure. Some investigators dispute the above statement, reporting complete removal of the urethra through a simple perineal incision (AHLERING and LIESKOVSKY 1988). Quite often, however, a small portion of the urethra, which eventually may become a site of clinical recurrence, is unavoidably left behind. The risk of incomplete resection of the urethra is increased even when only a few weeks have elapsed between the cystoprostatectomy and the secondary urethrectomy (STÖCKLE et al. 1990). Along with other authors, we therefore advocate secondary urethrectomy using a combined perineal and suprapubic approach, which provides the best possible chance of removing the entire urethra (BEEBE and PERSKY 1969).

The third reason for performing a primary urethrectomy is that, when a urethral recurrence is detected, the lesion is often locally advanced or has already metastasized (CLARK 1984). Not all authors, however, have the same pessimistic opinion about metachronous urethral transitional cell carcinoma that has been discovered by clinical examination, or urethral brushings, or washing cytology and endoscopy. A few authors have reported excellent treatment results after therapeutic urethrectomy for urethral recurrence detected during a very strict follow-up schedule (BEAHRS et al. 1984; HARDEMAN and SOLOWAY 1990). They showed that the treatment outcome in patients with urethral recurrence was very similar to that in patients who had undergone prophylactic urethrectomy (FAYSAL 1980). Most authors, however, have reported that the prognosis of a metachronous transitional cell carcinoma in the urethra is poor, often because of early hematogenous spread through the corpus spongiosum. Many patients with urethral recurrence will already have metastatic disease at diagnosis. The presence of metastatic disease will determine survival. This is particularly obvious when the survival of patients with urethral recurrence is reviewed. As in most other series, all of our patients diagnosed with a urethral recurrence died (CARPENTER 1989; CLARK 1984; CORDONNIER and SPJUT 1962; HENDRY et al. 1974; POOLE-WILSON and BARNARD 1971; RICHIE and SKINNER 1978; SCHELLHAMMER and WHITMORE 1976a; STÖCKLE et al. 1990; VAN POPPEL and BAERT 1991a; ZABBO and MONTIE 1984).

A fourth argument in favor of primary urethrectomy, therefore, could be the risk of poor patient compliance, since lifelong follow-up is necessary to diagnose an early urethral recurrence. Although most recurrences in the urethra occur early following radical surgery, they have been reported to occur up to 20 years after cystoprostatectomy (SCHELLHAMMER and WHITMORE 1976a). Since the number of urethral recurrences increases with time, patients who have an intact urethra should be informed of the need for a strict follow-up schedule.

The final argument favoring simultaneous urethrectomy is that an in continuity resection of the bladder and urethra better satisfies the requirements of oncological surgery by avoiding the transection of a tumor-containing viscus (SCHELLHAMMER and WHITMORE 1976a).

13.3
Arguments Against Prophylactic Urethrectomy

Despite the above arguments, urologists appear willing to find reasons why only a minority of their patients should undergo simultaneous urethrectomy. Some urologists fear extending the time of an already long radical procedure in order to perform simultaneous urethrectomy. Also, as already mentioned, some authors are convinced that a urethral recurrence can be detected early, permitting effective therapy.

A more important factor in the last 10 years has been availability of procedures for successful reconstruction of the urinary tract, with the use of bladder substitution techniques that are now routinely applied. A new trend towards potency-sparing cystectomy is also going against urethrectomy since it has been shown that resection of the urethra significantly impairs erectile function (KITAMURA et al. 1987; SCHLEGEL and WALSH 1987; TOMIC and

SJÖDIN 1992). Finally, it has been reported that simultaneous urethrectomy increases morbidity (FRAZIER et al. 1992) or gives rise to perineal discomfort and delayed mobilization and, therefore, carries an increased risk of thromboembolic complications (COUTTS et al. 1985).

13.4
Risk Factors for Urethral Recurrence

The arguments for and against the use of prophylactic urethrectomy restructure the question of its absolute and relative indications. It is, therefore, important to identify preoperatively those patients who are at risk of developing a recurrence in the remnant urethra. There is, at present, no prospective study on the use of prophylactic urethrectomy. The risk factors for metachronous urethral tumor recurrence have been identified on the basis of retrospective clinical studies.

Some authors have clearly demonstrated that the incidence of urethral recurrence after cystoprostatectomy is much higher (reaching 37%) in patients presenting with invasion of the bladder neck or of the prostatic urethra (FAYSAL 1980; HARDEMAN and SOLOWAY 1990). A much lower incidence of recurrence – 3%–7% has been found in patients with multiple tumors or those with multifocal carcinoma in situ (LEVINSON et al. 1990; HARDEMAN and SOLOWAY 1990; FAYSAL 1980; CLARK 1984). This incidence is only slightly higher than that reported after cystectomy for solitary tumors (3%–4%) (CLARK 1984; HARDEMAN and SOLOWAY 1990).

It is not disputed that prostate involvement is the most important factor predicting subsequent urethral recurrence. The resultant risk is much higher than that accompanying the presence of carcinoma in situ or multifocal tumors. It should, however, be clear that all patients with transitional cell carcinoma of the bladder are at risk for tumor recurrence in the remnant urethra.

Involvement of the urothelium of the ureters has also been described to be an indicator for eventual urethral involvement (FAYSAL 1980). It is, therefore, important to perform frozen sections of the ureters during surgery in order to recognize carcinoma in situ of the ureters. A survey on the possible effect of cigarette smoking on the incidence of bladder recurrences after partial cystectomy and on urethral recurrences after radical cystectomy showed that smokers present more often with urethral recurrence (CARPENTER 1989). This finding suggested the necessity of a simultaneous urethrectomy in patients who smoke.

13.5
Preoperative Assessment of the Prostatic Urethra

When the urethral involvement is the determining factor in the decision to perform a prophylactic urethrectomy or to leave the urethra behind (to be used for a bladder replacement), the assessment of the prostatic urethra before surgery is of great importance. The need for accurate sampling of the prostatic urethra was first suggested by prostate mapping studies which showed malignant changes in the prostatic urethra in 50%–70% of patients (MAHADEVIA et al. 1986; GU and LIANG 1991). In another extensive study, 4-mm step sections were performed in 84 cystoprostatectomy specimens. Thirty-six patients (43%) were found to have transitional cell carcinoma of the prostate. Of this group, 94% had prostatic urethra involvement and 6% had a normal prostatic urethra, but transitional cell carcinoma was present in the periurethral structures. This high incidence of involvement suggests that increasing the intensiveness of the search for prostate invasion results in an increased incidence of this diagnosis (WOOD et al. 1989a).

Not all patterns of prostatic urethral involvement present an equal risk for recurrence. The tumor involvement can be limited to the urethra or to the epithelium of the periurethral ducts or it may include the prostatic stroma. Duct and stromal invasion has been the most striking prognostic factor for subsequent urethral recurrence. Therefore, preoperative staging with transurethral and transrectal biopsy techniques has been advocated (HARDEMAN and SOLOWAY 1990).

Although several authors have confirmed the necessity of a thorough precystectomy assessment or rigorous screening of the prostatic urethra, the technique of endoscopic assessment has not always been described in detail. Random biopsies, either cold punch or resection biopsies of the prostatic urothelium, have been proposed. It is now agreed that transurethral resection biopsy of the prostate is necessary in order to screen for prostatic involvement and that this biopsy should be routinely performed in patients with bladder cancer. In most patients the prostatic urethra will appear normal cystoscopically. Concerning the extent of prostatic resection, it has been pointed out that an insufficient

or limited transurethral resection biopsy of the prostatic urethra could fail to detect prostatic involvement. Therefore, extensive biopsies are now advocated (WOOD et al. 1989b; HARDEMAN et al. 1988). Such biopsies will help to correctly diagnose the prostatic involvement in 90% of patients, as was shown in a detailed examination of cystoprostatectomy specimens (WOOD 1989b). This problem was further studied by SAKOMOTO et al. (1993), and it was demonstrated that transurethral resection random biopsies of the prostate may frequently fail to detect prostatic invasion. An appropriate transurethral resection sampling of the prostatic tissue at the 5 and 7 o'clock positions of the verumontanum portion proved necessary to detect any prostatic duct and acinar involvement.

13.6
Indications for Prophylactic Urethrectomy

The above-mentioned findings and considerations have certainly influenced the evolution of opinions as to the appropriate indications for prophylactic urethrectomy. In the past some authors have advocated routine urethrectomy in all patients undergoing cystectomy irrespective of the stage or the type of bladder tumor (CLARK 1984; STAMS 1974), whereas others have favored simultaneous urethrectomy only in the presence of the classical risk factors, including: (a) multifocal tumors, (b) the presence of diffuse carcinoma in situ, (c) involvement of the ureters, and (d) bladder neck or prostatic urethra involvement (SCHELLHAMMER and WHITMORE 1976a; RICHIE and SKINNER 1978; ZABBO and MONTIE 1984; POOLE-WILSON and BARNARD 1971; STÖCKLE et al. 1990; VAN POPPEL et al. 1989). One investigator has recommended routine cystoprostatourethrectomy in cigarette smokers (CARPENTER 1989). Another group of authors, however, have limited the indication for urethrectomy at the time of cystectomy to patients with tumor invasion of the urethra or carcinoma in situ in the prostatic urethra, demonstrated either by endoscopy or by pathologic examination of urothelial biopsies (AHLERING et al. 1984; BEAHRS et al. 1984; FAYSAL 1980; HARDEMAN and SOLOWAY 1990; RAZ et al. 1978; HICKEY et al. 1986; LEVINSON et al. 1990; LILIEN and CAMEY 1984; WOOD et al. 1989a). These authors consider multifocal disease and diffuse carcinoma in situ as low-risk factors for urethral recurrence when the prostate is not involved, and feel that such patients can be safely managed with close follow-up and without prophylactic urethrectomy.

Controversy remains as to the importance of the distinction between different depths of prostatic invasion. Some authors have strongly advocated prophylactic urethrectomy regardless of the depth of prostatic involvement (ZINCKE et al. 1985), while others have further studied this indication and recommended radical cystoprostatectomy and urethrectomy for those patients with ductal and stromal invasion only (MATZKIN et al. 1991).

All these considerations have led to consensus on at least one matter, namely that the urethra should never be left behind in patients with tumors invading the stroma of the prostate or when tumor is present in the membranous, bulbar, or pendular urethra (SKINNER et al. 1995).

13.7
Follow-up of the Remnant Urethra

As mentioned above, the entire urethra is at risk for tumor recurrence in all stages of transitional cell carcinoma of the bladder. Therefore, when the urethra is not removed and not used for a substitute bladder, it should be followed very closely.

Urethroscopy and urethrography are not very well suited for the early detection of urethral recurrence (RICHIE and SKINNER 1978). When these examinations are positive, patients will often have symptoms such as urethral discharge and are likely to have either locally advanced or metastatic disease. It has been shown that cytologic studies on urethral washings are very reliable, with high sensitivity and high specificity (HICKEY et al. 1986; WOLINSKA et al. 1977).

Urethral washing with 20 cc of saline is performed through a 10- to 14-French catheter inserted to the level of the proximal end of the urethra. The procedure is simple and not very uncomfortable for the patient (HICKEY et al. 1986). The use of lubricants is not allowed since they could render the cytologic interpretation more difficult. This cytologic examination has to be repeated every 6 months (or even more frequently in high-risk patients) for an indefinite period since urethral recurrences can occur after many years (SAROSDY 1992).

Some authors have relied on flow cytometry of urethral washings for early detection of urethral recurrence. It is clear that this method only detects nondiploid recurrent tumors (HERMANSEN et al. 1988).

No strict follow-up protocol has been proposed for patients who have undergone a bladder substitution. The reliability of the first voided urine cytology in evaluating urethral recurrence after bladder substitution is not known, and no prospective study is available on which mode of assessment is appropriate. Flexible endoscopy and cytology are the only diagnostic modalities available in this group of patients.

13.8
Technique of Prophylactic Urethrectomy

A prophylactic urethrectomy is recommended when a patient presents a urethral transitional cell carcinoma in conjunction with bladder cancer, when the patient is at high risk for urethral recurrence, or when the urethra is not used for bladder substitution.

13.8.1
Classical Urethrectomy

An incontinuity resection of the urethra en bloc with the bladder is advisable in order to avoid tumor cell spillage and local implantation (SCHELLHAMMER and WHITMORE 1976a). It is important to perform a total urethrectomy, including the urethral meatus and fossa navicularis. Although the glandular urethra is not lined by transitional cell epithelium but by stratified squamous epithelium, several authors have found recurrent tumors at this level after subtotal urethrectomy (SCHELLHAMMER and WHITMORE 1976b; ZABBO and MONTIE 1984; JOHNSON and GUINN 1970; CORDONNIER and SPJUT 1962; STÖCKLE et al. 1990; SAROSDY 1992; SHINKA et al. 1989). The classical technique, with the patient placed in a lithotomy position, uses a perineal incision (either transverse or longitudinal) through the bulbo-cavernosus muscle for the separation of corpus spongiosum and corpora cavernosa. The proximal urethra is dissected free after ligation of both bulbar arteries. The glandular urethra is removed through a second incision (WHITMORE and MOUNT 1970; BRENDLER et al. 1990). A suction drain and a compressive dressing are used in order to prevent bleeding and hematoma formation, which may lead to foreskin necrosis. Some authors recommend a resection of the foreskin at the time of urethrectomy (CLARK 1984).

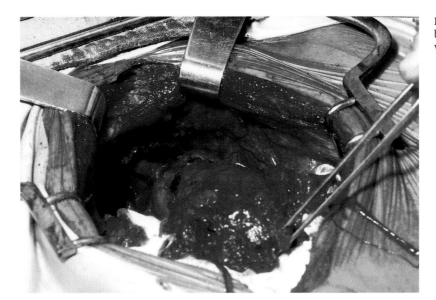

Fig. 13.1. Dissection of the membranous urethra through the pelvic floor

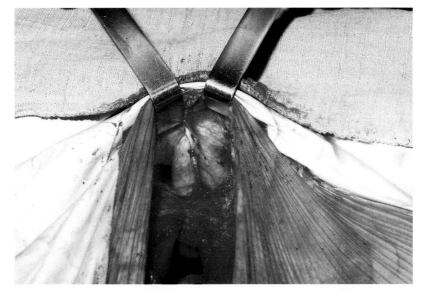

Fig. 13.2. Prepubic exposure of the penile shaft

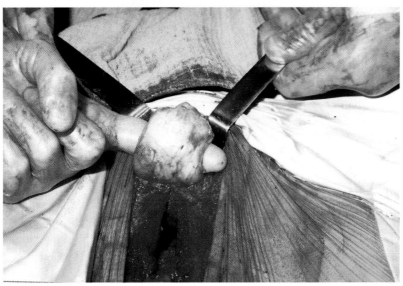

Fig. 13.3. Inversion of the penis dissected upon Buck's fascia

Fig. 13.4. Separation of the corpus spongiosum from the corpora cavernosa

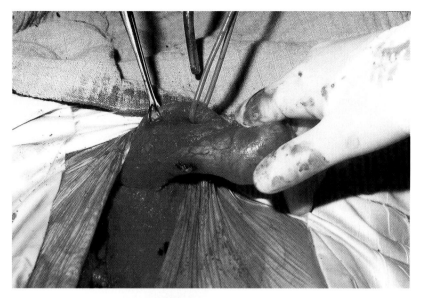

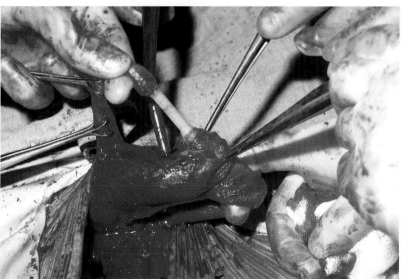

Fig. 13.5. Transection of the glandular urethra

The main disadvantages of perineal urethrectomy are the postoperative perineal pain and discomfort, hindering mobilization and increasing the risk of thromboembolic complications. Another disadvantage is the time required for the urethrectomy on top of an already time-consuming operation.

13.8.2
Prepubic Urethrectomy

In order to circumvent the above-mentioned disadvantages of classical urethrectomy, we have developed an alternative technique, namely prepubic urethrectomy. This technique has been extensively described (VAN POPPEL et al. 1989; VAN POPPEL and BAERT 1991a,b; VAN POPPEL 1993) and videotaped (VAN POPPEL and BAERT 1995). Since our report, one other author has described his experience with the use of this technique (ZHANG 1995).

After the radical cystoprostatovesiculectomy, the membranous urethra is dissected bluntly around the indwelling bladder catheter through the pelvic floor to reach the bulbous urethra. Only gentle traction is applied on the cystoprostatectomy specimen in order to avoid avulsion of the unsupported membranous urethra (Fig. 13.1). An attempt is made to get as

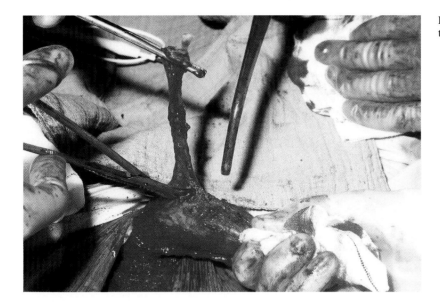

Fig. 13.6. Dissection of the urethra towards the bladder

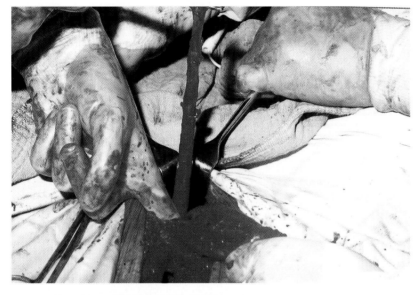

Fig. 13.7. Blunt dissection of the bulbous urethra

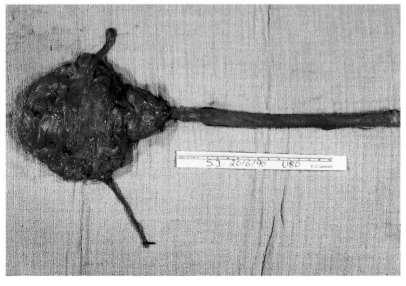

Fig. 13.8. In continuity removed cystoprostatourethrectomy specimen

far distally as possible in order to facilitate the prepubic dissection that is now started.

The skin incision can be extended caudally to the penile base. The penile shaft is exposed and encircled as close as possible to Buck's fascia (Fig. 13.2). It is then easy to bring the penile body into the hypogastric incision by simple traction and progressive invagination of the penile skin (Fig. 13.3). A longitudinal incision of Buck's fascia along the spongiocavernosus adhesion line is made and the corpus spongiosum is sharply dissected free of the corpora cavernosa (Fig. 13.4). The urethra is further dissected towards the glans penis. Inversion of the glans sometimes enables resection of the entire glandular urethra and urethral meatus (Fig. 13.5). Otherwise, a classical resection using a glandular incision is performed.

Then, the urethra is further separated from the corpus cavernosum towards the bladder (Fig. 13.6). This is accomplished with sharp and blunt dissection. The urethra is now nearly completely mobilized, but still fixed in its posterior aspect where the bulbar arteries enter the corpus spongiosum. Either these vessels can be visualized and clipped before transection, or they can be bluntly separated (Fig. 13.7). In the latter situation, hemorrhage can be stopped by the application of a short-lasting pressure or by oversewing. When the cystoprostatourethrectomy specimen is removed (Fig. 13.8), the pelvic floor is closed from the retropubic space with two or three large needle stitches that assure appropriate hemostasis. In the prepubic space, a suction drain is inserted that is immediately activated after eversion of the penile body into its skin and closure of the prepubic subcutaneous adipose tissue. The penis is wrapped in a compressive dressing that is not removed before 48 h, at which time the suction drain can also be withdrawn.

We started to perform prepubic urethrectomies in 1985 and have now used this technique in more than 180 patients. In three patients the prepubic hemostasis was a problem, as a consequence of which supplementary blood transfusion was given. Subcutaneous penile hematoma occurred when we first started to use the procedure, and required secondary foreskin resection. Scrotal hematoma is not uncommon but does not need any measures other than the postoperative application of a suspensory. On average the procedure takes no more than 15 min to complete. There is no need to place the patient in the lithotomy position, thus saving time and decreasing thromboembolic problems in the lower limbs.

Another disadvantage of the classical perineal urethrectomy, namely the perineal pain and discomfort, is avoided with the use of this new approach. Patients can be readily mobilized after 2 or 3 days, which also can be important in decreasing the number of postoperative venous complications after this type of pelvic surgery.

Urethrectomy via the prepubic approach is in our view an easy and safe way of achieving a simultaneous prophylactic urethrectomy. This is confirmed by the limited experience with this technique reported in another center (Zhang 1995).

13.9
Conclusions

All patients who undergo cystoprostatectomy for transitional cell carcinoma of the bladder are at risk of subsequent urethral recurrence. This risk is minimal (less than 4%) for some of these patients, e.g., those with low-grade muscle-invading solitary tumors located far from the bladder neck and without the presence of carcinoma in situ. In other patients the risk is unacceptably high (40%) and will necessitate simultaneous urethrectomy. This is needed in patients with high-grade tumors with invasion of the prostatic stroma. Most candidates for cystoprostatectomy have an intermediate risk of recurrence. Such patients are: (a) those with diffuse carcinoma in situ of the bladder, (b) those with carcinoma in situ or ductal invasion of the prostatic urethra, and (c) those with invasion of the bladder neck and involvement of the ureters. Before planning appropriate surgery, the tumor staging should include systematic biopsies of the bladder and transurethral resection biopsies at the verumontanum level of the prostatic urethra at the 5 and 7 o'clock positions.

One should remember that urethral recurrence may depend on the selection of the procedure to be performed by the urologist. The patient must be well informed about the risk of developing tumor recurrence with the use of a particular procedure in a specific clinical situation. Prophylactic urethrectomy is the only way to eliminate the mucosa with preclinical malignant changes. If such changes are not yet present, urethrectomy will eliminate an area of subsequent potential malignancy.

In patients with high-stage transitional cell carcinoma of the bladder, the 5-year survival is poor and urethral recurrence has often not had the time to occur. However, patients with lower stage disease whose urethra is left behind can survive long enough for the expression of urethral recurrence. It is very likely that this problem will increase in the future since more cystectomies will be curative and survival will be considerably longer.

Therefore, we are convinced that there is significant danger in the current tendency to offer patients bladder substitution after cystectomy. This attitude may increase the risk of urethral recurrence, which frequently necessitates secondary salvage surgery. The urologist who has to motivate the patient for cystectomy should not feel more comfortable when proposing a bladder replacement. It should be remembered that ileal conduit diversions are still well tolerated and that continent diversions in the umbilicus are an excellent and safe alternative. In the future, potency-sparing urethrectomy may gain in popularity and decrease the reluctance to perform prophylactic urethrectomy.

We believe that patients who are not considered for bladder replacement procedures should always undergo prophylactic urethrectomy. For those who could be candidates for bladder substitution, the advantages of the latter will have to be weighed against the risk of tumor recurrence. All patients in whom the urethra is retained after cystoprostatectomy will need lifelong follow-up with endoscopy and cytology.

Prepubic urethrectomy is an easy and safe procedure that entails less operative and postoperative morbidity than classical perineal urethrectomy.

Acknowledgements. We would like to express our gratitude to Agnes Goethuys for word processing and typing the manuscript.

References

Ahlering TE, Lieskovsky G (1988) Surgical treatment of urethral cancer in the male patient. In: Skinner D, Lieskovsky G (eds) Diagnosis and management of genitourinary cancer. Saunders, Philadelphia, pp 622–633

Ahlering TE, Lieskovsky G, Skinner DG (1984) Indications for urethrectomy in men undergoing single stage radical cystectomy for bladder cancer. J Urol 131:657–659

Ashworth A (1956) Papillomatosis of the urethra. Br J Urol 28:3–13

Beahrs JR, Fleming TR, Zincke H (1984) Risk of local urethral recurrence after radical cystectomy for bladder cancer. J Urol 131:264–266

Beebe DS, Persky L (1969) Urethral extension of vesical neoplasm. Surgery 66:687–690

Brendler LB, Schlegel PN, Walsh PC (1990) Urethrectomy with preservation of potency. J Urol 144:270–273

Carpenter AA (1989) Clinical experience with transitional cell carcinoma of bladder with special reference to smoking. J Urol 141:527–528

Carroll PR, Dixon CM (1992) Surgical anatomy of the male and female urethra. Urol Clin North Am 19:339–346

Clark PB (1984) Urethral carcinoma after cystectomy: the case for routine urethrectomy. J Urol (Paris) 90:173–179

Cordonnier JJ, Spjut HJ (1962) Urethral occurrence of bladder carcinoma following cystectomy. J Urol 87:398–403

Coutts AG, Grigor KM, Fowler JW (1985) Urethral dysplasia and bladder cancer in cystectomy specimens. Br J Urol 57:535–538

Faysal MH (1980) Urethrectomy in men with transitional cell carcinoma of the bladder. Urology 16:23–26

Frazier HA, Robertson JE, Paulson DF (1992) Complications of radical cystectomy and urinary diversion: a retrospective review of 675 cases in 2 decades. J Urol 148:1401–1405

Gowing NFC (1960) Urethral carcinoma associated with cancer of the bladder. Br J Urol 32:428–439

Gu F-L, Liang Y-C (1991) Involvement of prostatic urethra and duct in bladder cancer. A report of 40 cases of prostate mapping. Prog Clin Biol Res 370:169–178

Hardeman SW, Soloway MS (1990) Urethral recurrence following radical cystectomy. J Urol 144:666–669

Hardeman SW, Perry A, Soloway MS (1988) Transitional cell carcinoma of the prostate following intravesical therapy for transitional cell carcinoma of the bladder. J Urol 140:289–291

Hendry WF, Gowing NF, Wallace DM (1974) Surgical treatment of urethral tumors associated with bladder cancer. Proc R Soc Med 67:304–307

Hermansen DK, Badalament RA, Whitmore JF (1988) Detection of carcinoma in the postcystectomy urethral remnant by flow cytometric analysis. J Urol 139:304–306

Hickey DP, Soloway MS, Murphy WM (1986) Selective urethrectomy following cystoprostatectomy for bladder cancer. J Urol 136:828–830

Johnson DE, Guinn GA (1970) Surgical management of urethral carcinoma occurring after cystectomy. J Urol 103:314–316

Kitamura T, Moriyama N, Shibamoto K, Ueki T, Fukutani K, Kawabe K, Aso Y (1987) Urethrectomy is harmful for preserving potency after radical cystectomy. Urol Int 42:375–379

Levinson AK, Johnson DE, Wishnow KI (1990) Indications for urethrectomy in an area of continent urinary diversion. J Urol 144:73–75

Lilien OM, Camey M (1984) 25 years experience with replacement of the human bladder (Camey procedure). J Urol 132:886–891

Mahadevia PS, Koss LG, Irene JT (1986) Prostatic involvement in bladder cancer. Prostate mapping in 20 cystoprostatectomy specimens. Cancer 58:2096–2120

Matzkin H, Soloway MS, Hardeman S (1991) Transitional cell carcinoma of the prostate. J Urol 146:1207–1212

Melicow MM (1945) Tumors of the urinary drainage tract: urothelial tumors. J Urol 54:186–193

Poole-Wilson DS, Barnard RJ (1971) Total cystectomy for bladder tumors. Br J Urol 43:16–24

Raz S, McLorie G, Johnson S, Skinner DG (1978) Management of the urethra in patients undergoing radical cystectomy for bladder carcinoma. J Urol 120:298–300

Richie JP, Skinner DG (1978) Carcinoma in situ of the urethra associated with bladder carcinoma: the role of urethrectomy. J Urol 119:80–81

Sakomoto N, Tsuneyoshi M, Naito S, Kumazawa J (1993) An adequate sampling of the prostate to identify prostatic involvement by urothelial carcinoma in bladder cancer patients. J Urol 149:318–321

Sarosdy MF (1992) Management of the male urethra after cystectomy for bladder cancer. Urol Clin North Am 19:391–396

Schellhammer PF, Whitmore JF Jr (1976a) TCC of the urethra in men having cystectomy for bladder cancer. J Urol 115:56–60

Schellhammer PF, Whitmore JF Jr (1976b) Urethral meatal carcinoma following cystourethrectomy for bladder carcinoma. J Urol 115:61–64

Schlegel PN, Walsh PC (1987) Neuroanatomical approach to radical cystoprostatectomy with preservation of sexual function. J Urol 138:1402–1406

Shinka I, Uekado Y, Aoshi H (1989) Urethral remnant tumors following simultaneous partial urethrectomy and cystectomy for bladder cancer. J Urol 142:983–986

Skinner DG, Studer UE, Okada K, et al. (1995) Which patients are suitable for continent diversion or bladder substitution following cystectomy or other definitive local treatment? Int J Urol 2(Suppl 2):105–122

Stams UK, Gursel EO, Veenema RJ (1974) Prophylactic urethrectomy in male patients with bladder cancer. J Urol 111:177–179

Stöckle M, Gökcebay E, Riedmiller H, Hohenfellner R (1990) Urethral tumor recurrences after radical cystoprostatectomy: the case for primary cystoprostatourethrectomy? J Urol 143:41–43

Tomic R, Sjödin JG (1992) Sexual function in men after radical cystectomy with or without urethrectomy. Scand J Urol Nephrol 26:127–129

Van Poppel H (1993) Prophylactic prepubic urethrectomy strongly recommended. Urology Times 21:13

Van Poppel H, Baert L (1991a) Innovative technique for urethrectomy. Prepubic technique and results in 41 patients. Prog Clin Biol Res 370:147–150

Van Poppel H, Baert L (1991b) Präpubische Urethrektomie. Akt Urol 22:I–X

Van Poppel H, Baert L (1995) Prepubic urethrectomy. Video Urology Times, Advanstar Communications, New York, vol 8, program 1

Van Poppel H, Strobbe E, Baert L (1989) Prepubic urethrectomy. J Urol 142:1536–1537

Whitmore WF Jr, Mount BM (1970) A technique of urethrectomy in the male. Surg Gynecol Obstet 131:303

Wolinska WH, Melamed MR, Schellhammer PF (1977) Urethral cytology following cystectomy for bladder carcinoma. Am J Surg Pathol 1:225

Wood DP Jr, Montie JE, Pontes JE, Vanderbrug-Medendorp S, Levin HS (1989a) Transitional cell carcinoma of the prostate in cystoprostatectomy specimens removed for bladder cancer. J Urol 141:346–349

Wood DP Jr, Montie JE, Pontes JE, Levins HS (1989b) Identification of transitional cell carcinoma of the prostate in bladder cancer patients: a prospective study. J Urol 142:83–86

Zabbo A, Montie JE (1984) Management of the urethra in men undergoing radical cystectomy for bladder cancer. J Urol 131:267–268

Zhang GK (1995) Simultaneous prepubic urethrectomy with radical cystectomy for transitional cell carcinoma of the bladder. J Urol 153(Suppl):213A

Zincke H, Utz DC, Farrow GM (1985) Review of Mayo Clinic experience with carcinoma in situ. Urology 26(Suppl 4):39–43

14 Orthotopic Reconstruction Following Radical Cystectomy: the USC Experience

J.P. Stein and S.D. Boyd

CONTENTS

14.1
Introduction

Since the early 1900s, innovative surgeons have persistently pursued how best to replace the original bladder removed for either benign or malignant disease. As we enter the mid 1990s, the ultimate goals of lower urinary tract reconstruction have become more than simply the diversion of urine and protection of the upper urinary tract. Contemporary objectives of lower urinary tract reconstruction should include elimination of the need for a cutaneous stoma, urostomy appliance, or intermittent catheterization, while maintaining a more natural voiding pattern allowing volitional micturition through the intact native urethra. The advances in urinary diversion have been made in an effort to provide patients with a more normal life-style and an improved self-image following removal of the bladder.

14.2
History of Urinary Diversion

The first reported urinary diversion into a segment of a bowel was by Simon in 1852. He performed a ureterosigmoidostomy in a patient with exstrophy of the bladder by bringing the ureters, with the use of needles and large suture, and creating fistulas into the rectum. Although the patient subsequently died of sepsis, this marked the first reported attempt at urinary diversion. The following 100 years were marked by a continued search for better ways to reconstruct the lower urinary tract. Subsequently, over the past 45 years, the evolution of urinary diversion has developed along three distinct paths: a noncontinent cutaneous form of urinary diversion, a continent cutaneous form of urinary diversion, and most recently an orthotopic form of diversion to the native urethra.

Beginning in 1950, Bricker introduced the ileal conduit which established a reliable form of urinary diversion. This form of diversion remained, even until the early 1990s, the "gold standard" to which all other forms of urinary diversion were compared. Concurrent with Bricker's introduction of the ileal conduit, Gilchrist independently reported on the concept of a continent cutaneous form of diversion, utilizing the ileocecal valve as the continence mechanism, and the distal ileum as a catheterizable stoma (Gilchrist et al. 1950). However, Gilchrist's ileocecal reservoir garnered little support, in contrast to the Bricker ileal conduit.

The concept of a continent cutaneous diversion (introduced by Gilchrist) was eventually popularized by Kock (1971) and Skinner et al. (1984a,b) and revolutionized lower urinary tract reconstruction to a continent cutaneous form. This form of urinary diversion required catheterization of an abdominal

J.P. Stein, MD, Assistant Professor, Department of Urology, University of Southern California, USC/Norris Comprehensive Cancer Center, 1441 Eastlake Avenue, Los Angeles, CA 90033, USA
S.D. Boyd, MD, Professor, Department of Urology, University of Southern California, USC/Norris Comprehensive Cancer Center, 1441 Eastlake Avenue, Los Angeles, CA 90033, USA

stoma, and relieved patients from the need for an external urostomy appliance. CAMEY and LE DUC (1979) reported their pioneering work with orthotopic neobladders to the native urethra. This was a substantial accomplishment which demonstrated the feasibility of lower urinary tract reconstruction to the urethra, with reasonable continence rates, in carefully selected male patients following cystectomy.

Since 1982, we have been dedicated to the continued improvement of lower urinary tract reconstruction in patients undergoing cystectomy. We have employed the continent ileal reservoir as described by KOCK et al. (1982) as the primary form of urinary diversion at the University of Southern California. With increasing experience, and the aim of improving this form of diversion, we have subsequently attempted to reduce the incidence of late complications and the need for reoperation. During this period we have continuously updated our results and reported the complications associated with the KOCK ileal reservoir. Subsequently, a series of modifications have been made to continually refine this form of diversion (LIESKOVSKY et al. 1991; GINSBERG et al. 1991; STEIN et al. 1994a, 1996a).

From 1982 to 1986, the continent cutaneous KOCK ileal reservoir became the procedure of choice in all patients requiring urinary diversion at our institution (SKINNER et al. 1984a,b). Subsequently, in 1986 we began to perform orthotopic reconstruction to the urethra in carefully selected male patients undergoing cystectomy. Our initial clinical and functional experience with this form of diversion in men was excellent (SKINNER et al. 1991).

Prior to 1990, orthotopic reconstruction was limited to male patients and considered to be contraindicated in the female subject undergoing cystectomy. Reasons for this included the fact that the urethra was routinely removed during cystectomy as it was thought necessary to provide an adequate surgical cancer margin. In addition, it was believed that the female patient would be unable to maintain a continence mechanism if orthotopic diversion was performed. However, based on an extensive pathologic review of female cystectomy specimens removed for transitional cell carcinoma of the bladder, it was shown that the urethra could be safely preserved in the majority of women undergoing cystectomy (STEIN et al. 1995). This pathologic study provided criteria which helped to safely identify appropriate female candidates for orthotopic diversion following cystectomy for bladder cancer. In addition, anatomic dissection of the female pelvis

has provided a better understanding of the continence mechanism in women (COLLESELLI et al. 1994). These important discoveries provided a foundation on which to offer women lower urinary tract reconstruction to the urethra. Our initial clinical experience in women demonstrated outstanding functional results (STEIN et al. 1994b). This achievement marked another significant step forward in the evolution of lower urinary tract reconstruction.

It is our firm opinion that the orthotopic neobladder currently represents the most ideal form of urinary diversion available today, and should now be considered the gold standard with which other forms of diversion are compared. In fact, in 1993 at the Fourth International Consensus Conference on Bladder Cancer in Antwerp, Belgium, consensus opinion was that in the properly selected bladder cancer patient, urinary reconstruction to the urethra is the procedure of choice in most centers worldwide. We believe that this form of diversion can be safely performed on more than 90% of men, and nearly 80% of women undergoing cystectomy for bladder cancer. This chapter will focus on the indications for and the technique of orthotopic KOCK ileal neobladder construction in male and female patients.

14.3
Orthotopic Urinary Diversion

Although the optimal bladder substitute remains to be developed, the orthotopic neobladder most closely resembles the original bladder in both location and function. The orthotopic neobladder eliminates the need for a cutaneous stoma or for a cutaneous collection device. This form of diversion relies upon the intact rhabdosphincter continence mechanism, eliminating the need for the often plagued efferent continence mechanism of most continent cutaneous reservoirs and the need for intermittent catheterization. The majority of patients undergoing orthotopic reconstruction are continent and able to void to completion without intermittent catheterization (STEIN et al. 1994b; ELMAJIAN et al. 1996).

All orthotopic urinary reservoirs should have a large capacity, have a low pressure, be nonrefluxing (protecting the upper urinary tract), and have a nonabsorptive surface that allows the patient to volitionally void per urethra. The continence mechanism is maintained by the external striated sphincter muscle (rhabdosphincter muscle) of the pelvic floor, while voiding is accomplished by concomitantly increasing intra-abdominal pressure (Valsalva), along with relaxation of the pelvic floor.

The literature is replete with opinions on which bowel segment and/or reservoir is optimal for construction of the orthotopic neobladder. The small intestine, terminal ileum and cecum, large intestine, or a combination of these have all been utilized to construct a urinary reservoir. It is the authors' preference to use the small bowel (ileal reservoir) as it appears to offer less contractility, greater compliance, and improved continence rates compared with large bowel neobladders. There is evidence to suggest that the muscular-walled colon is less compliant than ileum, and may store urine at higher pressures than ileum (HINMAN 1988). In addition, several clinical studies have demonstrated that the urodynamic characteristics of ileum appear to be superior to those of the colon. BERGLUND et al. (1987) showed the superiority of ileal versus cecal reservoirs. LYTTON and GREEN (1989) demonstrated that ileal reservoirs accommodate larger volumes at lower pressures than right colon reservoirs. DAVIDSSON et al. (1992) evaluated the urodynamic profiles of neobladders constructed from ileum and the right colon and found that although the volume capacity was similar, the pressure at maximum capacity was much lower with the ileal reservoir. Furthermore, mucosal atrophy with less reabsorption of urinary constituents appears to be more reliable in small bowel than in large bowel reservoirs (NORLEN and TRASTI 1978). For these reasons, in addition to the ease with which the small bowel can be surgically manipulated, it is the author's preference to use ileum in the construction of the reservoir.

14.4
Patient Selection for Orthotopic Diversion

Two important criteria must be fulfilled when considering any patient for orthotopic lower urinary tract reconstruction. First, the external sphincter must remain intact to provide continence and to allow for conscious voiding per urethra. Second, the cancer operation must under no circumstance be compromised by the orthotopic reconstruction at the urethroenteric anastomosis, the retained urethra, or the surgical margins. If these two criteria can be safely met, the patient may then be considered for orthotopic reconstruction following cystectomy.

In general, all cystectomy patients are potential candidates for orthotopic reconstruction. Contraindications to this form of diversion include: a noncompliant patient with a mental or physical handicap, impaired renal function with a serum creatinine greater than 2.5 mg/dl, and the presence of inflammatory bowel disease. However, patients with an elevated serum creatinine secondary to ureteral obstruction should have the upper urinary tract decompressed (via a percutaneous nephrostomy tube) in order to recover and determine the baseline renal function prior to reconstruction.

Although controversy exists on the subject, patient age alone should not be a contraindication to orthotopic diversion. A differentiation between physiologic and chronological age should be made. In a recent review of 295 male patients undergoing orthotopic diversion, the overall percentage of patients with good and satisfactory continence was statistically similar in older (greater than 70 years) and younger age groups ($P < 0.001$) (ELMAJIAN et al. 1996). These findings underscore the notion that patient age alone should not preclude orthotopic urinary diversion. Furthermore, body habitus has not been an excluding factor for orthotopic reconstruction. In fact, the obese patient is an ideal candidate for this form of diversion, as the need to negotiate a thick abdominal wall for intermittent catheterization is eliminated.

14.4.1
Orthotopic Reconstruction

Most patients requiring lower urinary tract reconstruction undergo cystectomy for transitional cell carcinoma of the bladder. Despite progress in chemotherapeutic regimens, radical cystectomy remains the treatment of choice for high-grade, invasive bladder cancer. Furthermore, as the incidence of bladder cancer rises, patients requiring cystectomy and subsequent urinary diversion for transitional cell carcinoma of the bladder can also be expected to increase in number.

It is critical that when orthotopic diversion is performed in patients undergoing cystectomy for a pelvic malignancy, it is ensured that the cancer operation is not compromised by the reconstruction. Of particular concern is the risk of a urethral or pelvic recurrence. Urethral recurrences occur in approximately 10% of all male patients following cystectomy for bladder cancer (FREEMAN et al.

1994). The greatest risk factor for a urethral recurrence in men is tumor involvement of the prostate in the radical cystectomy specimen; prostatic stromal invasion is more ominous than either ductal or mucosal involvement. Traditionally, patients in whom orthotopic diversion was considered underwent precystectomy evaluation of the prostate by means of a deep transurethral biopsy at the 5 and 7 o'clock positions adjacent to the verumontanum. These sites have been found to be the most common areas of involvement of the prostatic urethra, ducts, and stroma with transitional cell carcinoma (SAKAMOTO et al. 1993; WOOD et al. 1989). Patients found to have any prostatic tumor involvement were previously excluded from orthotopic diversion, and routinely underwent urethrectomy at the time of cystectomy.

sion) in male patients include the presence of carcinoma in situ or overt carcinoma of the urethra as demonstrated on frozen section analysis of the distal cystectomy margin. En bloc urethrectomy is performed at the time of cystectomy in those male patients with preoperatively known urethral tumor involvement. A delayed urethrectomy is performed in patients with prostatic stromal tumor involvement demonstrated on final pathologic examination of the cystectomy specimen who have undergone a cutaneous form of urinary diversion. Those patients with prostatic stromal invasion demonstrated in the cystectomy specimen who have undergone an orthotopic diversion are closely monitored postoperatively with urethral wash cytology in order to detect recurrence. Given these criteria, approximately 90% of men can be considered appropriate candidates for orthotopic reconstruction.

14.4.2
Indications and Contraindications for Orthotopic Reconstruction

Recently, as a result of an extensive review of our experience with continent urinary diversion, we have modified the exclusion criteria for orthotopic diversion in men. The incidence of urethral recurrence in male patients undergoing an orthotopic form of diversion was evaluated, and compared to the urethral recurrence rate in men undergoing a cutaneous form of diversion (FREEMAN et al. 1996). Interestingly, the estimated probability of a urethral recurrence at 5 years following cystectomy was significantly increased in patients with a cutaneous diversion, compared to those undergoing an orthotopic diversion (10% vs 4% respectively, $P = 0.015$). Even those patients with high-risk pathology (prostate involvement) diverted by means of an orthotopic diversion had a lower probability of urethral recurrence compared to patients with similar pathology undergoing a nonorthotopic form of diversion: the 5-year risk of recurrence was 5% in the orthotopic group as against 24% in the nonorthotopic group ($P = 0.05$). Although the exact etiology is unknown, it has been suggested that the orthotopic form of diversion may provide some protective effect; for example it is possible that the mucous or some other secretory product of the intestine prevents the development of cancer in the retained urethra (CROCITTO et al. 1994).

We believe that the current indications for urethrectomy (contraindication to orthotopic diver-

14.4.3
Orthotopic Diversion in Females

Concerns regarding orthotopic diversion in the female patient arose from the fact that the pathologic implications of sparing the female urethra had not been well studied previously. In addition, urethrectomy was routinely performed in women without sound scientific data. In contrast to male patients with prostatic tumor involvement, risk factors that may predict urethral tumor involvement in women have only recently been identified. In an extensive retrospective analysis of female cystectomy specimens we have helped to define the incidence of carcinoma involving the bladder neck and urethra in women with transitional cell carcinoma of the bladder (STEIN et al. 1995). This pathologic study identified important risk factors for urethral tumor involvement which could help in the selection of appropriate female candidates for orthotopic reconstruction following cystectomy for bladder cancer.

A total of 67 consecutive female cystectomy specimens, removed for biopsy-proven transitional cell carcinoma of the bladder between 1982 and 1990, were pathologically reviewed (STEIN et al. 1995). Histologic evidence of tumor (carcinoma in situ or invasive carcinoma) involving the urethra was present in nine patients (13%). In all cases, tumor was confined to the proximal or mid-urethra, and in no patient was the distal urethra involved with tumor. Most importantly, all patients with carcinoma involving the urethra had concomitant tumor involving the bladder neck. A total of 17 patients (25%) had tumor involvement of the bladder neck; all patients with uninvolved bladder neck also had an uninvolved urethra. Tumors involving the bladder neck and urethra tended to be high grade and high stage, and to be more commonly associated with lymph node-positive disease.

In addition to bladder neck involvement, anterior vaginal wall involvement with tumor was also identified as a major risk factor for urethral tumor involvement. All patients with tumor extending into the anterior vaginal wall were also found to have bladder neck involvement, and 50% of these specimens also demonstrated urethral tumor involvement. However, if the bladder neck was histologically free of tumor, then no patient demonstrated any urethral or vaginal wall tumor.

This pathologic study suggested that female patients without tumor involvement of the bladder neck and anterior vaginal wall may be considered appropriate candidates for orthotopic diversion to the urethra. However, not all specimens with tumor involving the bladder neck demonstrated urethral tumor involvement. This is an important issue because although bladder neck involvement with tumor is a risk factor for urethral tumor involvement, approximately 50% of patients with tumor involving the bladder neck will have a urethra free of tumor. In this situation, the patient could be considered an appropriate candidate for orthotopic diversion: although bladder neck involvement with tumor is a risk factor for concomitant urethral tumor involvement, pathologic evaluation of the proximal urethra appears to be the most critical determinant for orthotopic diversion.

These pathologic guidelines were subsequently evaluated prospectively in 29 consecutive women undergoing orthotopic diversion following cystectomy for transitional cell carcinoma of the bladder (STEIN et al. 1996b). All 23 cystectomy specimens without tumor involvement of the bladder neck were also free of tumor at the urethra. A total of six specimens demonstrated tumor involvement at the bladder neck, with only one of these six specimens demonstrating any urethral tumor involvement. These results appear to support our previously established pathologic criteria which identify the bladder neck as a risk factor for urethral tumor involvement.

In addition, in this series of 29 women undergoing orthotopic reconstruction we found intraoperative frozen section analysis of the distal surgical margin (proximal urethra) to be an accurate and reliable method to evaluate the proximal urethra for urethral tumor involvement. Intraoperative frozen section analysis accurately evaluated the proximal urethra in all 29 specimens removed for transitional cell carcinoma, including 28 cases without tumor involvement and the one specimen with carcinoma in situ involving the proximal urethra. In all 29 cases the frozen section result was correctly confirmed on permanent section of the cystectomy specimen. Currently, we believe that intraoperative frozen section of the proximal urethra is the most decisive method to determine whether a female patient is an appropriate candidate for orthotopic diversion. Furthermore, because of the risk of injuring the continence mechanism through preoperative biopsy of the bladder neck and urethra, and the availability of a method confirmed to reliably evaluate the proximal urethra (intraoperatively), we now rely upon intraoperative frozen section analysis of the proximal urethra for proper patient selection among women in whom orthotopic lower urinary tract reconstruction is being considered. With proper selection, at least 80% of women undergoing cystectomy may be regarded as appropriate candidates for orthotopic reconstruction.

14.5
Preoperative Evaluation

As a result of our recent analysis of orthotopic reconstruction in men and women we have modified our recommendations with regard to preoperative evaluation. Preoperative biopsies of the prostate in men and of the bladder neck in women are no longer performed. Orthotopic diversion to the urethra is contraindicated only in patients with overt transitional cell carcinoma of the urethral margin on intraoperative frozen section analysis.

All patients in whom orthotopic diversion is considered should understand that if the bladder or pelvic tumor involves the proximal urethra (diagnosed on intraoperative frozen section analysis), then lower urinary tract reconstruction should not be performed. In this case, a cutaneous form of diversion should be performed based upon the patient's desires, as discussed preoperatively. It is therefore important to involve the enterostomal therapy nurse in the preoperative period, to mark for an appropriate cutaneous stoma, and to instruct the patient how to catheterize should it be necessary.

14.6
Radical Cystectomy

The technique of en bloc radical cystectomy (anterior exenteration) with bilateral pelvic lymphadenectomy has remained standard and is described elsewhere (SKINNER and LIESKOVSKY 1988). However, preparation of the anterior urethra in patients undergoing orthotopic diversion deserves specific mention. This portion of the procedure is critical in maintaining the continence mechanism, and to the successful outcome of the procedure.

We have recently modified our technique of anterior dissection in the region of the apex in men undergoing orthotopic diversion. These changes were made based upon the anatomic discoveries of the continence mechanism in women (COLLESELLI et al. 1994), along with the excellent functional results observed in female patients undergoing orthotopic diversion (STEIN et al. 1995).

Recent neuroanatomic and histologic studies of the female pelvis and urethra in fetal specimens have provided a better understanding of the female urethra and continence mechanism (COLLESELLI et al. 1994). These anatomic dissections have identified three layers of smooth muscle in the proximal two-thirds of the urethra. The innervation of this proximal urethral segment can be traced back to the pelvic plexus coursing along the lateral aspect of the uterus, vagina, and bladder neck. A gradual transition from intermingling smooth muscle to striated pelvic floor muscle can be identified in the mid to lower third portion of the urethra. This striated pelvic floor muscle, the so-called rhabdosphincter muscle, with its major portion on the ventral aspect of the urethra, is innervated from branches off the pudendal nerve that course along the pelvic floor posterior to the levator muscles. These findings suggest that preservation of the distal half of the urethral musculature, together with the corresponding nerve supply, is crucial in maintaining the continence mechanism in females. Furthermore, cystectomy with en bloc removal of the uterus and cervix effectively denervates the bladder neck and the proximal urethral sphincter mechanism, rendering them ineffective as a continence mechanism.

This unique anatomic study supports the complete removal of the bladder neck with transection of the proximal urethra just beyond the urethrovesical junction since continence is maintained solely by the rhabdosphincter muscle of the lower urethra. In addition, minimal dissection should be performed anterior to the proximal urethra, as such dissection could injure the pudendal innervation to the rhabdosphincter and possibly damage the continence mechanism.

14.6.1
Anterior Dissection in Males

In the male patient undergoing cystectomy and orthotopic diversion, no dissection should be performed along the pelvic floor anterior to the urethra. Currently, the dorsal venous complex is sharply transected without dividing the puboprostatic ligaments or without securing vascular control. Cephalad traction on the prostate elongates the proximal and membranous urethra, and allows the urethra to be skeletonized laterally by dividing the so-called lateral pillars, which are extensions of the rhabdosphincter. The anterior two-thirds of the urethra is divided, exposing the urethral catheter. The urethral sutures are then placed under direct vision. Six 2-zero polyglycolic acid sutures are placed equally spaced into the urethral mucosa and lumen anteriorly. The rhabdosphincter, the edge of which acts as a hood overlying the dorsal vein complex, is included in these sutures if the venous complex has been sharply incised. This maneuver serves to enhance urinary continence, and compresses the dorsal vein complex against the urethra for hemostatic purposes. The urethral catheter is then drawn through the urethrotomy, clamped on the bladder side, and divided. Cephalad traction on the bladder side with the clamped catheter occludes the bladder neck, prevents tumor spill from the bladder, and provides exposure of the posterior urethra. Two additional sutures are placed in the posterior urethra incorporating the rectourethralis muscle or distal Denonvilliers' fascia. The posterior urethra is then divided and the specimen removed. The urethral sutures are appropriately tagged to identify their location and placed under a towel until the urethroenteric anastomosis is performed. Bleeding from the dorsal vein is usually minimal at this point. If additional hemostasis is required, one or two anterior urethral sutures can be tied to stop the bleeding. Frozen section analysis of the distal urethral margin of the cystectomy specimen is then performed to exclude tumor involvement.

14.6.2
Anterior Dissection in Females

When developing the posterior vascular pedicles during the cystectomy in women, the posterior vagina is incised at the apex just distal to the cervix. This incision is carried anteriorly along the lateral and anterior vaginal wall, forming a circumferential incision. The anterior-lateral vaginal wall is then grasped with a curved Kocher clamp. This provides counter-traction, and facilitates dissection between the anterior vaginal wall and the bladder specimen. Development of this posterior plane and vascular pedicle is best performed sharply with the use of hemoclips, and carried just distal to the vesicourethral junction. Palpation of a previously placed Foley catheter balloon in the bladder assists in identifying this region. This dissection effectively maintains a functional vagina. Furthermore, an intact anterior vaginal wall helps support the proximal urethra through a complex musculofascial support system that extends from the anterior vagina. The vagina is then closed at the apex and suspended to Cooper's ligament to prevent vaginal prolapse or the development of an enterocele postoperatively.

Alternatively, in the case of a deeply invasive posterior bladder tumor, when there is concern to provide an adequate surgical margin, the anterior vaginal wall can be removed en bloc with the cystectomy specimen. After division of the posterior vaginal apex, the lateral vaginal wall serves as the posterior pedicle and is divided distally. This leaves the anterior vaginal wall attached to the posterior bladder specimen. Again, the Foley catheter balloon facilitates identification of the vesicourethral junction. The surgical plane between the vesicourethral junction and the anterior vaginal wall is then developed distally at this location. Dissection is carried downward just distal to the proximal urethra, while the remaining urethra distally is left intact with the anterior vaginal wall. Vaginal reconstruction by a clam shell (horizontal) or side-to-side (vertical) technique is required. Other means of vaginal reconstruction may include: a rectus myocutaneous flap, a detubularized cylinder of ileum, a peritoneal flap, or an omental flap. Regardless, a well-vascularized omental pedicle graft is placed between the reconstructed vagina and neobladder, and secured to the levator ani muscles to separate the suture lines and prevent fistulization.

It is important that no dissection be performed anterior to the urethra along the pelvic floor in women considering orthotopic diversion. This prevents injury to the rhabdosphincter region and corresponding innervation which is critical in maintaining the continence mechanism. Any dissection performed anteriorly may injure these nerves and compromise the continence status. Some reports suggest that a sympathetic nerve-sparing cystectomy is important in maintaining continence in these women. We have routinely sacrificed the autonomic nerves coursing along the lateral aspect of the uterus and vagina, and relied upon the pudendal innervation of the rhabdosphincter region. We have obtained excellent continence results in women undergoing orthotopic diversion with this approach (STEIN et al. 1996b). In fact, extensive fluorourodynamic studies in women undergoing orthotopic diversion have identified this rhabdosphincter region as the area which provides the continence mechanism in these women (GROSSFELD et al. 1996). It is possible that preservation of the sympathetic nerves may contribute to the high incidence of hypercontinence and urinary retention requiring continuous intermittent catheterization reported by HAUTMANN et al. (1996).

When the posterior dissection is completed (ensuring that dissection is just distal to the vesicourethral junction), a Statinsky vascular clamp is placed across the bladder neck. With gentle traction the proximal urethra is divided anteriorly, distal to the bladder neck and clamp. The anterior urethral sutures are placed as described in the male patient. The distal portion of the catheter is then drawn into the wound through the urethrotomy and divided. The Statinsky vascular clamp placed across the catheter at the bladder neck prevents any tumor spill from the bladder. Gentle cephalad tract on the clamped catheter allows placement of the posterior urethral sutures. The posterior urethra is then transected and the specimen is removed. Frozen section analysis is performed on the distal urethral margin of the cystectomy specimen to exclude tumor.

14.7
Construction of the Kock Ileal Neobladder

The Kock ileal neobladder is constructed from an approximately 61-cm segment of terminal ileum (Fig. 14.1). The reservoir portion of the neobladder is constructed from two 22- to 25-cm segments of distal

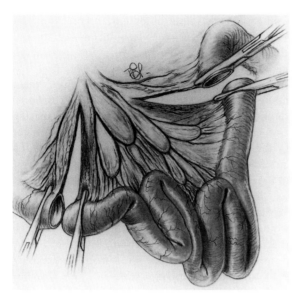

Fig. 14.1. The ileal segment used to construct the orthotopic Kock ileal neobladder. The distal mesenteric division is made approximately 20 cm proximal to the cecum along the avascular plane of Treves. A total length of 61 cm of ileum is required in the construction of the neobladder: two 22-cm segments for the reservoir portion of the pouch and a proximal 17-cm segment for the intussuscepted afferent nipple valve

ileum, while a single 17-cm segment of more proximal ileum is used to form the antireflux afferent nipple valve. The distal mesenteric division of the terminal ileum is performed along the avascular plane of Treves, between the ileocolic artery and the terminal ileal branches of the superior mesenteric artery, extending to the base of the small bowel mesentery. The proximal mesenteric division is short to ensure a broad vascular supply to the proximal ileal segment. Usually a 5-cm portion of proximal ileum is discarded proximal to the overall segment in order to ensure adequate mobility of the pouch and the small bowel anastomosis. The proximal end of the isolated ileal segment is closed with a running Parker-Kerr suture (3-0 chromic) and imbricated with a layer of 3-0 silk sutures. The small bowel continuity is reestablished with a standard small bowel anastomosis and the mesenteric trap closed.

The two isolated 22-cm ileal segments are positioned adjacent to one another in a "U" fashion with the apex directed caudally (Fig. 14.2a). They are sewn together along the serosa (side-to-side) approximately 1 cm from the mesentery with a 3-0 polyglycolic acid running suture. The ileum is opened just lateral to this serosal basting suture with electrocautery. The incised mucosa is approximated and oversewn the entire length with a 3-0 polyglycolic acid suture in two layers (Fig. 14.2a). This suture line forms the posterior wall of the reservoir.

Attention is then directed toward the 17-cm ileal segment and construction of the intussuscepted afferent nipple valve. Windows of Deaver are developed along the afferent limb mesentery adjacent to the serosa of this proximal 17-cm segment. The mesentery is divided away from the pouch, extending for 5–6 cm. This is best performed with electrocautery. This maneuver effectively strips the mesentery form the serosa of the ileum, ensuring that the mesentery is not incorporated into the intussuscepted nipple valve. Furthermore, this also helps prevent future prolapse or extussusception of the afferent nipple valve. One additional window of Deaver is created beyond the previously stripped mesentery, while preserving at least one vascular arcade in between. A 2.5-cm tetracycline-soaked piece of doubled polyglycolic acid mesh is then brought through this smaller window. This mesh will serve as an anchoring collar at the base of the nipple valve.

The intussuscepted antireflux afferent nipple valve is then created (Fig. 14.2b). The afferent nipple is intussuscepted by passing two Allis forcep clamps toward the anchoring collar, grasping the mucosa, and inverting the ileum into the pouch. This positions the mesh adjacent to the wall of the pouch at the base of the intussuscepted nipple. Next, two single rows of parallel 4.8-mm nonhemostatic staples (applied with a custom no-knife GIA 50 stapler), with the proximal four staples removed from each row, are applied to the medial and anterior aspects of the nipple (Fig. 14.3a). A third parallel staple line is applied (with a TA-55 stapling device) from outside the pouch between the posterior wall of the pouch along the mesenteric border and one layer of the intussuscepted nipple (Fig. 14.3b). The pinhole created by the TA-55 is oversewn from within the pouch to prevent formation of a fistula. This maneuver effectively fixes the afferent nipple valve to the posterior wall of the reservoir.

The anchoring mesh collar is fixed to the base of the afferent nipple valve. The mesh is circumferentially sutured to the serosa at the base of the nipple with 2-0 chromic. This helps prevent prolapse of the nipple valve.

The reservoir is closed by folding the ileum in the opposite direction back onto itself, creating a totally detubularized reservoir (Fig. 14.4). The anterior aspect of the pouch is closed in two layers with 3-0

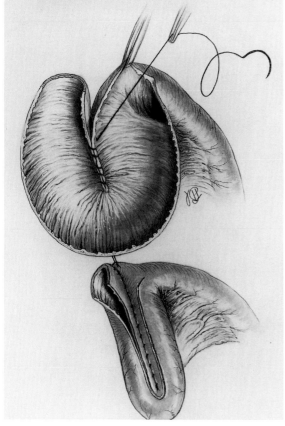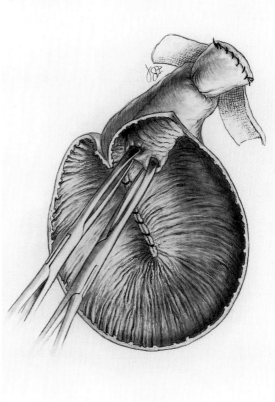

a   b

Fig. 14.2a,b. Creation of the pouch. **a** The two 22-cm segments are approximated in a "U" formation (directed toward the right lower quadrant) with a serosal basting suture 1 cm from the mesentery (*bottom*). The ileum is then opened with electrocautery adjacent to the basting suture line. The poste- rior wall of the reservoir is then sutured in two layers with a continuous 3-0 polyglycolic acid suture (*top*). **b** a 5- to 7-cm antireflux valve is created by intussusception of the afferent limb with Allis forcep clamps

polyglycolic acid sutures in a watertight fashion. It should be noted that the anterior suture line is stopped just prior to reaching the end of the right side, allowing easy entry of one finger. This is the most mobile and dependent portion of the reservoir and will be the portion of the reservoir anastomosed to the native urethra.

The ureteroileal anastomosis is then performed end-to-side with interrupted 4-0 polyglycolic acid sutures. We routinely stent the ureters with 8-French pediatric feeding tubes. These feeding tubes will be sutured to a 24-French hematuria catheter which is passed per urethra and positioned into the pouch. The urethral sutures are placed into the neobladder and tied down to form a tension-free, mucosa-to-mucosa, urethroileal anastomosis (Fig. 14.4). The pelvis is drained by a 1-inch Penrose drain for 3 weeks and removed along with the urethral catheter and stents at that time.

14.8
Results

14.8.1
Orthotopic Reconstruction in Men

We have recently updated our experience with orthotopic diversion in men (ELMAJIAN et al. 1996). From May 1986 through December 1993, 295 men aged 34–85 years (median age 66) underwent orthotopic reconstruction following cystectomy using the Kock ileal neobladder. The median follow-up in this group of patients was 3.6 years (range 0.4–8.5), with 95% of the patients followed up for at least 1 year.

There were three perioperative deaths for a mortality of 1.0%. Overall, 46 patients (15.7%) suffered a total of 52 early (less than 3 months postoperatively) complications; 21 were (7.2%) related to the

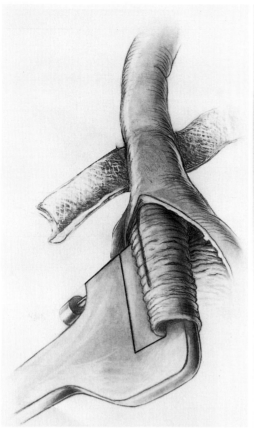
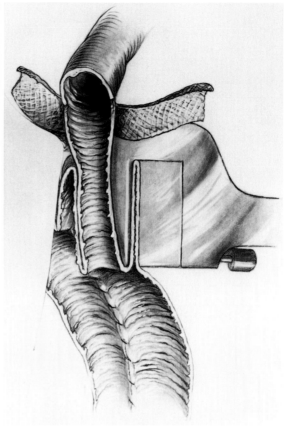

a   b

Fig. 14.3a,b. Fixation of the afferent limb. **a** Two rows of staples (with the distal four to six staples removed) are placed within the limb to stabilize the two leaves of the valve. **b** The valve is then fixed to the back wall from outside the reservoir. This fixes the intraluminal valve, which becomes more efficient as the reservoir fills, thus preventing reflux

orthotopic reservoir (pouch related), and 31 (10.6%) to the cystectomy (pouch unrelated). The most common early pouch-related complications included: a persistent urine leak in seven patients (2.4%), dehydration in six patients (2.0%), and urosepsis in five patients (1.7%). No patient required surgical revision for an early pouch-related complication. Forty-six late complications (greater than 3 months postoperatively) were reported in 40 patients (13.7%); 34 (11.6%) were pouch related, and 12 (4.1%) pouch unrelated. The most common late pouch-related complications included: Kock pouch stones in 12 patients (4.1%), afferent nipple stenosis in seven patients (2.4%), reflux in six patients (2.0%), and ureteroileal stenosis in four patients (1.4%). Of the 34 patients with pouch-related complications, 22 men required some form of surgical intervention, typically endoscopic to resolve the complication.

Daytime and nighttime continence in this group of men was reported as good (completely dry with-

out protection) or satisfactory (requiring no more than one pad during the day or night) in 87% and 86% of patients respectively. Over 95% of patients void not more than every 3–4h, with the majority of men voiding no more than every 4h. The majority (90%) of patients are able to void to completion, with only 10% of patients requiring some form of intermittent catheterization to empty their reservoir. Satisfaction is uniformly excellent in all patients.

14.8.2
Orthotopic Reconstruction in Women

Since 1990, 34 women aged 31–86 years (median age 66) have undergone orthotopic lower urinary tract reconstruction following cystectomy (Crocitto et al. 1994). The median follow-up in this group of patients is 21 months (range 7–53). The indication

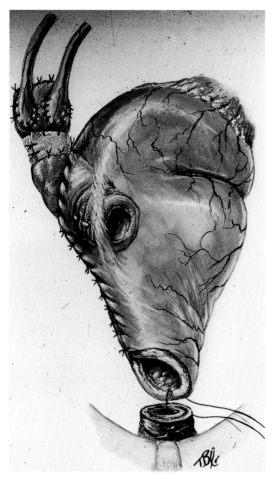

Fig. 14.4. After the afferent valve has been is constructed, the reservoir is completed by folding the ileum upon itself, and suturing it with 3-0 polyglycolic acid. The most dependent corner is left open for the urethral anastomosis. The urethroileal anastomosis is completed in a tension-free, mucosa-to-mucosa fashion with interrupted 2-0 polyglycolic acid sutures. Note that the ureteroileal anastomosis is completed prior to the urethral anastomosis

for cystectomy in 29 women (85%) was transitional cell carcinoma of the bladder. There were no perioperative deaths. Three patients (9%) suffered a total of four early complications: one pouch related (3%, urine leak), and three pouch unrelated. Late complications requiring rehospitalization or reoperation occurred in three patients (9%). However, only one of these late complications was pouch related, occurring in a women who developed a Kock pouch stone. To date there have been no urethral recurrences in this group of female patients.

Continence status was evaluable in 33 of the 34 patients. Complete daytime continence was reported by 28 of 33 (85%) women, and complete nighttime continence by 27 (82%) women. The ability to void to completion by the Valsalva maneuver and relaxation of the pelvic floor was reported by 28 (85%) patients. Only five patients require some form of intermittent catheterization to empty their neobladder. All patients are completely satisfied.

14.9
Discussion

The development of lower urinary tract reconstruction following cystectomy is a result of the persistent dedication of innovative and pioneering surgeons. No longer are the ultimate goals of urinary diversion simply to divert urine and to protect the upper urinary tract from significant damage; rather, there is the further aim of providing patients with the ability to volitionally void per urethra, in the hope of fostering a positive body and self-image.

Only a decade ago, the standard Bricker ileal conduit remained the primary form of urinary diversion in the United States. Patients were required to wear an external collecting device and were hampered by both a negative body image and the long-term renal morbidity secondary to reflux of infected urine (RICHIE et al. 1974; SHAPIRO et al. 1975). These unfortunate sequelae of cutaneous conduits stimulated the desire for improvement in lower urinary tract reconstruction, which ultimately led to the development of a continent cutaneous form of urinary diversion. This type of urinary diversion gained tremendous popularity in the early and mid 1980s, and resulted in a plethora of different forms of reconstruction incorporating various intestinal and/or colon segments.

A natural extension of the continent cutaneous form of urinary diversion was the orthotopic reservoir anastomosed directly to the native urethra. Orthotopic urinary diversion eliminated both the need for a cutaneous stoma and the often plagued continence mechanism (efferent limb), relying upon the intact external sphincter mechanism for continence. Orthotopic diversion initially became the ideal form of urinary reconstruction in carefully selected male patients undergoing cystectomy.

This form of lower urinary tract reconstruction was initially performed in selected male subjects, and was not considered technically possible in females as total urethrectomy was traditionally performed during the cystectomy. In addition, a lack of understanding of the continence mechanism in women dampened the enthusiasm for orthotopic reconstruction in females. However, with a better understanding of the continence mechanism in women, as well as the realization that the urethra can be safely preserved in selected female patients undergoing radical cystectomy, orthotopic lower urinary tract reconstruction has now become a viable form of diversion in women.

Overall, most male and female patients undergoing orthotopic diversion are continent, have the luxury of voiding every 4–6 h with excellent voided volumes, retain a more routine micturition pattern, avoid the need for a cutaneous stoma or external urostomy appliance, and live a more normal life-style with an improved self-image. Careful preoperative counseling for all patients in whom orthotopic lower urinary tract reconstruction is considered should include the possible need for clean intermittent catheterization in the rare patient unable to void with pelvic floor relaxation and Valsalva. In addition, all patients should understand the potential risk of a urethral recurrence, and the need for continued long-term surveillance of the retained urethra. Careful follow-up will be necessary to define the true risk of urethral or vaginal wall recurrence in women, and to diagnose urethral recurrences in all patients at an early curable stage. Presently, meticulous monitoring of the retained urethra includes careful palpation of the urethroenteric anastomosis on vaginal examination in women, and rectal examination in men. In addition, voided urine cytology should be performed on a regular basis in all patients at each follow-up visit.

14.10
Summary

The development of orthotopic lower urinary tract reconstruction has been a significant step in the continued progression of urinary diversion. We believe that the orthotopic reservoir should now be considered the gold standard against which other forms of diversion are compared. Orthotopic diversion can now be safely offered to both male and female patients undergoing cystectomy. With this form of diversion we hope that patients with bladder cancer, as well as their physicians, may be encouraged toward an earlier and more aggressive form of therapy with cystectomy, at a time when cure and ultimately survival are most likely.

References

Berglund B, Kock NG, Norlen L, Philison BM (1987) Volume capacity and pressure characteristic of the continent ileal reservoir used for urinary diversion. J Urol 137:29–34

Bricker EM (1950) Bladder substitution after pelvic evisceration. Surg Gynecol Obstet Am 30:1511–1521

Camey M, Le Duc A (1979) L'enterocystoplastie avec cystoprostatectomie totale pour cancer de la vessie. Ann Urol (Paris) 13:114

Colleselli K, Strasser H, Moriggl B, Stenzl A, Poisel S, Bartsch G (1994) Hemi-Kock to the female urethra: anatomical approach to the continence mechanism to the female urethra. J Urol 151:500A (abstract 1089)

Crocitto LE, Simpson J, Wilson TG (1994) Bladder augmentation in the prevention of cyclophosphamide induced hemorrhagic cystitis in the rat model. J Urol 151:379A (abstract 608)

Davidsson T, Poulsen AL, Hedlund H, et al. (1992) A comparative urodynamic study of the ileal and the colonic neobladder. Scand J Urol Nephrol 142(Suppl):143

Elmajian DA, Stein JP, Esrig D, et al. (1996) The Kock ileal neobladder: updated experience in 295 male patients. J Urol 156:920–925

Freeman JA, Esrig D, Stein JP, Skinner DG (1994) Management of the patient with bladder cancer. Urethral recurrence. Urol Clin North Am 21:645–651

Freeman JA, Tarter TA, Esrig D, et al. (1996) Urethral recurrence in patients with orthotopic ileal neobladders. J Urol 156:1615–1619

Gilchrist RK, Merricks JW, Hamlin HH, Rieger IT (1950) Construction of a substitute bladder and urethra. Surg Gynecol Obstet 90:752–760

Ginsberg D, Huffman JL, Lieskovsky G, Boyd S, Skinner DG (1991) Urinary tract stones: a complication of the Kock pouch continent urinary diversion. J Urol 145:956–959

Grossfeld GD, Stein JP, Bennett CJ, Ginsberg DA, Boyd SD, Lieskovsky G, Skinner DG (1996) Lower urinary tract reconstruction in the female using the Kock ileal reservoir with bilateral ureteroileal urethrostomy: update of continence results and fluorourodynamic findings. Urology 48:383–388

Hautmann RE, Paiss T, Petriconi R (1996) The ileal neobladder in women: 9 years of experience with 18 patients. J Urol 155:76–81

Hinman F Jr (1988) Selection of intestinal segments for bladder substitution: physical and physiological characteristics. J Urol 139:519–523

Kock NG (1971) Ileostomy without external appliances: a survey of 25 patients with intra-abdominal intestinal reservoir. Ann Surg 173:545–550

Kock NG, Nilson AE, Nilsson LO, Norlen LJ, Phillipson BM (1982) Urinary diversion via a continent ileal reservoir: clinical results in 12 patients. J Urol 128:468–476

Lieskovsky G, Boyd SD, Skinner DG (1991) Cutaneous Kock pouch urinary diversion. Probl Urol 5:256–262

Lytton B, Green DF (1989) Urodynamic studies in patients undergoing bladder replacement surgery. J Urol 141:1394–1397

Norlen L, Trasti H (1978) Functional behavior of the continent ileum reservoir for urinary diversion: an experimental and clinical study. Scand J Urol Nephrol Suppl 49:33

Richie JP, Skinner DG, Waisman J (1974) The effect of reflux on the development of pyelonephritis in urinary diversion: an experimental study. J Surg Res 16:256–261

Sakamoto N, Tsuneyoshi M, Naito S, Dumazawa J (1993) An adequate sampling of the prostate to identify prostatic involvement by urethelial carcinoma in bladder cancer patients. J Urol 149:318–321

Shapiro SR, Levowitz R, Colodney H (1975) Fate of 90 children with ileal conduit urinary diversion a decade later: analysis of complications, pyelography, renal function and bacteriology. J Urol 114:289

Simon J (1852) Ectopica vesicae (absence of the anterior walls of the bladder and pubic abdominal parietes): operation for directing the orifices of the ureters into the rectum; temporary success; subsequent death; autopsy. Lancet 2:568–569

Skinner DG, Lieskovsky G (1988) Technique of radical cystectomy. In: Skinner DG, Lieskovsky G (eds) Diagnosis and management of genitourinary cancer, vol I. Saunders, Philadelphia, pp 605–621

Skinner DG, Boyd SD, Lieskovsky G (1984a) Clinical experience with the Kock continent ileal reservoir for urinary diversion. J Urol 132:1101–1107

Skinner DG, Lieskovsky G, Boyd SD (1984b) Technique of creation of a continent internal ileal reservoir (Kock pouch) for urinary diversion. Urol Clin North Am 11:741–749

Skinner DG, Boyd SD, Lieskovsky G, Bennett C, Hopwood B (1991) Lower urinary tract reconstruction following cystectomy: experience and results in 126 patients using the Kock ileal reservoir with bilateral ureteroileal urethrostomy. J Urol 146:756–760

Stein JP, Huffman JL, Freeman JA, Boyd SD, Lieskovsky G, Skinner DG (1994a) Stenosis of the afferent anitreflux valve in the Kock pouch continent urinary diversion: diagnosis and management. J Urol 338–340

Stein JP, Stenzl A, Esrig D, et al. (1994b) Lower urinary tract reconstruction following cystectomy in women using the Kock ileal reservoir with bilateral ureteroileal urethrostomy: initial clinical experience. J Urol 152:1404–1408

Stein JP, Cote RJ, Freeman JA, et al. (1995) Lower urinary tract reconstruction in women following cystectomy for pelvic malignancy; a pathological review of female cystectomy specimens. J Urol 154:1329–1333

Stein JP, Freeman JA, Esrig D, et al. (1996a) Complications of the afferent anitreflux valve mechanism in the Kock ileal reservoir. J Urol 1579–1584

Stein JP, Grossfeld G, Freeman JA, et al. (1996b) Orthotopic lower urinary tract reconstruction in women using the Kock ileal neobladder: updated experience in 27 patients. J Urol 155:399A (abstract 353)

Wood DP Jr, Montie JE, Pontes JE, Levin HS (1989) Identification of transitional cell carcinoma of the prostate in bladder cancer patients: a prospective study. J Urol 142:83–85

15 Complications of Radical Cystectomy

L. Baert, A.-A. Elgamal, and H. Van Poppel

CONTENTS

L. Baert, MD, PhD, Professor and Chairman, Department of Urology, UZ Gasthuisberg, University Hospitals of Leuven, Herestraat 49, B-3000 Leuven, Belgium and Clinical Professor, Department of Urology and Radiation Oncology, University of Southern California, USC/Norris Comprehensive Cancer Center, 1441 Eastlake Avenue, Los Angeles, CA 90033, USA
A.-A. Elgamal, MD, PhD, Consultant Urologist and Research Associate, Department of Urology, UZ Gasthuisberg, University Hospitals of Leuven, Herestraat 49, B-3000 Leuven, Belgium
H. Van Poppel, MD, PhD, Professor, Department of Urology, UZ Gasthuisberg, University Hospitals of Leuven, Herestraat 49, B-3000 Leuven, Belgium

15.1 Introduction

Radical cystectomy in the male entails the en bloc removal of the bladder with its peritoneal covering, perivesical adipose tissue, distal ureteral segments, prostate gland and seminal vesicles, distal vas deferens and its ampulla, and pelvic lymph nodes. Removal of the urethra in continuity with the radical cystectomy specimen is indicated in patients with multicentric, primary carcinoma in situ and in patients with involvement of the bladder neck and/or prostatic urethra by transitional cell carcinoma (Freiha 1992). In the female, radical cystectomy is also known as anterior pelvic exenteration. This entails the en bloc removal of the bladder with its peritoneal coverings, the entire urethra including the external meatus, the uterus, fallopian tubes, and ovaries, the anterior vaginal wall, and the pelvic lymph nodes. In most cases, only the anterior third of the vagina is resected, leaving enough wall to reconstruct a functional vagina. However, the loss of a functional vagina is possible and every patient should be apprised of that possibility prior to the operation. In young, sexually active women whose tumors are located on the anterior wall or dome of the bladder and whose biopsy samples of the trigone and floor show no carcinoma, resection of the anterior vaginal wall may be avoided. Men and women should be carefully counseled regarding the potential loss of function of primary sex organs, loss of libido, and changes in activities and body image that may follow any radical cystectomy and urinary diversion operation.

Some surgeons prefer a limited dissection pelvic lymphadenectomy extending along the medial aspect of the external iliac vessels (Wishnow et al. 1987). Other surgeons believe that pelvic lymphadenectomy can be as extensive as to skeletonize the common, internal, and external iliac vessels circumferentially (Learner et al. 1993; Skinner 1982). Such single-stage pelvic lymphadenectomy with en bloc radical cystectomy can provide long-term free survival, particularly for patients with localized primary tumors and minimal metastatic nodal disease.

The incidence of complications following such a large operation as radical cystectomy remains substantial (MONTIE et al. 1995). Some complications may be relatively minor but still prolong hospitalization or subject the patient to additional pain or inconvenience. Therefore, most urologists would agree that, of all the operations in urologic oncology, cystectomy provides the most opportunities for "things to go wrong." The key point is the prevention or early detection of complications, which can minimize their impact.

15.2
Perioperative Care and Anesthetic Precautions

As in radical prostatectomy, we believe that a systematic regimen for perioperative care can be of value in preventing some common complications potentially associated with radical cystectomy (BAERT et al. 1996).

15.2.1
Preoperative Measures

Patients may be encouraged to donate, preoperatively, 1–2 units of blood for autologous transfusion. This can assure a safe blood transfusion by eliminating risks of antigenic sensitization or transmission of diseases. However, a minimum of 3 l of compatible blood should be reserved for the patient preoperatively.

Mechanical bowel preparation is substantial, and involves the sequential oral intake of macrogol (Kleanprep) in 5 l of saline during the evening prior to surgery. Neomycin and metronidazole can be added by oral intake, or in an enema on the morning of surgery, to enhance bowel cleansing. TANAKA et al. (1991) reported a significantly low (0%) incidence of postoperative infection in patients who had received mechanical bowel preparation as well as oral tobramycin–vancomycin prophylaxis before cystectomy and ileal urinary diversion.

Enoxaparin (Clexan) 40 mg s.c./12 h, which is a low-molecular-weight heparin substitute, is given on the evening before surgery. Skin preparation includes scrubbing with surgical soap and shaving the lower abdomen, pubis, scrotum, and perineum. The optimal stoma site can be marked, if cutaneous urinary diversion is planned.

15.2.2
Intraoperative Measures

Properly fitting elastic compression stockings are recommended for all patients to minimize the probability of intraoperative thromboembolic disease. A broad-spectrum antibiotic should be given before starting the operation as prophylaxis against potential infection. The use of prophylactic administration of antibiotics is important, and it is believed that administration in the 2 h before surgery is the most effective in reducing the risk of wound infection (CLASSEN et al. 1992). Patients are placed on the operating table in a supine position with gentle back extension in the Trendelenburg position to allow adequate venous drainage of the lower extremities. A 20-gauge urethral catheter is utilized, after wash of the urethra with polyvidon iodum (Iso-Betadine). This will help in the identification of the urethra during dissection.

Blood loss and transfusion requirements are expected to be markedly reduced when the deep dorsal venous complex is ligated in accordance with the reported recommendations on careful anatomic dissection of the dorsal vein complex (FITZPATRICK 1974; REINER and WALSH 1979). Because of the high propensity of transitional cells to implant on raw surfaces, it is extremely important to avoid opening the bladder during the operation and spilling its contents into the pelvic cavity. If spillage occurs, thorough irrigation with liters of distilled water or normal saline solution should be carried out (FREIHA 1992). Hypothermia is not uncommon during a cystectomy and urinary diversion; therefore, warming the patient might prevent potential clotting abnormalities.

15.2.3
Postoperative Measures

We have recommended the continuation of enoxaparin (Clexan) at 40 mg s.c./12 hourly, up to 10 days following the surgery, to guard against thromboembolic disease. Frequently repeated dorsiflexion exercises during the early postoperative period are mandatory. Early ambulation of the patient is highly recommended, with avoidance of a prolonged dependent position of the lower extremities. It is of importance to keep the patient properly hydrated to guard against hypercoagulability. Elastic stockings should be continued until the patient is fully ambulatory, however, their propensity to slip below the knee level and to act as tourniquets may promote thrombosis (BAERT et al. 1996).

Continuous care and follow-up of urine drainage in a closed sterile system are required to avoid infection or obstruction. In addition, special care must be taken in respect of the recovery of gastrointestinal tract motion.

15.2.4
Anesthetic Precautions

Safety and appropriate quality assurance should always be considered during catheterization, intubation, and blood transfusion. In the properly prepared patient, current techniques for anesthesia permit a wide range of surgical procedures in a hemodynamically stable subject with relatively rapid postoperative recovery of mental and physiologic function. Operative risk has been related to evidence of heart failure, recent infarction, preoperative rhythm disturbance, type of surgical procedure, age greater than 70 years, presence of "important" valvular aortic stenosis, and "poor general condition" (KILLIP 1992).

For most radical cystectomies, we prefer the use of combined general and lumbar epidural anesthesia to ensure better hemodynamic stability during the operation and early recovery period. This method allows for the possible use of the epidural catheter for patient-controlled analgesia. For induction anesthesia, we use the new hypnotic drug propofol, which is known for its minimal influence on postoperative nausea and vomiting. For the epidural anesthesia we use a combination of a local anesthetic (bupivacaine 0.16%) and a very low concentration of an opioid (sufentanil 1 µg/ml). The patient is monitored with electrocardiography, systemic arterial catheter, central venous catheter, pulmonary artery catheter, pulse oximeter, capnograph, central body temperature probe, and measurement of urine output. The new antiemetics alizapride and ondansetron are the drugs of choice for treatment of adverse effects (e.g.,

postoperative nausea or vomiting) of anesthetics on intestinal motility (BAERT et al. 1996).

15.3
Nonspecific Common Operative Complications

15.3.1
Bleeding

The one major intraoperative complication of radical cystectomy is excessive blood loss. Occasionally, bleeding from the dorsal vein complex may be excessive and require transfusion (FREIHA 1992). Bleeding may also arise during the control of the lateral bladder pedicles and dissection of bladder from the anterior rectal wall. Most of the bleeding encountered in the pelvis comes from veins and small arteries, and thus can be controlled temporarily with packing and manual pressure until a safe volume status is restored (MONTIE et al. 1995). Bleeding may also occur during dissection because of injury to the great vessels of the pelvis. It is of importance to repair the injury of such great vessels without compromising the lumen in order to avoid the serious and potentially life-threatening complications of arterial insufficiency of the lower extremities and venous obstruction with edema and risk of pulmonary embolism. The urologist should have no hesitation in obtaining an intraoperative consultation with a vascular surgeon for an opinion or assistance in the repair.

Bleeding may also occur because of rectal perforation and/or during intestinal pedicle dissection for the construction of a urinary diversion. There are insufficient data in the recent literature on the average blood loss and the incidence of transfusion during radical cystectomy and urinary diversion. However, this loss ranges from 1200 ml (AHLERING et al. 1989) up to significant hemorrhage requiring more than 10 units of blood transfusion (FRAZIER et al. 1992).

15.3.2
Cardiothoracic Complications

Considerable stress may be placed on the cardiovascular system in patients undergoing a cystectomy owing to the length of the operation, the intravenous administration of fluids, increased levels of antidi-uretic hormone which lead to relative oliguria, and the amount of blood loss that requires replacement by crystalloid and colloid solutions perioperatively. Silent cardiac ischemia can occur during cystectomy with excessive volume expansion. Thus the monitor-ing of workload and cardiac enzymes is appropriate in many cases intraoperatively and in the immediate postoperative period (MONTIE et al. 1995). Also, a history of ischemic heart disease or a recent infarction is an important cardiovascular risk factor that warrants correction preoperatively.

Prevention of postoperative chest complica-tions requires perioperative care of respiration and thromboembolic disease. Early ambulation, deep breathing, and chest physiotherapy are helpful sup-portive measures. Atelectasis must be aggressively treated and, if pneumonia does develop, appropriate antibiotics should be started in accordance with the results of sputum culture.

15.3.3
Thromboembolic Disease

Thromboembolic disease is a serious, potentially lethal complication of urologic and, in particular, pelvic surgery. Most patients undergoing radical cystectomy have an increased risk of deep vein thrombosis compared with the general surgical population. In patients undergoing pelvic surgery without thromboembolic prophylaxis, studies have demonstrated deep vein thrombosis rates as high as 51%, pulmonary embolism rates as high as 22%, and fatal pulmonary embolism rates as high as 2.6% (for review see KIBEL and LOUGHLIN 1995). Following radical cystectomy, the risk of thromboembolic com-plications is always present; nevertheless, the clinical diagnosis is not so frequent. These high rates have stimulated urologists to use various methods of pro-phylaxis to prevent thromboembolic complications (BAERT et al. 1996).

Of increasing concern is the risk of late thromboembolic complications. On average, late deep venous thrombosis is diagnosed 12–20 days postoperatively. Once prophylactic regimens are stopped, an existing nidus can propagate, since the hypercoagulable state may exist for as long as 3 weeks postoperatively. Therefore, it is advocated that postdischarge prophylaxis be applied in pelvic surgery patients to avoid facing increased numbers of late thromboembolic complications

following early hospital discharge (KIBEL and LOUGHLIN 1995).

15.3.4
Complications Related to Lymphatics

The generous utilization of hemoclips is recom-mended during lymphadenectomy in order to secure even the smallest lymphatics and to prevent the leakage of lymph (FREIHA 1992). Lymphocele may develop from excessive lymphatic drainage, parti-cularly in cases where the peritoneum is recon-structed in an attempt at closure. Little information is available on the incidence of lymphedema of the genitalia or lower extremities (FRAZIER et al. 1992; MONTIE and WOOD 1989; SKINNER et al. 1988). Lymphedema is seen more commonly when exten-sive pelvic lymphadenectomy is combined with preoperative radiation. Chronic lymphedema can be a disabling complication for the patient, and thera-peutic options are limited and often ineffective (MONTIE et al. 1995).

15.3.5
Long Hospitalization
and Socioeconomic Complications

Radical cystectomy with urinary diversion consti-tutes one of the most complex operations and is as-sociated with relatively high morbidity. Therefore, one of the main problems associated with this opera-tion is the lengthy hospitalization and the corre-sponding high potential cost. Recently, there has been a tendency to discharge patients early following radical cystectomy to avoid the financial drawbacks of lengthy hospital stay. KOCH et al. (1995) have de-signed and implemented a collaborative care path-way approach to standardize care and minimize inefficient medical practices in patients undergoing radical cystectomy and urinary reconstruction. They have identified nonessential procedures that do not influence patient comfort or morbidity and could safely be reduced. Through the implementation of their approach, total hospital charges were decreased by 37.5% (from $39 174 to $19 479), and hospital stay reduced from 12.7 to 10.3 days on average. There were also decreases in the duration of surgery, blood loss, intensive care unit use, and postoperative mor-bidity rates (KOCH et al. 1995).

15.4
Complications Related to the Gastrointestinal Tract

15.4.1
Nutrition, Gastric Decompression, and Ulcer Prophylaxis

As expected, malnourished patients with bladder cancer who are treated by radical cystectomy have greater operative morbidity, greater operative mortality, and more days of intensive care than their nutritionally normal counterparts (MOHLER and FLANIGAN 1987). However, nutritional support in the immediate perioperative period does little to alter operative complications. At least initially, most patients need total parenteral nutrition (TPN) after radical cystectomy. TPN support during the recovery period is required more often in patients with postoperative complications that delay return of normal bowel function. Accordingly it has been estimated that some of the recent decrease in operative mortality from cystectomy must be due to nutritional support instituted once a complication has developed (MONTIE et al. 1995).

Any type of urinary diversion following cystectomy usually requires gastric decompression until normal peristaltic activity returns and edema at the enterostomy resolves. Most surgeons apply a nasogastric tube, which is uncomfortable for patients if left in place for 4–5 days, until spontaneous return of bowel activity is evident (MONTIE et al. 1995). Nasogastric intubation is poorly tolerated and, therefore, we have advocated the percutaneous intraoperative gastrostomy tube for gastric decompression in all radical cystectomies. This percutaneous gastrostomy tube is easy and safe in application, is well tolerated, and offers patients maximal postoperative comfort compared with nasogastric intubation. In the immediate postoperative period, patients are allowed to drink small quantities, while gastric drainage is continued as long as postoperative ileus is present. When gastrointestinal peristalsis is restored, the tube is clamped and oral feeding can begin. When required, it can be used as a feeding gastrostomy tube. Moreover, the use of the percutaneous gastrostomy tube does not interfere with deep respiration and, consequently, reduces the incidence of infection and prevents pulmonary complications. This tube can be easily removed after 7–12 days postoperatively without causing any problems. At that time, patients have a normal breakfast and 2 h later the tube is flushed with saline and then quickly

removed (VAN POPPEL and BAERT 1991). Also, we have been systematically using H_2-blocking agents (e.g., cimetidine) as effective prophylaxis against ulcer formation postoperatively in all patients. An ulcer can occur as a result of stress from the operation, prolonged gastric decompression, and alteration of normal gastrointestinal bacteria flora. Therefore, the use of such prophylactic treatment is of importance.

15.4.2
Rectal Perforation

Historically, rectal injuries have been associated with high morbidity and mortality. However, most of these data have been based on injuries in which unprepared bowel, contaminated penetrating trauma, and delays in identification and repair of the rectal injuries contributed to a poor outcome. For the contemporary cystectomy, the conditions under which rectal injuries occur are more controlled. Patients have had preoperative bowel preparation and surgeons are able to promptly identify and repair the rectal laceration. The recent incidence of rectal perforation during cystectomy is 7% in nonirradiated patients; however, the incidence may increase to 27% in salvage cystectomy patients (KOZMINSKI et al. 1989). Small rectal injuries in well-vascularized, adequately prepared bowel can be repaired primarily with a low incidence of complications. Prior pelvic radiation is not an absolute contraindication to this treatment approach. For management of rectal perforation during pelvic surgery, see BAERT et al. (1996).

15.4.3
Intestinal Obstruction, Anastomotic Leak, and Fistula

The basic principles concerning the use of intestinal segments in urinary tract diversion and many of the related complications have previously been reviewed in detail (MCDOUGAL 1992b). Two of the most highly morbid complications resulting from this procedure, bowel obstruction and anastomotic leakage, are related to intestinal anastomosis. These complications are more common in continent urinary diversion. Urinary leakage remains the primary late complication and is the reason for reoperation in 10%–15% of the patients who require further surgery (SKINNER et al. 1988). Usually, it is due to a small pinhole fistula at the base of the diverted urinary pouch. It is hoped that meticulous closure of the intestinal segment, used as a reservoir, by the stapling device will further reduce the incidence of this complication. Absorbable staples have been used to construct a continent urinary reservoir in children. KIRSCH et al. (1996) found this to decrease operative time, cost, and blood loss, and none of the patients had reservoir stones during follow-up for up to 3 years. Reestablishment of bowel continuity is a substantial requirement for all methods of diversion. Therefore, a biofragmentable anastomosis ring (the Valtrac Bar) has been used for end-to-end reanastomosis of the distal and proximal bowel segments after resection. However, no significant difference in respect of bowel leakage, ileus, or obstruction was found when the technique was compared with stapled or sutured anastomosis (BUBRICK et al. 1991).

15.5
Complications Related to Cystectomy and Urinary Diversion

15.5.1
Stoma Complications

Competent stoma function is one of the most important requirements for patients who have undergone cystectomy and ileal conduit. A high frequency of stoma and peristomal complications has been attributed in previous studies to the absence of expert enterostomal therapy care (NORDSTRÖM and NYMAN 1991). The use of inadequate surgical technique, an ill-fitting appliance, and poor stomal hygiene have contributed to these complications.

Recent studies have emphasized the relevance of a skilled enterostomal nurse for the care and rehabilitation of ileal conduit patients. KLEIN et al. (1989) reported that only 8.5% of their patients had complications related to the stoma and/or peristomal skin. It is noteworthy that their patients were seen by both the surgeon and the enterostomal nurse at all follow-up visits. During the initial visit (4–6 weeks postoperatively) and on subsequent visits, the stoma and peristomal skin were inspected and the stoma was recalibrated for the exact fitting of the appliance in order to prevent urine leakage and skin complications. Optimal fitting of the collecting device and prompt treatment of peristomal skin infection minimized the early stomal complications. A rarely reported complication that developed in one of our patients was postoperative skin allergy to the stump of the collecting device; dermatologic care was required to overcome this hypersensitivity reaction.

Therefore, it is much better to start patient preparation preoperatively. It is important to take into account the impact of the patient's body habitus in the standing, sitting, and supine positions when choosing the stoma site; the style and manner of dressing might also be considered (GRUNE and TAYLOR 1996). Most commonly the selected site of stoma is in the right lower abdominal quadrant on a line between the anterior iliac spine and the umbilicus. Body creases and previous scars that may lead to difficulty in appliance application need to be avoided. The enterostomal therapist involved in the care can assist the patient in achieving realistic expectations through preoperative instruction in appliance use.

Stomal stenosis, which most often appears with flush stomas, is noted in approximately 5% of adult cases. Other late stomal complications that require revision include parastomal hernia (4%–14%), retraction (1%–2%), ischemia (1%), stenosis (4%–10%), prolapse (1%–2%), and poor location (KLEIN et al. 1989).

15.5.2
Incontinence

Numerous operative techniques have been developed in recent years for continent diversion wherein urine is emptied at intervals by patient self-catheterization. The most popular of these operations have been reviewed by BENSON and OLSSON (1992). The idea of having a continent cutaneous diversion is an old one in urologic surgery but KOCK et al. (1982) were the first to apply it successfully in the clinic. They adapted a technique of ileocystoplasty and added the principle of intussusception to prevent reflux and maintain continence. Initially, they reported their results in 12 patients who underwent urinary diversion via a continent ileal reservoir, emptied by intermittent patient self-catheterization through a cutaneous opening in the abdominal wall, for the efferent intussuscepted limb. Continence was achieved in all 12 patients, although a second procedure was necessary in seven patients due to a malfunction of the continence-providing valve (KOCK et al. 1982). Plication or tapering of the terminal ileal segment along with the ileocecal valve has provided the continence mechanism in the Indiana ileocecal reservoir. ROWLAND et al. (1987) reported satisfactory continence in 93% of their 29 patients (11 females and 18 males) operated on between 1982 and 1986. THÜROFF et al. (1988) used 10–15 cm of cecum and ascending colon and two ileal loops of the same length for construction of the Mainz urinary reservoir. They modified a technique involving the use of an intussuscepted continence nipple and used the umbilicus as a stomal site for continent urinary diversion. Of the 51 patients under intermittent catheterization, all but two were completely dry. Their initially reported problem of prolapse of the continence nipple was resolved after staple fixation of the nipple to the bowel wall and to the ileocecal valve was introduced.

Another variety of operative procedures has been developed for the provision of a low-pressure, high-capacity urinary pouch that allows male patients to initiate voiding by pelvic floor relaxation and the Valsalva maneuver. These operations were initiated and popularized by CAMEY and LE DUC (1979). Recent innovations have resulted in the creation of the urethral Kock Pouch, which is a low-pressure, low-volume nonrefluxing ileal reservoir connected to the male urethra and controlled by the external urethral sphincter (GHONEIM et al. 1987). Use of this appliance-free continent urethral Kock pouch appears to be the most popular diversion method among male patients undergoing radical cystectomy (BENSON and OLSSON 1992; ELMAJIAN et al. 1996; GHONEIM et al. 1992b; JAVADPOUR 1986; KOCK et al. 1989; SHAABAN et al. 1991; SKINNER et al. 1989, 1991).

It must be noted that the degree of continence is not uniformly defined and is subjectively assessed (MONTIE et al. 1995). Therefore, making comparisons between different studies is frequently difficult. In general, daytime continence has been obtained in 95% of men, whereas 70%–100% have nighttime continence. The reason for the increased incidence of nocturnal enuresis is related to ablation of the spinal reflex arc, which ensures external sphincter contractions. Additionally, external sphincter recruitment does not occur except under voluntary conscious control (JAKOBSEN et al. 1987).

GHONEIM et al. (1992b) have reported on a group of 185 men followed up after radical cystectomy and reconstruction of the urethral Kock pouch as a bladder substitute. In 117 of these patients the minimum follow-up was 1 year. Ninety-two percent of the patients were completely continent during the day, while 73% were fully continent at night. The use of imipramine hydrochloride (25 mg at bed time) resulted in an excellent response in eight of the 32

patients who suffered from variable degrees of bedwetting. An updated report on 195 men who underwent Kock ileal neobladder reconstruction at the University of Southern California has revealed an 87% incidence of good or satisfactory daytime continence and an 86% incidence at nighttime (ELMAJIAN et al. 1996). KHAFAGY et al. (1987) reported diurnal continence and nocturnal incontinence in 75.5% of 110 patients who underwent radical cystectomy and ileocecal bladder reconstruction. STUDER et al. (1995) found that the degree of urinary continence correlated well with the functional capacity of their ileal low-pressure bladder substitute. An increased capacity of the Studer bladder at 3–12 months postoperatively resulted in improved continence. Of 100 consecutive men, 92% were continent during the day 1 year postoperatively and 80% were continent at night 2 years postoperatively. BENSON et al. (1996) have retrospectively evaluated their experience with the Studer neobladder in 32 patients with a mean follow-up of 25 months (range 6–68). This study revealed a high success rate with regard to continence, the daytime and nighttime continence rates being 94% and 74%, respectively. KORAITIM and KHALIL (1992) reported 100% daytime continence and 40% nighttime continence in 23 patients who underwent nerve-sparing radical cystectomy with ileocecal neobladder substitution. They advocated preservation of the distal one-third of the prostatic capsule and the distal urethra, and tightening of the two levator ani muscles over the urethrocecal anastomosis.

KOCK and his associates (1988) reported a new method for urinary diversion to an augmented and valved rectum. This method was applied in 13 male and nine female patients, all of whom were continent during the day and dry at night. Reflux of the rectal contents to the colon and to the upper urinary tract was prevented by fashioning of an intussusception valve at the rectosigmoid junction. Further experience of GHONEIM et al. (1992b) with the augmented and valved rectum (modified rectal bladder) revealed continence during the day in all 57 women thus treated. Enuresis was noted in six patients, all of whom responded to imipiramine hydrochloride therapy.

HAUTMANN et al. (1996) have studied 18 women who underwent a nerve-sparing cystectomy with orthotopic bladder replacement. This ileal neobladder was connected to the proximal urethra or urethrovesical junction. At 3 months postoperatively, excellent continence was achieved in eight patients, while two had grade 1 stress incontinence and three were hyperincontinent. HAUTMANN et al. were unable to demonstrate any long-term advantage of the nerve-sparing and urethral support-sparing cystectomy technique as far as micturition was concerned. Of the patients treated and followed for a longer period, 70% developed hyperincontinence. STENZL et al. (1995) reported optimal postoperative results with regard to continence and voiding in five carefully selected women who underwent radical cystectomy and orthotopic neobladder reconstruction. They preserved the entire lateral vaginal wall and performed nerve-sparing dissection of the bladder neck and proximal urethra. Excellent treatment results were reported by STEIN et al. (1994) in 14 women who underwent cystectomy with reconstruction using the Kock ileal reservoir connected to the urethra.

15.5.3
Infection

Infection has been the single most common complication after cystectomy. Infection can be manifested as: (a) wound infection, (b) urinary tract infection, or (c) *Clostridium difficile* colitis.

The severity of wound infections ranges from cellulitis to gross infection or pelvic abscess. Each of these problems contributes to morbidity and prolongs hospital stay (MONTIE et al. 1995). Wound infection after cystectomy and urinary diversion has been reported in up to 28.6% of patients (TANAKA et al. 1991). The incidence of infection correlates well with the American Society of Anesthesiology risk score. Preoperative bowel preparation and prophylactic systemic antibiotics have dramatically decreased the risk of wound infection; however, the type of antibiotic used and timing of administration are of major importance (CLASSEN et al. 1992). The most commonly isolated bacteria are bacteroids, and most pelvic abscesses are associated with a large pelvic hematoma or urinary or fecal fistula. Closed suction drains contribute to a decrease incidence of pelvic abscesses and permit ease of nursing care, quantification of drainage, and minimization of introduction of infection.

Eighty percent of patients with conduit or continent diversion are bacteriuric with diverse bacterial flora. In addition, patients with colon and ileal conduit reflux are subject during the course of the diversion to a 15% incidence of acute pyelonephritis. On the other hand patients with a continent diversion have a 5%–20% incidence of septic episodes within 1 year of the reconstruction. The reasons underlying this incidence of infection are: (a) the decreased bacteriostatic activity of urine (with higher pH than normal), (b) the presence of an unimpaired reservoir of bacteria in the interposed bowel segment, (c) translocation of bacteria from the bowel lumen into urine and blood when the bowel segment is distended, and (d) unimpeded access to renal parenchyma in open system diversion (McDOUGAL 1992a).

A short course of antibiotic therapy such as that given for preoperative prophylaxis can induce *C. difficile* colitis. This can be induced by oral, parenteral, or topical therapy and by almost any antibiotic. The most common association, however, is with broad-spectrum antibiotics such as clindamycin, ampicillin, or cephalosporin. In addition *C. difficile* spores can be acquired by contact with other hospitalized patients or their environment and are commonly transmitted via the hands of hospital personnel. If untreated, pseudomembranous colitis due to overgrowth of *C. difficile* can lead to fever, severe diarrhea, hypovolemic shock, toxic dilatation of the colon, cecal perforation, hemorrhage, and possibly death. However, *C. difficile* colitis can also mimic the more common "benign" antibiotic-associated diarrhea. Diagnosis depends on sigmoidoscopy and/or stool tests for *C. difficile* toxins. If the results of these tests are positive, either oral metronidazole or vancomycin is recommended (FEKETY and SHAH 1993).

15.5.4
Sexual Dysfunction and Quality of Life

In the past all men undergoing radical cystectomy were expected to be impotent. More recently, however, the neuroanatomic approach to radical cystectomy has permitted preservation of sexual function in appropriately selected patients by avoiding injury to branches of the pelvic plexus that innervate the corpora cavernosa (SCHLEGEL and WALSH 1987). Important modifications in the surgical technique have been proposed to reduce the incidence of this morbidity in order to preserve the quality of life. However, impotence remains one of the important complications of cystectomy. Recently, SCHOENBERG et al. (1996) reviewed their 16-year experience in 101 patients who underwent nerve-sparing radical cystectomy for bladder cancer at the Johns Hopkins Hospital. They found that this technique did not compromise cancer control rates while it has improved the quality of life. As expected, recovery of sexual function correlated well with patient age. The incidence of potency following cystectomy was 62% in men in the fifth decade of life and 20% in those in the eighth decade of life. With preservation of the neurovascular bundle, potency could be maintained in 15 of 21 evaluable patients with an ileocolic neobladder by MARSHALL et al. (1991). KORAITIM and KHALIL (1992) reported erectile potency in half of their 32 surgically treated patients. All four patients treated by JAVADPOUR (1986) had preservation of potency following cystoprostatectomy. As in most patients who have undergone radical prostatectomy, impotence which follows cystectomy can be successfully managed with intracavernous injection of vasoactive medications and the use of a penile prosthesis (BAERT et al. 1996).

The overall impact of cystectomy and urinary diversion on the patient's life-style must be minimized (MONTIE et al. 1995). The negative effects on body image and life-style are the primary motivating factors for lower urinary tract reconstruction using an orthotopic bladder connected to the urethra (STEIN et al. 1994). Nevertheless, HAUTMANN et al. (1996) found that overall patient satisfaction, including sexual life, was good in 18 females who underwent nerve-sparing cystectomy with preservation of the proximal urethra for the formation of an orthotopic bladder.

Previous studies showed that after cystectomy and conduit diversion, 23% of patients did not resume their occupation (BABAIAN and SMITH 1991). Accidental leakage of urine, or fear of such leakage, was the most common negative psychological aspect of the ileal conduit. This was followed by factors related to altered body image. Female patients more often than males have considered body image-related factors to be the most negative aspect of the treatment outcome (NORDSTROM and NYMAN 1991). BOYD et al. (1987) compared the quality of life of ileal conduit patients and that of those with a continent cutaneous Kock reservoir. The ileal conduit patients had the poorer self-image, as defined by a decrease in sexual desire and in all forms of physical contact (sexual and nonsexual). The subset of patients who underwent conversion from conduit to continent pouch, however, were the most satisfied, and they were also physically and sexually most active.

15.5.5
Ureterointestinal Anastomotic Strictures

The development of ureterointestinal anastomotic stricture is a late complication that arises in up to 8.0% of patients with a reconstructed lower urinary tract following radical cystectomy (ELMAJIAN et al. 1996; RAZVI et al. 1996; VANDENBROUCKE et al. 1993). Most ureteroenteric strictures are discovered within a year after the original diversion procedure. Reasons for the development of such strictures include:

1. Compromised vascularity and ischemic changes of the mobilized distal ureteral segment
2. Inadequate technique of anastomosis
3. Inflammation
4. The presence of postradiation changes
5. Tumor recurrence

We believe that the incidence of stenosis can be decreased by careful dissection of the distal ureter with minimal mobilization, by application of mucosa-to-mucosa anastomosis without tension, and by positioning the butt end of the ileal conduit retroperitoneally. Any urinary tract infection should be promptly controlled. It is of major importance to exclude tumor recurrence since this may substantially influence the treatment decision. Traditionally, this complication has been managed by open surgical intervention including laparotomy incision and reimplantation of the vascularized ureter in the intestinal pouch. However, recent improvements in endourologic management have resulted in an effective alternative to open surgery.

Fluoroscopy and a wide selection of guide wires (e.g., a hydrophilic guide wire) and ureteral catheters are essential for endourologic management, which is a potentially complex procedure (RAZVI et al. 1996). Retrograde ureteral catheterization can be difficult and often is not successful. General anesthesia and placement of the patient in the prone position are required for antegrade stenting of a distal ureteral stenosis. A full-thickness incision of the stricture should be performed until fat or retroperitoneal tissue is identified. After completion of the endoureterotomy, a stent should be placed in the ureter. The use of a stent without side holes in the part traversing the intestinal portion of the diversion may be preferable since the optimal duration of stent placement remains unclear. Ureteroenteric anastomotic strictures may recur when treated by means of endoscopic balloon catheter dilation (SHAPIRO et al.

1988). Cornud et al. (1992) employed a technique for electroincision of strictured ureterointestinal anastomosis in a total of nine stenoses in seven patients. The operative time did not exceed 45 min and the procedure was performed without bleeding, fistula formation, or other major complications. All five patients reported by Kramolowsky et al. (1987) who had semirigid fascial or balloon dilatation alone had recurrence of the stricture. Dilatation in conjunction with percutaneous intraureteral incision of the stricture through a flexible choledochoscope-nephroscope resulted in short-term resolution of each of the four ureteroileal strictures.

We have compared endourologic management with open surgical repair in a previous report. Most of the eight nonmalignant stenoses that were treated by balloon dilation, endoscopic incision, or stenting by means of a double J ureteral catheter recurred following removal of the stent. By contrast, stricture reappeared in only one of the 11 patients treated with open surgery strictures (at 21 months after the open surgical revision) (Vandenbroucke et al. 1993). Kramolowsky et al. (1988) reported a success rate of 89% (eight of nine strictures) at an average follow-up of 33 months in patients treated by open surgical revision, and a 71% (five of seven strictures) success rate in those who underwent endourologic correction. Therefore, it was concluded that the lower morbidity, decreased cost, and shorter hospital stay associated with the endourologic approach make it preferable to open revision. For elderly patients who fail initial endoscopic revision and for patients with cancer recurrence, placement of an indwelling stent is a reasonable alternative. Nevertheless, less than 30% of the patients who develop anastomotic stricture will require open surgical revision.

15.5.6
Reflux

Most investigators agree that reflux of urine at the ureterocolic anastomosis is a serious complication that can result in deterioration of renal function within a short period. Nevertheless, there is no consensus on the necessity of prevention of reflux at the ureteroenteric anastomosis after cystectomy and urinary diversion (Skinner et al. 1995). Studer et al. (1995) found no significant reflux from their ileal low-pressure bladder substitute unless the reservoir was overfilled. They believed that even upon straining during voiding, the increased intra-abdominal

pressure will act equally on the reservoir and the ureters, without isolated increase in the pressure of the reservoir alone. However, short-term follow-up results are not sufficient for the long-term assessment of the impact on renal function. It is to be noted that deterioration of renal function in ileal conduit patients was rarely seen until patients were followed up for more than 5 years.

Most of the commonly used antireflux techniques can be effective in reflux prevention, but the tunnel techniques are known to have a higher incidence of late stenosis than the intussuscepted nipple valve technique (Ghoneim et al. 1992b; Shaaban et al. 1992a).

15.5.7
Stones

There is an increased incidence of urinary tract calculi following intestinal diversion. The pathophysiology of this process is unclear, but it is thought to be due to increased calcium excretion and the high incidence of urinary tract infection with urease-producing bacteria. These infections contribute to a high ammonia concentration in the renal pelvis, ureters, and diverted intestine (McDougal 1992a). Calculus formation in an ileal conduit or pouch often occurs when foreign bodies, such as sutures or staples, serve as a nidus for mineral condensation. The mucus produced by the intestine may also have a role as one of the factors in urolithiasis. Upper tract calculi (renal stones) have been seen in approximately 10% of patients with ileal conduit diversion if they were followed for more than 10 years. Their presence was associated with recurrent upper tract infection and/or obstruction leading to stasis (Montie et al. 1995). Intestinal pouches have a substantial risk for stone formation, the risk approaching 20% even in patients who were followed for a relatively short period (Ginsberg et al. 1991).

Recently the incidence of late pouch-related complications was studied in 295 men who underwent Kock ileal neobladder reconstruction and had a reported median follow-up of 3.6 years. Unexpectedly, this study revealed a low (4.1%) incidence of stone formation (Elmajian et al. 1996). Terai et al. (1996) found that stones developed in 7 of 54 patients (12.9%) who had the Indiana pouch as compared to 31 of 72 (43.1%) with a Kock pouch. The incidence of urolithiasis gradually increased with longer follow-up; at 5 years after surgery it was 16% for the former group and 34% for the latter group. In this comparative study, infrequent pouch irrigations were considered to be an important risk factor for the formation of urinary calculi. Prevention of reflux, chronic bacteriuria, and exposed metal staples has been considered important for the reduction of stone formation. Maintaining an adequate state of hydration, preventing stasis of concentrated urine, and ingestion of supplemental bicarbonate or citrate have been advocated as prophylaxis in patients with urinary diversions who exhibit metabolic acidosis, hypercalciuria, and hyperoxaluria (RAZVI et al. 1996). Etiologic factors such as persistent urinary tract infection, anastomotic stricture, and metabolic derangement may require attention prior to removal of upper urinary tract calculi. The size, number, and location of stones and the anatomy of the patient's collecting system must be considered before treatment with extracorporeal shockwave lithotripsy (ESWL). A large stone burden is best managed with the percutaneous antegrade approach. Antegrade percutaneous passage of a guide wire into the conduit or pouch may provide a means of attaining retrograde access to the ureter. This is essential for endoscopic treatment of upper tract calculi. Stone formation within an ileal conduit rarely requires intervention as most of these stones pass spontaneously. Calculi may be present within a diversion in patients who are asymptomatic, present with pain, present with incontinence, produce difficulty in catheterization, or have recurrent infections.

The management of distal calculi within a urinary diversion may be technically challenging because of the unfamiliar anatomy and the relative fragility of the intestinal diversion. ESWL has been used successfully to treat obstructive stones within the afferent portion of a Kock pouch (BOYD et al. 1988) and in an Indiana pouch (COHEN and STREEM 1994) without adverse effects on the pouch. However, despite stone fragmentation, endoscopic retrieval of the remaining fragments is often required to ensure a stone-free state.

The risk of recurrent stones is relatively high following the initial management of calculi in patients with a urinary diversion. COHEN et al. (1996) found that stones recurred in 8 of 25 patients (32%) after ESWL and/or percutaneous nephrolithotomy, the mean interval to recurrence being 27 months. The risk of new stone formation after 5 years was estimated to be 63% and was significantly greater in patients with recurrent bacteriuria after treatment.

15.6
Metabolic Abnormalities of Urinary Intestinal Diversion

Following radical cystectomy, a segment of intestine is most commonly used for bladder replacement, either as a conduit or as a storage pouch for urine. The incidence of metabolic complications is low when a small segment of ileum is used as a conduit (VAN POPPEL et al. 1994). Numerous complications may occur in the short- and long-term as a consequence of metabolic abnormalities. The incidence of these complications is to a large extent dependent on the segment of bowel used for diversion. Such complications are influenced by the degree of absorption of solutes across the bowel segment (MCDOUGAL 1992a). If the stomach is used in diversion, hypokalemic, hypochloremic metabolic alkalosis can occur. When the jejunum is used, hyponatremic, hypochloremic, hyperkalemic metabolic acidosis may occur. The electrolyte abnormality that commonly occurs with continent diversions using ileum and/or colon is hyperchloremic metabolic acidosis. The reported incidence of metabolic acidosis varies widely, from a low of 10% to a high of 65% (BOYD et al. 1989). The incidence of metabolic acidosis may be even higher in patients who undergo diversion with the use of colonic segments (KOCH et al. 1991). The severity of hyperchloremic acidosis associated with ureterosigmoidostomy is related to the surface area of colonic mucosa exposed to urine. Therefore the use of an isolated rectal bladder with terminal colostomy could decrease this problem. However, the rectal bladder was not found to be optimal since it was associated with a significant incidence of enuresis (GHONEIM and ASHAMALLAH 1974).

The surface of colonic mucosa exposed to urine could be decreased, resulting in a decreased rate of reabsorption, by the use of a modified rectal bladder in which an intussuscepted colorectal valve prevented reflux of urine from the rectum to the proximal colon (EL-MEKRESH et al. 1991; GHONEIM et al. 1992a). When exposed to urine, the ileal absorption of potassium is greater than that in the colon. Both of these segments secrete sodium and bicarbonate and reabsorb ammonia, ammonium, hydrogen ions, and chloride. Other electrolyte abnormalities seen in the clinic include hypokalemia, hypomagnesemia, hypocalcemia, hyperammonemia, and elevated blood urea and creatinine.

Alkalization with oral sodium bicarbonate and/or blockers of chloride transport are effective in restoring normal acid-base balance. Oral sodium citrate plus citric acid, bicitrate, or Shohl's solution provides an effective alternative treatment except for their taste, which is objectionable to patients. Chlorpromazine at 25 mg, given 3 times daily, or nicotinic acid at 400 mg, given 3 times daily, may be useful in limiting the degree of acidosis, decreasing the need for alkalizing agents, and avoiding excessive sodium load in patients with cardiac or renal disease. However, these agents are not sufficient when used alone and should be used with caution to prevent side-effects (McDougal 1992a).

Hypokalemia is more common in patients with ureterosigmoidostomy, whereas ileal conduit has no influence on total body potassium (Williams et al. 1967). When managing hypokalemia associated with hyperchloremic acidosis, the treatment must include replacement of potassium as well as correction of the acidosis with bicarbonate. Marked flaccid paralysis may develop if the acidosis is corrected without attention to potassium replacement.

Hypocalcemia and hypomagnesemia severe enough to cause symptoms are infrequent complications of urinary intestinal diversion. Hypocalcemia is a consequence of depleted body calcium stores and excessive renal wasting. Symptoms of hypocalcemia include irritability, tremors, tetany, and in severe cases convulsions. The well-known manifestations of hypocalcemia include positive Chvostek and Trousseau signs. Treatment of choice for hypocalcemia is calcium infusion given either parenterally or orally, depending on the severity of the hypocalcemia.

Chronic acidosis and serum abnormalities that affect calcium cause increased serum levels of sulfate and phosphate with increased excretion, and interfere with vitamin D metabolism. They work together to cause subtle alterations in bone content in the majority of patients with urinary intestinal diversion. Osteomalacia was observed after an extended period in patients with ureterosigmoidostomy and augmentation cystoplasty. Laboratory evaluation usually reveals a normal or depressed serum calcium level, normal or slightly depressed serum phosphate, and an elevated alkaline phosphatase level. Patients who have osteomalacia generally complain of pain in the weight-bearing bones. They often respond to treatment with bicarbonate but occasionally they may require supplemental vitamin D_3 and calcium to remineralize the bone (McDougal 1992a). A recent study (Tschopp et al. 1996) found no evidence of osteomalacia, osteoporosis, or significant metabolic acidosis in 14 patients with an ileal bladder substitute who were followed for a period of up to 8 years.

However, it is not known whether osteopenia would also be absent in the following patients:

1. Patients with poor renal function
2. Patients at risk for long-term functional or metabolic disturbances from their bladder substitute
3. Patients with orthotopic bladder substitutes constructed from long bowel segments

All intestinal segments used for urinary diversion have venous return that drains into the portal circulation directly into the liver. A marked increase in the absorption of ammonia may occur due to the increase in the load of ammonia in urine and by the action for urease enzyme of associated bacterial infection. The liver usually adapts rapidly to this change by increasing its capacity for ureagenesis. The hepatic reserve for ammonia clearance when liver function is normal prevents the occurrence of acute changes in serum ammonia level. In severe cases hyperammonemic encephalopathy has been reported. This condition is most common in patients with ureterosigmoidostomy and chronic liver disease. When hyperammonemia occurs, the patient should be suspected of having underlying liver disease or systemic bacteremia with or without associated obstruction of the urinary diversion (McDougal 1992a). The treatment of ammonegenic coma includes draining the obstructed intestinal diversion, with a rectal tube in the case of ureterosigmoidostomy or with a Foley catheter in patients with continent diversion. This drainage minimizes the length of exposure of the intestinal mucosa to urine. Systemic antibiotics are given to which urease-producing bacteria are known to be sensitive. The administration of oral neomycin and minimization of protein intake are essential to reduce the ammonia load from the enteric source. Additionally, oral or rectal lactulose may be given to combine with ammonia in the gut and prevent its absorption. In severe cases the treatment may consist of intravenously given arginine glutamate at 50 g in 11 5% dextrose.

15.7
Morphologic Changes and Malignant Transformation

Ileal and colonic mucosa undergo substantial morphologic changes when used to reconstruct the urinary tract in either conduit or reservoir fashion (Philipson et al. 1983). Carlén and associates

(1990) studied biopsy specimens from continent cecal urinary reservoirs and their ileal nipple valves in ten patients who were followed up for a period from 2 to 9 years. In the colonic mucosa, microvilli were found to be shorter and reduced in number when compared with the histologic picture at the time of reservoir construction. Mucosal edema and reduced numbers of goblet cells were found in six of the ten patients examined. In the nipple valve mucosa there were no microvillous changes. The presence of metaplastic formation of glycocalyceal bodies was interpreted as adaptation. Neurogenic processes, enterochromaffin cells, and Paneth cells were always well preserved in the cecal as well as the ileal mucosa. HALL et al. (1993) studied the functional changes of an ileal segment following 3 months of urinary diversion in rats. They confirmed the presence of prominent and consistent mucosal atrophy, evidenced by loss of microvilli with a decreased villi-to-crypt ratio. Despite these atrophic changes, intestinal segments continued to transport urinary solutes similarly to normal nondiverted segments. These investigators presented evidence to suggest that in the short term, atrophic structural changes did not decrease the absorptive capacity of the intestinal mucosa.

DAVIDSSON et al. (1996) studied the morphologic changes of the mucosa following ileocolocystoplasty in a rat model. Their findings were consistent with the previous reports. Moreover, they found that the intracellular ultrastructural changes in both colon and ileal mucosa were similar. Such atrophic changes were considered more likely to be due to deprivation of intraluminal content than to exposure to urine.

In the recent literature, there is mounting evidence that cancer may arise as a significant complication 10–20 years after urinary diversion to enteric mucosa. Carcinoma develops in the area of the stump where the urothelium is adjacent to the intestinal mucosa, even though the urine no longer comes into contact with the anastomosis. The highest incidence of cancer is found in cases where transitional cell epithelium is left in contact with colonic epithelium and both are bathed by feces and urine. The mean incidence of "urocolonic cancer" occurring at the ureterointestinal anastomosis in patients with ureterosigmoidostomy is 11%. Adenocarcinoma accounts for approximately 85% of all cases and transitional cell carcinoma accounts for 10%. However, the exact mechanisms involved in cancer development are not well understood. It is not known whether cancer arises from transitional epithelium or from

colonic epithelium (HUSMANN and SPENCE 1990; KALBLE et al. 1990; McDOUGAL 1992a; SHAABAN et al. 1992b; SOHN et al. 1990). In a study of 186 patients who underwent various uroenteric reconstruction procedures using bowel segments exposed to urine without fecal stream and who were followed up for more than 10 years, malignancy was diagnosed in only 2% (SHOKEIR et al. 1995). FILMER and SPENCER (1990) reviewed the recent literature for the incidence of malignancy in bladder augmentations and intestinal conduits. They found a high incidence of adenocarcinoma in ileocystoplasty patients, the findings being similar to those in ureterosigmoidostomy patients with regard to tumor location and histologic type. They hypothesized that infected urine bathing a suture line between enteric and transitional mucosa may lead to cancer formation; by contrast the incidence of cancer was insignificant in patients with intestinal conduit.

Therefore, long-term surveillance of all patients with urinary diversion is mandatory. Periodic endoscopy may be the most sensitive method for the detection of malignancy, and intravenous urography, computed axial tomography, and urine cytology are also helpful. Hematuria, ureteral obstruction, and abnormal cytology are the warning signs of cancer.

15.8
Renal Failure

It has been estimated that 20% of patients with ileal conduit who are followed up for a long period will show progressive deterioration of renal function. It is also known that about 6% of these patients will ultimately die of renal failure. Deterioration of renal function is less common (10%) in patients with nonrefluxing pouches. The incidence is greater in patients with ureterosigmoidostomy urinary diversion, 10%–20% of such patients being expected to die of renal failure within 15 years post-diversion (MONTIE et al. 1995). The mechanisms involved in post-urinary diversion renal failure include:

1. Chronic electrolyte abnormalities
2. Pyelonephritis
3. Ureterointestinal stenosis
4. Urolithiasis
5. Prolonged hemodynamic effects of reflux (KOCH et al. 1991)

A decrease in glomerular filtration rate, renal tubular changes due to obstruction or pyelonephritis, and hepatic disorders may substantially enhance the degree of deterioration in renal function seen with prolonged follow-up. Measures for the prevention of renal failure include strict evaluation of renal function before the diversion is performed. The presence of preexisting renal failure will tend to favor the use of conduit diversion rather than a retentive diversion. Additionally, the correction of metabolic disorders must be adapted to the intestinal segment used for diversion; administration of sodium bicarbonate and nicotinic acid or chlorpromazine will correct the hyperchloremic acidosis following the use of ileum or colon.

15.9
Mortality of Radical Cystectomy

Radical cystectomy as a surgical procedure for the treatment of invasive bladder cancer has been rapidly changing over the second half of this century. Earlier, the absence of a reliable method of diversion or storage of urine precluded a successful operation. Ureterosigmoidostomy then became feasible, but the inadequacy of bowel preparation, poor anesthesia, suboptimal perioperative care, and a lack of antibiotic therapy led to significant morbidity and mortality in up to 50% of patients (FREIHA 1992; BENSON and OLSSON 1992; MONTIE et al. 1995). In 1950, BRICKER reported a technique of cutaneous diversion with an ileal conduit for bladder substitution after pelvic exenteration. The use of this procedure sharply decreased mortality rates from cystectomy to 15%–20%. The absence of appropriate enterostomal therapy and inadequate collecting appliances commonly relegated the patients to a lifetime of leaking urine and suffering from constant odor. Nevertheless, the ease of construction of this diversion and the low incidence of complications led the Bricker ileal conduit to become the gold standard of urinary diversion. A combination of preoperative irradiation and subsequent cystectomy then emerged during the 1960s and 1970s. The results of the combined modality approach were initially reported to be better than those of surgery alone. During the same period, however, other series of cystectomy-treated patients were reported showing better treatment results than those obtained with the combined approach. This indicated that the survival benefit which was thought to be derived from preoperative irradiation was more likely due to better cystectomy, with a much lower mortality. Continued improvement in perioperative care and better patient selec-

tion contributed to further reduction in the operative mortality.

Contemporary reports show the incidence of operative mortality of radical cystectomy to range between 0% and 6%. GHONEIM et al. (1992b) reported no postoperative mortality in 185 men who underwent cystectomy and reconstruction of the urethral Kock pouch. MONTIE and WOOD (1989) reported a 0.4% mortality in 229 patients using alternative forms of urinary diversion. Among the 295 men who underwent radical cystectomy and urinary diversion by means of the Kock ileal neobladder at the University of Southern California, the operative mortality was only 1% (ELMAJIAN et al. 1996). BENSON et al. (1992) reported an operative mortality of 1.4% in 73 consecutive patients with continent or standard urinary diversion. In 1988, SKINNER et al. reported a 1.9% mortality in 531 men and women treated with radical cystectomy and continent diversion. The mortality was 2% in the last 100 consecutive cystectomies performed by FREIHA until 1992. STUDER et al. (1995) have also reported a 2% mortality in a group of 100 consecutive men with ileal bladder substitution. The mortality was 2.5% in 675 patients who underwent radical cystectomy at Duke University during the past two decades (FRAZIER et al. 1992). A recent report on 63 patients who underwent ureterosigmoidostomy showed a mortality of 3.2% (BISSADA et al. 1995), while it was 3.4% in 88 patients with an ileal conduit and preoperative irradiation (HENDRY 1986). AHLERING et al. (1989) reported a mortality of 5.5% in 55 radical cystectomy patients with an ileal conduit, a Kock pouch, or a modified Indiana pouch. Finally, SOLOWAY et al. (1994) reported a mortality of 6% in 130 patients who underwent radical cystectomy with adjuvant radiation or chemotherapy.

15.10
Conclusions

Radical cystectomy may be the most complex and difficult surgical procedure in uro-oncology due to the combined efforts at eradication of cancer from the pelvis and reconstruction of a "new" lower urinary tract. The prevalence of early and late postoperative complications correlates well with multiple parameters which include: (a) the patient's general condition, (b) the histologic characteristics of the tumor, (c) the clinical stage, (d) the use of preventive perioperative care procedures, (e) the skill of the surgeon, and (f) the type and suitability of the urinary diversion applied for reconstruction of the lower urinary tract. Ileal conduit has represented the gold standard of treatment of patients with multifocal tumors, carcinoma in situ, or tumors extending to the bladder neck or proximal urethra, with relatively minimal postoperative morbidity. Innovations in surgical techniques have provided both males and females with the opportunity for nerve-sparing radical cystectomy and continent bladder substitution which substantially improves their quality of life. Therefore, continent diversion merits more widespread utilization. There is a need, however, to await long-term treatment results which are not yet available. Advances in anesthesia, enteric anastomosis, endourology, and lithotripsy have reduced the incidence of reoperation and consequent complications. One may conclude that contemporary radical cystectomy has become a "mature" procedure which is efficient in controlling the localized bladder cancer and has achieved a significant decline in morbidity and a very low mortality.

References

Ahlering TE, Weinberg AC, Razor B (1989) A comparative study of the ileal conduit, Kock pouch and modified Indiana pouch. J Urol 142:1193–1196

Babaian RJ, Smith DB (1991) Effect of ileal conduit on patients' activities following radical cystectomy. Urology 37:33–35

Baert L, Elgamal AA, Van Poppel H (1996) Complications of radical prostatectomy. In: Petrovich Z, Baert L, Brady LW (eds) Carcinoma of the prostate. Innovations in management. Springer, Berlin Heidelberg New York, pp 139–156

Benson MC, Olsson CA (1992) Urinary diversion. In: Walsh PC, Retik AB, Stamey TA, Vaughan ED Jr (eds) Campbell's urology, 6th edn. Saunders, Philadelphia, pp 2654–2720

Benson MC, Slawin KM, Wechsler MH, Olsson CA (1992) Analysis of continent versus standard urinary diversion. Br J Urol 69:156–162

Benson MC, Seaman EK, Olsson CA (1996) The ileal ureter neobladder is associated with a high success and a low complication rate. J Urol 155:1585–1588

Bissada BK, Morcos RR, Morgan WM, Hanash K (1995) Ureterosigmoidostomy: is it a viable procedure in the age of continent urinary diversion and bladder substitution? J Urol 153:1429–1431

Boyd SD, Feinberg SM, Skinner DG, Lieskovsky G, Baron D, Richardson J (1987) Quality of life survey of urinary diversion patients: comparison of ileal conduits versus continent Kock ileal reservoirs. J Urol 138:1386–1389

Boyd SD, Everett RW, Schiff WM, et al. (1988) Treatment of unusual Kock pouch urinary calculi with extracorporeal shock wave lithotripsy. J Urol 139:805–806

Boyd SD, Schiff WM, Skinner DG, et al. (1989) Prospective study of metabolic abnormalities in patients with continent Kock pouch urinary diversion. Urology 33:85

Bricker EM (1950) Bladder substitution after pelvic evisceration. Surg Clin North Am 30:1511

Bubrick MP, Corman ML, Cahill CJ, Hardy G Jr, Carter Nance F, Shatney CH. The BAR Investigational Group (1991) Prospective, randomized trial of the biofragmentable anastomosis ring. Am J Surg 161:136–142

Camey N, Le Duc A (1979) L'entérocystoplastie avec cystoprostatectomie totale pour cancer de la vessie. Ann Urol 13:114

Carlén B, Willén R, Misson W (1990) Mucosal ultrastructure of continent cecal reservoir for urine and its ileal nipple valve 2–9 years after construction. J Urol 143:372

Classen DC, Evans RS, Pestotnik SL, Horn SD, Menlove RL, Burke JP (1992) The timing of prophylactic administration of antibiotics and the risk of surgical-wound infection. N Engl J Med 326:281–286

Cohen TD, Streem SB (1994) Minimally invasive endourologic management of calculi in continent urinary reservoirs. Urology 43:865–868

Cohen TD, Streem SB, Lammert G (1996) Long-term incidence and risks for recurrent stones following contemporary management of upper tract calculi in patients with urinary diversion. J Urol 165:62–65

Cornud F, Mendelsberg M, Chrétien Y, Helenon O, Bonnel D, Dufour B, Moreau JF (1992) Fluoroscopically guided percutaneous transrenal electroincision of ureterointestinal anastomotic strictures. J Urol 147:578–581

Davidsson T, Carlén B, Bak-Jensen E, Willén R, Månsson W (1996) Morphologic changes in intestinal mucosa with urinary contact – effects of urine or disuse? J Urol 156:226–232

Elmajian DA, Stein JP, Esrig D, et al. (1996) The Kock ileal neobladder: updated experience in 295 male patients. J Urol 156:920–925

El-Mekresh M, El-Din ABS, Fayed SM, Brevinge H, Kock NG, Ghoneim MA (1991) Bladder substitutes controlled by the anal sphincter: a comparison of the different absorption potentials. J Urol 146:970–972

Fekety R, Shah AB (1993) Diagnosis and treatment of Clostridium difficile colitis. JAMA 269:71–75

Filmer RB, Spencer JR (1990) Malignancies in bladder augmentations and intestinal conduits. J Urol 143:671–678

Fitzpatrick TJ (1974) Venography of the deep dorsal venous and valvular systems. J Urol 111:518

Frazier HA, Robertson JE, Paulson DF (1992) Complications of radical cystectomy and urinary diversion: a retrospective review of 675 cases in 2 decades. J Urol 148:1401–1405

Freiha FS (1992) Open bladder surgery. In: Walsh PC, Retik AB, Stamey TA, Vaughan ED Jr (eds) Campbell's urology, vol 3. Saunders, Philadelphia, pp 2750–2774

Ghoneim MA, Ashamallah A (1974) Further experience with the rectosigmoid bladder. Br J Urol 46:511

Ghoneim MA, Kock NG, Lycke G, El-Din ABS (1987) An appliance-free, sphincter-controlled bladder substitute: the urethral Kock pouch. J Urol 138:1150–1154

Ghoneim MA, Ashamallah AK, Mahran MR, Kock NG (1992a) Further experience with the modified rectal bladder (the augmented and valved rectum) for urine diversion. J Urol 147:1252–1255

Ghoneim MA, Shaaban AA, Mahran MR, Kock NG (1992b) Further experience with the urethral Kock pouch. J Urol 147:361–365

Ginsberg D, Hoffman JL, Lieskovsky G, et al. (1991) Urinary tract stones: a complication of the Kock pouch continent urinary diversion. J Urol 145:956–959

Grune MT, Taylor RJ (1996) Aspects of urinary diversion: the current role of conduits. AUA Update Series (lesson 21) 15:166

Hall MC, Koch MO, Halter SA, Dahlstedt SM (1993) Morphologic and functional alterations of intestinal segments following urinary diversion. J Urol 149:664–666

Hautmann RE, Miller K, Steiner U, et al. (1993) The ileal neobladder: 6 years experience with more than 200 patients. J Urol 150:40–45

Hautmann RE, Paiss T, de Petriconi R (1996) The ileal neobladder in women: 9 years of experience with 18 patients. J Urol 155:76–81

Hendry WF (1986) Morbidity and mortality of radical cystectomy (1971–78 and 1978–85). J R Soc Med 79:395–400

Husmann DA, Spence HM (1990) Current status of tumor of the bowel following ureterosigmoidostomy: a review. J Urol 144:607–610

Jakobsen H, Steven K, Stigsby B, et al. (1987) Pathogenesis of nocturnal urinary incontinence after ileocaecal bladder replacement. Continuous measurement of urethral closure pressure during sleep. Br J Urol 59:148–152

Javadpour N (1986) Cystoprostatectomy for bladder cancer with preservation of potency and no stoma. J Urol 136:1377

Kälble T, Tricker AR, Friedl P, Waldherr R, Hoang J, Staehler G, Möhring K (1990) Ureterosigmoidostomy: long-term results, risk of carcinoma and etiological factors for carcinogenesis. J Urol 144:1110–1114

Khafagy MM, El-Kalawy M, Ibrahim A, Safa M, Meguid HA, Bassioni M (1987) Radical cystectomy and ileocaecal bladder reconstruction for carcinoma of the urinary bladder. A study of 130 patients. Br J Urol 60:60–63

Kibel AS, Loughlin KR (1995) Pathogenesis and prophylaxis of postoperative thromboembolic disease in urological pelvic surgery. J Urol 153:1763–1774

Killip T (1992) Anesthesia and major noncardiac surgery. JAMA 268:252–253

Kirsch AJ, Olsson CA, Hensle TW (1996) Pediatric continent reservoirs and colocystoplasty created with absorbable staples. J Urol 156:614–617

Klein EA, Montie JE, Montague DK, et al. (1989) Stomal complications of intestinal conduit urinary diversion. Cleve Clin J Med 56:48–52

Koch MO, McDougal WS, Reddy PK, Lange PH (1991) Metabolic alterations following continent urinary diversion through colonic segments. J Urol 145:270–273

Koch MO, Seckin B, Smith JA (1995) Impact of a collaborative care approach to radical cystectomy and urinary reconstruction. J Urol 154:996–1001

Kock NG, Nilson AE, Nilsson LO, Norlén LJ, Philipson BM (1982) Urinary diversion via a continent ileal reservoir: clinical results in 12 patients. J Urol 128:469–475

Kock NG, Ghoneim MA, Lycke G, Mahran MR (1988) Urinary diversion to the augmented and valved rectum: preliminary results with a novel surgical procedure. J Urol 140:1375–1379

Kock NG, Ghoneim MA, Lycke G, Mahran MR (1989) Replacement of the bladder by the urethral Kock pouch: functional results, urodynamics and radiological features. J Urol 141:1111–1116

Koraitim M, Khalil R (1992) Preservation of urosexual functions after radical cystectomy. Urology 39:117–121

Kozminski M, Konnak JW, Grossman HB (1989) Management of rectal injuries during radical cystectomy. J Urol 142:1204–1204

Kramolowsky EV, Clayman RV, Weyman PJ (1987) Endourological management of ureteroileal anastomotic strictures: is it effective? J Urol 137:390–394

Kramolowsky EV, Clayman RV, Weyman PJ (1988) Management of ureterointestinal anastomotic strictures: comparison of open surgical and endourological repair. J Urol 139:1195–1198

Lerner SP, Skinner DG, Lieskovsky G, et al. (1993) The rationale for en bloc pelvic lymph node dissection for bladder cancer patients with nodal metastases: long-term results. J Urol 149:758–765

Marshall FF, Mostwin JL, Radebaugh LC, Walsh PC, Brendler CB (1991) Ileocolic neobladder post-cystectomy: continence and potency. J Urol 145:502–504

McDougal WS (1992a) Metabolic complications of urinary intestinal diversion. J Urol 147:1199–1208

McDougal WS (1992b) Use of intestinal segments in the urinary tract: basic principles. In: Walsh PC, Retik AB, Stamey TA, Vaughan ED (eds) Campbell's urology. Saunders, Philadelphia, pp 2595–2629

Mohler JL, Flanigan RC (1987) The effect of nutritional status and support on morbidity and mortality of bladder cancer patients treated by radical cystectomy. J Urol 137:404–407

Montie JE, Wood DP Jr (1989) The risk of radical cystectomy. Br J Urol 63:483–486

Montie JE, Pavone-Macaluso M, Tazaki H, et al. (1995) What are the risks of cystectomy and the advances in perioperative care? Int J Urol 2(Suppl 2):89–104

Nordström GM, Nyman CR (1991) Living with a urostomy. A follow up with special regard to the peristomal-skin complications, psychosocial and sexual life. Scand J Urol Nephrol 138(Suppl):247–251

Philipson BM, Kock NG, Jagenburg R, et al. (1983) Functional and structural studies of ileal reservoirs used for continent urostomy and ileostomy. Gut 24:392–398

Razvi HA, Martin TV, Sosa RE, et al. (1996) Endourologic management of complications of urinary intestinal diversions. AUA Update Series (lesson 22) 15:••

Reiner WG, Walsh PC (1979) An anatomical approach to the surgical management of the dorsal vein and Santorini's plexus during radical retropubic surgery. J Urol 121:198

Rowland RG, Mitchell ME, Bihrle R, Kahnoski RJ, Piser JE (1987) Indiana continent urinary reservoir. J Urol 137:1136–1139

Schlegel PN, Walsh PC (1987) Neuroanatomical approach to radical cystoprostatectomy with preservation of sexual function. J Urol 138:1402–1406

Schoenberg MP, Walsh PC, Breazeale DR, Marshall FF, Mostwin JL, Brendler CB (1996) Local recurrence and survival following nerve sparing radical cystoprostatectomy for bladder cancer: 10-year follow up. J Urol 155:490–494

Shaaban AA, Dawaba MS, Gaballah MA, Ghoneim MA (1991) Urethral controlled bladder substitution: a comparison between Parks S pouch and hemi-Kock pouch. J Urol 146:973–976

Shaaban AA, Gaballah MA, El-Diasty TA, Ghoneim MA (1992a) Urethral controlled bladder substitution: a comparison between the intussuscepted nipple valve and the technique of Le Duc as antireflux procedures. J Urol 148:1156–1161

Shaaban AA, Sheir KZ, El-Baz MA (1992b) Adenocarcinoma in an isolated rectosigmoid bladder: case report. J Urol 147:457–458

Shapiro MJ, Banner MP, Amendo MA, et al. (1988) Balloon catheter dilation of ureteroenteric strictures: long-term results. Radiology 168:385–387

Shokeir AA, Shamaa M, El-Mekresh MM, El-Baz M, Ghoneim MA (1995) Late malignancy in bowel segments exposed to urine without fecal stream. Urology 46:657–661

Skinner DG (1982) Management of invasive bladder cancer: a meticulous pelvic node dissection can make a difference. J Urol 128:34–36

Skinner DG, Lieskovsky G, Boyd SD (1988) Continent urinary diversion. 5-year experience. Ann Surg 208:337–344

Skinner DG, Lieskovsky G, Boyd S (1989) Continent urinary diversion. J Urol 141:1323–1327

Skinner DG, Boyd SD, Lieskovsky G, Bennett C, Hopwood B (1991) Lower urinary tract reconstruction following cystectomy: experience and results in 126 patients using the Kock ileal reservoir with bilateral ureteroilial urethrostomy. J Urol 146:756–760

Skinner DG, Studer UE, Okada K (1995) Which patients are suitable for continent diversion or bladder substitution following cystectomy or other definitive local treatment? Int J Urol 2(Suppl 2):105–112

Sohn M, Füzesi L, Deutz F, Lagrange W, Kirkpatrick JC, Braun JC (1990) Signet ring cell carcinoma in adenomatous polyp at site of ureterosigmoidostomy 16 years after conversion to ileal conduit. J Urol 143:805–807

Soloway MS, Lopez AE, Patel J, Lu Y (1994) Results of radical cystectomy for transitional cell carcinoma of the bladder and the effect of chemotherapy. Cancer 73:1926–1931

Stein JP, Stenzl A, Esrig D, et al. (1994) Lower urinary tract reconstruction following cystectomy in women using the Kock ileal reservoir with bilateral ureteroileal urethrostomy: initial clinical experience. J Urol 152:1404–1408

Stenzl A, Colleselli K, Poisel S, Feichtinger H, Pontasch H, Bartsch G (1995) Rationale and technique of nerve sparing radical cystectomy before an orthotopic neobladder procedure in women. J Urol 154:2044–2049

Studer U, Danuser H, Merz VW, Springer JP, Zingg EJ (1995) Experience in 100 patients with an ileal low pressure bladder substitute combined with an afferent tubular isoperistaltic segment. J Urol 154:49–56

Tanaka M, Matsumoto T, Ogata N, Masuda S, Kumazawa J (1991) Preoperative oral and postoperative parenteral antibiotic prophylaxis of wound infection in total cystectomy with ileal urinary diversion. Urol Int 47:44–47

Terai A, Ueda T, Kakehi Y, Terachi T, Arai Y, Okada Y, Yoshida O (1996) Urinary calculi as a later complication of the Indiana continent urinary diversion: comparison with the Kock pouch procedure. J Urol 155:66–68

Thüroff JW, Alken P, Riedmiller H, Jacobi GH, Hohenfellner R (1988) 100 cases of Mainz pouch: continuing experience and evolution. J Urol 140:283–288

Tschopp ABS, Lippuner K, Jaeger PH, Merz VW, Danuser H, Studer UE (1996) No evidence of osteopenia 5 to 8 years after ileal orthotopic bladder substitution. J Urol 155:71–75

Vandenbroucke F, Van Poppel H, Vandeursen H, Oyen R, Baert L (1993) Surgical versus endoscopic treatment of non-malignant uretero-ileal anastomotic strictures. Br J Urol 71:408–412

Van Poppel H, Baert L (1991) The percutaneous operative gastrostomy for gastric decompression in major urological surgery. J Urol 145:100–102

Van Poppel H, Vandeursen R, Baert L (1994) Bricker urinary diversion after cysto(prostato)urethrectomy. Still an acceptable diversion. Abstr. of the XIth Congress of the European Association of Urology, Berlin, July 13–16

Williams RE, Davenport TJ, Burkinshaw, et al. (1967) Changes in whole body potassium associated with uretero-intestinal anastomosis. Br J Urol 39:676

Wishnow KI, Johnson DE, Ro JY, Swanson DA, Babaian RJ, von Eschenbach AC (1987) Incidence, extent and location of unsuspected pelvic lymph node metastasis in patients undergoing radical cystectomy for bladder cancer. J Urol 137:408–410

Weinberg AC, Boyd SD, Lieskovsky G, Ahlering TE, Skinner DG (1988) The hemi-Kock augmentation ileocystoplasty: a low pressure anti-refluxing system. J Urol 140:1380–1384

16 Long-term Results of Brachytherapy with Iridium-192 Implants

H. Van Poppel, M. Van de Heuvel, Y. Lievens, E. Van Limbergen, L. Vanuytsel, and L. Baert

CONTENTS

16.1 Introduction

The recommended treatment for muscle-invasive transitional cell carcinoma of the bladder is radical surgery. It is, however, acknowledged that other treatment strategies can also be effective in selected patients. Transurethral resection (TUR), open partial cystectomy, radiotherapy, or combinations thereof have been shown to be effective in controlling local disease and extending survival, sometimes ultimately resulting in permanent tumor control.

Radiotherapy has become rather unpopular in urologic practice in the management of patients with bladder cancer. The only patients who are still routinely being referred for the treatment include those who refuse cystectomy, those who are in a poor general condition, those who need palliative therapy, and the occasional patient who may need adjuvant radiotherapy. Interstitial radiotherapy in patients with carcinoma of the bladder is infrequently used in the United States but it has gained some popularity in Europe. Although it has been used with good results, the combination of surgery and radiotherapy has never become a generally accepted therapeutic approach. The modern urologist seems to prefer radical surgery and bladder substitution procedures for locally invasive bladder cancer that does not involve the prostatic urethra. Continent diversions are used when the patient has to undergo simultaneous prophylactic urethrectomy. Bladder replacement, however, is a major surgical procedure and it is still not widely utilized even in some major medical centers, especially in the female patient. Bladder replacement is frequently associated with nocturnal enuresis and with the loss of sexual function, although a nerve-sparing cystectomy is feasible in properly selected patients.

Since quality of life has become a significant issue in cancer management, the novel approaches to bladder replacement and continent diversion are relevant and very important to the present-day urologist. The most important issue, however, remains cancer control and survival, with bladder preservation clearly being second in importance. A bladder-preserving approach is therefore judged to be reasonable only if survival is not jeopardized and if there is a high likelihood of achieving local tumor control (Koiso et al. 1995).

Transurethral resection (Solsona et al. 1992) or partial cystectomy (Sweeney et al. 1992) will control only a small proportion of carefully selected patients with a solitary primary lesion. The patients selected for these conservative surgical procedures have to present with lesions which are in an accessible location in the bladder and must not have associated carcinoma in situ. The combination of surgery with chemotherapy has also been reported to be effective in controlling tumor in properly selected patients, but radiation therapy is currently the standard bladder-preserving therapy (Koiso et al. 1995). Definitive radiotherapy was shown to be particularly effective in locally controlling the disease when the

H. Van Poppel, MD, PhD, Professor in Urology, M. Van Den Heuvel, MD, Resident in urology, Y. Lievens, MD, Resident in Radiotherapy, E. Van Limbergen, MD, PhD, Professor in Radiotherapy
L. Vanuytsel PhD, MD, Professor in Radiotherapy, Departments of Urology and Radiotherapy UZ Gasthuisberg, University Hospitals of Leuven, Herestraat 49, B-3000 Leuven, Belgium
L. Baert, MD, PhD, Professor and Chairman, Department of Urology, UZ Gasthuisberg, University Hospitals of Leuven, Herestraat 49, B-3000 Leuven, Belgium and Clinical Professor, Department of Urology and Radiation Oncology, university of Southern California, USC/Norris Comprehensive Cancer Center, 1441 Eastlake Avenue, Los Angeles, CA 90033, USA

tumor has previously been completely resected (SHIPLEY and ROSE 1985).

Interstitial radiotherapy makes it possible to deliver a high dose of radiation to a limited bladder volume within a short period of time. The permanent implantation of radioactive isotopes such as radon-222 and gold-198, as well as temporary implantation using radium-226, cesium-137, or iridium-192, has been used with varying success (GOSPODAROWICZ et al. 1995).

16.2
K.U. Leuven Experience with Iridium-192

16.2.1
Materials and Methods

The first patient who underwent brachytherapy in our clinic was treated in March 1983 and the last patient included in this report was treated in November 1990. During this period, 174 radical cystectomies were performed while 28 (14%) carefully selected patients had brachytherapy. As expected, most (24) of these patients were males. The mean age of the patients was 64 years (range 36–85 years).

The selection criteria used in this study were:

1. Solitary and histologically confirmed transitional cell carcinoma
2. A lesion diameter of less than 5 cm
3. Tumor not invading the bladder neck
4. No carcinoma in situ in random bladder biopsies.

Of the 28 patients treated, 12 (43%) had tumors localized to the mobile part of the bladder and 16 (57%) had tumor arising in the fixed part of the bladder. High-grade T1 lesions and muscle-invasive tumors but not transmurally extending T2 and T3 lesions were included.

Pretreatment work-up included urine cytology, intravenous urography, computerized axial tomography of the pelvis, cystoscopy, and complete TUR of the tumor. Tumor size ranged from 2 to 5 cm (mean 3.5 cm). The stage distribution was as follows: T1GIII in four (14%), T2GII in one (4%), T2GIII in 11 (39%), T3GII in three (11%), and T3GIII in nine (32%).

Prior to surgery, external beam radiotherapy was administered to the pelvis; the T1 patients received 10.5 Gy in three daily doses, while the T2 and T3 patients received 40 Gy in 20 equal fractions. All treatments were given using two opposed anteroposterior fields. The interval between radiotherapy and surgery was 2 weeks for T1 and 4–6 weeks for T2 and T3 patients. In nine (32%) patients in whom the TUR scar was suspected to contain residual tumor, a partial cystectomy was performed and two source carrier tubes were inserted. In the remaining 19 (68%) patients, in whom the TUR scar was not suspected to contain tumor, a simple implant with two or three carriers was performed, depending on the target volume (Fig. 16.1). Because

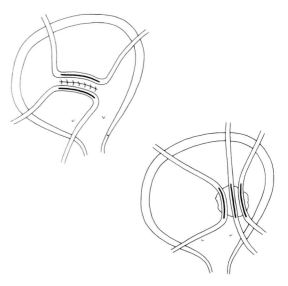

Fig. 16.1. Implantation of two carriers after partial cystectomy or of three carriers in a healthy looking scar

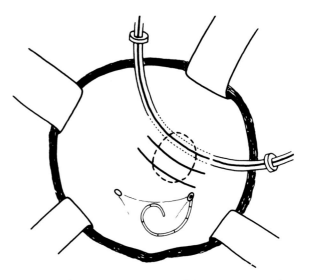

Fig. 16.2. Schematic representation of the operative site after placement of three line sources and insertion of a double J ureteral catheter

of the proximity of the ureteral meatus a ureteral reimplantation, far away from the pathologic zone, was performed in five (18%) patients. In three (11%) other patients a double J stent was inserted and remained in place for a period of 6 weeks (Fig. 16.2).

Just before surgery, a check cystoscopy was performed in order to determine a safe place for the cystotomy. Then, a staging lymph node dissection was undertaken. One study patient who had lymph node involvement diagnosed on frozen section was not treated by interstitial implantation but rather by external beam radiotherapy alone. The bladder was opened in a cystoscopically checked healthy area (Fig. 16.3). The target volume was evaluated by measuring the TUR scar and a safety margin of 1 cm was added (Fig. 16.4). The bladder wall was then pierced with a hollow needle of 1.6 mm in diameter (Fig. 16.5). A nylon guide was passed through this hollow needle (Fig. 16.6). The second and the third needles were then inserted (Fig. 16.7). Following removal of the needles, a carriertube was slipped over the nylon guide (Fig. 16.8). The guidewire was pulled backwards to the lateral end of the radiation source position and was fixed to the nylon tube by a metal button. In this position the guidewire serves as a stop for the radioactive iridium-192 wire that will be inserted through the other end of the nylon tube (Fig. 16.2). The exact length of the zone to be implanted was then determined and a metal dummy wire was slipped into the tube through the loading end, and also fixed by metal buttons. When all tubes were in place (Fig. 16.9), the bladder was closed after the insertion of the suprapubic catheter. The pelvis was drained with standard suction drains. The nylon tubes for the iridium-192 were brought through the abdominal wall and fixed to the skin in order to avoid their inadvertent dislocation (Fig. 16.10).

After 3–4 days of postoperative care in the urology unit, the patient care was taken over by the radiation oncologist. In the radiotherapy simulator room, orthogonal radiographs of the pelvis were obtained with the metal dummy wires in place (Fig. 16.11). These radiographs were necessary to establish the geometry for the implant dosimetry. Isodose curves were then generated with the assistance of a computer. The planned implant dose to be delivered depended on the preoperatively administered external beam radiotherapy. Following 10.5 Gy contribution from external beam radiotherapy, a dose of 65 Gy was given with the implant, while after 40 Gy, an implant dose of 25 Gy was prescribed. Depending on the prescribed dose and on the actual activity of the

iridium-192 wires, treatment duration varied from 24 to 80 h. After the prescribed radiation dose had been delivered, the implant was removed and the patient was returned to the urology service for further postoperative care.

The bladder drainage was removed after 2 weeks. Patients were closely followed up and urine cytology was obtained at 3-monthly intervals. The first cystoscopy was performed 6 months following the treatment and repeated at 3-monthly intervals. Intravenous urography and computerized tomography of the pelvis were performed at 1 year posttreatment and repeated annually. The mean follow-up was 6.9 years with a range from 1 to 12 years.

16.2.2
Results

16.2.2.1
Oncologic Results

Histologic examination of specimens obtained in the nine partial cystectomies showed only scar tissue in seven patients and persistent transitional cell carcinoma in two. Treatment results in these patients with shorter follow-up data have already been reported (VAN LIMBERGEN and VAN POPPEL 1989; VAN POPPEL et al. 1990, 1992).

Currently, 16 (57%) patients are alive with no evidence of disease and five (18%) have died of non-cancer-related causes without evidence of recurrent tumor at the time of death. Tumor progression has been noted in seven (25%) patients. One of these seven patients had superficial tumor recurrence, was treated with neodymium: YAG laser, and died because of cardiac disease without evidence of tumor recurrence. Three patients had a muscle-invasive local recurrence after brachytherapy for T3GIII tumor and underwent salvage cystectomy but died within 2 years of distant metastases. Two patients had systemic progression without local recurrence and one patient had an inoperable local recurrence. All of these three patients initially had T3GIII tumor and died of metastases within 16 months of interstitial implant; adjuvant chemotherapy was not attempted.

Local recurrence occurred in five (18%) study patients. One of these patients initially had a T1GIII transitional cell carcinoma. None of the 12 patients presenting with T2 tumors relapsed locally while four (33%) of the 12 T3 tumors showed local recurrence. Systemic relapse occurred in six (21%) pa-

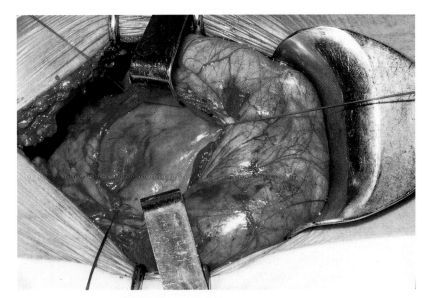

Fig. 16.3. Cystotomy showing the TUR scar at the posterior bladder wall

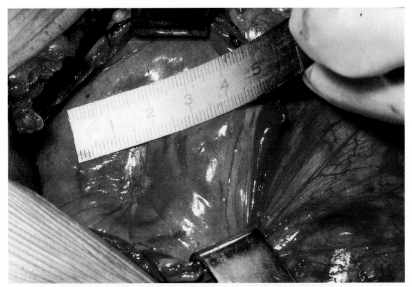

Fig. 16.4. Measurement of the area to be implanted with a safety margin of 1 cm around the scar

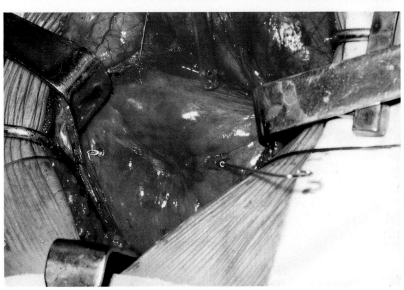

Fig. 16.5. Insertion of the first hollow needle

Fig. 16.6. Passage of the nylon wire through the needle

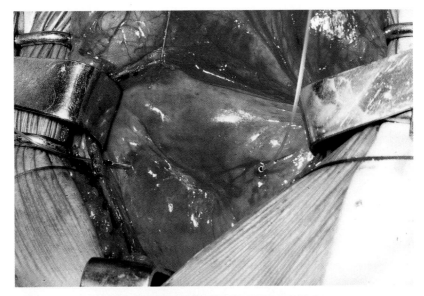

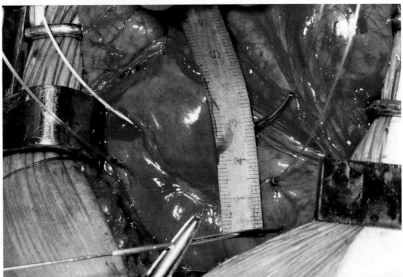

Fig. 16.7. Insertion of the third needle

Fig. 16.8. Slipping the nylon tube over the nylon wire

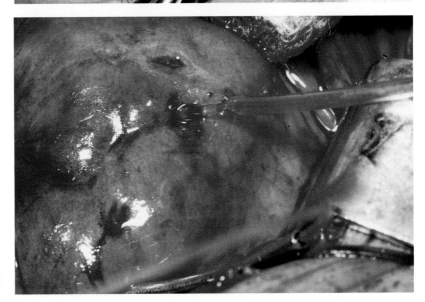

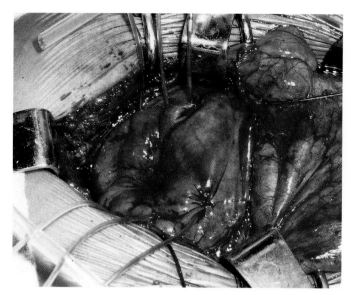

Fig. 16.9. Three tubes in place

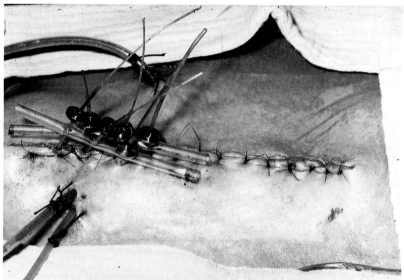

Fig. 16.10. Situation after wound closure showing the three tubes for iridium-192, a suprapubic bladder catheter, and two suction drains

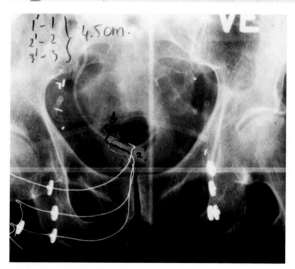

Fig. 16.11. Radiograph showing the placement of the metal dummy in the nylon tube

tients, all of whom initially presented with T3GIII tumors.

16.2.2.2
Complications

The mean hospital stay was 16 days. After hospital discharge all patients presented with transient radiocystitis which persisted for the first few postoperative weeks. One of these patients, however, had severe cystitis and bladder shrinking. This patient was finally treated with bilateral nephrostomies. The bladder, however, remained tumor free and the patient refused cystectomy and definitive urinary diversion.

Vesicocutaneous fistula was present in two (7%) patients. Bladder drainage for another 2 weeks was sufficient in resolving the leakage, as confirmed by a subsequently performed cystogram. After the implantation one patient developed a bladder neck stenosis of the left trigone and was treated by laser incision of the bladder neck.

Hydronephrosis occurred in three (11%) patients. One of these three patients had a ureteral re-implantation at the time of the iridium-192 implant. The other two had an implantation at a latero-posterior location and a temporary double J catheter was inserted. The hydronephrosis was asymptomatic and kidney function remained normal, so no other treatment was required.

16.3
Discussion

It was Marja Curie-Sklodowska, born in Warsaw in 1867, who gave her name to curietherapy. She was the first to use a small radium tube for the treatment of cancer. For her discoveries she received the Nobel prize in physics in 1904 and in chemistry in 1911. When Madame Curie died in Paris in 1934, DARGER (1931) had already used radium needles for the treatment of bladder cancer. The implantation technique with radium-226 needles and later with cesium-137 was further developed mainly in The Netherlands and in France. Initially most patients undergoing bladder implantation were treated with radium-226, but for personnel safety reasons this was replaced by cesium-137. With the development of artificial isotopes, particularly iridium-192, new implantation techniques were also developed. The afterloading technique with nylon tube implants was first used in France in 1971 (BOTTO et al. 1980).

The use of interstitial radiation in patients with bladder cancer is still most common in European countries. Few radiation oncologists, however, are familiar with this procedure and not all departments of radiotherapy have the necessary equipment for brachytherapy.

The main advantage of using iridium-192 wire implantation is the possibility of afterloading. During the implantation procedure only nonradio-active carriers are implanted under digital and visual monitoring, permitting accurate positioning. When the position of these carriers is found to be optimal, iridium-192 is afterloaded. The carriers used for this interstitial implantation are well tolerated by the tissues and vesico-cutaneous fistulas are much less frequent than with radium or cesium needle implants. Also, the removal of the radioac-tive sources and their carriers is possible without the need for anesthesia. The afterloading technique reduces the risk of radiation exposure for medical and nursing staff. Moreover protective shielding is easier with iridium-192, which is an isotope of lower photon energy than radium-226 or cesium-137.

Generally, patients with solitary T1, T2, and T3a tumors of a limited diameter (<5 cm) are accepted for interstitial radiation. In many cases, the brachytherapy is preceded by a course of external beam radiotherapy in order to prevent tumor recurrence in the incisional scar.

Published results of different series of bladder brachytherapy are not completely comparable since the radioactive sources and implantation techniques have changed so much over the past 80 years. There is also a selection bias, with some medical centers perform partial cystectomies while others never perform this procedure for invasive bladder cancer. Additionally, patient selection criteria and the follow-up process vary.

Most reports on interstitial radium therapy in patients with carcinoma of the bladder come from Rotterdam. The reported incidence of local control obtained in that medical center was 91% for T1 lesions, 84% for T2 lesions, and 72% for T3 lesions. In patients with T1GIII tumors a local control rate of 84% was obtained at 5 years (VAN DER WERF-MESSING and HOP 1981; VAN DER WERF-MESSING et al. 1983a,b). The experience with cesium-137 therapy came from two other Dutch medical centers, which reported 5-year actuarial local control rates of 82% for T1 and 74% for T2 and T3a tumors (BATTERMAN and TIERIE 1986; BATTERMAN and BOON 1988; DENEVE et al. 1992).

The most recent experience with iridium-192 came from different European centers and also from the United States. This experience can be summarized as follows: for category T1GIII tumors, bladder relapse rates of 15%–28% have been reported, with 5-year actuarial survival rates of 70%–80%. For T2 cancer relapse rates of 7%–32% and 5-year actuarial survival rates of 50%–76% have been noted (GERARD 1985; MAZERON et al. 1988; STRAUS et al. 1988; VAN LIMBERGEN and VAN POPPEL 1989; ROZAN et al. 1992; MOONEN et al. 1994; PERNOT et al. 1996). For T3a tumors, a bladder relapse rate of 28%–39% and a 5-year actuarial survival rate of 61%–72% have been reported (WIJNMAALEN and VAN DER WERF-MESSING 1986; GROSSMAN et al. 1993). Our own results reported here show similar success rates.

Interstitial radiotherapy in well-selected bladder cancer patients results in a high percentage of local control and excellent survival rates. It is, therefore, surprising that the application of interstitial radiotherapy remains restricted to a few centers. The best candidates for interstitial radiotherapy are those patients who are also candidates for bladder substitution, and since the latter has become more popular, many urologists prefer this solution. However, interstitial radiotherapy remains an excellent alternative treatment modality since preserving the bladder function is still an important goal when possible. In elderly patients who are not very fit for bowel surgery or in patients with a vascular prosthesis, in whom bowel surgery has to be avoided, brachytherapy can become the optimal therapeutic solution.

There is no difference in the efficacy of the different isotopes, but iridium-192 brachytherapy certainly has less complications and is easier to manage. Since 1990, we have nearly always performed a partial cystectomy (with ureteral reimplantation when necessary) and implanted two wires, without increasing the complication rates. The placement of two catheters makes the procedure easier and renders postoperative care simple.

16.4
Conclusion

Interstitial radiation is useful in patients with small (<5 cm) T1GIII, T2, or T3a bladder cancer without severe dysplasia on random biopsies. Modern brachytherapy using afterloading techniques with iridium-192 is safe, easy, less complicated, and as effective as previously used alternative techniques. Because the majority of patients treated with implantation are highly selected, the results are not directly comparable to those achieved by external beam radiotherapy or cystectomy.

Therefore, there is a need for prospective randomized trials comparing the different treatment strategies in the management of bladder cancer (GOSPODAROWICZ and WARDE 1992). However, it will be difficult to recruit sufficient numbers of patients for such trials unless urologic surgeons are prepared to consider the possibility that radical cystectomy may not be the best treatment for all patients with invasive bladder cancer.

Acknowledgements. Gratitude is expressed to Agnes Goethuys for her assistance in the word-processing and preparation of this manuscript.

References

Batterman JJ, Boon TA (1988) Interstitial therapy in the management of T2 bladder tumors. Endocurietherapie, Hyperthermia Oncol 14:1–6

Batterman JJ, Tierie AH (1986) Results of implantation for T1 and T2 bladder tumors. Radiother Oncol 5:85–90

Botto H, Perrin JL, Auvert J, Salle M, Pierquin B (1980) Treatment of malignant bladder tumors by iridium 192 wiring. Urology 16:467–469

Darget R (1931) La radium thérapie des tumeurs vésicales. Bull Soc Franç Urol 171–173

Deneve W, Lybeert ML, Goor C, Crommelin MA, Ribot JG (1992) T1 and T2 carcinoma of the urinary bladder: long term results with external, preoperative, or interstitial radiotherapy. Int J Radiat Oncol Biol Phys 23:299–304

Gérard JP (1985) La curiethérapie à l'Iridium dans le traitement conservateur des cancers infiltrants de vessie. J Urol (Paris) 91:139–143

Gospodarowicz MK, Warde P (1992) The role of radiation therapy in the management of transitional cell carcinoma of the bladder. Hematol Oncol Clin North Am 6:147–168

Gospodarowicz MK, Quilty PM, Scalliet P, et al. (1995) The place of radiation therapy as definitive treatment for bladder cancer. Int J Urol 2(Suppl 2):41–48

Grossman HB, Sandler HM, Perez-Tamayo C (1993) Treatment of T3a bladder cancer with iridium implantation. Urology 41:217–220

Koiso K, Shipley W, Keuppens F, et al. (1995) Int J Urol 2(Suppl 2):49–57

Mazeron JJ, Crook J, Chopin D, Abbou CC, Le Bourgeois JP, Auvert J, Pierquin B (1988) Conservative treatment of bladder carcinoma by partial cystectomy and interstitial iridium 192. Int J Radiat Oncol Biol Phys 15:1323–1330

Moonen LMF, Horenblas S, Van der Voet JCM, Nuyten MJC, Bartelinck H (1994) Bladder conservation in selected T1GIII and muscle invasive T2-T3a bladder carcinoma using combination therapy of surgery and iridium 192 implantation. Br J Urol 74:322–327

Pernot M, Hubert J, Guillemin F, et al. (1996) Combined surgery and brachytherapy in the treatment of some cancers of the bladder (partial cystectomy and interstitial iridium-192). Radiother Oncol 38:115–120

Rozan R, Albuisson E, Donnarieux D, et al. (1992) Interstitial iridium-192 for bladder cancer (a multicentric survey: 205 patients). Int J Radiat Oncol Biol Phys 24:469–477

Shipley WU, Rose MA (1985) Bladder cancer: the selection of patients for treatment by full dose irradiation. Cancer 55:2278–2284

Solsona E, Iborra I, Ricos JV, Monros JL, Dumont R (1992) Feasibility of TUR for muscle infiltrating carcinoma of the bladder: prospective study. J Urol 147:1513–1515

Straus KL, Littman P, Wein AJ, Whittington R, Tomaszewski JE (1988) Treatment of bladder cancer with interstitial iridium-192 implantation and external beam irradiation. Int J Radiat Oncol Biol Phys 14:265–271

Sweeney P, Kursh ED, Resnick MI (1992) Partial cystectomy. Urol Clin North Am 19:1701–1711

van der Werf-Messing B, Hop WCJ (1981) Carcinoma of the urinary bladder (category T1NxM0) treated either by radium implant or by TUR only. Int J Radiat Oncol Biol Phys 7:299–303

van der Werf-Messing B, Menon RS, Hop WCJ (1983a) Carcinoma of the urinary bladder category T2NxM0 treated by the combination of radium implant and external irradiation. Int J Radiat Oncol Biol Phys 9:177–180

van der Werf-Messing B, Menon RS, Hop WCJ (1983b) Cancer of the urinary bladder category T2, T3 (NxM0) treated by interstitial radium implant: second report. Int J Radiat Oncol Biol Phys 9:481–485

Van Limbergen E, Van Poppel H (1989) Bladder conserving treatment with interstitial implantation for invasive bladder cancer. Advances in Clinical Oncology, European School of Oncology, pp 179–184

Van Poppel H, Van Limbergen E, van der Schueren E, Baert L (1990) Interstitial radiotherapy for invasive bladder cancer. Abstr 5th Congress Eur Soc Surg Oncol

Van Poppel H, Van Limbergen E, Tan R, Baert L (1992) Longterm results of interstitial radiotherapy for invasive bladder cancer. Abstr Euro-American Conference on Urological Cancer, pp 42

Wijnmaalen A, van der Werf-Messing B (1986) Factors influencing the prognosis in bladder cancer. Int J Radiat Oncol Biol Phys 12:559–565

17 Bladder-Conserving Therapy for Invasive Bladder Cancer Using Transurethral Surgery, Chemotherapy, and Radiation Therapy with Patient Selection by Initial Treatment Response

W.U. Shipley, A.L. Zietman, D.S. Kaufman, A.F. Althausen, and N.M. Heney

CONTENTS

17.1 Introduction

The Fourth International Consensus Meeting on Bladder Cancer provided updated results of conservative surgery, radiation therapy, and systemic chemotherapy, each as monotherapy, as well as strategies of combined modality treatment with two or three of these modalities as reviewed by a panel of nine urologic oncologists (K. Koiso, W.U. Shipley, S. Keuppen, L. Baert, R.R. Hall, M. Hudson, S. Khoury, Y. Kubota, and H. Van Poppel). Based on this review, ten areas of consensus were reached:

1. The primary goal of bladder preservation treatment for a patient with muscle-invading bladder

cancer is survival; bladder preservation in the interest of quality of life is a secondary objective.

2. Only a small proportion of carefully selected patients may be cured by transurethral surgery alone or by partial cystectomy alone.

3. Radiation therapy is currently the standard bladder-preserving therapy against which all other bladder-preserving methods must be compared.

4. Systemic chemotherapy as monotherapy is inadequate and cannot be recommended.

5. The addition of cisplatin-containing systemic chemotherapy to radiation therapy or conservative surgery appears to improve local control. Whilst no multimodality therapeutic regimen has yet been shown to be clearly optimal with regard to local efficacy and minimization of toxicity, monotherapy for bladder-preserving treatment is probably not desirable as a routine approach.

6. Deferring the patient from immediate cystectomy does not appear to compromise survival nor does the addition of primary systemic chemotherapy appear to increase significantly the morbidity of cystectomy or radiotherapy.

7. All patients treated by bladder-preserving therapy must return to the urologist for regular cystoscopic follow-up so that additional therapy may be started at the earliest opportunity, if relapse occurs.

8. Bladder substitution will always be second best and is suboptimal compared with a normally functioning disease-free bladder.

9. If alternatives to cystectomy are not considered, little progress will be made in the treatment of muscle-invading bladder cancer.

10. Randomized phase III trials will have to be performed to establish the role of optimal combined modality treatment for bladder preservation but patient recruitment to such trials may prove difficult unless urologists are prepared to open their minds to the possibility that cystectomy

W.U. Shipley, MD, Head, Genitourinary Oncology Unit, Department of Radiation Oncology, Massachusetts General Hospital, Boston, MA 02114, USA
A.L. Zietman, MD, Genitourinary Oncology Unit, Department of Radiation Oncology, Massachusetts General Hospital, Boston, MA 02114, USA
D.S. Kaufman, MD, Medical Oncology Unit, Department of Medicine, Massachusetts General Hospital, Boston, MA 02114, USA
A.F. Althausen, MD, Department of Urology, Massachusetts General Hospital, Harvard Medical School, Boston, MA 02114, USA
N.M. Heney, MD, Department of Urology, Massachusetts General Hospital, Harvard Medical School, Boston, MA 02114, USA

may not be the best treatment for all patients with muscle-invading bladder cancer.

A bladder-conserving approach is only justified in a patient who is otherwise a cystectomy candidate when this approach has a high likelihood of achieving total eradication of tumor in the bladder. Selection criteria for these approaches may be either by initial favorable tumor factors such as size or the absence of ureteral obstruction or by the clinical complete response to induction therapy as judged by cystoscopic reevaluation. There is a lack of certainty in favorable prognostic factors for the achievement of local cure and thus these approaches inevitably do require both physician judgment (selection) and some patient risk. Close urologic surveillance is essential. Only those patients whose tumors show a clinical complete response to induction therapy are selected for bladder conservation. These "selected" patients then receive consolidation chemo-radiation therapy. Patients with less than a clinical complete response are advised to undergo cystectomy.

17.2
Radiation Therapy Alone

17.2.1
Historical Background

Many large series utilizing external beam radiation therapy alone without the use of favorable tumor selection factors were reported in the 1970s and 1980s with relatively similar results (Table 17.1) (Koiso et al. 1995; Jenkins et al. 1988; Shearer et al. 1988; Gospodarowicz et al. 1989; Mameghan et al. 1995). Those patients who were treated with radiation therapy alone were often inappropriate candidates for surgery. Despite that, a 20%–40% long-term cure rate was achieved with radiation therapy alone (Table 17.1). The total radiation doses used in these series varied from 60–65 Gy given in

1.8- to 2-Gy fractions 5 days a week (commonly done in North America) to 50–55 Gy given in 2.5 or 2.75 Gy per fraction (common in the United Kingdom). The clinical complete response rate, which is usually measured by a cystoscopic examination and biopsy 3–6 months after the completion of radiation therapy, ranged from 40% to 52%. Patients who did not respond completely to radiation were offered radical cystectomy if medically fit, or palliative management otherwise. Local tumor control rate at 5 years ranged from 35% to 45% for all patients. For those patients who achieved a clinical complete response the long-term local control rates were 45%–79%.

17.2.2
Modern Radiation Treatment Planning

As with other tumor sites, careful treatment planning is necessary to deliver the radiation to the clinical target volume accurately while limiting the radiation dose to normal tissue structures outside of the target volume. Careful documentation of the findings on cystoscopic and bimanual examination is necessary and should be combined with the information from computed tomography (CT) scan in an effort to document the full extent of the target volume of the primary tumor Cystogram at simulation is necessary to identify the mucosal surface of the bladder, while a CT scan is needed to provide information on the exterior bladder surface, extravesical tumor extension, and lymph node status. Using a cystogram alone without a planning CT scan may cause inadequate coverage of the bladder in up to 60% of patients (Larsen and Engelholm 1994; Rothwell et al. 1983). Bladder underdosing can occur during the course of external beam therapy, with up to 60% of the patients having more than 1.5 cm movement of at least one bladder wall relative to the isodose lines (Turner et al. 1994; Sur et al. 1993). Factors associated with bladder movement

Table 17.1. Results following external beam irradiation alone

Series	References	No. of patients	Clinical stage	5-Year survival	5-Year local bladder control
London Hospital	Jenkins et al. (1988)	182	T2–T3	40%	41%
U.K. Co-op Group	Shearer et al. (1988)	157	T3	23%	45%
Princess Margaret Hosp.	Gospodarowicz et al. (1989)	121	T2–T4a	40%	35%
Sydney, Prince of Wales	Mameghan et al. (1995)	342	T1–T4b	–	45%
Belgium/Netherlands Group	De Neve et al. (1995)	147	T2–T3	31%	35%

include large bladder size, a large residual tumor, or a primary tumor located at the base of the bladder. Advances in technology with three-dimensional dose planning systems and beam's eye views were found to be effective tools for treatment planning for bladder carcinoma (LARSEN and ENGELHOLM 1994). Treatment delivery accuracy is increased with real-time imaging systems (GILDERSLEVE et al. 1994). Most treatment policies call for the delivery of full dose to at least the whole bladder but we have advocated that the volume be reduced so that the final boost is delivered only to the primary tumor with an appropriate margin (SHIPLEY et al. 1986; MARKS and SHIPLEY 1992). The opinion of the Consensus Group at the Fourth International Consensus Meeting on bladder cancer was to recommend that the external beam radiation therapy volume encompass the bladder alone without any attempt to irradiate pelvic lymph nodes routinely (GOSPODAROWICZ et al. 1995). However, our institution and the RTOG continue to recommend an initial course of 40–45 Gy to the lymph nodes of the true pelvis plus the primary tumor target volume followed by a boost to the bladder and bladder tumor volume (KAUFMAN et al. 1993; TESTER et al. 1996). It should be noted that in these treatment approaches the radiation therapy is given concurrently with systemic cisplatin.

Interstitial implant has been used for early-stage bladder carcinoma for many years in Europe and will be reported in this book by van Poppel and colleagues (see Chap. 16). In the hands of experienced urologists and radiation oncologists, interstitial radiation for limited bladder cancer results in a high percentage of local control and excellent survival rates. Whether these favorable results are due to the delivery of a higher radiation dose to the tumor volume and than be achieved by external beam radiation or due to the thoughtful patient selection process is unclear. Thus it is not yet possible to conclude whether the brachytherapy approach offers any advantage over the more commonly and more easily used external beam radiation therapy.

Improved clinical complete response rates have been reported using accelerated fractionation schemes of external beam radiation therapy alone. The Royal Marsden Hospital treated patients with twice daily fractions of 1.8–2.0 Gy 5 days a weeks to doses between 57.6 and 64 Gy in up to 32 fractions over 26 days. Eighty-five patients were included in this study. Of 70 who had a cystoscopic reevaluation from 3 to 6 months following radiation therapy, 80% were found to be clinically complete responders (COLE et al. 1992; HORWICH et al. 1995). In a randomized trial done in the 1970s in 168 patients unsuited for cystectomy but with T2–T4 tumors, hyperfractionated external beam radiation therapy alone (1.0 Gy 3 times a day to a total dose of 84 Gy) was compared with conventional treatment of 2.0 Gy daily to 64 Gy. This study showed a significant survival benefit for hyperfractionation at 5 years (27% vs 18%), with a significant improvement in the complete response rate (41% vs 25%) but also a statistically insignificant increase in bowel complications (NASLUND et al. 1994). Taken together these results suggest that altered fractionation including both hyperfractionation and acceleration (shorter overall treatment times) should improve results over external beam radiation alone and such approaches are being tested by a phase III trial at the Royal Marsden Hospital (HORWICH et al. 1995).

Table 17.2. Muscle-invading bladder cancer: success rates of bladder preservation with monotherapy

Treatment	References	No. of evaluated series	Total no. of patients	% with bladder free of invasive recurrence
Transurethral resection alone[a]	HERR (1987) HENRY et al. (1988)	2	331	20%[b]
Radiation therapy alone[c]	JENKINS et al. (1988) SHEARER et al. (1988) GOSPODAROWICZ et al. (1989) MAMEGHAN et al. (1995) DE NEVE et al. (1995)	5	949	41%
Chemotherapy alone (cisplatin + methotrexate)[c]	HALL (1992)	1	27	19%

[a] Used selectively as monotherapy; most patients had cystecgtomy.
[b] Intravesical drug therapy often used for noninvasive recurrent tumors.
[c] No transurethral resection of tumor.

17.3
Rationale for Combined Modality Therapy

Cure of the bladder of a muscle-invading tumor is possible in some patients by conservative surgery alone, by radiation therapy alone, or by systemic chemotherapy alone, as shown in Table 17.2. However, the 20%–40% success rate of each individual therapy used unselectively must be considered a poor outcome relative to modern radical cystectomy, where the pelvic local control rates approach 90%. Several reports, mostly retrospective, have suggested that the combination of transurethral tumor resection with subsequent by radiation therapy or multidrug systemic chemotherapy achieved an improved rate of freedom from recurrence of tumor in the bladder and/or a higher clinical complete response rate on rebiopsy and reassessment of the cytology in bladder washings (SHIPLEY and ROSE 1985; HALL 1995; SHIPLEY et al. 1987; SCHER et al. 1989; SAUER et al. 1990). At about the same time, laboratory studies demonstrated that several cytotoxic agents, including cisplatin and 5-fluorouracil, are capable of sensitizing tumor tissue to radiation and increasing cell kill in a synergistic fashion (DURAND and VANDERBYL 1988; BEGG 1990; FLENTJE et al. 1991). Taken together, these studies framed the rationale for combined treatment approaches incorporated in conservative surgery by transurethral resection followed by concurrent chemotherapy and radiation. By reducing tumor bulk, conservative surgery likely reduces the dose of chemotherapy and radiation therapy required for complete tumor eradication in the urinary bladder. Thus in this potentially complementary and clinically feasible way, combinations of these three modalities provide higher complete response rates than any of the modalities alone (Table 17.3) and still allow for selection of bladder conservation by the initial response of the primary tumor to induction therapy.

17.4
Results of Combined Modality Therapy

Over the last 3 years four reports combining these modalities in clinically feasible regimens have strengthened the case for combined therapy for bladder preservation. These include results from the University of Erlangen in Germany (DUNST et al. 1994), the University of Paris (HOUSSETT et al. 1993), the Massachusetts General Hospital (KAUFMAN et al. 1993; KACHNIC et al. 1997), and the Radiation Therapy Oncology Group (RTOG) (TESTER et al. 1993, 1996) (Table 17.4). Three of these studies have

Table 17.3. Muscle-invading bladder cancer: complete response rates after monotherapies and combined modality therapies (modified from KOISO et al. 1995)

Treatment	References	No. of evaluated series	Total no. of patients	% clinical complete responses
Radiation therapy alone	JENKINS et al. (1988) GOSPODAROWICZ et al. (1989) QUILTY and DUNCAN (1986) SMAALAND et al. (1991)	4	721	45%
Chemotherapy alone	KEATING et al. (1989) KURTH et al. (1991) HALL and ROBERTS (1991) NAFFEZZINI et al. (1991) ROBERTS et al. (1991) FARAH et al. (1991)	6	301	27%
TURBT plus chemotherapy	SCHER et al. (1989) HALL et al. (1984) PROUT et al. (1990) PARSONS and MILLION (1991)	4	225	51%
TURBT plus chemo-radiotherapy	PARSONS and MILLION (1991) FUNG et al. (1991) TESTER et al. (1991) CERVAK et al. (1991)	4	218	71%

TURBT, Transurethral resection of tumor.

Table 17.4. Recent reports of survival and of survival with bladder preservation in patients treated by conservative surgery and concurrent chemotherapy plus radiation therapy

Series	Treatment	No. of patients	5-Year survival	5-Year survival with bladder preservation
SAUER et al. (1990) DUNST et al. (1994)	TURBT, concurrent cisplatin, and XRT	79	52%	41%
TESTER et al. (1996)	Concurrent cisplatin and XRT	42	52%	42%
TESTER et al. (1996)	MCV and concurrent cisplatin and XRT	91	62%[a]	44%[a]
KACHNIC et al. (1996)	TURBT, MCV, concurrent cisplatin, and XRT	106	52%	43%

XRT, External beam irradiation; MCV, methotrexate, cisplatin, vinblastine; TURBT, transurethral resection of tumor.
[a] Based on 4-year data.

Table 17.5. Recent reports of survival and of survival with bladder preservation in patients treated by conservative surgery and chemotherapy alone

Series	Treatment	No. of patients	5-Year survival	5-Year survival with bladder preservation
SROUGI and SIMON (1994)	M-VAC and partial cystectomy	30	53%	20%
STERNBERG et al. (1995)	TURBT + M-VAC but without cystectomy in 31 patients	64	–[a]	33%[a]
SCHER et al. (1989) SCHULTZ et al. (1994)	M-VAC and conservative surgery	111	48%	21%
GIVEN et al. (1995)	TURBT, MCV plus, in 49 patients (53%), concurrent cisplatin and XRT	93	51%	18%

XRT, External beam irradiation; MCV, methotrexate, cisplatin, vinblastine; M-VAC, methotrexate, vinblastine, adriamycin, cisplatin; TURBT, transurethral resection of tumor.
[a] Median follow-up 30 months at time of report.

included aggressive transurethral resection with radiation therapy and cisplatin-based chemotherapy (DUNST et al. 1994; HOUSSETT et al. 1993; KACHNIC et al. 1997), and three have incorporated selection for bladder conservation including those patients with a clinical complete response to induction chemo-radiation (HOUSSETT et al. 1993; KACHNIC et al. 1997; TESTER et al. 1993, 1996). As shown in Table 17.4, the overall survival at 5 years is 52%, which is similar to a prospective radical cystectomy series reporting patients with similar clinical stages and age (MARTINEZ-PINEIRO et al. 1995). Perhaps one of the reasons why the survival rates using transurethral resection and chemo-radiotherapy are better than reported rates with external beam radiation therapy is the recognition that patients who are at high risk for local failure can be identified early and cystectomy promptly performed. Cystoscopies were carried out 4–8 weeks following completion of chemo-radiotherapy and any patient with persistent

and invasive tumor was referred for salvage cystectomy before local regrowth (and a second chance for metastases) could occur.

Several recent reports on treatment by conservative surgery and chemotherapy alone provide evidence that radiation therapy considerably enhances the effectiveness of transurethral resection and systemic chemotherapy in maintaining the bladder free of tumor (SROUGI and SIMON 1994; STERNBERG et al. 1995; SCHULTZ et al. 1994; GIVEN et al. 1995). As shown in Table 17.5, the 5-year survival figures are equally high, all around 50%, because on recurrence the tumors are treated promptly with radical cystectomy. However the 5-year survival with bladder preservation is considerably lower, from 20% to 33% (cf. results in Table 17.4). Special mention is made of the report by Given and colleagues from the University of Florida (GIVEN et al. 1995), in which transurethral surgery and chemotherapy were used on all 93 patients but external beam radiation therapy with or without concurrent cisplatin was used in only 49 patients, with the result that only 18% of patients were surviving after 5 years with bladder preservation.

17.5
Recurrence of Superficial Bladder Tumors

Superficial bladder tumors may recur in 10%–30% of patients who have had bladder preservation following multimodality therapy (KAUFMAN et al. 1993; SCHER et al. 1989; SAUER et al. 1990; DUNST et al. 1994; HOUSSETT et al. 1993; KACHNIC et al. 1996; TESTER et al. 1993, 1996). The preserved bladder retains the biologic ability to form tumors (mainly carcinoma in situ) which are amenable to standard management using transurethral resection and intravesical drug therapy. Fifteen of the 21 patients in the Massachusetts General Hospital series who developed either a Ta tumor or a carcinoma in situ, amongst the 76 patients treated with bladder preservation, have been maintained in remission by transurethral resection and intravesical drug therapy for 15–49 months following the development of a new tumor (KACHNIC et al. 1997). Four of these patients have progressed to muscle-invading tumors requiring cystectomy and two have persistent superficial tumors managed conservatively. All patients treated by multimodality bladder-preserving therapies must be willing to undergo regular cystoscopic follow-up so that transurethral surgery, intravesical chemotherapy, or cystectomy can be used at the earliest opportunity, if necessary.

17.6
Tolerance of the Bladder to Modern Radiation Therapy With or Without Chemotherapy

The concern of the urologist that a conserved, irradiated bladder functions poorly has been answered by recent reports using modern radiation techniques (LYNCH et al. 1992). In the Erlangen experience only three cystectomies were necessary for bladder shrinkage amongst 192 preserved bladders, for an incidence of 1.6% (HOUSSETT et al. 1993). We reported excellent tolerance in a retrospective review of 21 women who were successfully treated by bladder conservation using chemo-radiation (KACHNIC et al. 1997). With a median follow-up of 56 months all patients were continent without dysuria or hematuria. Bladder function was improved or unchanged after treatment in 91% of the patients. No patient reported a compromise in bowel or sexual function. A recent update of the results in 106 patients treated consecutively at our institution with transurethral resection of tumor, and two cycles of methotrexate, cisplatin, and vinblastine chemotherapy, followed in 76 cases by concurrent cisplatin and full-dose radiation therapy to 64.8 Gy, shows that no patient has had to undergo cystectomy for shrinkage or bleeding (KACHNIC et al. 1996).

17.7
Conclusion

Bladder conservation trials report results by clinical stage, which may underestimate the extent of disease. Cystectomy-based trials are usually reported by pathologic staging and exclude approximately 15% of patients found at surgery to have metastatic nodal disease in the upper pelvis or higher. Despite the inability to exclude some patients with metastatic disease, survival following bladder-conserving treatment with transurethral resection, chemotherapy, and radiation has been reported to be similar to that in cystectomy-based series for patients of similar clinical stage and age, and such treatment also offers a 60%–70% chance of maintaining a normally functioning bladder. Because this approach has been shown to fail in about 30% of patients with clinical stage T2–T3b bladder cancers, additional methods are needed to identify these patients so a prompt cystectomy can be performed. Selection criteria include having a clinical complete response following induction with chemo-radiation, selection of only the most favorable patients (such as those with clinical T2 tumors or those in whom a visibly complete TURB was judged possible), or both.

Bladder-conserving therapy should be offered to selective patients with invasive bladder cancer as an effective alternative to radical cystectomy. Such treatment should be administered by experienced teams of urologists, medical oncologists, and radiation oncologists.

References

Begg A (1990) Cisplatin and radiation: interaction probabilities and other therapeutic possibilities. Int J Radiat Oncol Biol Phys 19:1183–1189

Cervak J, Cufer T, Maroit F, et al. (1991) Combined chemotherapy and radiotherapy in muscle-invasive bladder carcinoma. Complete remission results. ECCO 6:Abstract #561

Cole D, Durrant K, Robert J, et al. (1992) A pilot study of accelerated fractionation in the radiotherapy of invasive carcinoma of the bladder. Br J Radiol 65:792–798

DeNeve W, Lybeert ML, Goor C, et al. (1995) Radiotherapy for T2 and T3 carcinoma of the bladder: the influence of overall treatment time. Radiother Oncol 36:183–188

Dunst J, Sauer R, Schrott KM, et al. (1994) Organ-sparing treatment of advanced bladder cancer: a 10 year experience. Int J Radiat Oncol Biol Phys 30:261–266

Durand R, Vanderbyl S (1988) Response of cell populations in spheroids to radiation-drug combinations. NCI Monogr 6:95–100

Farah R, Chodak GW, Vogelzang NI, et al. (1991) Curative radiotherapy following chemotherapy for invasive bladder carcinoma (a preliminary report). Int J Radiat Oncol Biol Phys 20:413–417

Flentje M, Eble M, Haner U (1991) Additive effects of cisplatin and radiation in human tumor cells under toxic conditions. Radiother Oncol 24:60–63

Fung CY, Shipley WU, Young RH, et al. (1991) Prognostic factors in invasive bladder carcinoma in a prospective trial of preoperative adjuvant chemotherapy and radiotherapy. J Clin Oncol 9:1533–1542

Gildersleve J, Dearnaley DP, Evans PM, Law M, Rawlings C, Swindell W (1994) A randomized trial of patient repositioning during radiotherapy using a megavoltage imaging system. Radiother Oncol 31:161–168

Given RW, Parsosn JT, McCarley D, et al. (1995) Bladder-sparing multimodality treatment of muscle-invasive bladder cancer. A 5-year follow-up. Urol 46:499–505

Gospodarowicz MK, Hawkins MV, Rawling GA, et al. (1989) Radical radiotherapy for muscle invasive transitional cell carcinoma of the bladder: failure analysis. J Urol 142:1448–1453

Gospodarowicz MK, Quilty PM, Scalliet P, et al. (1995) The place of radiation therapy as definitive treatment of bladder cancer. Int J Urol 2:41–48

Hall RR (1992) Transurethral resection for transitional cell carcinoma. Urol 6:460–470

Hall RR (1995) Bladder preserving treatment: the role of transurethral surgery alone and with combined modality therapy for muscle-invading bladder cancer. In: Vogelzang NJ, Scardino PT, Shipley WU, Coffey DS (eds) Comprehensive textbook of genitourinary oncology. Williams and Wilkins, Baltimore, pp 509–513

Hall RR, Roberts JT (1991) Neoadjuvant chemotherapy, a method to conserve the bladder? ECCO 6:Abstract 144

Hall RR, Newling DWW, Ramsden PD, et al. (1984) Treatment of invasive bladder cancer by local resection and high dose methotrexate. Br J Urol 56:668–672

Henry K, Miller J, Mort M, Loening S, Fallon B (1988) Comparison of transurethral resection to radical therapies for stage B bladder tumors. J Urol 140:964–967

Herr HW (1987) Conservative management of muscle-infiltrating bladder cancer: prospective experience. J Urol 138:1162–1163

Horwich A, Pendlebury S, Dearnaley DP (1995) Organ conservation in bladder cancer. Eur J Cancer 31:208

Housset M, Maulard C, Chretien YC, et al. (1993) Combined radiation and chemotherapy for invasive transitional-cell carcinoma of the bladder: a prospective study. J Clin Oncol 11:2150–2157

Jenkins BJ, Blandy JP, Caulfield MJ, et al. (1988) Reappraisal of the role of radical radiotherapy and salvage cystectomy in the treatment of invasive bladder cancer. Br J Urol 62:343–346

Kachnic LA, Shipley WU, Griffin PP, Zietman AL, Kaufman DS, Althausen AF, Heney NM (1996) Combined modality treatment with selective bladder conservation for invasive bladder cancer: long-term tolerance in the female patient. Cancer J Sci Am 2:79–84

Kachnic LA, Kaufman DS, Griffin PP, Heney NM, Althausen AF, Zietman AL, Shipley WU (1997) Bladder preservation by combined modality therapy for invasive bladder cancer. J Clin Oncol 15:1022–1029

Kaufman DS, Shipley WU, Griffin PP, Heney NM, Althausen AF, Efird JT (1993) Selective bladder preservation by combined modality treatment of invasive bladder cancer. N Engl J Med 329:1377–1382

Keating J, Zincke H, Morgan WR, et al. (1989) Extended experience with neoadjuvant M-VAC chemotherapy for invasive transitional cell carcinoma of the urinary bladder. J Urol 141:244a

Koiso K, Shipley WU, Keuppen S, et al. (1995) The status of bladder preserving therapeutic strategies in the management of patients with muscle invasive bladder cancer. Int J Urol 2:49–57

Kurth K II, Splinter TA, Jacqmin D, et al. (1991) Transitional cell carcinoma of the bladder: a phase II study of chemotherapy in T3-4 NO MO of the EORTC GU group. In: Alderson AR, Oliver RT, Hanham IW, Bloom HJ (eds) Urological oncology dilemmas and developments. Wiley Liss, New York, pp 115–128

Larsen LE, Engelholm SA (1994) The value of 3-dimensional radiotherapy planning in advanced carcinoma of the urinary bladder based on computed tomography. Acta Oncol 33:655–694

Lynch WJ, Jenkins BJ, Fowler CG (1992) The quality of life after radial radiotherapy for bladder cancer. Br J Urol 70:519–521

Maffezzini M, Torelli T, Villa E, et al. (1991) Systemic preoperative chemotherapy with cisplatin, methotrexate, and vinblastine for locally advanced bladder cancer: local tumor response and early follow-up results. J Urol 145:741–743

Mameghan H, Fisher R, Mameghan J, et al. (1995) Analysis of failure following definitive radiotherapy for invasive transitional cell carcinoma of the bladder. Int J Radiat Oncol Biol Phys 31:247–254

Marks LB, Shipley WU (1992) Techniques for external irradiation of patients with invasive carcinoma of the urinary Bladder. In: Levitt SH (ed) Technologic: basis of radiotherapy: practical clinical applications, 2nd edn. Lea & Febiger, Philadelphia, chapter 22, pp 335–341

Martinez-Pineiro JA, Martin MG, Arocena NF, et al. (1995) Neoadjuvant cisplatin chemotherapy before radical cystectomy in invasive transitional cell carcinoma of the bladder: a prospective randomized phase III study. J Urol 153:964–973

Naslund I, Nilsson B, Littbrand B (1994) Hyper-fractionated radiotherapy of bladder cancer: a 10 year follow-up of a randomized clnical trial. Acta Oncol 33:397–402

Parsons JT, Million RR (1991) Bladder cancer. In: Perez CA, Brady IW (eds) Principles and practice of radiation oncology. Lippincott, Philadephia, pp 1036–1058

Prout GR, Shipley WU, Kaufman D, et al. (1990) Preliminary results in invasive bladder cancer with transurethral resection, neoadjuvant chemotherapy and combined pelvic irradiation plus cisplatin chemotherapy. J Urol 144:1128–1134

Quilty P, Duncan W (1986) Primary radical radiotherapy for T3 transitional cell cancer of the bladder: an analysis of survival and control. Int J Radiat Oncol Biol Phys 12:853–860.

Roberts JT, Fossa SP, Richards SB, et al. (1991) Results of Medical Research Council phase II study of low dose cisplatin and methotrexate in the primary treatment of locally advanced (T3 and T4) transitional cell carcinoma of the bladder. Br J Urol 68:162–168

Rothwell R, Ash D, Jones W (1983) Radiation treatment planning for bladder cancer: a comparison of cystogram localization with computed tomography. Clin Radiol 34:103–111

Sauer R, Dunst J, Altendorg-Hofmann A, et al. (1990) Radiotherapy with and without cisplatin in bladder cancer. Int J Radiat Oncol Biol Phys 19:687–691

Scher HI, Herr HW, Sternberg C, et al. (1989) Neoadjuvant chemotherapy for invasive bladder cancer. Experience with the MVAC regimen. Br J Urol 64:250–256

Schultz TK, Herr HW, Zhang ZF, et al. (1994) Neoadjuvant chemotherapy for invasive bladder cancer: prognostic factors for survival in patients treated with M-VAC with 5-year follow-up. J Clin Oncol 12:1394–1401

Shearer RJ, Chilvers CE, Bloom HJG, et al. (1988) Adjuvant chemotherapy in T3 carcinoma of the bladder. Br J Urol 62:558–564

Shipley WU, Rose MA (1985). Bladder cancer. The selection of patients for treatment of full-dose irradiation. Cancer 55:2278–2284

Shipley WU, Van der Schueren E, Kitagawa T, et al. (1986) Guidelines for radiation therapy in clinical research on bladder cancer. In: Denis L, Niijima T, Prout GR Jr, Schroder FH (eds) Developments in bladder cancer. EORTC Genitourinary Group monograph 3. Liss, New York, pp 109–121

Shipley WU, Prout GR Jr, Einstein AB, et al. (1987) Treatment of invasive bladder cancer by cisplatin and radiation in patients unsuited for surgery. JAMA 258:931–935

Smaaland R, Akslen LA, Tonder B, et al. (1991) Radical radiation treatment of invasive and locally advanced bladder carcinoma in elderly patients. Br J Urol 67:61–69

Srougi M, Simon SD (1994) Primary methotrexate, vinblastine, doxorubicin and cisplatin chemotherapy in bladder preservation in locally invasive bladder cancer: A 5-year follow-up. J Urol 151:593–597

Sternberg CN, Raghaven D, Ohi Y, et al. (1995) Neo-adjuvant and adjuvant chemotherapy in locally advanced disease: what are the effects on survival and prognosis. Int J Urol 2:75–87

Sur RK, Clinkard J, Jones WG et al. (1993) Changes in target volume during radiotherapy treatment of invasive bladder cancer. Clin Oncol 5:30–33

Tester W, Porter A, Heney J, et al. (1991) Neoadjuvant combined modality program with possible organ preservation for invasive bladder cancer. Proc Am Soc Clin Oncol 10:165

Tester W, Porter A, Asbell S, et al. (1993) Combined modality program with possible organ preservation for invasive bladder carcinoma: results of RTOG protocol 85–12. Int J Radiat Oncol Biol Phys 25:783–790

Tester W, Caplan R, Heaney J, et al. (1996) Neoadjuvant combined modality program with selective organ preservation for invasive bladder cancer: results of RTOG phase III trial 8802. J Clin Oncol 14:119–126

Turner S, Swindell R, Bowl N, Read G, Cowan RA (1994) Bladder movement during radiation therapy for bladder cancer: implication for treatment planning. Int J Radiat Oncol Biol Phys 30:199–200

18 Muscle-Invasive Bladder Cancer: Transurethral Resection and Radiochemotherapy as an Organ-Sparing Treatment Option

R. Sauer, S. Birkenhake, R. Kühn, C. Wittekind, P. Martus, J. Dunst, and K.M. Schrott

CONTENTS

18.1 Introduction

Up to 80% of all transitional cell carcinomas of the urinary bladder are found to be superficial at the time of diagnosis (Ta–T1). In spite of a 50% recurrence rate and a 10%–15% progression rate, these tumors can be controlled adequately by transurethral resection (TURB) and intravesical chemotherapy or immunotherapy. However, poorly differentiated T1 tumors and muscle-invasive tumors (>T2) require a more aggressive treatment approach.

Presently, radical cystectomy is considered the standard treatment for muscle-invasive as well as locally and regionally progressing bladder cancer. Perioperative mortality of less than 5% and local recurrence rates of 5%–10% (Pagano et al. 1991; Rhagavan et al. 1990; Skinner and Lieskovsky 1988; Stöckle et al. 1991; Whitmore et al. 1988; Wishnow et al. 1992) are frequently reported. Unfortunately, more than half of all cystectomized patients will die from their cancer as a consequence of occult widespread tumor metastases. Sophisticated techniques for urinary diversion do not alter the fact that cystectomy is still associated with severe long-term problems including social and psychosocial limitations and a considerable loss of quality of life. Therefore, the question arises as to whether primary cystectomy can be replaced by an organ-sparing comprehensive treatment for patients with a muscle-invasive cancer (Abradt et al. 1993; Blandy et al. 1980; Bloom et al. 1982; Chauvet et al. 1993; Cervak et al. 1993; Coppin et al. 1992; De Neve et al. 1995; Duncan and Quilty 1986; Dunst et al. 1994; Dunst 1991; Goodman et al. 1981; Miller and Johnson 1973; Quilty and Duncan 1985; Rebischung et al. 1992; Rotman et al. 1987; Russel et al. 1990; Sauer et al. 1990; Shearer et al. 1988; Shipley et al. 1987; Smaaland et al. 1991; Tester et al. 1993; Zietman et al. 1993). Cystectomy will then be reserved as the salvage treatment modality for nonresponding or recurrent tumors.

It has been the policy at the University of Erlangen-Nürnberg to use definitive radiotherapy (RT) with or without concurrent chemotherapy with platinum derivatives (CT) for invasive bladder cancer in a prospective protocol since 1982. Herein, we present our 14-year experience with a median follow-up time of 7.5 years.

R. Sauer, MD, Professor, Direktor der Universitäts-Strahlenklinik, Universitätsstrasse 27, D-91054 Erlangen, Germany

S. Birkenhake, MD, Universitäts-Strahlenklinik, Universitätsstrasse 27, D-91054 Erlangen, Germany

R. Kühn, MD, Privat-Dozent, Urologische Universitätsklinik, Maximiliansplatz 5, D-91054 Erlangen, Germany

C. Wittekind, MD, Professor, Direktor des Pathologischen Instituts der Universität Leipzig, Liebigstrasse 6, D-04103 Leipzig, Germany

P. Martus, MD, Privat-Dozent, Institut für Medizinische Dokumentation und Statistik der Universität, Waldstrasse 6, D-91054 Erlangen, Germany

J. Dunst, MD, Professor, Direktor der Universitäts-Strahlenklinik, Dryanderstrasse, D-06097 Halle/Saale, Germany

K.M. Schrott, MD, Professor, Direktor der Urologischen Universitätsklinik, Maximiliansplatz 5, D-91054 Erlangen, Germany

18.2
Patients and Methods

Between May 1982 and May 1996, a total of 333 patients with locally advanced bladder cancer were entered into the protocol if they fulfilled the following criteria: muscle invasive (pT2–4) or high-risk pT1 cancer (G3, associated Tis or Ta, tumor diameter ≥5 cm, residual and nonresectable tumor after TURB, multifocality, multiple recurrences), no distant metastases, and no prior pelvic irradiation (Table 18.1). Lymph node metastases (detected by computed tomography or ultrasound), multiple TURBs prior to (RT-CT), or poor general condition with contraindications for radical surgery were not exclusion criteria.

18.2.1
Treatment Protocol

Treatment was commenced by TURB aimed at maximal reduction of the tumor mass and complete resection (R0). The protocol scheme is depicted in Fig. 18.1. Residual tumor was assessed histologically by biopsies from all resection margins: R0 indicated microscopically complete TURB (i.e., curative resec-

tion), R1 microscopic tumor residual, R2 macroscopic tumor residual, and RX no adequate information about residual tumor. Systematic bladder mapping (at least six random biopsies) assessed the presence or absence of carcinoma in situ (Tis) or any accompanying dysplasias. T category and tumor grade were defined according to the TNM classification of 1992 (UICC). Routine clinical staging included radiographs of the chest, abdominal and pelvic computed tomography, and an isotope bone scan.

Radiotherapy was initiated 4–8 weeks after TURB using 10-MV photons and a four-field box technique with individually shaped portals. All treatment volumes received daily fractions of 1.8–2.0 Gy given 5 days/week. Between May 1982 and May 1990, the total dose to the level of true pelvis up to the L4/5 interspace was 45–46 Gy and to the whole bladder, 54–65 Gy. Since June 1990, the total dose and the treatment volume (Fig. 18.2) have been prescribed in relation to T category, grading, and residual tumor after TURB according to the regimens depicted in Table 18.2.

Since October 1985, CT has been given simultaneously with RT immediately before each treatment fraction on days 1–5 and 29–33. Cytotoxic treatment has consisted of cisplatin (25 mg/m^2) throughout the whole study except for the years 1990 and 1991, when carboplatin (65 mg/m^2) was given routinely. At present, carboplatin is restricted to those patients with congestive heart disease or elevated serum creatinine levels (>1.2 mg%) or decreased creatinine clearance (<50 ml/min).

One to 3 months after completion of RT-CT, remission was assessed by deep transurethral resection of the former tumor bed. In the case of histologically proven complete remission (CR), patients under-

Table 18.1. Distribution of patients by treatment

Treatment	Total treated	%	Evaluated	%
RT	128	38	98	29
RT + CT	205	62	184	55
Total	333	100	282	85

RT, Radiotherapy; RT + CT, radiotherapy and chemotherapy.

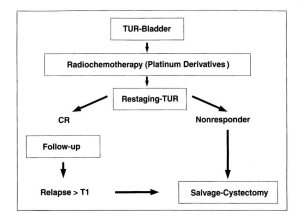

Fig. 18.1. Protocol scheme in patients with muscle-invasive cancer at Erlangen University, 1982–1996

Table 18.2. Prescribed radiation dose and treatment volume in relation to T category, grading, and residual tumor after TURB. Doses have been specified to the reference point according to ICRU report Nr. 50

Stage	Radiation dose (Gy)		
	Para-aortic region	True pelvis	Bladder
T1–3, G1–2, R0, N0	–	45	54
T1–3, G3, R0, N0	45	45	59.4
T1–3, G1–2, R1, N0	–	54	59.4
T1–4, G3, R1	45	54	59.4
All R2	45	54	59.4
All N+	45	54	59.4

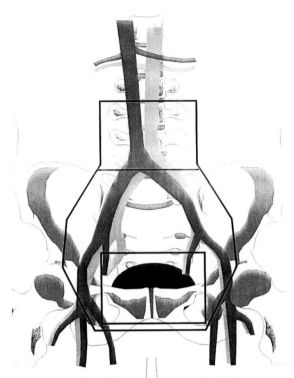

a

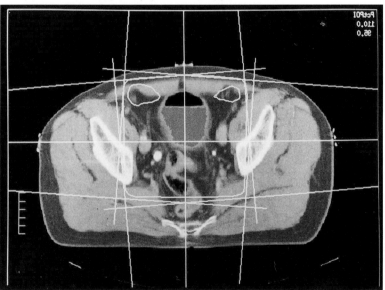

b

Fig. 18.2. a Field margins in the anterior-posterior projection for RT of pelvic and para-aortic lymph nodes with bladder boost. **b** Isodose plan of the four-field technique for irradiation of the pelvis. The 95% isodose line surrounds the treatment volume. Small areas anteriorly mark maximum dose of 110%

went follow-up at 3-month intervals. Follow-up consisted of: cystoscopy, biopsies of all suspected areas, and urine cytology. Superficial and well-differentiated and circumscribed tumor residuals or recurrences were treated by TURB and intravesical chemo- or immunotherapy. Patients with deeply infiltrating or poorly differentiated residual tumor (nonresponders or partial responders) or recurrences underwent immediate salvage cystectomy.

18.2.2
Patient Characteristics

Table 18.3 depicts the characteristics of 282 patients evaluable for this analysis: 98 patients received RT alone and 184 received RT-CT, either with cisplatin ($n = 115$) or with carboplatin ($n = 69$). Among these were 150 (53%) patients with tumors in the pT3 category and 125 (44%) with macroscopic tumor re-

Table 18.3. Important patient and tumor characteristics

Parameter	No.	%
Male	216	77
Female	66	23
Age (median and range), years	66 (31–93)	
pT categories		
T1	53	19
T2	54	19
T3	150	53
T4	25	9
R status after 1st TURB		
R0	55	19
R1	99	35
R2	125	44
Rx	3	2
Median follow-up (years)	7.5	

Table 18.4. Comparison of initial CR rates achieved with different treatment modalities

Treatment	Complete remission	
	No.	%
TURB alone	55	20
TURB + RT	56	57
TURB + RT + carboplatin	48	70
TURB + RT + cisplatin	78	85

Table 18.5. Prognostic factors for initial response. Endpoint is the histologically proven CR rate by restaging TURB

Factor	P values	
	Univariate	Multivariate
Age	<0.01	NS
pT category	<0.0001	<0.0001
Grading (1 and 2 vs 3 and 4)	0.030	NS
R status after 1st TURB	<0.0001	0.0003
RT vs RT-CT	0.0008	0.05
RT vs RT-CT (cisplatin)	0.0002	0.003
RT-CT (cisplatin) vs RT-CT (carboplatin)	0.025	0.020

sidual after TURB (R2). The 53 pT1 patients belonged to the high-risk group. The selection criteria for the 282 patients were as follows:

1. Transitional cell carcinoma
2. pT2–4
3. pT1 high risk (G3/4, associated Tis, R1–2, lymph node involvement, multiple TURBs)
4. ≥45 Gy radiation dose to the bladder and the true pelvis

Excluded from analysis were 12 patients with squamous cell carcinoma of the bladder and 39 patients with T1 G1–2 disease.

18.2.3
Statistics

All patients were followed up until August 1996. No patients were lost to follow-up. Median follow-up was 90 months, with a range from 4 to 187 months. Survival rates were calculated according to Kaplan-Meier; differences in survival were tested for statistical significance by the log rank test. The survival figures exclude intercurrent deaths (cause-specific survival) but are not corrected according to age. Multivariate analysis was performed using the Cox regression model.

18.3
Results

18.3.1
Rates of Complete Remission

Table 18.4 summarizes the rates of histologically proven complete remission following TURB alone,

TURB plus RT, and TURB plus RT-CT. TURB alone led to complete remission (i.e., R0 = curative resection) in 55 (20%: 55/282) of the patients. The corresponding figures with additional RT were 57% (56/98) and as high as 80% (145/181) after RT-CT. With a CR rate of 85%, RT in combination with cisplatin was superior to RT and carboplatin, which had a CR rate of 70% ($P = 0.02$).

The main prognostic factors for initial response (Table 18.5) were the pT category ($P < 0.001$) and the R status ($P = 0.0003$). In multivariate analysis, the RT-CT combination in general, and also RT-CT with cisplatin as compared with RT-carboplatin, retained an independent prognostic influence. Age was no longer of prognostic value.

18.3.2
Survival

For all 282 patients, the cause-specific survival rates were 52% (59%) and 43% (43%) at 5 and 10 years, respectively (age-corrected data in parentheses). Forty-three percent after 5 years and 35% after 10 years survived with a preserved and well-functioning bladder. Survival rates after RT were 40% at 5 years and 31% at 10 years, and 38% at 5 years and 29% at 10 years with a preserved bladder. Following RT-CT with concurrent cisplatin, the survival rates were 64% (69%) and 48% (51%) at 5 and 10 years.

Initial pT category, residual tumor after TURB (R status), and CT had a significant influence on cause-specific survival.

18.3.2.1
pT Category

Figure 18.3 depicts the survival curves according to the initial pT category. The 5-year survival rates were 77% for pT1 (*n* = 53), 55% for pT2 (*n* = 54), 48% for pT3 (*n* = 150), and 23% for pT4 tumors (*n* = 25). For muscle-invading tumors (pT2–4, *n* = 229), the cause-specific survival rates were 48% and 34% at 5 and 10 years (age-corrected rates: 54% and 39%, respectively).

18.3.2.2
R Status

The extent of residual tumor after TURB prior to RT/RCT was the most important prognostic factor for survival (Fig. 18.4), both in univariate and in multivariate analysis (Table 18.6). In R0 patients, the 5- and 10-year survival rates were 75% and 53%. The corresponding figures were 48% and 26% after R1 resection and 34% and 20% after R2 resection. Summarizing all analyzed prognostic factors, Table 18.6 shows that R status had a stronger impact on survival with and without preserved bladder than pT category and age. Patients with completely resected pT2-3 tumors with survival rates of 78% and 59% at 5 and 10 years had the best prognosis. In comparison, incompletely resected pT1 cancers had a prognosis comparable to nonresectable muscle-invading tumors despite the lower T category.

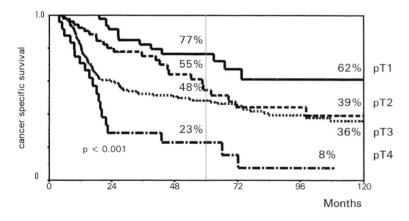

Fig. 18.3. Impact of pT category on cause-specific survival (*n* = 282)

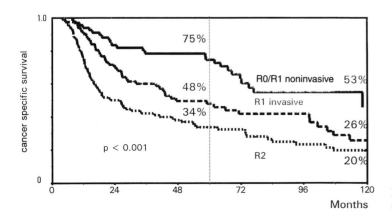

Fig. 18.4. Impact of R status on cause-specific survival (*n* = 278)

Table 18.6. Univariate and multivariate analysis of factors with impact on survival ($n = 282$); p values are shown

Parameter	Overall survival		Cancer-specific survival		Alive with bladder	
	Univ.	Multiv.	Univ.	Multiv.	Univ.	Multiv.
Age	<0.001	0.005	<0.005	0.002	<0.05	<0.05
pT category	<0.001	0.012	<0.0001	0.003	0.004	NS
R status after 1st TUR	<0.001	0.0003	<0.0001	0.003	<0.0001	<0.001
RT vs RT-CT	<0.01	NS	<0.01	NS	NS	–
RT vs RT-CT (cisplatin)	<0.01	NS	<0.02	NS	NS	–
RT-CT (carboplatin) vs RT-CT (cisplatin)	<0.05	NS	<0.05	NS	NS	–

18.3.2.3
Patient Age

Age had a significant impact on cancer-specific survival as well as on bladder preservation. The influence of age on cancer-specific survival was stronger than that of CT in both univariate ($P = 0.005$) and multivariate analysis ($P = 0.002$), and this was also true with regard to cystectomy-free survival ($P < 0.05$ in both univariate and multivariate analysis).

18.3.3
Simultaneous Chemotherapy

Administration of CT simultaneously with RT improved not only the initial response (rate of histologically confirmed complete responses), but also the cause-specific survival rates (Figs. 18.5, 18.6). For a detailed analysis, we selected patients ($n = 104$) who received "full chemotherapy," i.e., the prescribed dose of 25 mg/m^2 cisplatin or 65 mg/m^2 carboplatin during the first cycle and at least 75% during the second cycle. Sixty-four patients with cisplatin and 40 with carboplatin formed the study group. Fifty-seven patients with reduced dose were excluded,

along with 23 additional patients who received cisplatin plus 5-fluorouracil in a feasibility study.

Figure 18.5 shows the impact of concurrent CT on survival. For full-dose CT, reduced CT, and RT alone, cause-specific survival rates were 63%, 48%, and 40% at 5 years and 43%, 35%, and 31% at 10 years ($P < 0.05$). The difference in survival for patients with reduced CT and RT alone is not statistically significant. Patients who were treated between 1982 and 1985 by RT alone served as controls (historical control). The disease-free survival rates were 33% and 37% at 5 years and 28% and 21% at 10 years for RT alone and RT combined with CT, respectively (NS).

In addition, the type of CT had an impact on survival (Fig. 18.6). The cause-specific survival rates for patients receiving cisplatin and carboplatin were 64% and 54% at 5 years and 48% and 27% at 10 years, respectively ($P < 0.05$, univariate analysis).

18.4
Salvage Cystectomy

Salvage cystectomy because of residual or recurrent tumor after RT/RCT was performed in 69 patients (24%) and in 78 (23%) of the whole treatment group

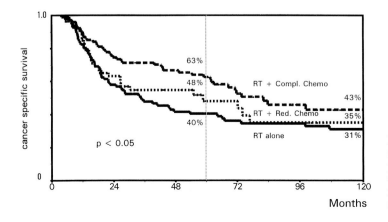

Fig. 18.5. Impact of RCT with cisplatin or carboplatin on cause-specific survival compared with RT alone ($n = 282$). Complete chemotherapy = full prescribed dose in the first cycle and ≥75% in the second cycle. *Red. chemo*, reduced chemotherapy

Fig. 18.6. Comparison of the impact of RT plus cisplatin (*Cis*) and RT plus carboplatin (*Carbo*) on cause-specific survival ($n = 282$)

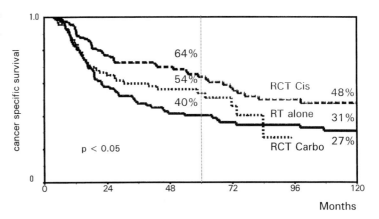

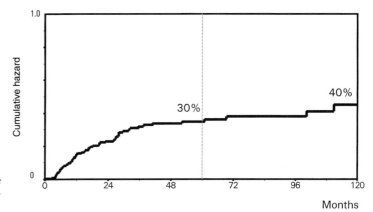

Fig. 18.7. Kaplan-Meier plot of cumulative probability of cystectomies following restaging TURB

(333 pts). The cumulative hazard rose during the first 3.5 years following treatment and remained constant over the next 8–10 years (Fig. 18.7). Seventy-nine percent of the long-term surviving patients (>5 years) were able to keep their own functional bladder. There was no improvement in cystectomy-free survival following CT.

For the majority of the patients with muscle-invasive recurrent or residual tumors, salvage cystectomy was still a curative treatment, with a 5-year survival rate of 34% (age-corrected rate: 40%). In nonresponders to RCT, an age-corrected 5-year survival rate of 38% was achieved. In cases with muscle-infiltrating recurrences, the corresponding figure was 40% (detailed data will be published soon).

18.5
Toxicity

There were two cases of gastrointestinal toxicity grade IV (WHO). One patient died after resection of

the damaged intestinal loop perioperatively. Three other patients underwent cystectomy because of bladder damage (two patients with shrinking bladder following multiple TURBs prior to RT, one patient with tumor bleeding during RT-CT). Some other patients had a reduced bladder capacity due to multiple TURBs prior to RT-CT. Typical acute radiation-induced side-effects, such as transient urocystitis and enteritis, were easily managed by symptomatic treatment alone. Ninety-four percent of the patients receiving CT experienced hematologic toxicity [grade I 29%, grade II 34%, grade III 30%, grade IV 1% (WHO)].

18.6
Discussion

Treatment strategies in oncology should include efforts to increase survival rates as well as to maintain a good quality of life. Radical cystectomy is of limited value in the treatment of occult tumor spread to the pelvis and retroperitoneum or in the prevention of systemic tumor cell dissemination. Despite R0 resection and pTN0 status, there is still a high death rate following radical cystectomy (JAKSE et al. 1985; JUNG and JAKSE 1996; PAGANO et al. 1991; RHAGAVAN et al. 1990; SHEARER et al. 1988; SKINNER and LIESKOVSKY 1988; STÖCKLE et al. 1991; WHITMORE et al. 1988; WISHNOW et al. 1992). On the other hand, cystectomy with some form of urinary diversion is associated with a considerable loss of quality of life. It has been suggested that cystectomy as the primary treatment option for bladder cancer should be replaced by an organ-sparing procedure with or without RT (ABRADT et al. 1993; BLANDY et al. 1980; CHAUVET et al. 1993; CERVAK et al. 1993; COPPIN et al. 1992; DE NEVE et al. 1995; DUNCAN and QUILTY 1986; DUNST et al. 1994; DUNST 1991; GOODMAN et al. 1981; GOSPODAROWICZ et al. 1989; HOUSSET et al. 1993; JAKSE et al. 1985; JAHNSON et al. 1991; KACHNIC et al. 1995; KAUFMAN et al. 1993; KOISO et al. 1995; MAMEGHAN et al. 1995; MARTINEZ-PINEIRO et al. 1995; MILLER and JOHNSON 1973; QUILTY and DUNCAN 1985; ROTMAN et al. 1987; RUSSEL et al. 1990; SAUER et al. 1990, 1996; SCHER et al. 1989; SELL et al. 1991; SHEARER et al. 1988; SHIPLEY et al. 1987; SMAALAND et al. 1991; TESTER et al. 1993; ZIETMAN et al. 1993).

During a 14-year period from 1982 through 1996, a total of 333 consecutive, nonselected patients with invasive bladder cancer were treated in a prospective nonrandomized trial. Patients treated between 1982 and 1985 by TURB plus postoperative RT served as a control group to estimate the efficacy of single-drug CT as an adjunct to RT. In 1990, both the RT dose and the treatment volume were adapted to tumor characteristics and postoperative tumor status (i.e., R status). Tumor dose was increased in patients with R1–2 status, poor grading, and lymph node involvement. During a 2-year period we tested carboplatin as an alternative to cisplatin in 69 patients. Since 1991, carboplatin has only been administered in patients in whom the use of cisplatin is contraindicated.

For the present analysis, we selected patients having muscle-invasive and high-risk T categories. Comparing the end results of our protocol, the 5-year survival rates were as high as in the best cystectomy sries for pT2–3a tumors, and were even better for pT3b–4 tumors (Table 18.7; PAGANO et al. 1991; RHAGAVAN et al. 1990; SKINNER and LIESKOVSKY 1988; STÖCKLE et al. 1991; WHITMORE et al. 1988; WISHNOW et al. 1992). The highest survival rates following primary cystectomy were reported from a multicenter study that randomized

Table 18.7. Survival rates reported in selected cystectomy series compared with the results of the Erlangen organ-sparing treatments

Tumor stage	University of Erlangen				Radical cystectomy[a]
	RT		RT-CT		% Survival
	No.	%	No.	%	
pT2	46	46	58	–	56–75
pT3a	43	33	54	40	26–78
pT3b	33	22	53	–	11–29
pT4	0	0	34	–	–
Total	122	100	199		

[a] JUNG and JAKSE (1996).

adjuvant MVAC CT versus radical cystectomy alone (STOCKLE et al. 1991). These findings confirm our treatment policy at the University of Erlangen-Nürnberg, which restricts cystectomy to those patients who fail after an RT-CT combination.

Major prognostic factors for initial response were the pT category, R status after TURB, CT, and RT-CT with cisplatin (Table 18.5). For cause-specific survival, pT category, R status, and age were of prognostic significance; the same was true for CT in the univariate analysis (Table 18.6). These factors have been discussed in detail elsewhere (DUNST et al. 1994; DUNST 1991). The prognostic significance of a residual tumor after primary TURB has been pointed out by SHIPLEY et al. (1987).

Transitional cell carcinoma is sensitive both to RT and to CT. Cisplatin, carboplatin, adriamycin, methotrexate, vinblastine, and 5-fluorouracil are effective single agents. Their combination with simultaneous RT will improve the cytotoxic effects by adding or potentiating antitumor effects; however, RT and CT have different spectra of toxicity. In our series, concurrent single-drug CT with cisplatin increased the CR rate from 57% (56/98) with RT alone to 85% (78/92) with RT-CT. Carboplatin appeared to be less effective, with a CR rate of 70% (48/69). The greater efficacy of RT-CT compared with RT alone has also been described by other groups (ABRADT et al. 1993; CHAUVET et al. 1993; CERVAK et al. 1993; FUNG et al. 1991; JAKSE et al. 1985; KAUFMAN et al. 1993; REBISCHUNG et al. 1992; ROTMAN et al. 1987; RUSSEL et al. 1990; TESTER et al. 1993; ZIETMAN et al. 1993). A randomized Canadian NCJ study found a markedly higher local remission rate after 2 years when using RT plus cisplatin rather than RT alone (COPPIN et al. 1992).

The impact of CT on long-term results remains questionable (DUNST et al. 1994; SCHER et al. 1989). The higher CR rate following RT-CT need not be translated into an improved disease-free survival and a definite benefit in overall survival (SAUER et al. 1996). On the contrary, we found that patients with CR following RT-CT experienced a higher frequency of muscle-invasive relapses, leading to a higher cystectomy rate, compared to patients with a CR after RT alone. It is very likely that the impact of RT-CT on cause-specific survival was a result of the high CR rate that followed salvage cystectomy in nonresponders (univariate analysis, $P < 0.01$). After incorporation of the variable R status into the final Cox model, RT-CT combination lost its prognostic significance with respect to the endpoint cause-specific survival.

18.7
Conclusions

Organ-sparing RCT for bladder cancer is safe and effective. One treatment-related death and one severe long-term complication were observed. Survival rates compared very favorably with those after primary radical cystectomy. In addition, 79% of the survivors retained their normal bladder function. Since R status after initial TURB was the strongest prognostic factor with respect to survival and initial response, R0 resection is recommended before starting RT or RT-CT. Our treatment schedule includes immediate cystectomy in cases of persistent tumor or invasive relapse. Major prognostic factors for initial response and survival were: patient age, pT category, and R status. Concurrent administration of cisplatin (or carboplatin) enhanced the CR rate by one-third (57% vs 80%). When CT was applied at a full dose, RT-CT after TURB also improved patients' survival, compared with RT alone. Cisplatin was superior to carboplatin in terms of CR rate and survival.

References

Abradt RP, Pontin AR, Barnes RD (1993) Chemotherapy versus radical irradiation plus salvage-cystectomy for bladder cancer severe late small bowel morbidity. Eur J Surg Oncol 19:279–282

Birkenhake S, Sauer R, Kühn R, Martus P, Wittekind C, Schrott KM (1997) Effekte der simultan zur Radiotherapie applizierten Chemotherapie bei der Primärtherapie des muskelinvasiven Blasenkarzinoms. Strahlenther Onkol 173:••–••

Blandy JP, England HR, Evans SJW, Hope-Stone HF, Mair GM, Mantell BS, Oliver RT (1980) T3 bladder cancer – the case for salvage cystectomy. Br J Urol 52:506–510

Bloom HJG, Hendry WF, Wallace DM, Skeot RG (1982) Treatment of T3 bladder cancer: controlled trial of pre-operation radiotherapy and radical cystectomy versus radical radiotherapy. Br J Urol 54:136–151

Cervak J, Cufer T, Kragelj B, Zakotnik B, Stanonik M (1993) Sequential transurethral surgery, multiple drug chemotherapy and radiation therapy for invasive bladder carcinoma: initial report. Int J Radiat Biol Phys 25:777–782

Chauvet B, Brewer J, Felix-Faire C, Davin JL, Viecet P, Rebrul F (1993) Combined radiation therapy and cisplatin for locally advanced carcinoma of the urinary bladder. Cancer 72:2213–2218

Coppin C, Cospordarowicz M, Dixon P (1992) Improved local control of invasive bladder cancer by concurrent cisplatin and preoperative or radical radiation. Proc Am Soc Clin Oncol 11:198–201

De Neve W, Lybeert ML, Goor C, Crommelin MA, Ribot JG (1995) Radiotherapy for T2 and T3 carcinoma of the bladder: the influence of overall treatment time. Radiother Oncol 36:183–188

Duncan W, Quilty W (1986) The result of a series of 963 patients with transitional cell carcinoma of the urinary bladder primarily treated by radical megavoltage X-tray therapy. Radiother Oncol 7:299–310

Dunst J, Sauer R, Schrott KM, Kühn R, Wittekind C, Altendorf-Hofmann A (1994) Organ sparing treatment of advanced bladder cancer. A 10 year experience. Int J Radiat Oncol Biol Phys 30:261–266

Dunst J (1991) Die Radiotherapie im interdisziplinären Behandlungskonzept des Harnblasenkarzinoms. Strahlenther Onkol 167:563–580

Fung CY, Shipley WU, Young RH, et al. (1991) Prognostic factors in invasive bladder carcinoma in a prospective trial of preoperative adjuvant chemotherapy and radiotherapy. J Clin Oncol 9:1533–1542

Goodman GD, Hilop TG, Elvord JM, Balfour J (1981) Conservation of bladder function in patients with invasive bladder cancer treated by definitive irriadiative and selective cystectomy. Int J Radiol Oncol Biol Phys 7:569–573

Gospodarowicz MK, Hawkins MV, Rawlings GA, et al. (1989) Radical radiotherapy for muscle invasive transitional cell carcinoma of the bladder: failure analysis. J Urol 142:1448–1454

Housset M, Maulard C, Chretien Y, et al. (1993) Combined radiation and chemotherapy for invasive transitional-cell carcinoma of the bladder: a prospective study. J Clin Oncol 11:2150–2157

Jahnson S, Petersen J, Westman G (1991) Bladder carcinoma – a 20 year review of radical irradiation therapy. Radiother Oncol 22:111–117

Jakse G, Frommhold N, Nedden D (1985) Combined radiation and chemotherapy for locally advanced transitional cell carcinoma of the urinary bladder. Cancer 55:1659–1664

Jenkins BJ, Caulfield MJ, Fowler CG, et al. (1988) Reappraisal of the role of radical radiotherapy and salvage cystectomy in the treatment of invasive (T2/T3) bladder cancer. Br J Urol 62:343–346

Jung P, Jakse G (1996) Bladder preservation in invasive locally confined bladder cancer. Onkologie 19:296–301

Kachnic LA, Kaufman DS, Zietman AI, et al. (1995) Selective bladder preservation by combined modality therapy for invasive bladder cancer. Int J Radiat Oncol Biol Phys 32(Suppl):271

Kaufman DS, Shipley WU, Griffin PP, Heney NM, Althanter AF, Eford JG (1993) Selective bladder preservation by combination treatment of invasive bladder cancer. N Engl J Med 329:1377–1381

Koiso K, Shipley W, Keuppens F, et al. (1995) The status of bladder-preserving therapeutic strategies in the management of patients with muscle-invasive bladder cancer. Int J Urol (Jpn) 2(Suppl 2):49–57

Mameghan H, Fisher R, Mameghan J, Brook S (1995) Analysis of failure following definitive radiotherapy for invasive transitional cell carcinoma of the bladder. Int J Radiat Oncol Biol Phys 31:247–254

Martinez-Pineiro JA, Gonzalez M, Arocena F, Flores N, Roncero CR, Portillo JA, Escudero A (1995) Neoadjuvant cisplatin chemotherapy before radical cystectomy in invasive transitional cell carcinoma of the bladder: a prospective randomized phase III study. J Urol 153:964–973

Miller LS, Johnson DE (1973) Megavoltage irradiation for bladder cancer. Cancer 10:771–782

Pagano F, Bassi P, Galetti TP (1991) Results of contemporary radical cystectomy for invasive bladder cancer: a clinicopathological study with emphasis on the inadequacy of the tumor, nodes and metastases classification. J Urol 145:45–49

Quilty PM, Duncan W (1985) Primary radical radiotherapy for T3 transitional cell cancer of the bladder: an analysis of survival and control. Int J Radiat Oncol Biol Phys 12:853–860

Rebischung JC, Vannetzel JM, Fournier F (1992) Cyclic concomitant chemoradiotherapy for invasive bladder cancer: phase 2 study with organ preservation. Proc Am Soc Clin Oncol 11:208–214

Rhagavan D, Shipley WU, Garnick MB, Russel PM, Richie JP (1990) Biology and management of bladder cancer. N Engl J Med 322:1129–1138

Rotman M, Macchia R, Silverstein R (1987) Treatment of advanced bladder cancer with irradiation and concomitant 5-fluorouracil infusion. Cancer 59:710–715

Russel KJ, Boileau MA, Higano C, et al. (1990) Combined 5-fluorouracil and irradiation for transitional cell carcinoma of the urinary bladder. Int J Radiat Oncol Biol Phys 19:693–699

Sauer R, Dunst J, Altendorf-Hofmann A, Fischer H, Bornhof C, Schrott KM (1990) Radiotherapy with and without cisplatin in bladder cancer. Int J Radiat Oncol Biol Phys 19:687–691

Sauer R, Birkenhake S, Martus P (1996) Efficacy of radiochemo-therapy with platin-derivatives compared to radiotherapy alone in organ sparing treatment of bladder cancer. Int J Radiat Oncol Biol Phys 36(Suppl):142

Scher H, Herr H, Sternberg C, et al. (1989) Neo-adjuvant chemotherapy for invasive bladder cancer. Experience with the M-VAC regimen. Br J Urol 64:250–256

Sell A, Jakobsen A, Nerstrom B, Sorensen BL, Steven K, Barlebo H (1991) Treatment of advanced bladder cancer category T2, T3 and T4a. A randomized multicenter study of preoperative irradiation and cystectomy versus radical irradiation and early salvage cystectomy for residual tumor. DAVECA protocol 8201. Danish Vesical Cancer Group. Scand J Urol Nephrol (Suppl) 138:193–201

Shearer RJ, Chilvers CE, Bloom HJ, Horwich A, Batiker H (1988) Adjuvant chemotherapy in T3 carcinoma of the bladder. Br J Urol 62:558–564

Shipley WU, Prout GR, Einstein AB, et al. (1987) Treatment of invasive bladder cancer by cisplatin and radiation in patients unsuited for surgery. JAMA 258:931–935

Skinner DG, Lieskovsky G (1988) Management of invasive and high grade bladder cancer. In: Diagnosis and management of genitourinary cancer. Saunders, Philadelphia, p 295

Smaaland R, Aksilen LA, Tonder B, et al. (1991) Radical radiation therapy of invasive and locally advanced bladder carcinoma in elderly patients. Br J Urol 67:61–69

Stöckle M, Riedmüller H, Hohenfellner R (1991) Radikale Zystektomie – oft zu spät? Therapieergebnisse der radikalen Zystektomie mit und ohne adjuvante oder induktive M-VAC Behandlung. In: Hartung R, Hübner W, Kropp W (ed) Urologische Beckenchirurgie. Springer, Berlin Heidelberg New York, pp 279–287

Tester W, Porter A, Asbell S, et al. (1993) Combined modality program with possible organ preservation for invasive bladder carcinoma: results of RTOG protocol 85-12. Int J Radiat Oncol Biol Phys 25:783–790

Whitmore WF, Batata MA, Thoneim MA, Grabstald H, Unal A (1988) Radical cystectomy with or without prior irradiation in the treatment of bladder cancer. J Urol 139:299A

Wishnow KI, Levinson AK, Johnson DE (1992) Stage B (T2/3aN0) transitional cell carcinoma of the bladder highly curable by radical cystectomy. Urology 39:1–9

Zietman AL, Shipley WU, Kaufman DS (1993) The combination of cisplatin based chemotherapy and radiation with treatment of muscle invading transitional cell cancer of the bladder. Int J Radiat Oncol Biol Phys 27:161–170

19 External Radiotherapy in the Treatment of Muscle-Invasive Transitional Cell Carcinoma of the Bladder

L. Vanuytsel and W. Van den Bogaert

19.1
Introduction

The enthusiasm for radiotherapy in the primary treatment of invasive bladder cancer has decreased over the last two decades for several reasons. If applied to full dose in an unselected patient population, the success of radiotherapy will be hampered by the inability to achieve and to maintain local control in a substantial number of patients. Secondly, the improvement in surgical management and peri- and postoperative care with the possibility of creating continent urinary diversions and sparing the neurovascular bundles has rendered radical surgery more acceptable for most patients. Thirdly, the recognition that invasive bladder cancer is often a generalized disease at the time of diagnosis has diverted attention from preoperative radiation to neo-adjuvant chemotherapy in an attempt to sterilize distant micrometastatic deposits.

During the past decade, however, several important studies have reaffirmed the potential role of radiotherapy in the treatment of invasive transitional cell carcinoma of the bladder. These issues will be discussed in this chapter.

19.2
Radiotherapy in the Primary Treatment

19.2.1
Radiotherapy as an Adjunct to Surgery

In 1988, Parsons and Million published a comprehensive review of the literature up to 1983 on preoperative radiotherapy in stage B2–C (T3) bladder carcinoma. They analyzed both retrospective and randomized studies and concluded that, when comparison of concomitantly treated series was performed, the addition of preoperative irradiation for clinical stage B2–C disease added approximately 15%–20% to the 5-year survival.

Preoperative radiotherapy had been abandoned by most centers by the mid 1980s since it was believed that the improved understanding of pelvic surgical anatomy and new surgical techniques had secured excellent local control and that additional local treatment would be superfluous (Skinner and Lieskovsky 1984; Wishnow and Dmochowski 1988). In addition, major attention was directed towards (neo-)adjuvant chemotherapy in an attempt to eradicate micrometastatic disease. The ultimate aim was to improve disease-free and overall survival.

Most modern surgical ($\pm$ neoadjuvant chemotherapy) series do not investigate the incidence of local recurrence as an endpoint (Pagano et al. 1991; Skinner et al. 1991; Stöckle et al. 1995). Data on the incidence of local recurrence are therefore scarce. Local recurrence in organ-confined invasive bladder cancer (pT2–pT3a) is rare, the rate certainly being less than 10% (Wishnow and Dmochowski 1988; Skinner and Lieskovsky 1984). In patients with tumors with an extravesical component (pT3b–pT4), reported recurrence rates vary between 10% (6/61 patients) (Wishnow and Dmochowski 1988) and 18% (9/50 patients) (Freiha et al. 1996). Data on local control after radical surgery in clinically staged patients are even harder to find. Pollack et al. (1995) analyzed the records of 240 patients with T2–

L. Vanuytsel, MD, Professor in Radiotherapy, Department of Radiotherapy, UZ Gasthuisberg, University Hospitals of Leuven, Herestraat 49, B-3000 Leuven, Belgium
W. Van den Bogaert, MD, Professor in Radiotherapy, Department of Radiotherapy, UZ Gasthuisberg, University Hospitals of Leuven, Herestraat 49, B-3000 Leuven, Belgium

T4 bladder carcinoma treated between 1984 and 1990. The 5-year actuarial local control rates after cystectomy were 93% for stage T2, 91% for stage T3a, 71% for stage T3b, and 56% for stage T4. The only factors that correlated well with freedom from distant metastasis, in a Cox multivariate analysis, were pathological stage ($P < 0.004$), local failure ($P < 0.007$), and lymph node status ($P < 0.03$). The 5-year actuarial incidence of freedom from distant metastasis for those with local control was 77%, compared to 29% for those with local failure ($P < 0.0001$). In 75% of cases, local failure occurred in the absence of or before the occurrence of distant metastatic disease.

Measures to improve local control in patients at high risk for local recurrence after radical surgery, i.e., T3b and T4 patients, could therefore have a favorable impact on disease-free and overall survival. However, the chemotherapy arsenal presently available seems to have little impact on local control as 85% of patients with T3b and T4 tumors in the M.D. Anderson series (POLLACK et al. 1995) received modern type adjuvant multiagent therapy and nevertheless had 5-year local recurrence rates of 29% and 44%, respectively.

The impetus to reconsider preoperative radiotherapy as a possible tool to improve local control and ultimately disease-free survival in patients with advanced bladder cancer comes from a second study of the M.D. Anderson group (COLE et al. 1995) comparing the outcome in terms of local control in patients with clinical stage T2–T4 disease treated with either preoperative radiotherapy and radical cystectomy or radical cystectomy alone. The first group, 301 patients, with a median follow-up of 91 months, was treated between 1976 and 1983. The later group, 220 patients with a median follow-up of 54 months, was treated between 1985 and 1990. For patients with tumors clinically confined to the bladder, T2–T3a patients, no differences in actuarial local control were observed. However, for patients with T3b disease actuarial local control at 5 years for the group with the combined treatment was 91% versus 72% for the group with cystectomy alone ($P < 0.003$). There was also a trend for improved disease-free (59% vs 47%) and overall survival (52% vs 40%) at 5 years for the group receiving preoperative radiation treatment. Although the comparison is retrospective, it is likely that any biases would favor the cystectomy-only group, as this group had the advantage of more modern imaging and surgical techniques and the majority of patients received

multiagent chemotherapy, i.e., 56% overall and 80% of stage T3 patients versus none in the preoperative radiation group. Moreover, both groups were treated by the same group of surgeons and prognostic factors were equally balanced.

In view of these data, and the low toxicity of preoperative irradiation when delivered with four fields to 40 or 50 Gy in 2-Gy daily fractions, preoperative radiation treatment should be considered as adjuvant to surgery ($\pm$ chemotherapy) in clinical stage T3b disease, as it may impact on local control, and ultimately on disease-free and overall survival. Local control should be a prospectively recorded endpoint in any phase II/III trial on adjuvant treatment in bladder cancer.

19.2.2
Full-Dose Radiotherapy

In 1986, DUNCAN and QUILTY reported the results in a series of 963 patients with bladder carcinoma treated with curative intent by radical radiotherapy between 1971 and 1982. This series is quite unique in that selection bias was minimal as it was the policy of the department and referring surgeons for patients with invasive bladder cancer to be treated primarily by radiotherapy. Patients were treated to total doses ranging from 55.0 Gy to 57.5 Gy in 20 fractions over 4 weeks. Five-year survival rates were 40% for T2, 26% for T3, and 12% for T4 tumors. Although these were clinically staged patients with undoubtedly more advanced disease stage for stage than those patients reported in surgical series, results are far from optimal and lower than can be achieved with radical surgery. The main problem is the inability to achieve and maintain a clinical complete remission in a significant proportion of patients. At first follow-up cystoscopy 3–6 months after treatment, complete tumor regression is achieved in only about 45% of patients treated (DUNCAN and QUILTY 1986; GOSPODAROWICZ et al. 1989). Moreover, a substantial number of patients will recur locally during follow-up.

As local tumor control is a prime condition for disease-free and overall survival, it is clear that radical radiation treatment should only be offered to patients with a high probability of maintained local control. In recent years several authors have looked in detail, using multiple regression analysis, at the factors correlated with initial local regression and maintained control (GOSPODAROWICZ et al. 1989;

QUILTY et al. 1986; POLLACK et al. 1994). Their conclusions may be summarized as follows. Factors independently associated with initial response are stage, clinical perivesical extension (T3b, T4), tumor size, clinical complete transurethral resection, ureteral obstruction on intravenous pyelography (IVP), and hemoglobin level. Moreover, it should be noted that an important factor for achieving local control has gained little attention in the literature, i.e., complete coverage of the tumor by the radiation treatment fields. LARSEN and ENGELHOLM (1994) compared the three-dimensional computed tomography based treatment plans of 110 patients with the conventional cystogram-based plans and found inadequate coverage of the target volume in 50% of patients with conventional planning. Other authors have obtained similar results (for a review, see LARSEN and ENGELHOLM 1994).

Factors which independently correlate with durable local control are: initial complete remission, T-stage, tumor grade, hemoglobin level, and associated carcinoma in situ. Factors independently linked with overall survival are: local control, age, complete transurethral resection, stage, tumor size, and hemoglobin level.

The importance of completeness of transurethral resection for the incidence of local control and overall survival was first recognized by SHIPLEY et al. (1985) and has been confirmed by several other authors in large series (DUNST et al. 1994; POLLACK et al. 1994).

High-dose radiation therapy, i.e., 66–70 Gy delivered in daily 2-Gy fractions over 6.5–7 weeks, offers a reasonable chance for long-term survival in patients with T2–T3a transitional cell carcinoma of the bladder, smaller than 5 cm, preferentially completely resected by endoscopic means, without associated carcinoma in situ, with normal IVP findings, and with a hemoglobin level equal or more than 12 g/dl. Well-selected patients within this group should be considered for combined treatment with conservative surgery and/or interstitial therapy (see Chap. 16). However, patients who do not fulfill these criteria should not be offered radiotherapy as the only treatment when cure is aimed for.

It is hoped that factors predictive for tumor radiosensitivity at the molecular level will become available to guide, in combination with the more traditional criteria listed above, the selection of patients who are appropriate candidates for radical irradiation. Until now, such factors are still on the laboratory bench (SHIPLEY 1996).

19.2.3
Nonstandard Radiation Schedules

Few radiobiological data exist to guide the design of nonstandard fractionation schedules. In an analysis of the clinical literature, MACIEJEWSKI and MAJEWSKI (1991) estimated the tumor dose necessary to control 50% (TCD_{50}) of T2–T3 bladder carcinomas to be about 63 Gy in 5 weeks. Extension of treatment beyond 5 weeks would, in order to maintain 50% control, necessitate a dose increment of 0.36 Gy/day to compensate for clonogenic repopulation of the tumor. Repopulation was judged to start around week 5, with a calculated potential doubling time of 5–9 days. Based on these results it was suggested that overall treatment time should be about 40 days. It should not exceed this period to avoid potential accelerated tumor clonogenic repopulation but, on the other hand, it should not be shorter either, since evidence is lacking for further reduction of the TCD_{50} with shorter treatment times while the incidence and severity of acute reactions would rise substantially (KLEINEIDAM and DUBBEN 1992; MACIEJEWSKI and MAJEWSKI 1992).

Hyperfractionation schedules are based on the linear quadratic model of cell response to radiation which predicts that, with decreasing fraction size, late-reacting tissues are spared to a larger extent than acute-reacting tissues and tumors (FOWLER 1989). Using fraction sizes smaller than the standard 2 Gy, it is possible to deliver total doses higher than the standard 66–70 Gy. In this way the radiobiological effect on the tumor and acutely reacting tissues can be increased, while the late effects are kept constant or increased to a lesser degree. A Swedish prospective trial (EDSMYR et al. 1985; NÄSLUND et al. 1994), initiated in 1971, randomized patients with stage T2–4 transitional cell carcinoma of the bladder between hyperfractionation, 1 Gy 3 times a day to a total dose of 84 Gy, and conventional treatment, 2 Gy once a day to a total dose of 64 Gy. A split-course schedule was used, with a treatment-free interval of 2 weeks in the middle of treatment; absolute numbers of overall survival and local control were low, possibly due to repopulation. However, with 10-year follow-up, this study showed superior overall survival ($P < 0.003$), initial local complete response ($P < 0.01$), and local control (not significant at 10 years due to the small number of patients) for the hyperfractionation arm. No increase in the incidence or severity of late complications was observed. Late effects comparable to those of standard treatment were also reported in a Radiation Therapy Oncology Group (RTOG) phase I–II escalation study, delivering 1.2 Gy twice a day with total doses ranging between 60.0 Gy and 69.6 Gy (Cox et al. 1988).

Accelerated fractionation aims at reducing the negative impact of accelerated tumor clonogenic repopulation. Overall treatment time is shortened by delivering more than one standard fraction per day. If total dose is not reduced and if sufficient time between fractions is observed (a minimum of 6–8 h), accelerated fractionation will result in an increased frequency and severity of acute side-effects, but, in principle, not in an increase of late normal tissue injury, which depends little on overall treatment time (Fowler 1989). Several feasibility studies on accelerated radiation treatment in bladder cancer have been published. Two reports have observed, as expected, an increase in acute reactions without an increase in late complications (Plataniotis et al. 1994; Cole et al. 1992). It should be noted, however, that the number of patients was small and the median observation time short. This could well lead to an underestimation of the incidence of late complications (Lievens et al. 1996).

Of special interest is a two-step study performed by the Amsterdam group of Moonen et al. (1997). They reduced the overall treatment time of their conventional schedule of 66 Gy in 2-Gy fractions over 6.5 weeks to 5 weeks (step one: 15 patients) and then to 4 weeks (step 2: 25 patients). Tolerance for the 5-week schedule (median follow-up time 35 months) was excellent with no severe late side-effects. However, side-effects were common in the 4-week schedule (median follow-up 28 months). The acute bowel toxicity was markedly increased, leading in some patients to persistent late bowel complications. Severe late bladder complications were also prominent, with an actuarial incidence of 31% at 3 years. One pilot study on accelerated radiation in 86 patients with bladder cancer, delivering 57.5–64 Gy in 32 fractions in 28 days, has only been reported in abstract form (Pendlebury et al. 1994). In this study, too, late gastrointestinal and bladder toxicity was pronounced. Consequential late complications as seen in the bowel in the Amsterdam study (Moonen et al. 1997) result from severe acute mucosal reactions. They have been reported both in the clinical (Withers et al. 1995) and in the experimental setting (Dubray and Thames 1994). The authors of the latter study expressed their concern about the possible danger of hyperfractionation treatment with too short interfraction intervals and of acceler-

ated irradiation with too short overall treatment times.

In conclusion, if one wants to deviate from the standard fractionation schedule of 66–70 Gy in daily fractions of 2 Gy over 6.5–7 weeks, it seems reasonable, based on the data presented, to adopt a schedule with an overall treatment time close to 5 weeks, using some type of hyperfractionation with a biological effective dose (Fowler 1989) for late tissues close to that of a standard schedule, and observing an interfraction interval of 8 h or more. Preferentially, as there is clear promise for improved survival, such schedules should actively be investigated in prospective phase II/III trials.

19.3
Radiotherapy for Palliation of Local Disease

In patients suffering from symptomatic bladder cancer, but unfit for surgery or standard radiotherapy due to age, poor performance status, or extensive disease, hypofractionation radiation schedules have been applied, whereby a small number of large fractions is used. The aim is to palliate symptoms while minimizing the treatment burden, in terms of both treatment days and acute and late side-effects.

Fossa (1991) prospectively evaluated a schedule delivering 10 treatments of 3 Gy each, given over a period of 2 weeks. No symptom improvement, as assessed by patient questionnaire, was achieved. Salminen (1992) obtained complete symptom relief in 43% of patients, using a schedule of 30 Gy in six fractions, two fractions a week. Acute gastrointestinal toxicity and late gastrointestinal and urinary toxicity were marked, probably due in part to the AP-PA treatment technique. Rostom et al. (1996) performed a prospective dose-searching study. In a first group 36–39 Gy was delivered in six fractions over 35 days, while a second group received 34.5 Gy in the same number of fractions over 39 days. Treatment was given with a three- or four-field technique. Nearly 75% of patients had complete regression of their urinary symptoms. Acute tolerance was very good in both groups; persistent late bowel and bladder reactions were seen only in the first group. Use of a hypofractionation schedule similar to that used in the second group therefore seems worthwhile when symptomatic relief is sought in patients unfit or unsuitable for more aggressive treatment with curative intent.

19.4
Conclusions

Radiotherapy continues to play its role through the whole spectrum of muscle-invasive transitional cell carcinoma of the bladder. In well-selected T2–T3a patients, full-dose radiotherapy can offer a substantial probability for cure in patients unfit or unwilling to undergo surgery. Nonstandard fractionation schedules should actively be investigated as they bear the promise of improved disease-free survival without increase in late side-effects and as they could be more optimally integrated in combined treatment schedules. In more advanced T3b–T4 disease, the role of preoperative radiotherapy (± adjuvant chemotherapy) should be reappraised. Randomized trials to assess its impact on local control and ultimately on overall survival seem justified.

Moreover, radiotherapy together with chemotherapy and conservative surgery is an integral part of organ-sparing treatment schedules (see Chap. 17).

References

Cole CJ, Pollack A, Zagars GK, Dinney CP, Swanson DA, von Eschenbach AC (1995) Local control of muscle-invasive bladder cancer: preoperative radiotherapy and cystectomy versus cystectomy alone. Int J Radiat Oncol Biol Phys 32:331–340

Cole DJ, Durrant KR, Roberts JT, Dawes PJTK, Yosef H, Hopewell JW (1992) A pilot study of accelerated fractionation in the radiotherapy of invasive carcinoma of the bladder. Br J Radiol 65:792–798

Cox JD, Guse C, Asbell S, Rubin P, Sause WT (1988) Tolerance of pelvic normal tissues to hyperfractionated radiation therapy: results of protocol 83-08 of the Radiation Therapy Oncology Group. Int J Radiat Oncol Biol Phys 15:1331–1336

Dubray BM, Thames HD (1994) Chronic radiation damage in the rat rectum: an analysis of the influences of fractionation, time and volume. Radiother Oncol 33:41–47

Duncan W, Quilty PM (1986) The results of a series of 963 patients with transitional cell carcinoma of the urinary bladder primarily treated by radical megavoltage X-ray therapy. Radiother Oncol 7:299–310

Dunst J, Sauer R, Schrott KM, Kühn R, Witteking C, Altendorf-Hofmann A (1994) Organ-sparing treatment of advanced bladder cancer: a 10 year experience. Int J Radiat Oncol Biol Phys 30:261–266

Edsmyr F, Andersson L, Esposti PL, Littbrand B, Nilsson B (1985) Irradiation therapy with multiple small fractions per day in urinary bladder cancer. Radiother Oncol 4:197–203

Fossa SD (1991) Pelvic palliation radiotherapy of advanced bladder cancer. Int J Radiat Oncol Biol Phys 20:1379

Fowler JF (1989) The LQ formula and progress in fractionated radiation therapy. Br J Radiol 62:679–694

Freiha F, Reese J, Torti FM (1996) A randomized trial of radical cystectomy versus radical cystectomy plus cisplatin, vinblastine and methotrexate chemotherapy for muscle invasive bladder cancer. J Urol 155:495–500

Gospodarowicz MK, Hawkins NV, Rawlings GA, et al. (1989) Radical radiotherapy for muscle invasive transitional cell carcinoma of the bladder: failure analysis. J Urol 142:1448–1454

Kleineidam M, Dubben HH (1992) Overall treatment time in the radiotherapy of transitional cell cancer of the bladder. Radiother Oncol 23:270

Larsen LE, Engelholm SA (1994) The value of three-dimensional radiotherapy planning in advanced carcinoma of the urinary bladder based on computed tomography. Acta Oncol 33:655–659

Lievens Y, Vanuytsel L, Rijnders A, Van Poppel H, van der Schueren E (1996) The time course of development of late side effects after irradiation of the prostate with multiple fractions per day. Radiother Oncol 40:147–152

Maciejewski BA, Majewski S (1991) Dose fractionation and tumour repopulation in radiotherapy for bladder cancer. Radiother Oncol 21:163–170

Maciejewski BA, Majewski S (1992) Two or three component dose-time curves for bladder cancer. Radiother Oncol 23:271

Moonen L, van der Voet H, Horenblas S, Bartelink H (1997) A feasibility study of accelerated fractionation in radiotherapy of carcinoma of the urinary bladder. Int J Radiat Oncol Biol Phys

Näslund I, Nilsson B, Littbrand B (1994) Hyperfractionated radiotherapy of bladder cancer. A ten year follow-up of a randomized clinical trial. Acta Oncol 33:397–402

Pagano F, Bassi P, Galettie TP, Meneghini A, Milani C, Artibani W, Garbeglio A (1991) Results of contemporary radical cystectomy for invasive bladder cancer: a clinicopathological study with an emphasis on the inadequacy of the tumor, nodes and metastases classification. J Urol 145:45–50

Parsons JT, Million RR (1988) Planned preoperative irradiation in the management of clinical stage B2-C (T3) bladder carcinoma. Int J Radiat Oncol Biol Phys 14:797–810

Pendlebury S, Dearnaley DP, Wynne C, Horwich A (1994) Accelerated fractionation (AF) for bladder cancer. Radiother Oncol 32(S1):S143 (abstract)

Plataniotis G, Michalopoulos E, Kouvaris J, Vlahos L, Papavasiliou C (1994) A feasibility study of partially accelerated radiotherapy for invasive bladder cancer. Radiother Oncol 33:84–87

Pollack A, Zagars GK, Swanson DA (1994) Muscle-invasive-bladder cancer treated with external beam radiotherapy: prognostic factors. Int J Radiat Oncol Biol Phys 30:267–277

Pollack A, Zagars GK, Cole CJ, Dinney CPN, Swanson DA, Grossman HB (1995) The relationship of local control to distant metastasis in muscle invasive bladder cancer. J Urol 154:2059–2064

Quilty PM, Kerr GR, Duncan W (1986) Prognostic indices for bladder cancer: an analysis of patients with transitional cell carcinoma of the bladder primarily treated by radical megavoltage X-ray therapy. Radiother Oncol 7:311–321

Rostom AY, Tahir S, Gershuny AR, et al. (1996) Once weekly irradiation for carcinoma of the bladder. Int J Radiat Oncol Biol Phys 35:289–292

Salminen E (1992) Unconventional fractionation for palliative radiotherapy of urinary bladder cancer. Acta Oncol 31:449–454

Shipley WU (1996) Translational research in bladder cancer. Int J Radiat Oncol Biol Phys 35:411–412

Shipley WU, Rose MA, Perrone TL, Mannix CM, Heney NM, Prout GR Jr (1985) Full-dose irradiation for patients with invasive bladder carcinoma: clinical and histological factors prognostic of improved survival. J Urol 134:679–683

Skinner DG, Lieskovsky G (1984) Contemporary cystectomy with pelvic node dissection compared to preoperative radiation therapy plus cystectomy in management of invasive bladder cancer. J Urol 131:1069–1072

Skinner DG, Daniels JR, Russel CA, et al. (1991) The role of adjuvant chemotherapy following cystectomy for invasive bladder cancer: a prospective comparative trial. J Urol 145:459–467

Stöckle M, Meyenburg W, Wellek S, et al. (1995) Adjuvant polychemotherapy of nonorgan-confined bladder cancer after radical cystectomy revisited: long-term results of a controlled prospective study and further clinical experience. J Urol 153:47–52

Wishnow KI, Dmochowski R (1988) Pelvic recurrence after radical cystectomy without preoperative rediation. J Urol 140:42–43

Withers HR, Peeters LJ, Taylor JMG, et al. (1995) Late normal tissue sequelae from radiation therapy for carcinoma of the tonsil: patterns of fractionation study of radiobiology. Int J Radiat Oncol Biol Phys 33:563–568

20 Chemotherapy Before Definitive Treatment for Locally Advanced Bladder Cancer

F. Calabrò and C.N. Sternberg

CONTENTS

20.1
Introduction

Bladder cancer is one of the most common malignancies in Western society, especially among cigarette smokers. The incidence is slowly rising, with 52 900 new cases predicted in the United States in 1996 (Devesa et al. 1995; Parker et al. 1996). Although most cases are superficial at presentation, a substantial portion of these subsequently progress, while some 20% are invasive at the time of initial presentation.

Despite aggressive locoregional treatment with radical cystectomy and pelvic lymphadenectomy or radical radiotherapy (RT), up to 50% of patients with locally advanced, muscle-invasive bladder cancer may relapse. Invasive bladder cancer must, therefore, be regarded as a systemic disease. Distant metastases usually occur within 2 years of the initial

diagnosis (Prout and Griffin 1979; Sternberg 1995a). Known prognostic factors for relapse after cystectomy include depth of invasion, involvement of adjacent viscera (perivesicular fat, vascular invasion, prostate, vagina), and presence of lymph node metastases. A recent series of 261 surgically staged patients has confirmed these data. Overall 5-year actuarial survival rate was 54%. The 5-year survival for muscle-invasive organ-confined disease (pT2 and pT3a) without lymph node involvement approached 70%. With extravesical extension, 5-year survival was 22% for patients with T3b disease and 27% for patients with T4 disease without lymph node involvement. All stage pT4 and pT3 cancer patients with positive lymph nodes died within 3 years. Overall 5-year survival of patients with positive lymph nodes was 4%, compared with 60% for those without lymph node involvement (Pagano et al. 1991). Tumor stage and presence of lymph node involvement were the two most important prognostic factors in a multivariate analysis (Pagano et al. 1996).

Results with definitive RT have been somewhat discouraging and frequently difficult to interpret. An analysis of studies published from 1975 to 1994 reveals that only 50%–60% of the patients are free of residual disease at the first follow-up. An additional 40%–50% of patients fail locally with longer follow-up. Overall 5-year survival ranges from 16%–40% (Pollack and Zagars 1996). It should be noted that randomized trials have not been performed comparing RT and surgery. Patients in surgical series are pathologically staged whereas those in RT series are only clinically staged. It is known that clinical staging substantially underestimates the stage of disease, making direct comparisons between trials rather difficult. In addition, patients in RT series are generally elderly and in poorer medical condition than patients who are surgical candidates.

Preoperative RT has been evaluated in a number of randomized trials, which have failed to demonstrate an improvement in patient outcome when comparison is made with patients treated by radical

F. Calabrò, MD, Department of Medical Oncology, San Raffaele Scientific Institute, Via E. Chianesi 53, I-00144 Rome, Italy

C.N. Sternberg, MD, FACP, Chief, Department of Medical Oncology, San Raffaele Scientific Institute, Via E. Chianesi 53, I-00144 Rome, Italy cystectomy alone (MAMEGHAN and FISHER 1989; SKINNER and LIESKOVSKY 1984).

Improvements in surgical techniques, perioperative care, and early diagnosis have led to an increase in survival owing to stage migration of 10%–20% per stage (FEINSTEIN et al. 1985). In fact, tumors are found earlier than in the past and are generally smaller, with fewer deeply invasive tumors. The frequency of presence of a palpable mass has diminished, and the incidence of pN+ has decreased (HERR 1992).

Nonetheless, because of the poor cure rates associated with conventional treatments such as surgery and RT, and the frequent development of metastatic disease despite aggressive locoregional treatment, it has been assumed that occult distant micrometastases are present at the time of initial diagnosis. This has led to the search for new approaches to patient management. Response rates of 40%–70% with combination chemotherapy regimens have led to investigation of their use for locally invasive disease in combination with conventional modalities, either as neoadjuvant or classic adjuvant therapy.

20.2
Neoadjuvant Chemotherapy

20.2.1
Rationale

Neoadjuvant chemotherapy is directed at the possibility of systemic disease in patients with apparently localized disease. This approach has several potential advantages over postoperative adjuvant chemotherapy. First, neoadjuvant chemotherapy provides earlier exposure of potential micrometastases to chemotherapy. Second, an objective response to chemotherapy in the primary lesion provides important in vivo evidence that the therapy being used has antitumor activity and suggests that the tumor at remote sites will be sensitive as well. In contrast, if the primary lesion does not respond, the likelihood of success of the initial chemotherapy regimen in eradicating micrometastases would seem to be greatly diminished. This provides an early opportunity to consider alternative approaches. Third, significant regression of the primary tumor may allow local management to be tailored to the individual patient. Surgery may be technically easier because of reduced tumor bulk. A more conservative surgical procedure may be considered, or RT may be admin-

istered in lieu of surgery. The use of chemotherapy prior to RT may permit better delivery of drugs than is possible after RT, which may alter the vascular bed. Furthermore, the reported toxicity associated with neoadjuvant chemotherapy has been much lower than in patients with metastatic disease because these patients generally have operable disease and a better performance status (STERNBERG 1995a).

20.2.2
Chemotherapy in Bladder Cancer

Significant advances have been made in the treatment of patients with urothelial tract tumors. The most active chemotherapeutic agents for advanced disease are cisplatin (30% response rate with 95% CI of 25%–35%), methotrexate (30% response rate with 95% CI of 25%–35%), vinblastine (16% response rate and 95% CI of 8%–24%), and doxorubicin (17% response rate and 95% CI of 12%–22%) (STERNBERG et al. 1995b). Other new active single agents include paclitaxel (42% response rate and 95% CI 23%–63%) and gemcitabine (29% response rate) (BISSET and KAYE 1993; ROTH et al. 1994; STADLER et al. 1996; LORUSSO et al. 1996).

In the past decade, many cisplatin-based combination chemotherapy regimens such as M-VAC (methotrexate, vinblastine, adriamycin, and cisplatin) CISCA (cyclophosphamide, adriamycin, and cisplatin), CM (cisplatin, methotrexate), and CMV (cisplatin, vinblastine, and methotrexate) have shown significant antitumor activity in patients with advanced, metastatic urothelial cancer (STERNBERG et al. 1988; LOGOTHETIS et al. 1985; HARKER et al. 1985; STOTER et al. 1987). CM regimens have been evaluated in various sequencing schedules in order to avoid delayed methotrexate renal excretion from cisplatin-induced nephrotoxicity. Following the initial promising report by Stoter, the overall response rate in 166 cases culled from the literature is 15% complete response (CR) and 32% partial response (PR) (YAGODA 1987). In another popular regimen, CMV, the initial study reported 26% CR persisting 44 weeks and 26% PR (HARKER et al. 1985). CISCA has been given in varied doses and schedules and has produced 12% CR and 27% PR rates (LOGOTHETIS et al. 1985; SCHWARTZ et al. 1983).

Seven randomized studies have compared single-agent chemotherapy with a cisplatin-containing combination regimen. Most trials have shown a benefit in terms of response (STERNBERG 1995b). Medical oncologists have accepted the results of an international trial which demonstrated the superiority of cisplatin-containing combination therapy (M-VAC) over single-agent cisplatin in terms of both response and survival (LOEHRER 1992).

M-VAC combination therapy has been extensively evaluated following the initial reports from Sloan Kettering Memorial Hospital (STERNBERG et al. 1985, 1988). When compared to CISCA, M-VAC was superior in attaining response and in terms of survival (LOGOTHETIS et al. 1990). In metastatic disease, chemotherapy has been shown to be more effective against lymph node disease than against visceral metastases. In the Memorial Sloan-Kettering Hospital series, median survival was 33 months for patients with lymph node disease versus 12 months for patients with metastatic visceral disease. In the M.D. Anderson trial of M-VAC versus CISCA, 71% of patients with lymph node disease responded, versus 40% of patients with visceral disease. M-VAC was superior to CISCA in terms of both response and survival. Chemotherapy can also lead to complete responses in the bladder. This provides a rationale for using chemotherapy for locally invasive disease, which has a high probability of occult nodal metastases.

20.2.3
Nonrandomized Neoadjuvant Chemotherapy Trials

In 1990, SCHER et al. reviewed 43 published trials comprising more than 1000 patients who received neoadjuvant therapy. These trials were for the most part not randomized, and were notable for the differences in case selection, chemotherapy schedules, response criteria, and small patient numbers. There was heterogeneity in the extent of disease and variable proportions of patients completed treatment programs. Recognizing the limitations of these series, most studies demonstrated tumor downstaging in 50%–70% of patients, with clinical CR in 22%–43%. More recently, an international consensus conference has updated the review and drawn some important conclusions concerning neoadjuvant chemotherapy trials (STERNBERG et al. 1995a).

Most important is the recognition that response to chemotherapy is an extremely important prognostic factor for survival. SPLINTER et al. (1992a) evaluated 147 patients from eight centers treated with several neoadjuvant chemotherapy regimens

followed by radical or partial cystectomy. Five-year survival was 75% in patients who had downstaging of the primary tumor to pT0 or superficial disease versus only 20% for patients with residual muscle infiltrating disease ($\geq$ pT2) after chemotherapy. Similar results were obtained in Rome with neoadjuvant M-VAC. Patients who responded to chemotherapy with downstaging to clinical or pathologic T0 or superficial disease had a 5-year survival rate of 69%, compared to only 24% in patients with residual muscle-infiltrating disease (STERNBERG et al. 1993, 1995b). At the Sloan Kettering Memorial Hospital, univariate analysis of patients treated with neoadjuvant M-VAC found initial stage, ureteral obstruction, and a palpable mass to be the only significant pretreatment prognostic factors. In multivariate analysis, initial stage and post-chemotherapy pathologic stage were the only two significant prognostic factors. An association between post-chemotherapy downstaging and survival was observed for patients with extravesical disease at the start of treatment. In this subset, 5-year overall survival was 54% for patients with downstaging versus 12% for those without downstaging. Notably, the type of surgical procedure performed (none versus partial or radical cystectomy) and the time of post-chemotherapy surgery did not affect outcome (SCHULTZ et al. 1994).

In the majority of neoadjuvant chemotherapy trials, a difference was found between clinical (T) and pathologic (P) staging. These inconsistencies, which vary between 30% and 50%, complicate the assessment of neoadjuvant chemotherapy trials. In a review of 90 cases thought to be T0 to Tis after neoadjuvant chemotherapy and transurethral resection of the bladder (TURB), invasive tumors $\geq$pT2 were discovered in 32% (HERR 1990). This is not surprising, in view of the fact that most cystectomy series have reported staging errors (under- or overstaging) in 30%–50% of patients (HERR 1990, SMITH 1982). The overall accuracy of TURB in the EORTC was 88% (4 of 35 patients were understaged) (SPLINTER et al. 1992b), while at Sloan Kettering Memorial Hospital in New York it was 77% (14 of 60 patients were understaged) (SCHER et al. 1990). In Italy, the accuracy was 79% (8 of 29 patients were understaged) when comparing the results of TURB and cystectomy after M-VAC (STERNBERG et al. 1993, 1995b). Before recommending bladder preservation to a patient, this 30% clinical staging error must be seriously taken into consideration.

Neoadjuvant chemotherapy may also be given by intra-arterial administration. This approach has the advantage of increasing the local concentration of drugs. Intra-arterial chemotherapy has been frequently used in Japan and occasionally in the United States and Europe (NAITO et al. 1995; CHECHILE et al. 1990). Although preliminary data regarding intra-arterial neoadjuvant chemotherapy have shown some activity against transitional cell carcinoma of the bladder, it remains to be proven whether this type of therapy increases the efficacy of chemotherapeutic agents. The comparative efficacy of intra-arterial chemotherapy has never been tested. Therefore, this method cannot presently be considered routine. Further studies are required to define the role of this route of administration.

For patients with invasive bladder cancer, data from nonrandomized trials suggest that neoadjuvant chemotherapy can produce downstaging of the primary tumor. Pretreatment tumor stage and size, together with the clinical or pathologic response, are probably the most important prognostic factors for survival. These trials have illustrated the problems in interpreting response following neoadjuvant chemotherapy, due to the inconsistencies between clinical and pathologic staging. The inaccuracies of clinical staging, common also in other solid tumors, may confound the interpretation of results. Whether or not neoadjuvant chemotherapy has an effect on survival can only be answered in the context of well-controlled randomized trials (STERNBERG et al. 1995a).

20.2.4
Randomized Neoadjuvant Chemotherapy Trials

The results of several randomized trials have been published, while others are still in progress. Most trials have been closed without demonstrating a difference in survival due to neoadjuvant chemotherapy. This does not mean that there is no difference, only that insufficient numbers of patients

may have been entered in order to demonstrate a difference (STERNBERG et al. 1995b). Randomized neoadjuvant chemotherapy trials are reviewed in Table 20.1.

In a prospective randomized trial of 122 patients from Spain comparing cystectomy and neoadjuvant single-agent cisplatin prior to cystectomy, no difference in overall survival was demonstrated. In this trial, single-agent cisplatin, no longer considered as the best standard treatment, was given. Disease-free interval was significantly prolonged by chemotherapy. The authors did note a survival advantage in patients whose tumor was downstaged (MARTINEZ PINEIRO et al. 1995).

The largest study is that of the European Organization for Research and Treatment of Cancer (EORTC) and Medical Research Council (MRC) conducted from November 1989 to July 1995. Neoadjuvant CMV was given in the investigational arm followed by either radical cystectomy or full-dose external beam RT or preoperative RT and cystectomy. The standard arm consisted of definitive treatment alone, without neoadjuvant chemotherapy. The trial has enrolled 975 patients with G3T2, T3 or T4a, N0/Nx, M0 bladder cancer. The study, conducted in 89 institutions in 16 countries, was designed to detect a 10% increase in survival (from 50% to 60%). Cystectomy was planned in 484 patients, RT in 414, and combined treatment in 77. At a median follow-up of 29 months, no difference in overall survival was observed between patients receiving and those not receiving neoadjuvant CMV. Overall 2-year survival was 63% versus 60%. An 8% difference in metastatic progression (58% vs 50%) was seen in favor of the patients who had received neoadjuvant chemotherapy. Among 392 patients who underwent cystectomy, 33% in the CMV arm compared to 12% who did not receive CMV had pT0 in the cystectomy specimen, indicating a 21% pathologic complete response rate due to the chemotherapy. Toxicity was acceptable in this multicenter

Table 20.1. Randomized trials of neoadjuvant chemotherapy

Study group	Investigational arm	Standard arm	Patients	Results
EORTC/MRC	CMV/RT or Cyst	RT or Cyst	975	No difference
USA Intergroup	M-VAC/Cyst	Cyst	266 (298)	Ongoing
Spain (Cueto)	DDP/Cyst	Cyst	121	No difference
Italy (GISTV)	M-VEC/Cyst	Cyst	104	No difference
Italy (GUONE)	M-VAC/Cyst	Cyst	–	Ongoing
Nordic	ADM-DDP/PT/Cyst	RT/Cyst	325	15% difference in T3–T4a

RT, Radiation therapy; Cyst, cystectomy; CMV, cisplatin, methotrexate, vinblastine; M-VAC, methotrexate, vinblastine, adriamycin, cisplatin; DDP, cisplatin; M-VEC, methotrexate, vinblastine, epirubicin, cisplatin; ADM, adriamycin.

study, and delay in cystectomy did not result in an increase in unresectable patients. Longer follow-up will be required (HALL 1996a).

Contrasting results were obtained from another neoadjuvant chemotherapy trial. The Nordic Cooperative Bladder Cancer Study Group conducted a randomized trial of two cycles of neoadjuvant cisplatin and doxorubicin prior to a short course of preoperative RT followed by radical cystectomy, compared to RT and cystectomy alone. Neoadjuvant chemotherapy significantly reduced the death rate from cancer in patients with muscle-invasive T3–T4a disease ($P = 0.03$), although the level of significance for the whole trial, including patients with G3T1, was not significant ($P = 0.1$). In this trial 325 patients with G3T1, T2–4, Nx, M0, were entered. Whereas no advantage was seen for patients with superficial disease or T2, at 5 years a 15% difference in overall survival and a 20% difference in cancer-specific survival was observed for patients with pT3–T4 (MALMSTROM et al. 1996). A subsequent Nordic cystectomy trial II was initiated in 1991. This trial will only include patients with stage T2–T4a tumors. There is no preoperative RT. Three cycles of neoadjuvant CM will be evaluated.

The American phase III Intergroup Trial has been evaluating three cycles of neoadjuvant M-VAC chemotherapy. The trial is coordinated by the Southwest Oncology Group (SWOG) with collaboration of the Eastern Cooperative Oncology Group (ECOG) and the Cancer and Leukemia Group B (CALGB). It has been designed to evaluate neoadjuvant M-VAC and cystectomy versus cystectomy alone. The group plans to randomize 298 patients. Unlike the EORTC/MRC, the policy of these investigators has been to report results only after 50% of the patients have died. Accrual has been slow, with trial accrual for many years. A similar trial is ongoing in Northern Italy. The results of these trials coupled with those of the Nordic cystectomy trial II should further clarify the role of an anthracycline in cisplatin-containing combination chemotherapy.

LOGOTHETIS (1996) compared two cycles of neoadjuvant M-VAC prior to cystectomy and three cycles of adjuvant M-VAC to cystectomy followed by five cycles of adjuvant M-VAC. No survival benefit was demonstrated for either arm, although a high rate of downstaging of the primary tumor was noted after two cycles of neoadjuvant M-VAC. Inconsistencies between clinical and pathologic staging were demonstrated (LOGOTHETIS 1996).

Finally, a meta-analysis of randomized trials evaluating neoadjuvant chemotherapy failed to reveal a survival advantage in favor of neoadjuvant chemotherapy (overall hazard ratio of 1.02). However, this analysis included many trials in which single-agent chemotherapy, no longer considered optimum treatment, was used (GHERSI et al. 1995).

Randomized and nonrandomized trials have demonstrated the feasibility of administering neoadjuvant chemotherapy, with an overall response rate of about 70% and pathologic complete responses of 20%–30% in the primary muscle-invasive tumor. Response to neoadjuvant chemotherapy is an extremely important prognostic factor. Although patients who respond to initial chemotherapy are often reported as having an improvement in survival, the literature does not currently support these claims. Neoadjuvant chemotherapy may, however, be of interest in terms of bladder preservation.

20.3
Bladder Preservation

20.3.1
Neoadjuvant Chemotherapy and Bladder Preservation

The complications of cystectomy and urinary diversion have been recently outlined (FRAZIER 1992). In a series of 675 patients, the operative mortality was 2.5%. Of these 675 patients, 32% had immediate postoperative complications and 27% had long-term complications. There are two major reasons why patients refuse cystectomy: loss of sexual function and the ileal conduit (urostomy). Alternative approaches include bladder substitution and bladder preservation.

Several different methods of bladder substitution with continent diversion to the urethra are now in vogue. This type of surgery may achieve normal voiding through the urethra and avoid a urostomy. Not all patients with invasive bladder cancer are, however, candidates for bladder substitution. Only recently have selected women been offered this alternative (HAUTMANN and PAISS 1996; CANCRINI et al. 1995). Men who need a urethrectomy, or those undergoing salvage cystectomy after RT, are not candidates for bladder substitution, although many urologists suggest that orthotopic bladder substitution is equivalent to retaining one's bladder. It seems to be better for patients if they can retain their own bladder which is tumor free. There are three modalities of bladder preservation following neoadjuvant chemotherapy: partial cystectomy, TURB, and RT.

20.3.2
Partial Cystectomy

The role of partial cystectomy has been reconsidered in the era of neoadjuvant chemotherapy. Candidates for partial cystectomy following neoadjuvant chemotherapy are those who: (a) attain a clinical CR or significant clinical PR to neoadjuvant chemotherapy; (b) have solitary lesions in favorable anatomic locations (dome and anterior lateral walls of the bladder); (c) have no history of previous or recurrent infiltrative bladder cancer; (d) have no carcinoma in situ (CIS), and (e) have good bladder capacity (SROUGI and SIMON 1994; STERNBERG 1995b).

At Sloan Kettering Memorial Hospital, 111 candidates for radical cystectomy received four cycles of neoadjuvant M-VAC. Twenty-six patients with a favorable response to chemotherapy at restaging TURB underwent partial cystectomy. At a median follow-up of 6.9 years, survival was 65%, including 14 (54%) with an intact, functional bladder. Of the 26 patients, 19 had pT0 or superficial disease after chemotherapy. Pathologic response was correctly predicted by the post M-VAC TURB in 88% of cases. Twelve patients (46%) developed bladder recurrence, which was invasive in five (18%) and superficial in seven (26%). Patients with no tumor or noninvasive tumor in their surgical specimen had a 5-year survival rate of 87%, compared with a rate of 30% in patients with residual invasive cancer (HERR 1994).

In Rome, 12 of 65 patients with monofocal lesions who responded to chemotherapy underwent partial cystectomy after three cycles of neoadjuvant M-VAC. Prior to chemotherapy, six patients had been T3b, two were T3a, and four were T2. After chemotherapy, eight patients were downstaged to pT0, one had pTis, two had pT1, and one had minimal downstaging to pT2. At a median follow-up of 55+ (16–80+) months, eight of 12 (67%) patients are alive, seven (58%) with a functioning bladder. Five-year survival for these patients is 67% (STERNBERG et al. 1995c).

SROUGI and SIMON (1994) reported 30 patients who underwent three to four cycles of neoadjuvant M-VAC. Fourteen patients (47%) had a clinical CR and 16 (53%) had a PR or no response (NR). In all 14 patients with a CR the bladder was preserved. After 5 years 10/14 patients (71%) had recurrent disease; eight underwent radical cystectomy and two who had superficial disease were treated conservatively with intravesical therapy. At 5 years 6/14 (43%) have retained their bladder. Of 14 clinical CR patients, five (36%) had a partial cystectomy. Four of 16 patients who had a PR or NR underwent partial cystectomy. After 5 years two patients had bladder recurrence and underwent salvage radical cystectomy and two patients died of metastatic disease. Eleven of 14 CR patients (79%) were disease-free at 5 years, and 4/16 patients (25%) were disease-free at 5 years in the PR or NR group.

These series suggest that in selected cases partial cystectomy following neoadjuvant chemotherapy may be appropriate, with survival similar to that obtained with radical surgery. Selected patients whose tumors show significant tumor reduction may benefit from partial cystectomy. Patients with recurrent disease, extension to the prostatic urethra, or reduced bladder capacity are not candidates for partial cystectomy. Partial cystectomy can be successfully performed in patients with initial monofocal lesions who respond to neoadjuvant chemotherapy (SROUGI and SIMON 1994; STERNBERG 1995b; HERR 1994). Selected patients may be those with initial, small T3 tumors. Such an approach appears to offer local control equivalent to that attained by radical cystectomy. The combination of neoadjuvant chemotherapy and partial cystectomy requires longer follow-up in larger trials prior to any definitive statements regarding its efficacy (STERNBERG and PANSADORO 1996).

20.3.3
Transurethral Resection of the Bladder

In several series TURB has been shown to be therapeutic in patients who have undergone complete tumor resection. In selected patients with superficial T2 muscle-infiltrating tumors, TURB has been used as definitive treatment and has yielded essentially equivalent survival to radical cystectomy, the 5-year survival rate being 50%–70% (BARNES et al. 1967; STERNBERG and PANSADORO 1996). In Herr's series patients with T2 disease underwent a second staging TURB after referral to the Sloan Kettering Memorial Hospital. If the second TURB demonstrated T0 in the biopsy specimen, patients were observed and did not undergo radical cystectomy. At a follow-up of 5.1 years (range 3–7), 30 of 45 (65%) patients were disease-free. Some had a repeat TURB and intravesical therapy (HERR 1987). Fewer data exist about patients with more invasive disease, but TURB is generally considered to be inadequate treatment for patients with T3a or T3b, with 23% and 7% 5-year survival rates respectively (FAIR 1992).

Some series have reported survival in 20%–40% of cases treated by TURB (HERR 1987; BARNES et al. 1967; O'FLYNN et al. 1975; HENRY et al. 1988; OJEA et al. 1989; SOLSONA et al. 1994; STERNBERG and PANSADORO 1996). In a Spanish study 77 patients with T2 disease were treated by TURB alone. Forty-three of 77 (59%) patients were free of disease, 33 (45%) after a single TURB and 10 following repeated TURB. Five-year survival was 72% (OJEA 1989). SOLSONA et al. (1994) from Spain recently reported two consecutive series of patients with muscle-invasive (T2–T3a) bladder tumors that were treated by TURB alone. In the first series of 59 patients with >5 years follow-up, disease-free survival was 78%, with bladder preservation in 24 (41%) patients. In a second series, with >3 years follow-up, survival was 88% with a 69% rate of bladder preservation (35 of 51 patients). In another series, 5-year survival was evaluated in 114 patients treated with either TURB, preoperative RT and radical cystectomy, or radical cystectomy alone. In this nonrandomized retrospective study, similar survival rates and time to development of metastases were found among all of the groups (HENRY et al. 1988).

When neoadjuvant chemotherapy is integrated with TURB, results seem to be even better. At Sloan Kettering Memorial Hospital, 26 of 95 (28%) patients were disease-free with a functional bladder after neoadjuvant M-VAC (SCHER et al. 1990). Patients underwent multiple TURBs before and during chemotherapy. The impact of repeated TURB may be an important explanation for the good results in these patients. M-VAC plus TURB was maximally effective in patients with smaller lesions.

In Rome a stratified TURB was performed on all patients prior to and after three cycles of neoadjuvant M-VAC. Of 65 patients, 32 had TURB and did not undergo pathologic staging. Thirteen (42%) patients are tumor-free, and have had no recurrences. Twenty-three of the 32 (72%) patients are alive. Twenty of 32 (63%) have maintained an intact bladder. The median survival has not yet been reached. The 5-year survival rate is 65%. In this study, response to chemotherapy was the most important prognostic factor. Patients who had downstaging of the tumor to superficial disease or T0 after neoadjuvant chemotherapy have not yet

reached the median survival, with a 5-year survival rate of 69%. In contrast, patients who had muscle-infiltrating disease (>T2) after chemotherapy had a 5-year survival rate of 24%. In this series patients were selected for bladder sparing based on response to chemotherapy (STERNBERG et al. 1995b).

In the previously mentioned Brazilian study (SROUGI and SIMON 1994), patients were treated with neoadjuvant M-VAC followed by bladder-sparing surgical revaluation and followed up for at least 5 years. Biopsies were obtained by open surgery in 11 patients, and TURB in 19 patients. Five-year disease-free survival was greater in the CR group (79%) than in the PR or NR group (25%). These data emphasize the importance of close surveillance after bladder preservation, since 71% of patients had local recurrences.

HALL (1996b) has advocated an extensive TURB with dissection to the fat plus systemic chemotherapy as an alternative to cystectomy. He recommends removal of all visible and palpable tumor, including that which has extended into the perivesical fat and connective tissue. With cisplatin and methotrexate, 31/54 (57%) patients with T2–T3b tumors remained disease-free at 3 years and retained their bladders. For patients with T3 tumors 3-year survival was 79%.

Recently, two protocols were used for 46 patients with muscle-invasive disease. Protocol A consisted of TURB for diagnostic and debulking purposes, followed by two or three cycles of M-VAC or CMV chemotherapy. Patients with no or minimal disease underwent pelvic RT and nonresponders had cystectomy. Protocol B was identical to protocol A, but patients did not receive RT if they had a CR after chemotherapy. Twenty-two of 27 patients in protocol A had no or minimal disease at evaluation and received RT; 14 of them have no evidence of disease and have retained their bladder. In protocol B, 12 of 19 patients had no tumor at TURB, and seven remain with no evidence of disease with bladder preservation. Event-free survival at five years is 41% and 42% for groups A and B respectively. Both treatments achieved similar results in terms of survival and bladder preservation (VILLARONGA et al. 1996). This type of study, though not randomized and very preliminary, may suggest that the addition of RT after neoadjuvant chemotherapy does not provide any additional advantage.

A TURB demonstrating the absence of muscle-invasive disease after chemotherapy may select a subset of patients who can be managed with close surveillance in an attempt at bladder preservation.

As several pilot studies suggest, there is a group of patients with muscle-invasive bladder cancer who can be cured by the combination of a thorough endoscopic resection and systemic chemotherapy, without cystectomy or RT. As in the case of partial cystectomy, candidates for neoadjuvant chemotherapy and TURB alone may be those patients with T2 and smaller T3 tumors.

20.3.4
Radiotherapy

Radiotherapy has traditionally been used as a means of retaining an intact bladder. However, with the exception of countries such as Canada and England, RT has been used less frequently than surgery. With RT alone, only 20%–40% of patients are cured and preserve their bladder free of disease. In addition, at least 24% of patients may experience long-term morbidity. Significant prognostic factors for local curability are absence of ureteral obstruction, papillary histology, and visibly complete tumor resection by TURB prior to RT (GOSPODAROWICZ et al. 1991; SHIPLEY et al. 1995).

Neoadjuvant chemotherapy plus RT has been proposed by several investigators to preserve the bladder. Several of the known chemotherapeutic agents which have activity in bladder cancer also have the property of radiosensitization, including cisplatin, 5-fluorouracil, doxorubicin, paclitaxel, and mitomycin C. Cisplatin and 5-fluorouracil have most frequently been used concurrently with RT. Table 20.2 reviews the results attained with an integrated approach of neoadjuvant chemotherapy and RT.

In a series of 70 patients treated with neoadjuvant cisplatin followed by RT, 5-year actuarial survival was 40% (WALLACE et al. 1991). A randomized trial conducted by the National Cancer Institute of Canada demonstrated that chemoradiation, with concurrent cisplatin and RT, yielded statistically significantly better local tumor control than RT alone. No survival benefit was, however, seen (COPPIN et al. 1992).

Several other single-arm nonrandomized studies with synchronous chemotherapy and RT have been published (KAUFMANN 1993; HOUSSET et al. 1993; TESTER et al. 1993, 1996; SHIPLEY et al. 1995). In these reports more than 50% of patients have achieved tumor control with excellent survival compared to historical controls, an invalid method of statistical analysis.

In an update of a study from Boston, neoadjuvant MCV (CMV) chemotherapy was followed by external beam RT and cisplatin. Only patients who achieved a CR to initial chemotherapy and intermediate-dose RT were spared cystectomy. The planned therapy was TURB, followed by two cycles of MCV chemotherapy, plus two additional courses of cisplatin in combination with RT (4000 cGy). If tumor was found on cystoscopic reevaluation, immediate cystectomy was advised. If no tumor was found, a boost to 6480 cGy plus an additional dose of cisplatin was given. The 52% actuarial overall 5-year survival is similar to that achieved by others who employed radical cystectomy, compared with historical controls (a flawed method of statistical comparison). Multivariate analysis of the rate of bladder preservation without recurrence of invasive tumor revealed that the presence or absence of hydronephrosis was the only significant prognostic factor (SHIPLEY et al. 1995).

In another study, 29 patients with muscle-invasive bladder cancer underwent two to four cycles of neoadjuvant M-VAC followed by either RT (15

Table 20.2. Trials of neoadjuvant chemotherapy and radiotherapy

Author	Chemotherapy	Patients	CR (%)	Bladder preservation (%)	Survival rate (%)
Shipley	MCV/DDP c	106	70	43	52 (5 year)
Housset	5-FU/DDP c	54	74	NA	59 (3 year)
Tester	MCV/DDP c	92	79	60	62 (4 year)
Vogelzang	M-VAC	29	31[a]	55	70 (5 year)
Abratt	CMV	18	67	44	61 (3 year)
Kuten	CMV	56		23	68 (2 year)
Rifkin	MCV ± A	91	57	52	63 (2 year)

DDP c, cisplatin given concurrently with radiotherapy; MCV, methotrexate, vinblastine, cisplatin; M-VAC, methotrexate, vinblastine, adriamycin, cisplatin; A, adriamycin.
[a] Response to M-VAC alone.

patients) or radical cystectomy (11 patients), or no local therapy (three patients). The response rate was 69% to M-VAC with 31% attaining CR and 38% a PR. A functional bladder was attained in 55% of responding patients (VOGELZANG et al. 1993). In a study from Florida, 94 patients were treated with a bladder-sparing strategy. All patients had TURB, two to three cycles of CMV or M-VAC, and radiotherapy for selected cases. At a median follow-up period of more than 5 years, relapse-free survival was 49%. Of importance, the study selected patients who were poor surgical candidates and who had advanced T4 tumors. RT (6480 cGy) was offered to only 49 patients. The rate of bladder preservation was disappointingly low, only 18%. Hydronephrosis at presentation was a negative prognostic factor. Patient selection factors must be seriously considered in the interpretation of this trial (GIVEN et al. 1995).

Data on 224 patients treated with three different protocols were analyzed: RT >60 Gy (143 patients), low-dose RT followed by cystectomy (25 patients), or chemotherapy followed by definitive RT or surgery. Two-year survival was 63% for patients who received only RT, 72% for those undergoing cystectomy, and 68% for the neoadjuvant chemotherapy group. This was not a randomized study; however, 23% of patients treated with neoadjuvant chemotherapy were alive with intact bladder at 2 years (KUTEN et al. 1995).

In a recent review, prognostic factors for bladder relapse and distant failure following definitive RT, with or without neoadjuvant chemotherapy, were analyzed (MAMEGHAN 1995). The 342 patients with invasive bladder cancer fell into distinct prognostic groups determined by three independent factors: ureteric obstruction, tumor multiplicity, and T stage. These factors provided estimated risks of bladder relapse at 5 years which ranged from 34% to 91%. Knowledge of these prognostic factors can help in the selection of patients more suited for bladder preservation by definitive RT.

Bladder preservation can be successful only if a durable CR is attained. The true success of bladder preservation by integrated approaches of chemotherapy plus RT must be evaluated in randomized trials. Toxicities associated with RT are not insignificant and include decreased bladder function, cystitis, hematuria, and adhesions. Thus, attempts at bladder preservation with neoadjuvant chemotherapy and RT should evaluate not only the efficacy but also the toxicity of these combined modalities.

Neoadjuvant chemotherapy and bladder preservation is feasible and may be effective treatment, particularly for patients with smaller T2–T3a lesions. Other factors, such as the presence or absence of CIS in the prostatic urethra, bladder capacity, general medical conditions, and performance status of the patient will always affect the decision to employ chemotherapy or immediate surgery. Whether or not RT should be added to bladder-preserving treatments is still to be determined. Follow-up of patients who have retained their bladders after neoadjuvant chemotherapy requires close surveillance because of the risk of development of new tumors. Preliminary data seem to suggest that bladder preservation may be possible in 40%–50% of successfully managed patients with the combination of chemotherapy and TURB, partial cystectomy, or RT. The current situation is that there have been a paucity of randomized controlled trials to define the true value of these integrated therapies. Thus, it is presently impossible to draw definitive conclusions on the efficacy of bladder-preserving approaches.

20.4
Future Prospects

Since M-VAC was conceived in 1983, it has remained the gold standard against which new treatments have been measured (STERNBERG et al. 1985). Ongoing research is being undertaken to evaluate the effects of dose escalation of M-VAC (STERNBERG and DE MULDER 1992). However, long-term follow-up reveals that only 17%–20% of patients with metastatic disease are cured by combination chemotherapy (STERNBERG et al. 1989; SAXMAN et al. 1996). New active agents that can be incorporated into combination regimens must be found. Several drugs such as paclitaxel, gallium nitrate, ifosfamide, and gemcitabine have demonstrated activity.

Paclitaxel (taxol) is one of the most active single agents in the treatment of advanced bladder cancer. When given at a dosage of 250 mg/m^2 by 24-h continuous infusion, 11 of 26 (42%) of previously untreated patients responded, with seven (27%) achieving a CR (ROTH et al. 1994). The combination of paclitaxel, methotrexate, and cisplatin has been used in the salvage setting after M-VAC: of 25 heavily pretreated patients with metastatic urothelial malignancies, ten (40%) had a PR (TU et al. 1995). Studies incorporating these new agents into combination regimens are ongoing, with the goal of providing a regimen that has superior efficacy. The combination of vinblastine, ifosfamide, and gallium nitrate (VIG) likewise was extremely active, with a 67% response in unpretreated patients (DREICER et al. 1996; EINHORN et al. 1994). 5-Fluorouracil in continuous infusion with interferon-α, and cisplatin (FAP) produced a 61% response rate in patients who had failed M-VAC (LOGOTHETIS et al. 1992). An attempt by the EORTC to corroborate these results is underway, while M-VAC and FAP are being compared at the M.D. Anderson Cancer Center.

Many active agents and combinations are available, and further improvement in neoadjuvant chemotherapy will hopefully become possible. The heterogeneous nature of bladder cancer and the various therapeutic options provide a constant challenge to the clinician in planning appropriate management to avoid over- and undertreatment. Thus the ability to determine the metastatic phenotype of a given cancer and its sensitivity to chemotherapy would be highly beneficial to the patient and might allow the oncologist to tailor therapy and to optimize results of treatment combinations. The development of reliable noninvasive tests to predict clinical behavior and treatment outcome will represent a major advance.

The rapidly increasing understanding of the biology of bladder cancer, with respect to factors controlling its growth and predictors of response, is paving the way to future advances in the management of urothelial cancers. Techniques have been developed that have refined evaluation of certain histologic parameters such as ploidy, nuclear morphometry, and apoptosis. Aneuploidy, as determined by flow cytometry, has been associated with poorer survival in both low-stage and high-stage cancers although correlation may be better for low stages (LIPPONEN 1994). A high rate of cell division, as determined by immuno-histochemical staining with cell cycle-related proteins such as Ki-67 and PCNA, was detected in higher stage tumors and was associated with reduced survival. Again, this association is stronger for superficial bladder cancers (LIPPONEN et al. 1992). High tumor vascularity was a strong predictor of lymph node metastasis in one study (JAEGER et al. 1995), and of survival in another (DICKINSON et al. 1994). A recent study has shown that overexpression of the c-myc protein in urothelial cells is associated with high proliferation (LIPPONEN 1995).

Inactivation of the retinoblastoma RB tumor suppressor gene is thought to be an important step in cancer progression. Logothetis studied 43 patients with locally advanced bladder cancer and found that patients whose tumors had lost RB expression had a lower 3-year survival, suggesting that loss of RB expression is a prognostic factor in patients with advanced bladder cancer (TAKAHASHI et al. 1991).

Several large series have shown that abnormal p53 expression is found more frequently in higher grade and higher stage bladder tumors and is a predicator of poor outcome. ESRIG et al. (1995) investigated the role of p53 overexpression in 243 patients who underwent radical cystectomy. p53 overexpression was the sole independent predictor of poor outcome (75% vs 37%, $P < 0.001$) and decreased 5-year survival. Two preliminary reports examining the prognostic importance of the combination of altered p53 and RB expression suggest that mutation of the p53 and RB genes have independent and synergistic roles in the development of bladder cancer (ESRIG et al. 1995; LERNER 1995). These results have, however, been contradicted (VET 1995; JAHNSON 1995; GLICK 1996).

E-cadherin is an epithelial cell adhesion molecule associated with differentiation and is lost in many types of cancer. Several recent studies have shown an association between increased bladder cancer stage and a decrease in E-cadherin expression at the cell border. The c-erbB-2 oncogene encodes a cellular surface protein that shows significant sequence homology with EGFr and initially was identified as a transforming gene. Amplification of c-erbB-2 gene has been observed in bladder cancers. Several studies report that high expression of c-erbB-2 protein is associated with higher stage, increased metastasis, and poorer survival (SATO et al. 1992).

Although the prognostic and diagnostic usefulness of many of these markers in invasive bladder cancer remains to be fully evaluated, alterations in the biology and genetics of cells no doubt contribute to the processes of invasion and metastases and are likely to provide important, useful information for future identification and management of the patient with invasive bladder cancer.

20.5
Conclusions

Locally advanced bladder cancer represents a heterogeneous spectrum of diseases with different biologic and clinical behavior. It varies with respect to invasive potential, propensity for metastases, and sensitivity to chemotherapy. The data currently available from nonrandomized and randomized trials have not definitively established the precise role of neoadjuvant chemotherapy and its real impact on survival. Even if neoadjuvant chemotherapy does not improve survival, preliminary data suggest that bladder preservation may be possible in patients successfully managed by the combination of chemotherapy and TURB or partial cystectomy, and that such combined therapy will hopefully lead to better patient management.

References

Barnes RW, Bergmann RT, Hadley HL, Love D (1967) Control of bladder tumors by endoscopic surgery. J Urol 97:864–868

Bissett D, Kaye SB (1993) Taxol and taxotere – current status and future prospects. Eur J Cancer 29A:1228–1230

Cancrini A, Decarli P, Fattahi H, Pompeo V, Cantiani R, Vonheland M (1995) Orthotopic ileal neobladder in female patients after radical cystectomy: 2-year experience. J Urol 153:956–958

Chechile G, Montie J, Pontes JE, Bukowski RM (1990) Neoadjuvant intra-arterial chemotherapy in locally advanced bladder cancer. Prog Clin Biol Res 353:153–161

Coppin C, Gospodarowicz M, Dixon P, et al. for the NCI-Canada Clinical Trials Group K, Ontario (1992) Improved local control of invasive bladder cancer by concurrent cisplatin and preoperative or radical radiation (abstract). Proc Am Soc Clin Oncol 11:198

Devessa SS, Blot WJ, Stone BJ, Miller BA, Tarone RE, Fraumeni JF Jr (1995) Recent cancer trends in the United States. J Natl Cancer Inst 87:175–182

Dickinson AJ, Fox SB, Persad SA, et al. (1994) Quantification of angiogenesis as an independent predictor of prognosis in invasive bladder cancer. Br J Urol 74:762–766

Dreicer R, Propert KJ, Roth BJ, Einhorn LH, Loehrer PJ (1996) Vinblastine, ifosfamide, and gallium nitrate (VIG), an active new regimen in advanced carcinoma of the urothelium: a phase II trial of the Eastern Cooperative Oncology Group (E5892). Cancer

Einhorn LH, Roth BJ, Ansari R, Dreicer R, Gonin R, Loehrer PJ (1994) Phase II trial of vinblastine, ifosfamide, and gallium nitrate combination chemotherapy in metastatic urothelial carcinoma. J Clin Oncol 12:2271–2276

Esrig D, Shi SR, Bochner B, et al. (1995) Prognostic importance of p53 and Rb alterations in transitional cell carcinoma of the bladder (abstract). J Urol 153:536A

Fair WR. Organ Conservation in deeply invasive bladder tumors: a valid approach. World J Urol 1992:8–10

Feinstein AR, Sossin DM, Wells CR (1985) The Will Rogers phenomenon: stage migration and new diagnostic techniques as a source of misleading statistics for survival in cancer. N Engl J Med 312:1604–1608

Frazier HA, Robertson JE, Paulson DF (1992) Complications of radical cystectomy and urinary diversion: a retrospective review of 675 cases in 2 decades. J Urol 148(5):1401–1405

Ghersi D, Stewart LA, Parmar MKB (1995) Does neoadjuvant cisplatin-based chemotherapy improve the survival of patients with locally advanced bladder cancer? A meta-analysis of individual patient data from randomized clinical trials. Br J Urol 75:206–213

Given RW, Parsons JT, McCarley D, Wajsman Z (1995) Bladder-sparing multimodality treatment of muscle-invasive bladder cancer: a five-year follow-up. Urology 46:499–505

Glick AB, Weinberg WC, Wu IH, Quan W, Yuspa SH (1996) Transforming growth factor beta 1 suppresses genomic instability independent of a Gl arrest, p53 and Rb. Cancer Res 56(16):3645–3650

Gospodarowicz MK, Ryder WK, Keen CW (1991) Bladder cancer: long term follow-up results of patients treated with radical radiation. J Clin Oncol 3:155–161

Hall RR, for the MRC Advanced Bladder Cancer Working Party, EORTC GU Group, NCI Canada, Norwegian Bladder Cancer Group, Australian Bladder Cancer Study Group, Club Urologica Espanol, and FinBladder (1996a) Neoadjuvant CMV chemotherapy and cystectomy or radiotherapy in muscle invasive bladder cancer. First analysis of MRC/EORTC intercontinental trial. Proc Am Soc Clin Oncol 15:Abstract 612–244

Hall RR (1996b) The role of transurethral surgery alone and with combined modality therapy. In: Vogelzang NJ, Scardino PT, Shipley WU, et al. (eds) Comprehensive textbook of genitourinary oncology. William & Wilkins, Baltimore, pp 509–513

Harker W, Meyers FJ, Freiha FS, et al. (1985) Cisplatin, methotrexate, and vinblastine (CMV): an effective chemotherapy regimen for metastatic transitional cell carcinoma of the urinary tract a Northern California Oncology Group study. J Clin Oncol 3:1463–1470

Hautmann RE, Paiss T (1996) Does the option of the ileal neobladder stimulate patient and physician decision towards earlier cyctectomy? (abstract) J Urol 155:437A

Henry K, Miller J, Mari M, Loening SJ, Falow B (1988) Comparison of transurethral resection to radical therapies for stage B bladder tumors. J Urol 140:964–967

Herr HW (1987) Conservative management of muscle-infiltrating bladder cancer: prospective experience. J Urol 138:1162–1163

Herr HW (1990) The role of surgery in initial staging and follow up. In: Splinter TAW, Scher HI (eds) Neoadjuvant chemotherapy in invasive bladder cancer. Progress in clinical and biological research. Wiley-Liss, New York, pp 34–43

Herr HW (1992) Staging invasive bladder tumors. J Surg Oncol 51:217–220

Herr HW (1994) Uncertainty, stage and outcome of invasive bladder cancer. J Urol 152:401–402

Herr HW, Whitmore WF Jr, Morse MJ, Sogani PC, Russo P, Fair WR (1990) Neoadjuvant chemotherapy in invasive bladder cancer: the evolving role of surgery. J Urol 144:1083–1088

Herrada J, Dieringer P, Logothetis CJ (1996) Characterization of patients with androgen-independent prostatic carcinoma whose serum prostate specific antigen decreased following flutamide withdrawal. J Urol 155:620–623

Housset M, Maulard C, Chretien Y, et al. (1993) Combined radiation and chemotherapy for invasive transitional cell carcinoma of the bladder: a prospective study. J Clin Oncol 11:2150–2157

Jaeger TM, Weidner N, Chew K, et al. (1995) Tumor angiogenesis correlates with lymph node metastasis in invasive bladder cancer. J Urol 154:69–71

Jahnson S, Risberg B, Karlsson MG, Westman G, Bergstrom R, Pedersen J (1995) p53 and rb immunostaining in locally advanced bladder cancer: relation to prognostic variables and predictive value for the local response to radical radiotherapy. Eur Urol 28:135–142

Kaufman DS, Shipley WU, Griffin PP, Heney NM, Althausen AF, Efird JT (1993) Selective bladder preservation by combination treatment of invasive bladder cancer. N Engl J Med 329(19):1377–1382

Kuten A, Liu L, Glicksman AS (1995) Organ and functional preservation in the management of genitourinary cancer: bladder, prostate, and penis. Cancer Investig 13:108–124

Lerner EC, Qian Y, Hamilton AD, Sebti SM (1995) Disruption of oncogenic K-Ras4B processing and signaling by a potent geranyl geranyl transferase I inhibitor. J Biol Chem 270(45):26770–26773

Lipponen PK (1995) Expression of c-myc protein is related to cell proliferation and expression of growth factor receptors in transitional cell bladder cancer. J Pathol 175:203–210

Lipponen PK, Aaltomaa S (1994) Apoptosis in bladder cancer as related to standard prognostic factors and prognosis. J Pathol 173:333–339

Lipponen PK, Eskelinen MJ, Jauhiainen K, Harju E, Terho P, Haapasalo H (1992) Prognostic factors in WHO grade 2 transitional-cell bladder cancer (TCC); a novel two-grade classification system for TCC on mitotic index. J Cancer Res Clin Oncol 118:615–620

Loehrer P, Einhorn LH, Elson PJ, et al. (1992) A randomized comparison of cisplatin alone or in combination with methotrexate, vinblastine, and doxorubicin in patients with metastatic urothelial carcinoma: a Cooperative Group Study. J Clin Oncol 10:1066–1073

Logothetis CJ, Samuels ML, Ogden S, Dexeus FH, Swanson D, Johnson DE, von Eschenbach A (1985) Cyclophosphamide, doxorubicin and cisplatin chemotherapy for patients with locally advanced urothelial tumors with or without nodal metastases. J Urol 134:460–464

Logothetis CJ, Swanson D, Amato R, et al. (1996) J Urol 154(4):1241

Logothetis C, Xu HJ, Ro J, et al. (1992) Altered expression of the retinoblastoma protein and known prognostic variables in locally advanced bladder cancer. J Natl Cancer Inst 84:1256–1261

Logothetis CJ, Dexeus F, Finn L, Sella A, Amato RJ, Ayala AG, Kilbourn RG (1990) A prospective randomized trial comparing CISCA to MVAC chemotherapy in advanced metastastic urothelial tumors. J Clin Oncol 8:1050–1055

Logothetis C, Dieringer P, Ellerhorst J, Amato R, Sella A, Zukiwsi A, Kilbourn R (1992) A 61% response rate with 5-fluorouracil, interferon-α 2b and cisplatin in metastatic chemotherapy refractory transitional cell carcinoma (abstract). Proc Am Assoc Cancer Res 33:221

Lorusso V, Amadori D, Antimi M, et al. (1996) Studio di fase II sulla gemcitabine nel carcinoma vescicale. Abstract Book, Soc Ital Urol Oncol 17–18

Malmstrom PU, Rintala E, Wahlqvist R, Hellstrom P, Hellsten S, Hannisdal E (1996) Five year follow up of a prospective trial of radical cystectomy and neoadjuvant chemotherapy. Nordic Cystectomy Trial I. J Urol 155:1903–1906

Mameghan H, Fisher R (1989) Invasive bladder cancer. Prognostic factors and results of radiotherapy with and without cystectomy. Br J Urol 63:251–258

Mameghan H, Fisher R, Mameghan J, Brook S (1995) Analysis of failure following definitive radiotherapy for invasive transitional cell carcinoma of the bladder. Int J Radiat Oncol Phys 31(2):247–254

Mameghan H, Sandeman TF (1991) The management of invasive bladder cancer: a review of selected Australian studies in radiotherapy, chemotherapy and cystectomy. Aust N Z J Surg 61:173–178

Martinez Pineiro JA, Gonzalez Martin M, Arocena F, et al. (1995) Neoadjuvant cisplatin chemotherapy before radical cystectomy in invasive transitional cell carcinoma of the bladder: prospective randomized phase III study. J Urol 153:964–973

Naito S, Kuroiwa T, Ueda T, Hasuo K, Masuda K, Kumazawa J (1995) Combination chemotherapy with intra-arterial cisplatin and doxorubicin plus intravenous methotrexate and vincristine for locally advanced bladder cancer. J Urol 154:1704–1709

O'Flynn JD, Smith JD, Hanson JS (1975) Transurethral resection for the assessment and treatment of vesical neplasms. A review of 800 consecutive xases. Eur Urol 1:38–40

Ojea A, Nogueira-March JL, Figueiredo L, Jamardo D (1989) Tratamiento conservador con reseccion transuretral del cancer de vejiga estadio T2 estudio retroespectivo. ACTAS Urol Esp 13:441–443

Pagano F, Bassi P, Galetti TP, Meneghini A, Milani C, Artibani W, Garbeglio A (1991) Results of contemporary radical cystectomy for invasive bladder cancer: a clinicopathological study with an emphasis on the inadequacy of the tumor, nodes and metastases classification. J Urol 145:45–50

Pagano F, Bassi P, Drago GL, Piazza N, Abatangelo A, Spinadin R, Pappagallo GL (1996) A multivariate statistical analysis on 369 radical cystectomies for bladder cancer: old an new issues (abstract). J Urol 155:628A

Parker SL, Tong T, Bolden S, Wingo PA (1996) Cancer statistics, 1996. CA Cancer J Clin 65:5–27

Pollack A, Zagars GK (1996) Radiotherapy for stage T3b transitional cell carcinoma of the bladder. Sem Urol Oncol 14(2):86–95

Pollack A, Zagars GK (1996) Semin Urol Oncol 14:86–95

Prout GR Jr, Griffin PP (1979) Bladder cancer as a systemic disease. Cancer 3:2532–2539

Roberts JT, Hall RR (1994) The role of chemotherapy in the treatment of bladder cancer. In: Neal DE (ed) Tumours in urology: biology and clinical management. Springer, London Berlin Heidelberg New York, pp 79–90

Roth BJ, Dreicer R, Einhorn LH, et al. (1994) Significant activity of paclitaxel in advanced transitional cell carcinoma of the urothelium: a phase II trial of the Eastern Cooperative Oncology Group. J Clin Oncol 12:2264–2270

Rowinsky EK, Donehower RC (1995) Drug therapy: paclitaxel (taxol). N Engl J Med 332:1004–1014

Sato K, Maryiama M, Mori S, et al. (1992) An immunohistologic evaluation of c-erb-B2 gene products in patients with urinary bladder carcinoma. Cancer 70:2493–2498

Saxman SB, Loehrer PJ, Propert K, et al. (1996) Long term follow-up of phase III intergroup study of MVAC vs cisplatin in metastatic urothelial carcinoma (abstract). Proc Am Soc Clin Oncol 15:248

Scher H, Herr H, Sternberg C, et al. (1990) M-VAC (methotrexate, vinblastine, adriamycin and cisplatin) and bladder preservation. In: Splinter TAW, Scher HI (eds) Neoadjuvant chemotherapy in invasive bladder cancer. Progress in clinical and biological research. Wiley-Liss, New York, pp 179–186

Schultz PK, Herr HW, Zhang Z, et al. (1994) Neoadjuvant chemotherapy for invasive bladder cancer: prognostic factors for survival of patients treated with M-VAC with 5 years follow-up. J Clin Oncol 12:1394–1401

Schwartz S, Yagoda A, Natale RB, Watson RC, Whitmore WF, Lesser M (1983) Phase II trial of sequentially administered cisplatin, cyclophosphamide and doxorubicin for urothelial tract tumors. J Urol 130:681–684

Shipley WU, Kaufman DS, Zietman AL, Griffin PP, Heney NM, Althausen AF (1995) Selective bladder preservation by combined modality therapy for invasive bladder cancer (abstract). Eur J Cancer 31A Suppl 5:S239

Shipley WU, Rose MA (1985) The selection of patients for treatment by fulldose irradiation. Cancer 55:2278

Simon SD, Srougi M (1990) Neoadjuvant M-VAC chemotherapy and partial cystectomy for treatment of locally invasive transitional cell carcinoma of the bladder. In: Splinter TAW, Scher HI (eds) Neoadjuvant chemotherapy in invasive bladder cancer. Progress in clinical and biogical research. Wiley-Liss, New York, pp 169–174

Skinner DG, Lieskovsky G (1984) Contemporary cystectomy with pelvic node dissection compared to preoperative radiation therapy plus cystectomy in the management of invasive bladder cancer. J Urol 131:1069–1072

Smith JA, Whitmore WF, Jr (1981) Salvage Chemotherapy for bladder cancer after failure of definitive irradiation. J Urol 125:643

Solsona E, Iborra I, Ricos JV, Monros JL, Dumont R, Casanova JL (1994) Feasibility of transurethral resection for muscle infiltrating carcinoma of the bladder: prospective study, after 5 years of minimum follow-up. Proc Eur Assoc Urol, XIth Congress 224 (abstract 429)

Splinter TA, Scher HI, Denis L, et al. (1992a) The prognostic value of the pathological response to combination chemotherapy before cystectomy in patients with invasive bladder cancer. European Organization for Research on Treatment of Cancer – Genitourinary Group. J Urol 147:606–608

Splinter TAW, Pavone-Macaluso M, Jacqmin D, European Organization for Research and Treatment of Cancer Genitourinary Group (1992b) Phase II study of chemotherapy in stage T3-T4N0–xM0 transitional cell carcinoma of the bladder: evaluation of clinical response. J Urol 148:1793–1796

Srougi M, Simon SD (1994) Primary methotrexate, vinblastine, doxorubicin and cisplatin chemotherapy and bladder preservation in locally invasive bladder cancer. J Urol 151:593–597

Stadler WM, Kuzel TM, Raghavan D, Roth B, Vogelzang NJ, Levine EL, Dorr FA (1996) A phase II study if gemcitabine (gem) in bladder cancer (BC) (abstract). Ann Oncol 7:58

Sternberg CN (1995a) The treatment of advanced bladder cancer. Ann Oncol 6:113–126

Sternberg CN (1995b) Bladder preservation: a prospect for patients with urinary bladder cancer. Acta Oncol 34:589–597

Sternberg CN, De Mulder PHM (1992) A phase II/III trial iof high dose M-VAC chemotherapy + G-CSF versus classic M-VAC in advanced urothelial tract tumors. EORTC protocol 30924

Sternberg CN, Pansadoro V (1996) Transitional cell carcinomas of the urinary tract: bladder preserving treatments: chemotherapy and conservative surgery. In: Vogelzang NJ, Scardino PT, Shipley WS, et al. (eds) Comprehensive textbook of genitourinary onoclogy. Williams and Wilkins, Chicago, pp 30C:522–533

Sternberg CN, Yagoda A, Scher HI, et al. (1985) Preliminary results of methotrexate, vinblastine, adriamycin and cisplatin (M-VAC) in advanced urothelial tumors. J Urol 133:403–407

Sternberg CN, Yagoda A, Scher HI, et al. (1988) M-VAC (methotrexate, vinblastine, doxorubicin and cisplatin) for advanced transitional cell carcinoma of the bladder. J Urol 139:461–469

Sternberg C, Yagoda A, Scher HI, et al. (1989) Methotrexate, vinblastine, doxorubicin and cisplatinum for advanced transitional cell carcinoma of the urothelium: efficacy and patterns of response and relapse. Cancer 64:2448–2458

Sternberg C, Arena M, Calabresi F, et al. (1993) Neo-adjuvant M-VAC (methotrexate, vinblastine, adriamycin and cisplatin) for infiltrating transitional cell carcinoma of the urothelium. Cancer 72:1975–1982

Sternberg CN, Raghavan D, Ohi Y, et al. (1995a) Neo-adjuvant and adjuvant chemotherapy in locally advanced disease: what are the effects on survival and prognosis?. Int J Urol 2:76–88

Sternberg CN, Pansadoro V, Lauretti S, et al. (1995b) Neo-adjuvant M-VAC (methotrexate, vinblastine, adriamycin and cisplatin) chemotherapy and bladder preservation for muscle infiltrating transitional cell carcinoma of the bladder. Urol Oncol 1:127–133

Sternberg C, Pansadoro V, Lauretti S, et al. (1995c) Neo-adjuvant M-VAC chemotherapy and bladder preservation for muscle infiltrating transitional cell carcinoma (TCC) of the bladder (abstract). Eur J Cancer 31A Suppl 5:S239

Stoter G, Splinter TA, Child JA, et al. (1987) Combination chemotherapy with cisplatin and methotrexate in advanced transitional cell cancer of the bladder. J Urol 137:663–667

Takahashi R, Hashimoto T, Xu HJ, et al. (1991) The retinoblastoma gene functions as a growth and tumor suppressor in human bladder carcinoma cells. Proc Natl Acad Sci USA 88:5257–5261

Tester W, Porter A, Asbell S, et al. (1993) Combined modality program with possible organ preservation for invasive bladder carcinoma: results of RTOG protocol 85-12. Int J Radiat Oncol Biol Phys 25:783–790

Tester W, Caplan R, Heaney J, et al. (1996) Neoadjuvant combined modality program with selective organ preservation for invasive bladder cancer: results of Radiation Therapy Oncology Group phase II trial 8802. J Clin Oncol 14:119–126

Tu SM, Hossa E, Amato R, Kilbourn R, Logothetis CJ (1995) Paclitaxel, cisplatin and methotrexate combination chemotherapy is active in treatment of refractory urothelial malignancies. J Urol 154:1719–1722

Vet JA, Bringuier PP, Schaafsma HE, Witjes JA, Debruyne FM, Schalken JA (1995) Comparison of p53 protein-overexpression with p53 mutation in bladder cancer: clinical and biologic aspects. Lab Invest 73(6):837–843

Vieweg J, Whitmore WF Jr, Herr HW, Sogani PC, Russo P, Sheinfeld J, Fair WR (1994) The role of pelvic lymphadenectomy and radical cystectomy for lymph node positive bladder cancer. Cancer 74:3020–3028

Villaronga A, Orlando M, Chacon RD, Pedruzzi R, Signori H (1996) Can trans-urethral resection (TUR) and chemotherapy (CT) alone be effective treatment for muscle invasive bladder cancer? (abstract). Proc Am Soc Clin Oncol 15:258

Vogelzang NJ, Moormeier JA, Awan AM, et al. (1993) Methotrexate, vinblastine, doxorubicin and cisplatin followed by radiotherapy or surgery for muscle invasive bladder cancer: the University of Chicago experience. J Urol 149:753–757

Waehre H, Ous S, Klevmark B, Kwarstein B, Urnes T, sen TE, Fossa SD (1993) A bladder cancer multi-institutional experience with total cystectomy for muscle invasive bladder cancer. Cancer 72:3044

Wallace DM, Raghavan D, Kelly KA, et al. (1991) Neo-adjuvant (pre-emptive) cisplatin therapy in invasive transitional cell carcinoma of the bladder. Br J Urol 67:608–615

Yagoda A (1987) Chemotherapy of urothelial tract tumors. Cancer 60:574–585

21 Continuous Infusion Chemotherapy and Irradiation in the Treatment of Advanced Bladder Carcinoma

M. Rotman, H. Aziz, D. Schwartz, J. Cirrone, A. Schulsinger, K. Choi, and R. Macchia

CONTENTS

21.1 Introduction

Despite the extensive surgery involved in radical cystectomy in the treatment of muscle-invading bladder carcinoma, the procedure is unable to provide a 5-year survival rate of more than 26%–40% (Montie et al. 1984; Polle-Wilson and Barnard 1971). Patients thus treated suffer from loss of bladder function, the need for constant maintenance of the associated urinary diversion, and loss of sexual function and its accompanying psychological trauma. Although the use of preoperative radiation therapy has added another 10%–15% (Batata et al. 1981; Bloom et al. 1982; Vieti et al. 1971) to the 5-year survival rate, loss of bladder function and loss of sexual function remain problems that cannot be ignored. Thus, there has been a continued search for a therapeutic solution that would allow sparing of the bladder without compromising survival in patients with invasive tumors.

Radiation alone for T3 carcinoma of the bladder produces 5-year survival rates of not more than

M. Rotman, MD, Professor and Chairman, H. Aziz, MD, D. Schwartz, MD, J. Cirrone, MD, A. Schulsinger, MD, K. Choi, MD, Department of Radiation Oncology, SUNY Health Sciences Center @ Brooklyn, 450 Clarkson Avenue, Brooklyn, NY 11203, USA
R. Macchia, MD, Department of Urology, SUNY Health Sciences Center @ Brooklyn, 450 Clarkson Avenue, Brooklyn, NY 11203, USA

20%–38% (Hope-Stone et al. 1981; Miller and Johnson 1973; Quilty and Duncan 1986). The European (Blandy et al. 1980) and Canadian (Goodman et al. 1982) practice of initially treating muscle-invading carcinoma, such as stages T3a and T3b, with curative radiation, however, has provided an insight into bladder preservation when there is a significant tumor response and downstaging to p0. In the Blandy et al. (1980) series, patients who achieved p0 status after curative radiation therapy had a 5-year survival of 56%, and retained their bladders. It seemed, therefore, that if the rate of pathologic downstaging to p0 could be enhanced by increasing the radiation response, not only would the rate of bladder preservation increase, but survival would not be adversely affected and perhaps more patients would survive.

The radiosensitizing effect of 5-fluorouracil (5-FU) has been known since 1958 (Heidelberger et al. 1958) as a result of experimental work on rodent tumors and tissue cultures. In the 1960s, Stein and Kaufman (1966) demonstrated enhanced tumor regression when treating bladder cancer with preoperative irradiation and bolus 5-FU. Rotman et al. (1990) attempted to increase the complete response rate by using concomitant continuous intravenous infusion of 5-FU as a radiosensitizer in the treatment of advanced muscle-invasive bladder carcinoma.

21.2 Study Patients

From 1980 to 1990, a total of 25 patients with invasive bladder carcinoma were evaluated and accepted for treatment using concomitant 5-FU intravenous infusion and irradiation at the State University of New York, Health Science Center at Brooklyn. Twenty of the 25 patients (80%) were males and five (20%) were females. Their ages ranged from 45 to 95 years, the median age being 72 years. These patients either had refused surgery or were unacceptable for radical surgery. All patients had computed tomographic scans to demonstrate that their disease was confined to the pelvis. In addition, all patients underwent blood chemistry determinations, chest radiography, intravenous pyelography, bone scans, and liver function tests. Initially, patients were staged according to the Jewett Marshall system (JEWETT and STRONG 1946), with later conversion to the American Joint Committee TNM system (BEAHRS et al. 1983).

21.2.1
Tumor Stage and Grade

According to the TNM system (BEAHRS et al. 1983), one patient had stage T1 and seven patients had T2 tumors, while the numbers of T3a, T3b, and T4a tumors were nine, six, and two, respectively (Table 21.1). Most of these patients had poor prognostic features. Of the 25 patients, 22 (88%) were diagnosed as having transitional cell carcinoma. Of these, only two or 9% had grade 2 disease, while the other 20 (91%) were diagnosed as having either grade 3 or grade 4 disease. Three of the 25 patients (12%) had squamous cell carcinoma. Further breakdown of the patients according to additional prognostic factors (Table 21.2) showed 8/25 or 32% to have more than 50% involvement of the bladder. Seven of the 25 patients (28%) had between 25% and 50% of the circumferential wall of the bladder involved with tumor, while 10/25 (40%) had hydronephrosis. Sixteen of the patients (64%) had gross residual disease remaining after transurethral resection (TUR) at the time of irradiation.

21.2.2
Treatment Schedule

All patients received irradiation on the 4-MV linear accelerator. The initial treatment consisted of irra-

Table 21.1. TNM stages in the 25 patients with invasive bladder carcinoma who were accepted for treatment with concomitant 5-FU infusion and irradiation

TNM stage	No. of patients	%
T1	1/25	4
T2	7/25	28
T3a	9/25	36
T3b	6/25	24
T4a	2/25	8
		100

Table 21.2. Prognostic factors in the 25 study patients

Prognostic factors	No. of patients	%
Histology		
Squamous cell carcinoma	3/25	12[a]
Transitional cell carcinoma	22/25	88
Transitional cell carcinoma grade		
II	2/22	9
III or IV	20/22	91
Extent of involvement		
>50% of bladder	8/25	32
25%–50%	7/25	28
<25%	10/25	40
Hydronephrosis	8/25	32
Gross residual disease	16/25	64

[a] Excluded from analysis of survival.

diation of the entire pelvis via a four-field box technique giving a total dose of 4140–5040 cGy in 4.5–5 weeks at 180 cGy per fraction. The bladder was then boosted to 2000–2500 cGy in 2.5–3 weeks using a skip arc technique, giving a total dose of 6500 cGy. One patient received an iridium interstitial implant that delivered 3000 cGy to the tumor bed after the pelvic dose of 4140 cGy. Concomitant 5-FU infusion at a dose of $1000 \, mg/m^2/24 \, h$ was given for 120 h each in weeks 1, 4, and 7 or 2, 5, and 8 of treatment. In addition, 9% of patients also received mitomycin C as a 10-mg intravenous bolus on day 1 of radiation therapy.

21.3
Treatment Results

After excluding the three patients with squamous cell carcinoma, 22 patients with transitional cell carcinoma were evaluated for response and survival. Four to 6 weeks following completion of treatment, all patients underwent cystoscopy and biopsy for the evaluation of response.

21.3.1
Response Rate

In the group of patients with more superficially invasive tumors, i.e., stages T1 and T2, six of eight or 75% had an initial complete response (Table 21.3), while in the group with more deeply invading tumors, i.e., stages T3a, T3b, and T4 10/14 or 71% achieved a complete response. Thus, in both

Table 21.3. Complete pathologic responses achieved

Complete pathologic response	No. of patients	%
Initial		
T1 or T2	6/8	75
T2a, T3b, or T4a	10/14	71
Total initial response	16/22	73
With TUR and intravesical BCG/ mitomycin for residual disease		
T3a, T3b, or T4a	3/14	21
Overall complete response	19/22	86

Table 21.4. Survival rate according to tumor stage[a]

Stage	No. of patients	5-year survival (%)[b]
T1 or T2	6/8	75
T3a, T3b, or T4a	5/12	41
All stages	11/20	55

[a] Two patients were excluded due to development of distant metastases during treatment.
[b] Calculated by life table method.

of these groups of patients, the rate of initial response was 71%–75%. Three patients who had superficial residual disease and/or positive cytologic findings responded to repeated TUR and instillation of mitomycin C or BCG; thus, overall complete response was achieved in 19/22 or 86% of patients. Two patients who had deep muscle-invading residual disease underwent salvage cystectomy.

21.3.2
Survival

Two patients were excluded from survival analysis as they showed measurable metastatic disease during or soon after the completion of treatment. Thus 20 patients were available for survival analysis. The adjusted overall 5-year survival of patients (all tumor stages) was 55%. The 5-year survival of patients with superficial tumors (T1 or T2) was much higher, at 80%, than the rate for patients with deeply invasive tumors (T3a, T3b, or T4a), i.e. 41% (Table 21.4). The difference in survival rate between the two groups was further confirmed by comparing the survival of stage T2 and stage T3a patients: among the former patients the minimum survival was 72 months, as compared to a mean survival of 52 months in the latter patients ($P < 0.001$). The

relationship between survival and grade of the disease is unclear mainly due to the disproportionately small number of patients with low-grade disease (2 vs 18 with high-grade disease). The presence of hydronephrosis showed a trend toward a poor prognosis, but again, due to the small number of patients, the findings did not reach statistical significance ($P = 0.22$).

21.3.3
Pattern of Failure

A total of 11/20 patients (55%) from both groups have died. Seven patients died due to metastatic disease and most of them had deep muscle-invading disease. Three patients died of intercurrent disease and one from regional disease. All patients who died did so within 2 years of diagnosis.

Bladder preservation was achieved in the majority of patients. Of the nine patients who survived, seven retained their bladders and only two underwent salvage cystectomy. Seventy percent of the patients who died of metastatic disease or intercurrent disease also retained their bladders to the end.

21.4
Treatment Complications

Complications were classified according to the grading system of RTOG/ECOG for early and late morbidity. Twenty-one of the 22 patients (95%) experienced grade I/II diarrhea, managed with conservative treatment. Nine of 22 (41%) patients developed grade II cystitis, while 2/22 (9%) had grade III hematuria. Only one patient had grade IV toxicity. Hematologic toxicity was less common, as only two patients had a low white blood count below 2.5 during the second infusion. Grade I or II mucositis was seen in only three patients, requiring the dose of 5-FU to be reduced in one patient. The rate of late complications was low. Two patients had recurrent symptoms of dysuria and cystitis and responded to treatment. One elderly patient developed proctitis with chronic low-grade bleeding associated with persistent thrombocytopenia. This patient required a colostomy for cure of his symptoms. He refused reanastomosis after bleeding had stopped. He died 2 years later at the age of 91 from a heart attack during his 6th year of follow-up.

21.5
Discussion

In the United States, radical cystectomy is still the standard method of treatment for muscle-invading carcinoma of the bladder. It is surprising that this radical procedure is well accepted even though the rate of distant metastases is in the range of 40%–50% within the first 2 years (PROUT et al. 1979; RAGHAVAN et al. 1990), with a disappointing 5-year survival rate in the range of 26%–40% (MONTIE et al. 1984; POOLE-WILSON and BARNARD 1971). As stated above, the addition of preoperative radiation therapy has enhanced the 5-year survival rate of patients undergoing radical cystectomy by about 10%–15% (BATATA et al. 1981; BLOOM et al. 1982; VIETTI et al. 1971). The improved results achieved with preoperative radiation therapy and cystectomy are encouraging, but the procedure still entails the loss of bladder and sexuality. Most importantly, with preoperative irradiation and cystectomy, there has been only a slight decrease in the rate of distant metastases. The use of postoperative irradiation (MILLER and JOHNSON 1973), while adding to the morbidity, does not produce a worthwhile increase in the survival rate.

In certain European countries, bladder carcinoma has been first treated with a curative dose of radiation, with salvage cystectomy reserved for local failures. In spite of recent improvements in treatment techniques, survival rates following radiation alone in patients with muscle-invading disease have been disappointingly low, in the range of 20%–38% (HOPE-STONE et al. 1981; MILLER and JOHNSON 1973; QUILTY and DUNCAN 1986). Further efforts by the RTOG to improve survival rates with the addition of radiosensitizers such as misonidazole (RTOG 81-05) and high LET neutron radiation (RTOG 77-05/81-10) have proved disappointing. Similarly, the use of hyperfractionated radiation has yielded no appreciable increase in survival (RTOG 83-08).

The results of treatment with curative doses of irradiation delivered to patients with T2 and T3 tumors in the series of BLANDY et al. (1980) from London Hospital and of GOODMAN et al. (1982) from Canada (EAPEN et al. 1989) do, however, provide valuable information. BLANDY et al. (1980) found poor nonresponders and responders to be two distinct groups of patients. The 5-year survival rate in the radiosensitive complete-responder group was 56% and allowed for bladder preservation, as compared to a 17.5% survival for the group with residual disease that required salvage cystectomy. It appears,

therefore, that if the rate of complete pathologic response is increased, the number of bladder preservations would increase with a corresponding, albeit, small increase in survival. To achieve this goal, multidrug systemic chemotherapy alone was employed, first alone and later concurrently with irradiation.

At the Memorial Sloan-Kettering Hospital in New York, in a series of locally advanced bladder carcinomas, the use of M-VAC (methotrexate, vincristine, adriamycin, and cisplatin) provided a complete clinical response rate of 48%. Using M-VAC a complete clinical response rate of 32% was reported at the University of Chicago and at the Mayo Clinic. The use of MCV (methotrexate, cisplatin, and vinblastine) at Massachusetts General Hospital and CMV by the Northern California Oncology Group (NCOG) yielded complete response rates of 52% and 50%, respectively. At the M.D. Anderson Hospital, CISCA (cisplatin, cytoxan, and adriamycin) was utilized with a complete clinical response rate of 48% in locally advanced bladder carcinomas (SHIPLEY et al. 1984). The multidrug combinations were often too toxic for this usually elderly group of patients. Further, the effect of chemotherapy on local control was often not sustained or was incomplete. SCHER et al. (1989) demonstrated that 40% of the patients who were reported to have obtained complete clinical response still had local disease as demonstrated after partial or total cystectomy.

While multidrug chemotherapy was being investigated at the above institutions for the treatment of advanced bladder carcinoma and metastatic disease, the concomitant use of 5-FU with radiation was being investigated at our institution in the treatment of bladder carcinoma (ROTMAN et al. 1990). The selection of 5-FU was based on its known radiosensitizing effect. It also shows activity against bladder carcinoma, with associated relatively mild to moderate hematologic and gastrointstinal toxicities. In 1958, HEIDELBERGER et al. demonstrated the radiosensitizing effect of 5-FU in rodents, and this effect was confirmed by using cultures (BAGSHAW 1961). In 1963, WOODRUFF et al. actually demonstrated the radiosensitizing effect of 5-FU in the treatment of bladder carcinoma. In 1968, STEIN and KAUFMAN showed enhanced tumor regression in surgically treated bladders. Later, VIETTI et al. (1971), using mouse leukemia cells, further confirmed the radiosensitizing effect of 5-FU and its relationship to time of administration. The timing of delivery and the required concentration of the drug were very nicely and importantly evaluated by

BYFIELD et al. in 1977. The exact mechanism of the radiosensitizing effect of 5-FU is not known. The cellular presence of 5-FU may inhibit de novo synthesis of DNA by binding thymidylate synthetase. Defective RNA synthesis may also occur as a result of it being taken as an RNA precursor nucleotide. VIETTI et al. (1971) also suggested that the presence of 5-FU may produce further radiosensitization as a result of inhibition of repair of sublethal damage due to radiation.

Studies by MOERTEL et al. (1969) and Lo et al. (1976) employed bolus use of 5-FU and irradiation. In these early combined regimens of 5-FU and irradiation, 5-FU was given by bolus until myelosuppression had occurred. Lack of clinical benefit and myelotoxicity led to a steady decline in the use of bolus 5-FU and radiation. Later, BYFIELD et al. (1977) showed that maximum radiosensitization can best occur when the drug is given by infusion. Byfield et al. defined radiosensitization as a "state of cellular condition that develops gradually in 24 hours or more of continuous 5-FU exposure after each radiation exposure." These observations indicated that for radiosensitization to occur, 5-FU should be slowly infused throughout the period of irradiation.

CHABNER in 1982 and LOCKICH in 1984 explained that most chemotherapeutic agents are active in the DNA synthetic phase of the cell cycle. Since most cytotoxic agents have a short plasma half-life when administered by bolus injection, exposure to the drugs is limited to a small fraction of the tumor cell cycle; by contrast, with continuous infusion chemotherapy, tumor cells would have prolonged exposure to the drug. Following a randomized trial, SEIFERT et al. (1975) supported the contention that the radiosensitizing effects of 5-FU are greatest when the drug is infused rather than given as a bolus. When peak drug levels are avoided, so is extreme systemic toxicity.

The results of treatment in this group of patients with their host of poor prognostic factors seem satisfactory. Although most of the 25 patients in our series presented with bulky infiltrating disease, six had more than 50% of the bladder involved, eight had hydronephrosis, and 16 had gross residual disease following TURBT, their complete response rate (urine cytology negative) within 6 months was 62.5%. The final complete response rate of 86% was achieved after three patients underwent further treatment with TUR and intravesical BCG or mitomycin. It is noteworthy that in our series a prior TUR was not required to achieve a similar complete response rate, as was mentioned by SHIPLEY et al. (1984). RUSSEL et al. (1988), using 5-FU infusion and a concomitant radiation dose of 4000 cGy, demonstrated a complete response rate of 76%. It appears that the complete response rate obtained with the use of infusion 5-FU and concomitant radiation is twice that of irradiation alone when compared to the achievement of p0 status in the preoperative series. Bladder preservation, a major goal of our study, was achieved in the majority (17/20) of patients. Salvage cystectomy was necessary in only two cases.

As stated above, the 5-year survival rate for the patients with more superficial tumors (T1 and T2) was 75%, while for deep muscle-invading tumors (T3a, T3b, T4a) the corresponding rate was 41%, a figure 15%–20% higher than that reported using radiation or surgery alone. The high complete response rate in the patients with more advanced tumors was disappointingly not translated into a higher survival rate due, we believe, to the presence of occult metastatic disease at the time of treatment. The vast majority of our patients who died of metastatic disease did so within 2 years of their treatment. Multidrug adjuvant therapy, i.e., M-VAC or MCV, may be required to treat micrometastatic disease present at the time of diagnosis of the bladder tumor. In 1993, KAUFMAN et al. from Massachusetts General Hospital reported on a series of 53 patients with stages T2 to T4NxMo who were treated with initial TUR followed by two cycles of MCV and then concurrent bolus cisplatin 70 mg/m^2 1 day prior to a course of irradiation of 4000 cGy. The cisplatin was repeated on day 21. Those patients who obtained a complete response or were unsuitable for surgery then proceeded to a bladder-saving consolidative dose of 6480 cGy with cisplatin. Ten patients who did not achieve a complete response and were suitable for surgery underwent a radical cystectomy. At the median follow-up of 48 months, 45% were alive and free of tumor. Bladder preservation was achieved in 58% of patients.

EAPEN et al. (1989) reported on the use of intra-arterial infusion of cisplatin (bilateral hypogastric arteries) 3 weeks prior to irradiation and concomitantly during the first week of irradiation. The complete response rate was 90% at 2–3 years of follow-up. There was also a corresponding increase in survival.

ARCANGELI et al. (1996) recently reported on a phase 1–2 trial at an International Meeting in Rome in 1996 and again at the American Society for Therapeutic Radiology and Oncology (ASTRO) meeting in

Los Angeles, 27–30 October 1996, in which a series of invasive bladder carcinomas (15 T2, 16 T3, and 1 T4) were treated with or without an initial two cycles of MCV followed by concomitant protected venous infusion of cisplatin and 5-FU and irradiation. Treatment consisted of three 100-cGy fractions per day of irradiation, at 5 h intervals 5 days per week to a small pelvic volume to a dose of 5000 cGy in 3.5 weeks, followed by a boost dose of 2000 cGy to the bladder in 1.5 weeks. During irradiation, both cisplatin and 5-FU were given through separate tubing in a protracted infusion at $5 mg/m^2$ per day and $220 mg/m^2$ per day, respectively. A complete response rate of 91% was obtained in a series of 32 patients, with a 3-year cystectomy-free survival rate of 80%. High-grade toxicity was uncommon, while low-grade diarrhea and leukopenia were present in a limited number of patients.

21.6
Conclusions

Treatment with concomitant continuous infusion of 5-FU and radiation produces an excellent 5-year survival rate of 75% in T1 and T2 transitional carcinoma. The rate of 5-year survival in patients with deep muscle-invading carcinomas is 41%, due not to locoregional residual or local recurrent disease, but rather to development of metastatic disease. Bladder preservation is achieved in the majority of patients. The presence of micrometastases in advanced cases at the time of treatment may require upfront multidrug chemotherapy (MCV) in order to improve survival rates.

References

Arcangeli G, Tirindelli-Danesi D, Mecozzi, A, Saracino B, Cruciani E (1996) Combined hyperfractionated irradiation and protracted infusion chemotherapy in invasive bladder cancer with conservative intent. Phase I study. Int J Radiat Oncol Biol Phys 36:314

Bagshaw MA (1961) Possible role of potentiators in radiation therapy. Am J Roentgenol 85:822

Batata MA, Chi FCH, Hilaris BS, et al. (1981) Preoperative whole pelvis versus true pelvis irradiation and/or cystectomy for bladder cancer. Int J Radiat Oncol Biol Phys 7:1349

Beahrs OH, Henson DE, Hutter DE, Myers MH (eds) (1983) American Joint Committee on cancer manual for staging for cancer, 3rd edn. Lippincott, Philadelphia

Blandy JP, England HR, Evans SJ, et al. (1980) T3 bladder cancer, the case for salvage cystectomy. Br J Urol 52:506

Bloom HJ, Hendry WF, Wallace DM, et al. (1982) Treatment of T3 bladder cancer. Controlled trial of preoperative radiotherapy and radical cystectomy versus radical radiotherapy. Second report and review (for the Clinical Trial Group Inst. of Urology). Br J Urol 54:136

Byfield JE, Chan, P, Seagren SL (1977) Radiosensitization of 5-FU: molecular origins and clinical scheduling implications. Proc Am Assoc Cancer Res 18:74

Chabner B (1982) Pharmacologic principles of cancer treatment. Saunders, Philadelphia

Eapen L, Stewart D, Danjoix D, et al. (1989) Intraarterial cisplatin and concomitant radiation for locally advanced bladder cancer. J Clin Oncol 7:230–233

Goodman GB, Hislop TG, Elwood JM, et al. (1982) Conservation of bladder function in patients with invasive bladder cancer treated by definitive irradiation and selective cystectomy. Int J Radiat Oncol Biol Phys 7:569

Heidelberger C, Greishbach L, Montag B, et al. (1958) Studies in fluorinated pyrimidine. II. Effects of transplanted tumor. Cancer Res 18:305–317

Hope-Stone HF, Blandy JP, Oliver RTD, et al. (1981) Radical radiotherapy and salvage cystectomy in the treatment of invasive carcinoma of the bladder. In: Oliver RTD, Hendry WF, Bloom HJ (eds) Bladder cancer: principles of combination therapy. Butterworth, London, pp 127–138

Jewett HJ, Strong GH (1946) Infiltrating carcinoma of the bladder: relation of depth of penetration of the bladder wall to incidence of local extension and metastases. J Urol 55:366

Kaufman DS, Shipley WU, Griffin PP, et al. (1993) Selective bladder preservation by combination treatment of invasive bladder cancer. N Engl J Med 329:1377

Lo TCM, Wiley AL, Ausfield FJ, et al. (1976) Combined radiation therapy and 5-fluorouracil for advanced squamous cell carcinoma of the oral cavity and oropharynx: a randomized study. Radiology 126:229

Lockich JJ (1984) Infusion chemotherapy for cancer. Current Concepts Oncol 6:3

Miller LS, Johnson DE (1973) Megavoltage irradiation for bladder cancer: alone, postoperative or preoperative? Genit Cancer 10:771

Moertel CG, Childs DS, Reitemeier RJ, et al. (1969) Combined 5-fluorouracil and supervoltage radiation therapy of locally unresectable gastro-intestinal cancer. Lancet II:865

Montie JE, Straffon RA, Stewart BH (1984) Radical cystectomy without radiation therapy for carcinoma of the bladder. J Urol 131:477

Poole-Wilson DS, Barnard RJ (1971) Total cystectomy for bladder tumors. Br J Urol 43:16

Prout GR, Griffin PP, Shipley WU (1979) Bladder carcinoma as a systemic disease. Cancer 43:2532

Quilty PM, Duncan W (1986) Primary radical radiotherapy for T3 transitional cell cancer of the bladder. An analysis of survival and control. Int J Radiat Oncol Biol Phys 12:853

RTOG 77-05/81-10: Phase I, II, study comparing the value of neutrons alone, mixed beam and preoperative mixed beam in bladder carcinoma. RTOG, Philadelphia, Pa

RTOG 81-05: Phase I/II study on the value of combining misonidazole and radiotherapy in the treatment of bladder cancer. RTOG, Philadelphia, Pa

RTOG 83-08: Randomized phase II study to evaluate hyperfractionated radiation for locally advanced carcinoma of the bladder. RTOG, Philadelphia, Pa

Raghavan D, Shipley WU, Garnick MB, et al. (1990) Biology and management of bladder cancer. N Engl J Med 322:1129

Rotman M, Aziz H, Porrazzo M, et al. (1990) Treatment of advanced transitional cell carcinoma of the bladder with irradiation and concomitant 5-fluorouracil infusion. Int J Radiat Oncol Biol Phys 18:1131

Russel KJ, Boileau MA, Ireton RC, et al. (1988) Transitional cell carcinoma of the urinary bladder; histologic clearance with combined 5-FU chemotherapy and radiation therapy. Preliminary results of bladder preservation study. Radiology 167:845

Scher H, Hess H, Sternberg C, et al. (1989) Neoadjuvant chemotherapy for invasive bladder cancer. Experience with M-VAC regimen. Br J Urol 64:250

Seifert P, Baker LH, Reed ML, et al. (1975) Comparison of continuous infused 5-Fu with bolus injection in treatment of patients with colo-rectal adenocarcinoma. Cancer 36: 123–128

Shipley WU, Coombs LJ, Einstein AB, Jr, et al. (1984) National Bladder Cancer Collaborative Group: cisplatin and full dose irradiation for patients with invasive bladder carcinoma: a preliminary report of tolerance and local response. J Urol 132:899

Shipley WU, Kaufman D, Griffin P, et al. (1992) Radio-chemotherapy for invasive carcinoma of the bladder. In: Vaeth JM (ed) Radiotherapy/chemotherapy interaction in cancer therapy. Karger, Basel

Stein JJ, Kaufman JJ (1968) Treatment of carcinoma of the bladder with special reference to the use of preoperative radiation therapy combined with 5-FU. Am J Roentgenol Radium Ther Nucl Med 102:519–529

Van der Werf-Messing BHP, Friedal GH, Menon RS, et al. (1982) Carcinoma of the urinary bladder T3NXMO treated by preoperative irradiation followed by simple cystectomy. Int J Radiat Oncol Biol Phys 8:1849

Vietti J, Eggerding F, Valeriote F (1971) Combined effect of radiation and 5-fluorouracil on survival of transplanted leukemia cells. J Natl Cancer Inst 47:865

Woodruff MW, Murphy WT, Hodson JM (1963) Further observations on the use of combination 5-fluorouracil and supervoltage irradiation therapy in the treatment of advanced carcinoma of the bladder. J Urol 90:747

22 Postoperative Chemotherapy for Bladder Carcinoma

F.S. Freiha

CONTENTS

22.1
Introduction

Postoperative chemotherapy is also referred to as adjuvant chemotherapy. In this chapter we will discuss the results of cystectomy alone for invasive bladder cancer, the rationale for postoperative chemotherapy, the chemotherapeutic agents most commonly used, and the results of chemotherapy following cystectomy.

22.2
Cystectomy

Cystectomy remains the treatment with the best rates of cure for patients with invasive bladder cancer. until recently, and because of the drawbacks of cystectomy, namely the need for a urostomy and impotence, patients and their treating physicians were reluctant to accept the operation and often delayed treatment or chose less effective therapy, thus

F.S. Freiha, MD, Professor and Chief, Urologic Oncology, Department of urology, Stanford University Medical Center, 300 Pasteur Drive, Room S-287, Stanford, CA 94305, USA

jeopardizing cure. With the advent of potency-preserving surgical techniques, continent diversion, and bladder substitution, eliminating the need for a urostomy, cystectomy has become a more acceptable operation to both the patient and his treating physician.

With better imaging techniques and the use of laparoscopic lymph node biopsies, the accuracy of clinical staging continues to improve and assigned clinical stages now reflect more accurately the pathologic stages.

How good is cystectomy? Table 22.1 lists the 5-year disease-free survival results of selected recent series of cystectomy only for the different pathologic stages of bladder cancer. Patients with diseases confined to within the wall of the bladder (stages P2 and P3a) do very well with cystectomy alone. Added therapy to improve on these results and show a statistically significant benefit in survival will require large numbers of patients in prospective randomized trials which, at present, are not available.

The prognosis of patients with more advanced local disease treated only with cystectomy remains poor and needs improvement. The 5-year disease-free survival for patients whose tumors had invaded through the bladder wall (P3b) is 50% at best and for those with involvement of adjacent organs (P4) it is 30%. Furthermore, the 5-year disease-free survival for patients with regional lymph node metastases is 7%–36% (Stockle et al. 1986; Lerner et al. 1993; La Plante and Brice 1973; Dretler et al. 1973; Smith and Whitmore 1981; Skinner et al. 1982). It is in this group of patients that preoperative or postoperative chemotherapy may be beneficial.

The great majority of failures of cystectomy occur at distant sites. In 1979 Prout et al. reported on 151 patients treated with cystectomy: 50 failed, 37 at distant sites and 13 locally in the pelvis. Boileau et al., in 1980, reported on 159 patients treated with 50 Gy to the pelvis followed 6 weeks later by cystectomy: there were 53 recurrences, 40 at distant sites and 13 locally. In 1988 Wishnow and Dmoshowski reported on 178 patients treated by cystectomy only:

Table 22.1. Five-year survival rates (%) according to the P stage of patients treated with cystectomy only

Authors	P2	P3a	P3b	P4
MATHUR et al. (1981)	88	57	40	–
MONTIE et al. (1981)	50	63	29	–
SKINNER and LIESKOVSKY (1988)	82	69	29	–
FREIHA (1990)		83	47	64[a]
WISHNOW et al. (1992)		82	–	–

[a] Patients with involvement of the prostate only.

there were 46 recurrences, 36 at distant sites, five in the pelvis, and five at both distant sites and in the pelvis. In patients with disease limited to the bladder wall (stages P2 and P3a, No), WISHNOW et al. (1992) had 13 recurrences among 71 patients treated with cystectomy only: ten at distant sites and three locally in the pelvis.

In 1990, BRENDLER et al. reported on 76 patients treated by nerve-sparing cystectomy to preserve potency: there were 15 failures, 12 at distant sites and three locally in the pelvis. This unique report dispels the fear that nerve-sparing techniques may jeopardize the curative nature of cystectomy by increasing the rate of positive margins and local recurrence.

22.3
The Rationale for Postoperative Chemotherapy

There are several reasons for the use of postoperative chemotherapy:

1. Because the majority of failures after cystectomy occur at distant sites, it is believed that clinically undetectable micrometastases must be present at the time of cystectomy.
2. The availability of effective combination chemotherapy for metastatic transitional cell carcinoma which can be used adjuvantly.
3. The chemotherapy is administered at a time of minimal residual disease (micrometastases) and after the bulk of the tumor has been removed.
4. Treatment can be determined on the basis of pathologic rather than clinical staging, thus more accurately identifying and treating those patients who are at a higher risk of failure and avoiding unnecessary and potentially toxic therapy for those who may never need it.
5. Treatment does not delay delivery of a potentially curable therapy (cystectomy), especially in pa-

tients whose cancers may not be chemosensitive and may progress during treatment.

22.4
Chemotherapy

The information in this section was compiled from different sources (YAGODA 1983; CHABNER and MYERS 1989; Physicians Desk Reference 1995). The most effective single agents against metastatic transitional cell carcinoma are first discussed, followed by consideration of combination chemotherapy.

22.4.1
Cisplatin

Cisplatin or cis-diamminedichloroplatinum (CDDP) is a heavy metal complex that functions as an alkylating agent by inhibiting DNA. Its action is not specific to any phase of the cell cycle. More that 90% of an intravenously administered dose is bound to plasma proteins and is concentrated in the liver, kidneys, and small and large intestines. Its serum half-life is approximately 70 h. It is secreted primarily, but incompletely, in the urine, and about 35% of an administered dose is excreted in the urine within 5 days. Hydration, diuretics, and/or mannitol may increase the urinary excretion and reduce the serum half-life and, therefore, the toxicity of cisplatin.

There are several toxicities associated with the intravenous use of cisplatin. Nephrotoxiciity is dose related and cumulative. It is secondary to renal tubular damage and may be reduced by good hydration and the use of diuretics and mannitol. With prolonged use (three or four cycles), most patients experience some degree of renal insufficiency that may be permanent. Twenty-four-hour creatinine clearance is determined before each treatment. At Stanford University, cisplatin is not given to patients whose creatinine clearance is less than 45 cc/min and is given at half dose to those with a clearance of 45–60 cc/min.

Ototoxicity in the form of tinnitus and loss of hearing in the high-frequency range are not uncommon side-effects. Deafness is extremely rare. Patients who experience any degree of ototoxicity should be monitored frequently with audiograms. It is not known whether ototoxicity is reversible. If a hearing loss at 4000–8000 Hz range is significant, treatment should be discontinued. Neurotoxicity in the form of peripheral neuropathy manifested by numbness of the fingers and toes and, although less likely, gait imbalance, is not uncommon. It is usually reversible but it may be several months to a few years before the symptoms disappear.

Myelosuppression is seen in 25%–30% of patients. It can be more frequent and quite severe if cisplatin is used in combination with other myelosuppressive drugs. The nadir of myelosuppression is seen between the 2nd and 3rd weeks after treatment.

Nausea and vomiting occur in almost all patients and can be so severe that cisplatin has to be administered under heavy sedation with antiemetics. These symptoms start within 2 h of treatment and last for about 24 h. Occasionally, the nausea a nd vomiting continue for a few days and, in rare cases, a week.

Other toxicities include: hypomagnesemia and electrolyte disturbances secondary to renal tubular damage; hyperuricemia; Raynaud's phenomenon, especially if cisplatin is used in combination with vinblastine and bleomycin; heart failure, mainly due to overhydration, which is a necessary situation with the use of cisplatin; and alopecia, anorexia, and weight loss.

The dosage of cisplatin for transitional cell carcinoma is 70–100 mg/m^2 intravenously every 3 weeks. The schedule of administration differs among institutions. Some give 20 mg/m^2 every day for 5 consecutive days, whereas others give the entire dose over 10–20 min. At Stanford University, cisplatin is given over a 4-h period. The patients is admitted to the hospital and after a 12-h period of hydration to achieve a urine output of at least 150 cc/h, 100 mg/m^2 cisplatin is administered intravenously over 4 h under sedation with antiemetics, which are continued for another 24 h. Intravenous hydration is continued for a day. The patient is discharged if the nausea and vomiting are under control. This schedule requires a 2-day hospital admission.

Treatment is repeated in 3 weeks if the white blood count is higher than 3000, the platelet count is higher than 100 000, and the creatinine clearance is more than 60 cc/min. Cisplatin is withheld if the creatinine clearance drops below 45 cc/min and is given at half dose (50 mg/m^2) if the clearance is between 45 and 60 cc/min. Patients should be closely monitored for electrolyte abnormalities, especially hypomagnesemia and hyperuricemia, and for any evidence of ototoxicity.

In single-agent trials, patients with metastatic transitional cell carcinoma treated with 70–100 mg/ m^2 of cisplatin achieve a 30% response rate: complete (CR) and partial (PR) (YAGODA et al. 1976; MERRIN 1978; HERR 1980; SOLOWAY et al. 1981).

22.4.2
Methotrexate

Methotrexate is an antimetabolite that inhibits dihydrofolic acid reductase, which reduces dihydrofolates to tetrahydrofolates. The latter are used in the synthesis, repair, and replication of DNA. The action of methotrexate is specific to the S-phase of the cell cycle.

Fifty percent of an intravenously administered dose is bound to plasma protein. This binding can be easily dissociated by various compounds such as sulfonamides, tetracyclines, salicylates, chloramphenicol, and phenytoin, which can increase the toxicity of methotrexate by increasing the serum concentration of the unbound drug.

Methotrexate is metabolized in the liver and intracellularly to polyglutamated forms, which can be readily converted back to methotrexate. These polyglutamated forms diffuse into body fluids and effusions, where they can remain for extended periods and be converted back to methotrexate, thus prolonging contact time with tissues and increasing toxicity. Therefore, use of methotrexate may be contraindicated in patients with severe edema, ascites, or any form of effusion. The half-life of methotrexate is 8–15 h. It is excreted primarily by the kidneys. About 85% of an intravenously administered dose is excreted in the urine, unchanged, within 24 h. Delayed clearance of methotrexate significantly increases its toxicity, and, therefore, it should not be administered concomitantly with drugs, such as cisplatin, that decrease the glomerular filtration rate.

The major toxicities of methotrexate are myelosuppression, stomatitis, and mucosal ulcerations, which can lead to significant gastrointestinal bleeding. Other, less common side-effects include liver damage, pneumonitis, renal failure, and alopecia. All these toxicities can be enhanced if there is interference with renal clearance and protein binding of methotrexate, or if the drug is sequestered in fluid third spaces. Leucovorin calcium, a chemically reduced derivative of folic acid, reduces the toxicity of methotrexate and rescues damaged cells by competitively inhibiting methotrexate.

The dose of methotrexate for transitional cell carcinoma is 30–40 mg/m^2 intravenously each week. In single-agent trials responses of 15%–50% have been reported depending on the dose and on the extent of disease. Most responses are partial and short-lived, with a median duration of 6 months (ALTMAN et al. 1972; HALL et al. 1974; TURNER et al. 1977; NATALE et al. 1981).

22.4.3
Vinblastine

Vinblastine sulfate is one of the vinca alkaloids that exert their antitumor effect by inhibiting mitosis and arresting cell growth in metaphase. After intravenous administration of vinblastine sulfate, a triphasic serum decay pattern occurs that ranges from a few minutes to 24 h. Tissue binding is rapid and readily reversible. Most of the drug is excreted in the bile and less in the urine and the feces.

The major toxicity is myelosuppression, with the nadir in white blood cell count occurring 5–10 days after drug administration. Recovery is rapid. Other side-effects include alopecia, parathesias due to peripheral neuropathy, muscle and joint pains, constipation and intestinal ileus, and nausea and vomiting, all of which are rapidly reversible.

The dose of vinblastine sulfate in transitional cell carcinoma is 4–6 mg/m^2 intravenously every week. Patients with biliary tract obstruction should not receive the drug. The response rate to vinblastine as a single-agent treatment is 18%, and the average duration of response is only 4 months (BLUMENREICH et al. 1982). Because of its low toxicity, vinblastine can be used with other cytotoxic agents in combination chemotherapy.

22.4.4
Doxorubicin

Doxorubicin is an anthracycline antibiotic isolated from *Streptomyces peucetius*. It binds to DNA and inhibits nucleic acid synthesis. It can affect all phases of the cell cycle and is, therefore , not cell specific. Intravenous administration results in rapid tissue binding and plasma clearance. It is primarily excreted in the bile, and only 5% of an administered dose is cleared by the kidneys. Biliary obstruction and impaired liver function may be contraindications for its use.

Side-effects of doxorubicin include myelosuppression, occurring 10–14 days after administration

with rapid recovery within 3 weeks, and also nausea and vomiting, anorexia, loss of weight, alopecia, mucositis, and cardiomyopathy, which is the most serious and irreversible of the toxicities. The cardiac toxicity is dose related and occurs at a total dose of 550 mg/m^2 or more. Patients who have received mediastinal irradiation may not even be able to tolerate total doses higher than 400 mg/m^2. Weekly doxorubicin administration may reduce the cardiac toxicity and allow for use of a higher dose of the drug.

The dose of doxorubicin in transitional cell carcinoma ranges from 30 to 75 mg/m^2 intravenously every 3 weeks. Patients with a history of prior extensive irradiation or with minimal hepatic dysfunction should be started at the lower dose schedule. Every patient should receive a comprehensive cardiac evaluation before treatment with doxorubicin. When it is used in single-agent trials, doxorubicin results in 13%–23% response rates, and the average duration of response is 4 months (O'BRYAN et al. 1973; YAGODA et al. 1977a).

22.4.5
Cyclophosphamide

Cyclophosphamide is an alkylating agent that is transformed in the liver to its active metabolites, which interfere with rapidly proliferating cancer cells. Although its mode of action is not well known, it is believed to involve crosslinking of DNA. The maximum concentration of the metabolites of cyclophosphamide in the plasma occurs 2–3 h after intravenous administration. More than 60% of these metabolites are bound to plasma proteins. Most of the drug and its metabolites are excreted in the urine.

The major side-effects of cyclophosphamide and its metabolites are hemorrhagic cystitis and leukopenia. Most cases of hemorrhagic cystitis are transient and self-limiting with adequate hydration and frequent voidings to minimize contact time between the drug and the bladder mucosa. With prolonged use of cyclophosphamide, hemorrhagic cystitis may become a significant and serious complication requiring surgical intervention. Recovery from leukopenia is rapid and occurs in 7–10 days. Other side-effect include nausea and vomiting, pulmonary fibrosis, hemorrhagic pericarditis, and myocarditis. Cyclophosphamide may potentiate the cardiac toxicity of doxorubicin.

The dose of cyclophosphamide for transitional cell carcinoma is $650 \, mg/m^2$ intravenously every week, and the response to its use as a single agent varies from 7% to 35% (YAGODA et al. 1977b; SOLOWAY and MURPHY 1979).

Combination chemotherapy is more effective than single-agent chemotherapy (GAGLIANO 1980). Because cisplatin is the most effective of the single agents, it has been combined with two or three of the others. The most commonly used cisplatin-based combination chemotherapy are CMV (cisplatin, methotrexate, vinblastine), M-VAC (methotrexate, vinblastine, doxorubicin, cisplatin) and CISCA (cisplatin, cyclophosphamide, doxorubicin).

22.4.6
CMV

CMV was developed at Stanford University in the late 1970s. Cisplatin is given on day 2 at a dose of $100 \, mg/m^2$. Methotrexate $30 \, mg/m^2$ and vinblastine $4 \, mg/m^2$ are given on days 1 and 8. Treatment is repeated every 21 days. The initial results in 50 evaluable patients with metastatic transitional cell carcinoma showed a complete response rate of 28% and a partial response rate of 28% for a total response rate of 56% (HARKER et al. 1985). A recent update of this study showed a durable complete response rate of 23% (MILLER et al. 1993).

22.4.7
M-VAC

M-VAC combination chemotherapy was developed at Memorial Sloan-Kettering Cancer Center. Methotrexate $30 \, mg/m^2$ is given on day 1. Approximately 24 h later and after adequate hydration, vinblastine $3 \, mg/m^2$, adriamycin $30 \, mg/m^2$, and cisplatin $70 \, mg/m^2$ are given on day 2. Identical doses of methotrexate and vinblastine are repeated on day 15 and 22. Treatment is repeated every 28 days. Initial experience with M-VAC in 67 patients showed a complete response rate of 35% and a partial response rate of 40%, for an overall response rate of 75% (STERNBERG et al. 1985). A more recent update in 83 patients with either nodal or distant metastasis revealed a complete response rate of 37% (STERNBERG et al. 1988). The group of patients who achieved a complete response included some who were rendered complete responders by surgical excision of

residual disease after M-VAC chemotherapy. An additional 30% of patients had a partial response, for an overall response rate of 67%.

22.4.8
CISCA

CISCA was developed at the M.D. Anderson Cancer Center. Cisplatin $70 \, mg/m^2$ is given on day 2, and cyclophosphamide $650 \, mg/m^2$ and adriamycin $50 \, mg/m^2$ are given on day 1. Treatment is repeated every 3 weeks. The results in 97 previously untreated patients with disseminated and/or unresectable transitional cell carcinoma showed a complete response rate of 36% and a partial response rate of 16%. Patients with local nodal disease only repsonded more favorably than those with visceral metastasis (45% vs 20%) (LOGOTHETIS 1988).

22.5
Results of Postoperative Chemotherapy

There are relatively few studies of adjuvant chemotherapy for bladder cancer. Their results are summarized below.

The first report of the effects of postoperative chemotherapy was that of LOGOTHETIS et al. (1988). This was a retrospective analysis of three groups of patients treated with cystectomy. Group I ($n = 71$) comprised patients with a high risk of recurrency who received postoperative chemotherapy with CISCA. Group II ($n = 62$) comprised patients with a high risk of recurrence who never received chemotherapy and group III ($n = 206$), patients with a low risk of recurrence who never received chemotherapy. High risk is defined as the presence of stages P3b or P4, microvascular or microlymphatic invasion in the primary tumor, and/or pelvic lymph node metastases. At 2 years posttreatment there was a significant disease-free survival benefit in group I compared ot group II (70% vs 76%) (LOGOTHETIS et al. 1988).

SKINNER et al. (1991) reported on a prospective randomized adjuvant study also using CISCA chemotherapy. Patients with P3b, P4, and/or N1 disease were randomized postoperatively either to receive four cycles of CISCA or to be observed without further therapy. There was a significant difference in the 3-year diseases-free survival between the two groups, favoring the chemotherapy group

(70% vs 46%). Furthermore, the median survival was also significantly different: 4.3 years for the chemotherapy group and 2.4 years for the observation group.

STOCKLE et al. (1992) reported on a controlled prospective adjuvant chemotherapy trial, randomizing patients after cystectomy to receive M-VAC or M-VEC (in which epirubicin is substituted for doxorubicin) or observation. The study was terminated prematurely for ethical reasons because an interim analysis of the first 49 patients revealed a significant advantage in favor of those patients randomized to receive chemotherapy. Of 18 patients who received adjuvant chemotherapy only three showed disease progression, compared to 18 of 23 in the observation group.

In a radomized, prospective study comparing neoadjuvant and adjuvant M-VAC chemotherapy, LOGOTHETIS et al. (1996) found no difference in either disease-free survival or overall survival between the two groups of patients. At 31.7 months, the overall survival was 60% for the neoadjuvant group and 63% for the adjuvant group. The disease-free survival was 49% in the neoadjuvant group and 52% in the adjuvant group. Tolerance to treatment was not significantly different between the two treatment groups. Their results suggest that, although no difference in survival was observed, neoadjuvant M-VAC may be effective in increasing the resectability rate. They also observed that the clinical stage was reliable predictor of the pathologic findings at surgery (pathologic stage) (LOGOTHETIS et al. 1996).

WEI et al. (1996) treated 56 patients with high risk of recurrence of bladder cancer following cystectomy with an average of 4.63 cycles of CMV chemotherapy. They observed a median actual survival of 44 months and the 1- and 3-year survival probabilities were 92% and 50%, respectively. Grade 3 and 4 toxicities were minimal. Unfortunately, this was not a randomized study and little can be learned form the results.

The Stanford study reported by FREIHA et al. in 1996 is unique because it is the only prospective randomized study comparing immediate adjuvant treatment to delayed treatment at relapse with the same chemotherapy. It also evaluates the effects of treatment at the first indication of recurrence. Fifty patients with stage P3b, P4, and/or N1 disease were randomized after cystectomy either to receive immediately four cycles of CMV chemotherapy or to be observed and treated with CMV chemotherapy at the first evidence of recurrence. There were 25 patients in each arm. Freedom from relapse was 48% in the immediate treatment arm and 25% in the observation arm. This difference was statistically significant at a P value of 0.01. However, when the overall survival was evaluated there was no significant difference between the two treatment groups. This was probably because of the ability of CMV chemotherapy to cure a certain percentage of patients with metastatic disease, a fact which was previously observed (HARKER et al. 1985; MILLER et al. 1993).

Patients in the observation arm who suffered disease recurrence required much more treatment than just four cycles of CMV chemotherapy. Some needed as many as six cycles of chemotherapy and others required surgery to resect residual disease after chemotherapy.

The following is a recent update of the Stanford study. It includes patients who were still on treatment or were not followed long enough when the study was closed. There were 29 patients in the immediate treatment arm and 28 in the observation and delayed treatment arm. All patients were followed for a minimum of 30 months from the date of cystectomy. The median follow-up is 6 years. Freedom from relapse and disease-free survival were 41% (12/29) and 45% (13/29) in the immediate treatment arm compared to 21% (6/28) and 29% (8/28) in the observation and delayed treatment arm, respectively. Although there seems to be a trend towards a lower rate of recurrence and a higher rate of survival among patients who were immediately treated following cystectomy, none of these differences are statistically significant. The lack of significant difference in the incidence of freedom of recurrence and survival may be explained on the basis of the small number of patients in each arm and the ability of chemotherapy to cure a certain percentage of patients who relapse after cystectomy.

If the patients with regional lymph node metastasis are analyzed separately, the results are as follows: there were 21 patients in the immediate treatment arm and 18 in the observation and delayed treatment arm. Freedom from relapse and disease-free survival were 43% (9/21) and 43% (9/21) in the immediate treatment arm compared to 17% (3/18) and 28% (5/18) in the observation and delayed treatment arm, respectively. Again, none of these differences are statistically significant, indicating that cystectomy alone can cure a certain percentage of patients with regional lymph node involvement (17%) and that chemotherapy can cure a certain percentage of patients who suffer disease recurrence after cystectomy.

22.6
Conclusion

Locally advanced bladder cancer is a systemic disease and any local treatment is apt to fail. Chemotherapy, whether given before or after cystectomy, may improve disease-free survival for a certain percentage of patients. The advantage of adjuvant chemotherapy is that it is given to those patients whose disease is accurately staged and who are determined, by pathologic criteria, to be at high risk of failure.

Although the majority of the studies cited here show an advantage to postoperative chemotherapy when compared to no treatment, the Stanford study, which includes a group of patients randomized to observation only and treatment upon recurrence, fails to show a statistically significant benefit to adjuvant chemotherapy. Because of that, adjuvant chemotherapy cannot be considered standard treatment until further studies similar to the Stanford trial are conducted with a sufficiently large number of patients.

References

Altman CC, McCaque NJ, Ripepi AC, et al. (1972) The use of methotrexate in advanced bladder cancer. J Urol 108:271–273

Blumenreich MS, Yagoda A, natale RB, et al. (1982) Phase II trial of vinblastine sulfate for metastatic urothelial tract tumors. Cancer 50:435–437

Boileau MA, Johnson DE, Chan RC, Gonzales MO (1980) Bladder carcinoma: results with preoperative radiation therapy and radical cystectomy. Urology 16:569–576

Brendler CB, Steinberg GD, Marshall FF, Mostwin JL, Walch PC (1990) Local recurrence and survival following nerve-sparing radical cystoprostatectomy. J Urol 144:1137–1141

Chabner BA, Myers CE (1989) Clinical pharmacology of cancer chemotherapy. In: Devita VT Jr, Helman S, Rosenberg SA (eds) Cancer: principles and practice of oncology. Lippincott, Philadelphia, pp 349–395

Dretler SP, Ragsdale BD, Leadbetter WF (1973) The value of pelvic lymphadenectomy in the surgical treatment of bladder cancer. J Urol 109:414–418

Freiha F (1990) Treatment options for patients with invasive bladder cancer. Monogr Urol 11:34–42

Freiha F, Reese J, Torti F (1996) A randomized trial of radical cystectomy versus radical cystectomy plus cisplatin, methotrexate and vinblastine chemotherapy for muscle invasive bladder cancer. J Urol 155:495–500

Gagliano OR (1980) Adriamycin vs. adriamycin plus ciplatinum in transitional cell bladder carcinoma: a SWOG study. Proc Am Assoc Cancer Res 21:347

Hall RR, Bloom HJG, Freeman JE, et al. (1974) Methotrexate treatment for advanced bladder cancer. Br J Urol 46:431–436

Harker WG, Meyers FJ, Freiha FS, et al. (1985) Cisplatin, methotrexate and vinblastine (CMV): an effective chemotherapy regimen for metastatic transitional cell carcinoma of the urinary tract. A Northern California Oncology Group Study. J Clin Oncol 3:1463–1468

Herr H (1980) Diamminedichloride platinum II in the treatment of advanced bladder cancer. J Urol 123:953–955

La Plante M, Brice M III (1973) The upper limits of hopeful application of radical cystectomy for vesical carcinoma: does nodal metastasis always indicate incurability? J Urol 109:261–265

Lerner SP, Skinner DG, Lieskovsky G, et al. (1993) The rationale for en bloc pelvic lymph node dissection for bladder cancer patients with nodal metastasis: long term results. J Urol 149:758–761

Logothetis CJ (1988) The role of chemotherapy in the management of invasive bladder cancer. Eur Urol 14 (Suppl 1):19–23

Logothetis CJ, Johnson DE, Chong C, et al. (1988) Adjuvant chemotherapy of bladder cancer: a preliminary report. J Urol 139:1207–1210

Logothetis C, Swanson D, Amato R, et al. (1996) Optimal delivery of perioperative chemotherapy: primary results of a randomized prospective, comparative trial of preoperative and postoperative chemotherapy for invasive bladder cancer. J Urol 155:1241–1245

Mathur VK, Krahn HP, Ramsey EW (1981) Total cystectomy for bladder cancer. J Urol 125:784–788

Merrin C (1978) Treatment of advanced bladder cancer with Cis-diamminedichloroplatinum (II NSC 119875): a pilot study. J Urol 119:493–495

Miller RS, Freiha FS, Reese JH, Ozen H, Torti FM (1993) Cisplatin, methotrexate and vinblastine plus surgical restaging for patients with advanced transitional cell carcinoma of the urothelium. J Urol 150:65–69

Montie J, Straffon RA, Steward BH (1981) Cystectomy with or without radiation therapy: a 20 year analysis. In: Proceedings of the 77th Annual Meeting of the American Urological Association, Kansas City.

Natale RB, Yagoda A, Watson RC (1981) Methotrexate: an active drug in bladder cancer. Cancer: 47:1246–1249

O'Bryan RM, Luce JK, Talley RW, et al. (1973) Phase II evaluation of adriamycin in human neoplasia. Cancer 32:1–5

Physicians Desk Reference (1995) 49th edn. Medical Economics, Montvale, N.J.

Prout GR Jr, Griffith PP, Shipley WU (1979) Bladder carcinoma as a systemic disease. Cancer 43:2532–2539

Skinner DG, Lieskovsky G (1988) Management of invasive high-grade bladder cancer. In: Skinner D, Lieskovsky G (eds) Diagnosis and management of genito-urinary cancer. Saunders, Philadelphia, pp 295–312

Skinner DG, Tift JP, Kaufman JJ (1982) High dose, short course preoperative radiation therapy and immediated single stage radical cystectomy with pelvic node dissection in the management of bladder cancer. J Urol 127:671–677

Skinner DG, Daniels JR, Russell CA (1991) The role of adjuvant chemotherapy following cystectomy for invasive bladder cancer: a prospective comparative trial. J Urol 145:459–464

Smith JA, Whitmore WF Jr (1981) Regional lymph node metastasis from bladder cancer. J Urol 126:591–594

Soloway MS, Murphy WM (1979) Experimental chemotherapy of bladder cancer: systemic and intravesical. Semin Oncol 6:168–172

Soloway MS, Ikand M, Ford K (1981) Cis-diamminedichloroplatinum (II) in locally advanced and metastatic
  urothelial cancer. Cancer 47:476–481
Sternberg CN, yagoda A, Scher HI, et al. (1985) Preliminary
  results of M-VAC (methotrexate, vinblastine, doxorubicin
  and cisplatin) for transitional cell carcinoma of the
  urothelium. J Urol 133:403–409
Sternberg CN, Yagoda A, Scher HI, et al. (1988) The role of
  chemotherapy in the management of invasive bladder cancer. Eur Urol 14(Suppl 1) 24–28
Stockle M, Alken P, Engelmann U, Jacobi GH, Riedmiller H,
  Hohenfellner R (1986) Radikale Zystecktomie–oft zu spat?
  Akt Urol 17:234–239
Stockle M, Meyenberg W, Wellek S, et al. (1992) Advanced
  bladder cancer (stages pT3b, pT4a, pN1 and pN2): improved survival after radical cystectomy and 3 adjuvant
  cycles of chemotherapy. Results of a controlled prospective
  study. J Urol 148:302–308
Turner AG, Hendry WF, Williams GB, et al. (1977) The treatment of advanced bladder cancer with methotrexate. Br J
  Urol 49:673–678

Wei CH, Hsieh RK, Chiou TJ, Chen KK, Chang LS, Chen PM
  (1996) Adjuvant methotrexate, vinblastine and cisplatin
  chemotherapy for invasive transitional cell carcinoma:
  Taiwan experience. J Urol 155:118–121
Wishnow KI, Dmoshowski R (1988) Pelvic recurrence after
  radical cystectomy without preoperative radiation. J Urol
  140:42–43
Wishnow KI, Levinson KA, Johnson DE, et al. (1992) Stage B
  (P2/3a/No) transitional cell carcinoma of the bladder is
  highly curable by radical cystectomy. Urology 39:12–16
Yagoda A (1983) Chemotherapy for advanced urothelial cancer. Semin Urol 1:60–68
Yagoda A, Watson RC, Gonzales-Vitale JC, et al. (1976) Cis-
  dichloro-diammine platinum (II) in advanced bladder
  cancer. Cancer Treat Rep 60:917–923
Yagoda A, Watson RC, Whitmore WF Jr, et al. (1977a)
  Adriamycin in advanced urinary tract cancer. Cancer
  39:279–284
Yagoda A, Watson RC, Grabstald E, et al. (1977b) Adriamycin
  and cyclophosphamide in advanced bladder cancer. Cancer Treat Rep 61:97–101

23 Management of Patients with Pelvic Recurrence Following Radical Cystectomy

S.C. Formenti

23.1 Introduction

Although muscle-invasive transitional cell carcinoma of the bladder is notorious for early distant spread, there is a subset of patients in whom the first site of failure after radical cystectomy is local, within the pelvis. In the last 20 years, improved diagnostic and surgical techniques have contributed to improvement of local control rates, which has been reflected in better overall survival (SKINNER and LIESKOVSKY 1984; SCHOENBERG et al. 1996). This impact on survival has generated interest in further optimizing local control since it is conceivable that a limited number of patients can benefit from more aggressive local treatment. Accordingly, POLLACK et al. (1995) specifically examined the relationship between local failure and distant metastases and survival in 240 cystectomy patients. In multivariate analysis using Cox proportional hazard models with 15 different factors and local failure, the authors found only local failure to be independently predic-

S.C. FORMENTI, MD, Associate Professor, Department of Radiation Oncology and Medicine, University of Southern California, USC/Norris Comprehensive Cancer Center, 1441 Eastlake Avenue, Los Angeles, CA 90033, USA

tive of distant metastases (POLLACK et al. 1995). Based on these findings, both more extensive surgery and the addition of radiotherapy to surgery have been explored.

The use of en bloc pelvic lymph node dissection at the time of radical cystectomy has been studied by LERNER et al. (1993). In a retrospective review of 613 patients who underwent curative pelvic lymphadenectomy with en bloc radical cystectomy, 132 (22%) patients were identified with pathologically proven nodal metastases. In this group of 132 patients, those with less than six metastatic lymph nodes survived significantly longer than those with six or more lymph nodes, and node-positive patients with limited tumor burden (stage Pis, P1, P2, and P3a) survived longer than those with stage P3b or more. This last finding is consistent with the fact that the incidence of lymph node metastases is related to the depth of invasion of the primary tumor (SKINNER 1982). The most important finding of the study was a 20% actuarial 10-year survival rate for node-positive patients, supporting the use of node dissection with curative intent in those patients (LERNER et al. 1993). The same study challenged the concept that the majority of patients who present with nodal metastases tend to have relapses at the initial sites of clinical tumor involvement (DIMOPOULOS et al. 1994; STERNBERG et al. 1989). In fact, only 15 of 89 patients (17%) with tumor recurrence in Lerner's series (17%) had local pelvic recurrence as the first site of recurrence.

The addition of radiotherapy to surgery has also been explored with the intent of optimizing local control to improve overall survival. The underlying rationale is the potential for a moderate dose of radiotherapy to sterilize micrometastatic foci. Controversy exists regarding the real effect of preoperative radiotherapy; results from several nonrandomized studies of preoperative radiotherapy are conflicting, probably due to different patient selection or radiation dose selection (SMITH et al. 1982; SPERA et al. 1988; COLE et al. 1995; SKINNER and LIESKOVSKY 1984).

The NSABP conducted a prospective randomized study that has provided us with a better understanding of this issue. The study randomized 475 patients with invasive bladder cancer (clinical stages T2–4) to preoperative radiotherapy (45 Gy in 28–32 days) versus no radiotherapy. A second randomization after surgery assigned patients to 17 days of 5-fluorouracil or to a placebo. This study generated invaluable pathologic information on the effect of radiotherapy on invasive bladder cancer. In fact, the specimen obtained at the time of cystectomy demonstrated pathologically complete remissions (no detectable tumor) in 34% of the irradiated patients, compared to 9% of the nonirradiated patients (the lack of detectable tumor was due to complete tumor removal by the biopsy procedure before final surgery). In other words, radiotherapy eradicated the tumor in one-quarter of the patients so treated. Furthermore, when no tumor was found in the surgical specimen, survival in the irradiated series was superior when compared to both the nonirradiated tumor series ($P < 0.05$) and the irradiated tumor series ($P = 0.06$) (SLACK et al. 1977). These findings support the hypothesis that radiotherapy may have an impact on selected patients with tumors that are intrinsically more radiosensitive, with this impact being favorably reflected in the survival rate. In the future, a better understanding of tumor genetics may make it possible to identify, before radiotherapy, the subset of patients that will most benefit from preoperative treatment (ESRIG et al. 1994).

23.2
Patterns of Pelvic Recurrence

Any recurrence within the operative field, including the penis, perineum, wound, and lower abdomen, is considered a pelvic recurrence. Pelvic recurrences after radical cystoprostatectomy are still a difficult challenge to the oncologist. Their incidence is easily underestimated since patients in whom recurrence takes the form of distant metastases generally do not have radiologic studies of the pelvis to document persistent local control after cystectomy; potential synchronous pelvic recurrences are thus censored. Moreover, the precise pattern of failure after radical cystoprostatectomy is poorly documented and very much depends on the thoroughness of the postoperative follow-up. A protocol of routine testing of urine cytology is able to detect curable urethral recurrences, while semestral pelvic imaging may identify presymptomatic pelvic recurrences. In current

urologic practice, the latter is less often applied, probably because of the disappointing results achieved in the management of pelvic recurrences. As a consequence, these recurrences are usually detected because of clinical symptoms that have led to radiographic evaluation. At that stage they are usually incurable, with only a few anecdotal reports of salvaged patients.

Ten to 30% of patients who develop distant metastases are found also to have local recurrence; for most it is impossible to estimate whether the first site of recurrence was in the pelvis. Conversely, in the majority of patients, a symptomatic recurrence in the pelvis as the first site of recurrence heralds metastatic spread, making palliation the most rational approach. Whenever local recurrence occurs, the clinical course is characterized by severe morbidity with rapid deterioration of quality of life.

An exception to this clinical course is represented by cytologically diagnosed urethral recurrences, which are highly curable and, if properly managed, have no negative impact on overall survival. Since their origin, prognosis, and management are completely different, we shall discuss urethral recurrences separately from the other pelvic recurrences that occur following radical cystoprostatectomy. Furthermore, in this chapter, when reference is made to pelvic recurrences, I shall be alluding to nonurethral recurrences.

23.3
Urethral Recurrence

Urethral recurrence occurs in approximately 10% of patients who have undergone radical cystoprostatectomy for muscle-invasive bladder cancer.

The nature of recurrence after radical cystoprostatectomy has been the subject of controversy for many years. Since primary transitional cell carcinoma (TCC) of the urethral mucosa is a rare disease, it is conceivable that these relatively frequent metachronous tumors represent an expression of the original bladder carcinoma. Hypotheses on their origin include the seeding of the urothelium from the upstream tumor, metastasis, or new manifestation of the multicentric defect of the transitional cell epithelium which led to the original bladder carcinoma. The last-mentioned seems to be the most plausible theory. First of all, they are not associated with the presence of positive margins in the cystectomy specimen, making it unlikely to be a surgical miss. On the other hand, they display the geographic pattern of skip lesions randomly occurring throughout the full length of the anterior urethra. Moreover, they may arise years after definitive treatment of the bladder tumor (FREEMAN et al. 1994). Their description as "urethral recurrences" is probably inaccurate since it implies failure of the surgical management of the original tumor (FREEMAN et al. 1994). The typical multicentricity of TCC of the bladder suggests that these tumors probably are just another occurrence of TCC in the remaining urothelium. In the future, molecular biology will disclose the nature of the underlying genetic changes and could provide us with a definite understanding of these tumors. Until then, they will remain somehow inappropriately classified as "recurrences," since they cannot be considered surgical failures.

The identification of significant prognostic factors for urethral recurrence has modified surgical management and the protocol of patient follow-up after radical cystoprostatectomy. Prostatic urethra involvement is the strongest predictor for urethral recurrence (ASHWORTH 1956; HARDEMAN and SOLOWAY 1990; LEVINSON et al. 1990; TOBISU et al. 1991). TCC involvement of the prostate is much more common in men undergoing cystectomy for bladder cancer than was previously appreciated. The incidence of TCC in the prostate was reported to be 29%–43% in men whose cystoprostatectomy was analyzed by step-sectioning reconstruction (MONTIE et al. 1990; REESE et al. 1992). Sixteen to 71% of patients with anterior urethral recurrence had prostatic urethral involvement in the cystectomy specimen. Not all patients with prostate TCC develop urethral TCC; however, the absence of prostate TCC selects individuals with a low risk (1%–4%) for urethral TCC. The more extensive the involvement of the prostate by TCC, the greater the risk for urethral TCC: stromal invasion carries the highest risk, diffuse ductal extension is next, and purely prostatic urethral carcinoma in situ (CIS) has the least risk.

23.4
Management of Urethral Recurrence

Evaluation of the urethra following cystectomy should be performed by urethral wash cytology at 6-month to yearly intervals and must be continued for an indefinite period of time. Since most urethral recurrences are noted in the first 2–3 years after cystectomy, follow-up of the urethra needs to be most diligent during this period. When the recur-

rence is discovered by urethral washing and only CIS is present, patient outcome is excellent (HARDEMAN and SOLOWAY 1990). By contrast, if the diagnosis of urethral recurrence is prompted by symptoms such as pain or urethral bleeding, invasion is commonly present and survival is poor. Thus, the surgeon needs to actively search for urethral TCC; fortunately, urethral washing is easy to perform and accurate in making the diagnosis (WOLINSKA et al. 1977). It is performed with the use of a small catheter passed to the end of the urethra to flush 20–30 ml of sterile saline solution. The fluid draining around the catheter is then collected for cytologic examination. If cytology yields suspicious findings, it should be followed by urethroscopy. The first urethral wash is scheduled 4–8 weeks after cystectomy and periodically thereafter with decreasing frequency. An individual receiving an orthotopic reservoir to the urethra can be monitored by voided urine cytology. Urethral washing can also be performed by having the patient tighten the voluntary external sphincter during the flushing of the urethra. Figure 23.1a exemplifies the cytology and Fig. 23.1b documents the confirmatory biopsy findings in a patient with presymptomatic urethral recurrence.

Once the recurrence has been documented the management generally consists in total urethrectomy (AHLERING and LIESKOVSKY 1988). Potency-sparing urethrectomy has been reported as part of nerve-sparing cystoprostatectomy (BRENDLER et al. 1990), with two patients remaining potent following urethrectomy in which the neurovascular bundles were protected in the membranous urethra and the bulbous arteries were individually ligated. These preliminary data need confirmation in larger series. Asymptomatic patients diagnosed on the basis of cytology alone probably need no further staging and should proceed immediately to urethrectomy. Conversely, symptomatic patients or those presenting with a palpable mass may benefit from a pelvic computed tomographic scan to assess tumor extension to the pelvis or inguinal lymph nodes. Some patients who have synchronous distant metastases may be spared surgical excision, avoiding the morbidity of urethrectomy.

Experience with nonsurgical approaches to urethral recurrence is limited and such approaches should be considered experimental. There is little documentation of the use of intraurethral chemotherapy or immunotherapy in the anterior urethra (WITJES et al. 1991).

Systemic chemotherapy regimens, which have shown objective benefit in patients with metastatic

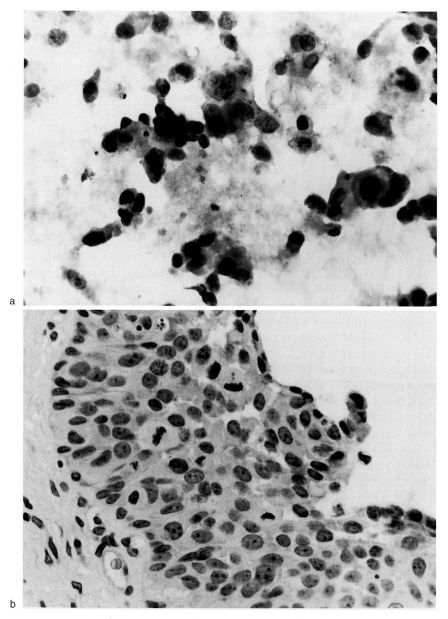

Fig. 23.1. a Urethral washing showing severe urothelial atypia with recurrent TCC. The cells show high nuclear/cytoplasmic ratios, hyperchromasia, coarse chromatin, variation in nuclear size and shape, and molding. (Courtesy of Dr. Sue Ellen Martin) Papanicolaou stain, ×400. **b** In the same patient the cytologic findings were confirmed by a biopsy of the urethra showing transitional cell carcinoma in situ. (Courtesy of Dr. Sue Ellen Martin) H & E stain, ×400

TCC, are reserved for patients with urethral recurrence who also have evidence of distant metastases (SCHER et al. 1988; STERNBERG et al. 1989; MOORE et al. 1990; SHINKA et al. 1989; STOCKLE et al. 1990). Radiation therapy plays an important palliative role for symptomatic relief in patients with unresectable urethral recurrences (HENDERSON et al. 1984).

23.5
Impact of Urethral Recurrence on Survival

It is difficult to determine conclusively whether urethral recurrence is an independent factor affecting survival. Before routine cytologic screening, it is likely that many of the advanced, symptomatic recurrences did indeed affect survival. Several reports have documented that symptomatic recurrences affect survival. The majority of patients in whom a symptomatic recurrence took place were dead within 2 years (CORDONNIER and SPJUT 1962; POOLE-WILSON and BERNARD 1971; SCHELLHAMMER et al. 1977; CLARK 1984). Several authors have found patient survival to correlate with the degree of invasion in the urethrectomy specimen, with survival ranging from 56 months for P0 lesions to only 5.1 months for invasive tumors (HARDEMAN and SOLOWAY 1990; HICKEY et al. 1986; HENDRY et al. 1974). Interestingly, BEAHRS et al. (1984) found that eliminating the urethral recurrence group from all patients with cystectomy for bladder cancer did not statistically improve the overall survival rate (49.6% vs 47.5% and 40.5% vs 37.8% at 5 and 10 years, respectively), in contrast to nonurethral recurrence, which was the parameter most affecting survival (BEAHRS et al. 1984).

In summary, survival appears to be independent of the occurrence of superficial urethral recurrences and appears to depend primarily on the pathology of the initial bladder cancer specimen. Whether an invasive urethral recurrence directly impacts on survival is still unsettled. It is conceivable that invasion beyond the lamina propria of the urethra spreads through the vascular spaces of the corpus spongiosum, allowing metastatic dissemination. It is clear that routine use of postcystectomy urethral cytology is the best measure to assure that the majority of recurrences are found at a still curable, superficial stage.

23.6
Other Pelvic Recurrences: Incidence and Characteristics

Unlike urethral recurrences, most other pelvic recurrences occur within 2 years after cystectomy. The surgical series that have attempted to document pelvic failure rates have reported incidences that range from 5% to 37% (HERR 1985). Several factors account for this variability. First of all, both surgery and postoperative care have rapidly evolved and results from series of patients treated in the 1950s are not comparable to the results of contemporary series. Second, as mentioned before, meticulousness and extent of the clinical assessment at the time of metastatic disease also influence the range of incidence. Third, it is difficult to compare results since some of the reported series included the use of preoperative radiotherapy. Furthermore, among the series of irradiated patients, different radiation doses and different fractionation regimens were used. Radiation dose appears to be an important factor in reducing local failure rates. For instance, in the University of Pennsylvania experience among the several radiation regimens explored, 500 cGy on the day prior to surgery with postoperative radiotherapy reserved for patients with either involved resection margins or advanced stage or high-grade tumors was as effective as the other regimens tested, but had fewer complications (SPERA et al. 1988). There is some suggestion that 40–50 Gy preoperatively, followed by cystectomy for high-grade or muscle-invasive tumors, may reduce the local recurrence rate to approximately 5% (KUBAN et al. 1990). However, in the last 15 years several series have reported that modern surgery alone, without the use of radiotherapy, is able to limit the incidence of pelvic recurrence to 5%–6%; as a consequence preoperative radiotherapy may have become obsolete (SKINNER and LIESKOVSKY 1984; SCHLEGEL and WALSH 1987; MONTIE et al. 1984; WISHNOW and DMOCHOWSKI 1988).

Pelvic failure after cystectomy is poorly documented: only a few series describe in detail the pattern of pelvic recurrences. WISHNOW and DMOCHOWSKI (1988) described ten patients with pelvic recurrences among a series of 178 consecutive patients. Half of the patients had synchronous distant metastases. The initial symptoms were pain in two patients, constipation in two, bleeding in two, and edema, priapism, tenesmus, and bowel obstruction in one patient each (WISHNOW and DMOCHOWSKI 1988). GREVEN et al. (1992) retrospectively analyzed 83 patients who were treated by cystectomy alone (without adjuvant or preoperative treatment). They reported that 13 of 83 patients had local recurrences, resulting in the 5-year actuarial local recurrence rate of 18%. It is of note that most of the pelvic recurrences in this study were detected because of the clinic symptoms (GREVEN et al. 1992). Neither histologic grade nor clinical stage was a predictor of local recurrence. Pathologic stage was the only significant predictor of pelvic recurrence ($P = 0.01$), with 15% of pT1, 18% of pT3a, 51% of pT3b, and 20% of pT4a tumors recurring in the pelvis. The interval from surgery to local recurrence ranged from 3 to 62 months with a median of 9 months. None of the patients with pelvic recurrences survived, and the median survival from diagnosis was 4 months (range 1–50 months). In neither series was the management of the recurrences described.

23.7
Diagnosis and Management

Probably the most successful approach to pelvic recurrences after cystectomy is their prevention by optimizing the initial local treatment. In fact, no effective salvage treatment is available for pelvic recurrences or metastases. Detection of asymptomatic pelvic recurrences after cystectomy, unfortunately, almost never translates into curability; nevertheless, it has a dramatic impact on quality of life. This detection of asymptomatic recurrence allows for the early application of therapy, reducing the well-known morbidity which is associated with a local recurrence. Thus, periodic evaluation of the pelvis following cystectomy is of value. In addition, patients most likely to respond to systemic treatment are those with a good performance status and, thus, earlier detection of metastases could be beneficial. Most recurrences become evident within the first 2 years after surgery, and follow-up is concentrated during this period. Physical examination of the pelvis, with digital rectal examination in men and pelvic examination in women, should be part of standard follow-up after cystectomy. Computed tomography of the pelvis may provide imaging of the sites of local recurrence not accessible by physical examination.

Surgical excision of recurrences within the pelvis are occasionally attempted. The reports of surgical treatment, however, are anecdotal and no patient series have been reported in the literature. Similarly, radiation is often used as a palliative measure to relieve pelvic pain or bleeding. The most frequently used radiation treatment schedules consist of 30 Gy in ten fractions. Chemotherapy plays a role in managing pelvic failures and compared to the experience acquired with other regimens previously used, substantial improvement is evident in the results of systemic chemotherapy with multidrug cisplatin-based regimens such as M-VAC (SCHER and NORTON 1993). Unfortunately, most of the durable complete responses have been noted in patients presenting with soft-tissue metastases at diagnosis and not after cystectomy.

23.8
The USC Experience

23.8.1
Urethral Recurrences

Recently, we have reviewed the pattern of urethral recurrences among 416 male patients treated at the University of Southern California (USC) (TARTER et al. 1995). The incidence of urethral recurrence among 248 patients who had undergone cutaneous urinary diversion was compared to that in 168 patients who had undergone Kock ureteroileal urethrostomy. The two groups of patients were of comparable age, but the median follow-up of the cutaneous diversion patients was longer (8.5 years compared to 3.5 years). The cutaneous diversion group had 27 urethral recurrences (10.9%) and the Kock urethrostomy group had four (2.4%) recurrences. Kaplan-Meier estimates of time to recurrence were used and the log rank test for censored data was applied to test for statistical significance. The probability of urethral recurrence at 5 years was found to be 12% in the cutaneous diversion group versus 5% in the Kock urethrostomy group ($P = 0.014$). Interestingly, none of the 12 patients with prostatic invasion in the Kock urethrostomy group had disease recurrence, compared to 6 of 24 patients (33%) in the cutaneous diversion group. Similarly, a lower incidence of urethral recurrence was found among the patients with CIS within the Kock urethrostomy group: the 5-year probability of urethral recurrence for CIS was only 4%, compared to 12.7% in the cutaneous diversion group. These findings suggest that patients undergoing reconstruction with a Kock urethrostomy have a lower risk of urethral recurrence than patients receiving cutaneous urinary diversion after cystectomy for TCC of the bladder. Prophylactic urethrectomy should be considered in patients with high-risk pathologic features who undergo cutaneous diversion .

23.8.2
Pelvic Recurrences

The medical records of 1065 patients treated by means of radical cystectomy with en bloc lymph node dissection between August 1971 and July 1995 were reviewed. This cohort of patients included 238 females and 827 males. Two hundred and thirty-eight patients (22.4%) had recurrence documented in the medical records; 175 patients recurred with distant metastases without evidence of local recurrence. Sixty-two patients had evidence of local recurrence (5.8%). In 40 (3.8%) patients, the diagnosis of local recurrence was synchronous with that of distant metastatic disease.

In 22 patients (2%), however, local recurrence alone was the initial disease site at recurrence. These patients comprised eight females and 14 males with a median age of 64 (range 23–84 years). Among the females, the most common site of recurrence was the vagina (six patients), one patient had local recurrence in pelvic nodes and another in the abdominal wall. Among the male patients, local recurrence was reported as pelvic in seven patients, in the pelvic nodes in four patients, in the abdominal wall in one patient, in the rectal wall in one patient, and in the penis in the last patient. For the entire group the median time from surgery to local recurrence was 14 months (range 3–33 months); the majority of recurrences occurred within 24 months (6/8 among the female patients and 18/22 among the male patients). Despite the fact that five patients underwent surgical excision of the metastatic site, 11 patients received radiotherapy and 13 received chemotherapy. Only one (4.5%) patient is alive without disease at 50 months following therapy. For the entire group of 22 patients, median survival from the detection of local recurrence was 9 months (range 2–50 months).

23.9
Conclusion

In conclusion, the USC experience confirmed that local recurrences following cystectomy are accompanied by a poor prognosis in the majority of patients.

References

Ahlering TA, Lieskovsky G (1988) Surgical treatment of urethral cancer in the male patient. In: Skinner DG, Lieskovsky G (eds) Diagnosis and management of genitourinary cancer. Saunders, Philadelphia, pp 627

Ashworth A (1956) Papillomatosis of the urethra. Br J Urol 28:3

Beahrs JR, Fleming TR, Zincke H (1984) Risk of local urethral recurrence after radicaly cystectomy for bladder cancer. J Urol 131:264

Brendler CB, Schlegel PN, Walsh PC (1990) Urethrectomy with preservation of potency. J Urol 144:270

Clark PB (1984) Urethral carcinoma after cystectomy. The case for routine urethrectomy. J Urol (Paris) 90:173

Cole CJ, Pollack A, Zagars GK, Dinney CP, Swanson DA, von Eschenbach AC (1995) Local control of muscle-invasive bladder cancer. Preoperative radiotherapy and cystectomy versus cystectomy alone. Int J Radiat Oncol Biol Phys 32:331–340

Cordonnier JJ, Spjut HJ (1962) Urethral occurrence of bladder carcinoma following cystectomy. J Urol 87:398

Dimopoulos MA, Finn L, Logothetis CJ (1994) Pattern of failure and survival of patients with metastatic urothelial tumors relapsing after cisplatinum-based chemotherapy. J Urol 151:598–601

Esrig D, Elmajian D, Groshen S, et al. (1994) Accumulation of nuclear p53 and tumor progression in bladder Cancer. N Engl J Med 331:1259–1264

Faysal MH (1980) Urethrectomy in men with transitional cell carcinoma of bladder. Urology 16:23

Freeman JA, Esrig D, Stein JP, Skinner DG (1994) Management of the patient with bladder cancer. Urol Clin North Am 21:645–651

Greven KM, Spera JA, Solin LJ, Morgan T, Hanks G (1992) Local recurrence after cystectomy alone for bladder carcinoma. Cancer 69:2767–2770

Hardeman SW, Soloway MS (1990) Urethral recurrence following radical cystectomy. J Urol 144:666–669

Henderson RH, Parsons JT, Morgan L, Million RR (1984) Elective ilioinguinal lymph node irradiation. Int J Radiat Oncol Biol Phys 10:811–819

Hendry WF, Gowing NFC, Wallace DM (1974) Surgical treatment of urethral tumors associated with bladder cancer. Proc R Soc Med 67:304

Herr HW (1985) Preoperative irradiation with and without chemotherapy as adjunct to radical cystectomy. Urology 25:127

Hickey DP, Soloway MS, Murphy WM (1986) Selective urethrectomy following cystoprostatectomy for bladder cancer. J of Urol 136:828

Kuban DA, El-Mahdi AM, Schellhammer PF (1990) Patterns of recurrence and prognosis in bladder carcinoma treated by preoperative radiation and cystectomy (abstract). Proc Am Radium Soc 15

Lerner SP, Skinner DG, Lieskovsky G, et al. (1993) Rationale for en bloc pelvic lymph node dissection for bladder cancer patients with nodal metastases: long-term results. J Urol 149:758–765

Levinson KA, Johnson DE, Wishnow KI (1990) Indications for urethrectomy in an era of continent urinary diversion. J Urol 144:73–75

Montie JE (1994) Follow-up after cystectomy for carcinoma of the bladder. Urol Clin North Am 21:639–643

Montie JE, Straffon RA, Steward BH (1984) Radical cystectomy without radiation therapy for carcinoma of the bladder. J Urol 131:477–482

Montie JE, Wood DP Jr, Venderberg Mendendort S (1990) The significance and management of transitional cell carcinoma of the prostate. Semin Urol 8:262–268

Moore AS, Cardona A, Shapiro W (1990) Cisplatin (cisdiamminedichloroplatinum) for treatment of transitional cell carcinoma of the urinary bladder or urethra: a retrospective study of 15 dogs. J Vet Intern Med 4:148

Pollack A, Zagars GK, Cole CJ, Dinney CPN, Swanson DA, Grossman HB (1995) The relationship of local control to distant metastasis in muscle invasive bladder cancer. J Urol 154:2059–2064

Poole-Wilson DS, Bernard RJ (1971) Total cystectomy for bladder tumors. Br J Urol 43:16

Reese JH, Freiha FS, Gelb AB (1992) Transitional cell carcinoma of the prostate in patients undergoing radical cystoprostatectomy. J Urol 147:92–95

Schellhammer PF, Bean MA, Whitmore WF Jr (1977) Prostatic involvement by transitional cell carcinoma: pathogenesis, patterns, and prognosis. J Urol 118:399–403

Scher HI, Norton L (1993) Chemotherapy for urothelial tract malignancies: breaking the deadlock. Semin Surg Oncol 8:316–342

Scher HI, Yagoda A, Herr HW (1988) Neoadjuvant MVAC (methotrexate, vinblastine, doxorubicin and cisplatin) for extravesical urinary tract tumors. J Urol 139:475

Schlegel PN, Walsh PC (1987) Neuroanatomical approach to radical cystoprostatectomy with preservation of sexual function. J Urol 138:1402–1406

Schoenberg MP, Walsh PC, Breazeale DR, Marshall FF, Mostwin JL, Brendler CB (1996) Local recurrence and survival following nerve sparing radical cystoprostatectomy for bladder cancer: 10-year follow-up. J Urol 155:490–494

Shinka T, Uekado Y, Aoshi H (1989) Urethral remnant tumors following simultaneous partial urethrectomy and cystectomy for bladder carcinoma. J Urol 142:983

Skinner DG (1982) Management of invasive bladder cancer; a meticrlous pelvic node dissection can make a difference. J Urol 128:34

Skinner DG, Lieskovsky G (1984) Contemporary cystectomy with pelvic node dissection compared to preoperative radiation therapy plus cystectomy in management of invasive bladder cancer. J Urol 131:1069–1072

Slack NH, Bross IDJ, Prout GR (1977) Five-year follow-up results of a collaborative study of therapies for carcinoma of the bladder. J Surg Oncol 9:393–405

Smith JA Jr, Batata M, Grabstald H, Sogani PC, Herr H, Whitmore WF (1982) Preoperative irradiation and cystectomy for bladder cancer. Cancer 49:869–873

Soloway Hardeman SW, Soloway MS (1990) Urethral recurrence following radical cystectomy. J Urol 144:666–669

Spera JA, Whittington R, Littman P, Solin LJ, Wein AJ (1988) A comparison of preoperative radiotherapy regimens for bladder carcinoma. Cancer 61:255–262

Sternberg CN, Yagoda A, Scher HI (1989) Methotrexate, vinglastine, doxorubicin, and cisplatin for advanced transitional cell carcinoma of the urothelium: efficacy and patterns of response and relapse. Cancer 64:2448

Stockle M, Gokcebay E, Riedmiller H (1990) Urethral tumor recurrences after radical cystoprostatectomy: the case for primary cystoprostatourethrectomy? J Urol 143:41

Tarter TH, Freeman JA , Chen SC, Esrig D (1995) Urethral recurrences in patients with ileal neobladders. Proceedings of the American Urological Association Ninetieth Annual Meeting, Volume 153, Abstract#342

Tobisu KI, Tanaka Y, Mizutani T (1991) Transitional cell carcinoma of the urethra in men following cystectomy for bladder cancer: multivariate analysis for risk factors. J Urol 146:1551–1554

Wishnow KI, Dmochowski R (1988) Pelvic recurrence after radical cystectomy without preoperative radiation. J Urol 140:42–43

Witjes JA, Debruyne FM, vander-Meijden AP (1991) Treatment of carcinoma in situ of the urethra with intraurethral instillations of bacillus Calmette-Guerin: case report and review of the literature. Eur Urol 20:170

Wolinska WH, Melamed MR, Schellhammer PF (1977) Urethral cytology following cystectomy for bladder carcinoma. Am J Surg Pathol 1:225–234

24 Management of Patients with Failure Following Definitive Radiotherapy

B.H. Bochner and S.D. Boyd

CONTENTS

24.1
Introduction

The therapeutic efficacy of all definitive treatments of clinically localized, invasive bladder cancer centers on its ability to control the local-regional disease and relieve symptoms. Various approaches using single or integrated therapy have been reported (BLANDY et al. 1980; BATATA et al. 1981; SMITH and WHITMORE 1981; ABRATT et al. 1984; HOPE STONE et al. 1984; SCHAEFFER et al. 1984; SHIPLEY et al. 1985; MATTHEWS et al. 1987; ROTMAN et al. 1987; VILLAR et al. 1987; ZINCKE et al. 1988; NISSENKORN et al. 1990; PIZZOCARO et al. 1990; ABRATT et al. 1991; KRAGELJ et al. 1992; ABRATT et al. 1993a; KAUFMAN et al. 1993; ABRATT et al. 1994; HERR and SCHER 1994; SROUGI and SIMON 1994; GIVEN et al. 1995; ORSATTI et al. 1995), with several different strategies demonstrating similar survival outcomes. Surgical intervention consisting of radical cystectomy and pelvic lymph node dissection has been the treatment of choice, particularly with physicians in the United States. Definitive local-regional treatment with radical radiation therapy is also widely used as primary therapy, definitive treatment after chemosensi-

B.H. BOCHNER, MD, Fellow, Urologic Oncology, Department of Urology, University of Southern California, USC/Norris Comprehensive Cancer Center, 1441 Eastlake Avenue, Los Angeles, CA 90033, USA
S.D. BOYD, MD, Professor, Department of Urology, University of Southern California, USC/Norris Comprehensive Cancer Center, 1441 Eastlake Avenue, Los Angeles, CA 90033, USA

tization, and neoadjuvantly prior to cystectomy ar. The ongoing desire to develop effective bladder-sparing therapies has led to several treatment regimens which take advantage of these multimodality approaches.

Radiation therapy alone as primary treatment for invasive bladder cancer has previously demonstrated long-term cure rates of 20%–30% (MILLER and JOHNSON 1973; GOFFINET et al. 1975; WALLACE and BLOOM 1976). Newer protocols involving combination therapy with transurethral resection and chemotherapy have reported greater success. Despite these improvements, patients treated on bladder salvage protocols remain at significant risk for treatment failure. These failures may be a result of: (a) incomplete response to therapy, (b) recurrent tumor that has regrown at the site of initial resection, (c) de novo formation of new tumor at other locations within the bladder, and (d) severe, refractory local symptoms (intractable irritability, radiation cystitis) that arise as a complication of therapy requiring cystectomy and urinary diversion.

24.2
Identification of Radiation Failures

Established protocols using primary radiation therapy will require follow-up endoscopic inspection of the bladder within 1–3 months after the completion of initial therapy. At that time careful evaluation for the response to treatment is sought. Prior detailed mapping of the bladder, obtained at the time of initial cystoscopy, is invaluable during this evaluation to aid in the identification of all previous sites of disease, as well as to direct accurate follow-up biopsies for post-therapy staging. Saline washings of the bladder are used as an adjuvant method to identify disease that may not be visually identified (carcinoma in situ) at cystoscopy. Bimanual examination under anesthesia is an essential aspect of staging that must be performed in all patients with residual, recurrent, or de novo disease. It must be recognized, however, that the fibrosis induced by radical radiation may preclude an accurate examination. Fibrotic scar that has become fixed may not be clinically discriminated from recurrent or residual disease. This difficulty is highlighted by findings from the M.D. Anderson series in which the clinical diagnosis was correct in only 26 of 62 patients (SWANSON et al. 1981). Thirty-one percent of patients were clinically understaged and 23% were clinically overstaged. Pathologic evaluation of biopsy material may offer the only accurate and objective evidence of residual disease. Characterization of disease in the pelvis and at distant sites requires the use of serum biochemical evaluation, chest x-ray, bone scan, and radiographic imaging of the pelvis and abdominal cavities (computerized tomography, magnetic resonance imaging). These studies play a central role in evaluation the response to the initial therapy and identifying recurrent disease that presents during the follow-up period. The feasibility of surgical resection can be determined or, alternatively, the patient eliminated as a candidate for further definitive local treatment if evidence of metastatic disease is identified. Patients found to have a complete response to initial therapy should undergo regular surveillance with cystoscopy and urinary cytology. Late recurrence of disease or the formation of new tumors has been found in patients many years after initial successful treatment.

Despite pathologic evidence of disease eradication, as many as 5% of patients treated with radical radiation therapy will experience intractable symptoms of irritation, hematuria (radiation cystitis), frequency, and urgency. Numerous local therapies have been tried in an attempt to alleviate symptoms; however, patients may require cystectomy and urinary diversion as the only effective therapy.

24.3
Operative Considerations

Early experience with salvage cystectomy was disappointing, demonstrating a high operative morbidity and mortality (EDSMYR et al. 1971; LUND 1978). Radiation-induced changes to the abdominal wall, bowel and ureters were responsible for a high percentage of the problems seen after salvage surgery. As experience with salvage cystectomy has grown, a better understanding of the radiation-induced changes to the surrounding abdominal and pelvic structures led to alterations in surgical technique which have significantly improved its safety. Following radical radiation therapy, a desmoplastic reaction within the pelvis and retroperitoneum takes place, obliterating normal surgical tissue planes. Tissue edema and cellular destruction gives way to an infiltration with subsequent fibrosis and loss of normal tissue elasticity. Available information suggests that tissue fibrosis is a direct result of tissue ischemia occurring as a result of endothelial cell damage and vascular occlusion (ANTONAKOPOULOS et al. 1982, 1984; STEWART 1986; RUBIN and WASSERMAN 1988). These changes play a particularly important role in the posterior dissection of the bladder and anterior rectal surface. As the normal plane separating these structures is obliterated, selective use of an initial perineal approach, as recommended by CRAWFORD and SKINNER (1980), to facilitate freeing of the bladder in the deep pelvis with completion of the cystectomy through the abdomen has been advocated in order to prevent rectal injury. Management of an injury to the rectum should consist in primary repair with the creation of a proximal diverting colostomy. Delayed healing of the irradiated rectum necessitates proximal diversion of the fecal stream to prevent tissue breakdown and leakage with subsequent pelvic abscess formation. While we have found the abdominal-perineal approach very useful in selected cases, others have reported that only a rare patient requires such a combined approach. The desmoplastic reaction frequently creates a fibrotic sheath covering the pelvic lymphatics, restricting or preventing skeletonization of the pelvic vasculature and removal of the pelvic lymph node packet (obturator; common, internal and external iliac). As the amount of time between completion of radiation therapy and cystectomy increases, so may the degree of fibrosis.

Prior to the recent popularization of the continent urinary diversion, the standard urinary tract reconstruction after cystectomy consisted of the ileal conduit. Current standard urinary tract reconstruction after cystectomy involves some form of continent urinary diversion in all but those patients with severely compromised renal function or debilitating illness (SKINNER and LIESKOVSKY 1988). The selection of the proper intestinal segment for reconstruction will substantially alleviate the operative morbidity associated with salvage cystectomy. The presence of severe radiation enteritis precludes the use of affected intestinal segments. The use of transverse colon for conduit formation or other intestinal segments for continent diversion or reconstruction may become necessary if the terminal ileum or other segments are severely affected (SCHMIDT et al. 1975). Although the use of stomach is an appealing alternative, most experience with this type of diversion has been in children. Limited information is available for the use of gastric segments in adults; however, several potential shortcomings have reserved this option to be reserved for highly selected cases (ADAMS et al. 1988; McDOUGAL 1992; LOCKHART et al. 1993).

24.4
Operative Outcome

Initial experience with surgical resection of radical radiation failures was characterized by operative complication rates of 44%–66% and mortality as high as 15%–33% (EDSMYR et al. 1971; LUND 1978). These data led many to question the rationale and wisdom of surgery after radiation failure. Most contemporary salvage cystectomy series, however, report significantly improved overall operative performance and decreased morbidity and mortality, reflecting the increased experience of urologic surgeons. Current experience with salvage procedures demonstrates mortality rates of 0%–11%, not dissimilar to rates found in nonirradiated patients undergoing primary cystectomy (BLANDY et al. 1980; CRAWFORD SKINNER 1980; SMITH and WHITMORE 1981; SWANSON et al. 1981).

Recent advances in surgical technique, anesthesia, and postoperative care have made the continent and orthotopic urinary reservoirs the diversions of choice with most urologic surgeons. Patient satisfaction surveys have indicated that continent diversions are more readily accepted than noncontinent types of diversions which require an appliance for urinary storage (BOYD et al. 1987). Previously, the use of long intestinal segments in irradiated patients was thought to carry a significantly increased risk of postoperative complications. Radiation-induced ischemic changes to the ureter and bowel were thought to be responsible for the high percentage of ureterointestinal anastomotic leaks, infection, and wound dehiscence. We have analyzed our experience with continent diversion (Kock pouch) in patients undergoing cystectomy for radiation failure or intractable symptoms associated with high-dose, radical radiation therapy (AHLERING et al. 1988). Forty-two patients who had received at least 4500 cGy of preoperative external beam radiation therapy were compared with 44 nonirradiated patients. Thirty-four patients were referred for radia-

tion failure and underwent radical cystectomy and Kock pouch urinary diversion without pelvic lymphadenectomy. Of the irradiated group, 24 (57%) had received 6000 cGy or more. A total of 31 nonirradiated patients underwent cystectomy and Kock pouch formation with a pelvic lymph node dissection and served as our control population. An additional eight patients who had received preoperative radiation and 13 control patients underwent conversion of an existing ileal conduit to a continent Kock pouch reservoir. Cystectomy and Kock pouch formation were performed using standardized techniques that have previously been described. Meticulous intraoperative management of the ureter was performed, including excision of all distal ureteral segments demonstrating radiation changes, preservation of the medial ureteral blood supply, creation of a spatulated, mucosa to mucosa anastomosis, and placement of ureteral stents bridging the new anastomoses. Although the ureter has demonstrated a relative resistance to the damaging effects of radiation, 1%–3% of patients treated with brachytherapy for gynecologic malignancies experience ureteral strictures/fibrosis (PEREZ et al. 1984; MONTANA and FOWLER 1989; PARLIAMENT et al. 1989). Pelvic radiation for bladder cancer is associated with a lower incidence of ureteral ischemia but must be carefully evaluated at the time of surgery to avoid the use of portions of the distal ureter that appear compromised. Using healthy segments of ureter out of the field of prior radiation will assure a watertight ureterointestinal anastomosis and prevent early urinary leakage, pelvic abscesses, sepsis, and long-term stricture disease.

Our comparison revealed no significant differences between the irradiated and control groups with respect to operative time, intraoperative blood loss, and transfusion requirements. This correlates well with other published series in which no significant difference in intraoperative performance or postoperative hospital recovery time was identified (SMITH and WHITMORE 1981; SWANSON et al. 1981). Instances of prolonged hospitalization were due to diarrhea and urinary leakage (11% controls, 20% irradiated patients; $P = 0.29$). These were the only significant postoperative complications in our series. No correlation was found between the degree of radiation received ($<$ or $>$ 6000 cGy) and the formation of a urinary leak. No pelvic abscesses, fascial dehiscence, or pulmonary emboli were observed in either group. In contrast, three large series of salvage cystectomies ($n = 179$) revealed a 22% rate of wound complications (14% infection, 8% wound dehiscence), 6% ureteroileal leaks, and 3% pulmonary emboli. Early complications have consisted primarily of wound problems (infections, dehiscence) and infections secondary to ureterointestinal leakage. Late complications have varied widely in reported series; most commonly, they have consisted of fistula formation, intestinal obstructions, and ureterointestinal anastomotic strictures.

As our experience with orthotopic, neobladder reconstruction increased, it clearly became our diversion of choice in most men and selected women undergoing radical cystectomy for malignant disease. In a review of 295 men undergoing Kock ileal neobladder reconstruction, eight patients who had received ≥5500 cGy of external beam radiotherapy were included (ELAMJIAN et al. 1996). Overall these patients did as well as their nonirradiated counterparts, although the small number of these patients prevents a detailed comparison. Continence in these patients was similar to the entire population, suggesting that orthotopic diversion can be an acceptable alternative in these patients. It has been our philosophy to favor orthotopic reconstruction to the urethra with a Kock ileal neobladder and simultaneous or subsequent placement of an artificial urinary sphincter for patients with marginal preoperative continence or patients who do not develop an acceptable level of urinary control after reconstruction. Those patients who have undergone such a treatment program have reported a high level of satisfaction, preferring their current status to a nonorthotopic diversion.

The placement of any prosthetic material into previously irradiated tissues carries an added risk for subsequent problems (RADOMSKI and HERSCHORN 1992). Poor wound healing secondary to ischemic changes to the surrounding tissues and impaired immune responses are thought to be responsible for episodes of device erosion and infection. To date none of our patients who have undergone salvage cystectomy and orthotopic urinary reconstruction have developed a sphincter erosion-infection. We have previously evaluated our experience with artificial urinary sphincter placement in patients who had undergoing pelvic surgery for a genitourinary cancer (MARTINS and BOYD 1995). One hundred and forty-five AMS 800 artificial sphincters had been placed with only 13 patients experiencing an erosion or infection. Of these 13 patients, seven (54%) had undergone pelvic irradiation (mean dose 4500 cGy). Overall, the risk of infection or erosion in patients with prior radiation is slightly increased compared with nonirradiated patients. However, proper care

and placement of the device, including meticulous handling of the tissues at the time of surgery, prolonged inactivation (6–12 weeks) of the device after implantation to allow for complete healing, and avoidance of traumatic catheterizations once the device is activated should lead to an acceptable postoperative result.

24.5
Patient Survival

As previouly stated, initial reports from early series showed poor overall survival in patients undergoing salvage surgery after radiation failure. LUND (1978) reported a 50% survival at 1 year in 101 patients treated by salvage cystectomy. Similarly EDSYMR et al. (1971) reported only 16 of 35 patients alive 1 year after surgery. Data from several series demonstrate that only 8%–33% of patients who demonstrate an incomplete response to radiation therapy undergo salvage cystectomy (WALLACE and BLOOM 1976; BLANDY et al. 1980; GOODMAN et al. 1981; GOSPODAROWICZ et al. 1989). Follow-up data thus represent a highly selected group of patients who experience a treatment failure. The selection criteria appear to differ with each individual study. More contemporary series have reported a 35%–40% overall 5-year survival for these selected patients undergoing cystectomy after radiation failure (BLANDY et al. 1980; SMITH and WHITMORE 1981; SWANSON et al. 1981; CRAWFORD and SKINNER 1982; ABRATT et al. 1993b; DUNST et al. 1994). Our most recent series of 36 patients undergoing salvage cystectomy and lower urinary tract reconstruction demonstrated a 36% 5-year overall survival (Fig. 24.1) These patients had received ≥5500 cGy of external beam radiation therapy prior to surgery for treatment failure.

Several features have been found to be associated with long-term outcome. BLOOM and co-workers (1982) found that age at the time of cystectomy significantly affected outcome. Men <60 years of age enjoyed an improved survival compared with men age >60. Pathologic stage after cystectomy has also been found to correlate with survival. Patients with superficial lesions do better than patients found to have locally advanced lesions. JOHNSON (1983) found a 60% 5-year survival in patients with superficial lesions; this dropped to below 30% for patients with pathologically advanced disease. Likewise, CRAWFORD and SKINNER (1980) found 10 of 16 patients (63%) with disease involving only the mucosa

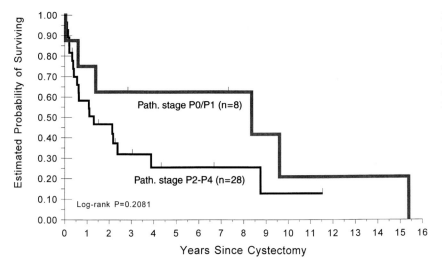

Fig. 24.1. Overall patient survival for 36 patients with superficial (P0–P1) or advanced transitional cell carcinoma of the bladder (P2–P4) undergoing salvage cystectomy and urinary reconstruction

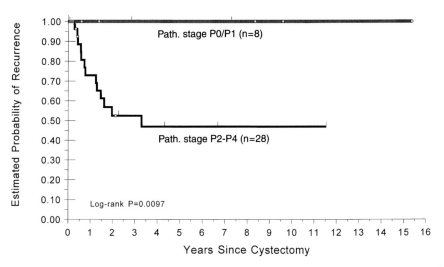

Fig. 24.2. Disease recurrence for 36 patients with superficial (P0–P1) or advanced transitional cell carcinoma of the bladder (P2–P4) undergoing salvage cystectomy and urinary reconstruction

to be alive at 5 years, as compared to 4 of 21 patients (19%) with involvement of the muscularis (P2 or greater). Smith and Whitmore (1981) found a 9% 5-year survival in patients with tumor involving adjacent structures, compared to 26% for patients with P3 tumors. Swanson et al. (1981) reported a 43% overall survival in their series of 62 patients. They found that patients with "advanced" disease (≥P3 lesions) behaved similarly, demonstrating a 30% 3-year survival. This was significantly worse than the 3-year survival – 90% – in patients with pathologically superficial disease. We also found pathologic stage to an accurate predictor of patient outcome after salvage cystectomy. Patients with disease confined to the lamina propria demonstrated a 63% 5-year survival, compared to a 26% 5-year survival for patients

whose tumors were P2 or greater (Fig. 24.1). We further found that pathologic stage could serve as a predictor of disease recurrence (Fig. 24.2). Thirteen of 28 patients (47%) with invasive disease (P2–P4) had disease recurrence by 5-years, compared to none of eight patients whose disease did not spread beyond the lamina propria (≤P1) ($P = 0.01$). Four patients were found to have disease recurrence only in the pelvis, four to have metastatic disease only, and two to have both local and distant disease. The local recurrence rate in this series is similar to that in other reported series (Whitmore and Batata 1984; Gospodarowicz et al. 1989). Some have suggested that survival is related to the timing of cystectomy, a reflection of the rapidity of disease recurrence (Dunst et al. 1994). Dunst et al reported a 46% 5-

year survival in patients undergoing cystectomy ≥9 months after primary therapy, compared to a 16% 5-year survival in patients receiving surgery <9 months from initial treatment. Others have not confirmed these findings (SMITH and WHITMORE 1981).

24.6
Conclusion

As further integrated therapies for bladder cancer undergo clinical evaluation, an increasing number of options will become available for the treatment of invasive bladder cancer. Bladder-sparing protocols involving various combinations of transurethral resection of tumor, chemotherapy, and radiation will increase as more effective agents are identified. Patients who fail to respond to these strategies will continue to be remain potential candidates for curative local therapy by salvage cystectomy. Current surgical techniques offer an acceptable level of operative morbidity and mortality in carefully selected patients.

It now appears that the extent of residual disease at the time of cystectomy is the most important prognostic indicator of failed radiation therapy. Clearly there is a subgroup of patients with advanced stage disease who are destined to do poorly with respect to long-term survival. Our inability to accurately predict pathologic stage from clinical preoperative evaluations limits our ability to select patients who will most benefit from salvage surgery.

References

Abratt RP, Barnes DR, Hammond JA, Sarembok LA, Tucker RD, Williams AM (1984) Radical irradiation and misonidazole for T2 grade III and T3 bladder cancer: 2 year follow-up. Int J Radiat Oncol Biol Phys 10:1719–1720

Abratt RP, P Craighead P, Reddi VB, Sarembock LA (1991) A prospective randomised trial of radiation with or without oral and intravesical misonidazole for bladder cancer. Br J Cancer 64:968–970

Abratt RP, Pontin AR, Barnes RD (1993a) Chemotherapy, radical irradiation plus salvage cystectomy for bladder cancer-severe late small bowel morbidity. Eur J Surg Oncol 19:279–282

Abratt RP, Wilson JA, Pontin AR, Barnes RD (1993b) Salvage cystectomy after radical irradiation for bladder cancer-prognostic factors and complications. Br J Urol 72:756–760

Abratt RP, Pontin AR, Barnes RD (1994) Neo-adjuvant chemotherapy and radical irradiation for locally advanced bladder cancer-a phase 2 study. Eur J Surg Oncol 20:576–579.

Adams MC, Mitchell ME, Rink RC (1988) Gastrocystoplasty: an alternative solution to the problem of urological reconstruction in the severely compromised patient. J Urol 140:1152–1156

Ahlering TE, Kanellos A, Boyd SD, Lieskovsky G, Skinner DG, Bernstein L (1988) A comparative study of perioperative complications with Kock pouch urinary diversion in highly irradiated versus nonirradiated patients. J Urol 139:1202–1224

Antonakopoulos GN, Hicks RM, Hamilton E, Berry RJ (1982) Early and late morphological changes (including carcinoma of the urothelium) induced by irradiation of the rat urinary bladder. Br J Cancer 46:403–416

Antonakopoulos GN, Hicks RM, Berry RJ (1984) The subcellular basis of damage to the human urinary bladder induced by irradiation. J Pathol 143:103–116

Batata MA, Chu FC, Hilaris BS, Whitmore WF, Kim YS, Lee MZ (1981) Bladder cancer in men and women treated by radiation therapy and/or radical cystectomy. Urology 18:15–20

Blandy JP, England HR, Evans SJ, et al. (1980) T3 bladder cancer the case for salvage cystectomy. Br J Urol 52:506–510

Bloom HJ, Hendry WF, Wallace DM, Skeet RG (1982) Treatment of T3 bladder cancer: controlled trial of pre-operative radiotherapy and radical cystectomy versus radical radiotherapy. Br J Urol 54:136–151

Boyd SD, Feinberg SM, Skinner DG, Lieskovsky G, Baron D, Richardson J (1987) Quality of life survey of urinary diversion patients: comparison of ileal conduits versus continent Kock ileal reservoirs. J Urol 138:1386–1389

Crawford ED, Skinner DG (1980) Salvage cystectomy after irradiation failure. J Urol 123:32–34

Crawford ED, Skinner DG (1982) Re: salvage cystectomy for bladder cancer after failure of definitive irradiation. J Urol 127:96

Dunst J, Sauer R, Schrott KM, Kuhn R, Wittekind C, Altendorf Hofmann A (1994) Organ-sparing treatment of advanced bladder cancer: a 10-year experience. Int J Radiat Oncol Biol Phys 30:261–266

Edsmyr R, Moberger G, Wadstrom L (1971) Carcinoma of the bladder: Cystectomy after supervoltage therapy. Scand J Urol Nephrol 5:215–221

Elmajian DA, Stein JP, Esrig D, et al. (1996) The Kock ileal neobladder: Updated experience in 295 male patients. J Urol 156:920–925

Given RW, Parsons JT, McCarley D, Wajsman Z (1995) Bladder-sparing multimodality treatment of muscle-invasive bladder cancer: a five-year follow-up. Urology 46:499–504

Goffinet DR, Hislop TG, Elwood JM (1975) Bladder cancer: Results of radiation therapy in 384 patients. Radiology 117:149

Goodman GB, Hislop TG, Elwood JM, Balfour J (1981) Conservation of bladder function in patients with invasive bladder cancer treated by definitive irradiation and selective cystectomy. Int J Radiat Oncol Biol Phys 7:569–573

Gospodarowicz MK, Hawkins NV, Rawlings GA, et al. (1989) Radical radiotherapy for muscle invasive transitional cell carcinoma of the bladder: failure analysis. J Urol 142:1448–1453

Herr HW, Scher HI (1994) Neoadjuvant chemotherapy and partial cystectomy for invasive bladder cancer. J Clin Oncol 12:975–980

Hope Stone HF, Oliver RT, England HR, Blandy JP (1984) T3 bladder cancer: salvage rather than elective cystectomy after radiotherapy. Urology 24:215–320

Johnson DE (1983) Salvage cystectomy. Semin Urol 1:53–59

Kaufman DS, Shipley WU, Griffin PP, Heney NM, Althausen AF, Efird JT (1993) Selective bladder preservation by combination treatment of invasive bladder cancer. N Engl J Med 329:1377–1382

Kragelj B, Jereb B, Kragelj L, Stanonik M (1992) Concurrent vinblastine and radiation therapy in bladder cancer. Cancer 70:2885–2890

Lockhart JL, Davies R, Cox C, McAllister E, Helal M, Figueroa TE (1993) The gastroileoileal pouch: an alternative continent reservoir for patients with short bowel, acidosis and/or extensive pelvic radiation. J Urol 150:46–50

Lund F (1978) cystectomy following full course irradiation. In: Pavone-Macaluso M, Smith PH, Edsmyr F (eds) Bladder tumors and other topics in urologic oncology. Plenum Press, New York, pp 287–289

Martins FE, Boyd SD (1995) Post-operative risk factors associated with artificial urinary sphincter infection-erosion. Br J Urol 75:354–358

Matthews PN, Minton MJ, Haw M, Philip PF (1987) The role of partial cystectomy in the treatment of recurrent invasive bladder cancer following radiotherapy. Br J Urol 60:132–135

McDougal WS (1992) Metabolic complications of urinary intestinal diversion. J Urol 147:1199–1208

Miller LS, Johnson DE (1973) Megavoltage irradiation for bladder cancer: Alone, postoperative or preoperative? Seventh National Cancer Conference Lippincott, Philadelphia, p 771

Montana GS, Fowler WC (1989) Carcinoma of the cervix: analysis of bladder and rectal radiation dose and complications. Int J Radiat Oncol Biol Phys 16:95–100

Nissenkorn I, Baniel J, Slucker D, Servadio C, Winkler H (1990) Comparison between short-course high-dose preoperative irradiation with immediate radical cystectomy and salvage cystectomy after full-dose irradiation. Eur Urol 18:23–26

Orsatti M, Curotto A, Canobbio L, et al. (1995) Alternating chemo-radiotherapy in bladder cancer: a conservative approach. Int J Radiat Oncol Biol Phys 33:173–178

Parliament M, Genest P, Girard A, Gerig L, Prefontaine M (1989) Obstructive ureteropathy following radiation therapy for carcinoma of the cervix. Gynecol Oncol 33:237–240

Perez CA, Breaux S, Bedwinek JM, Madoc Jones H, Camel HM, Purdy JA, Walz BJ (1984) Radiation therapy alone in the treatment of carcinoma of the uterine cervix. II. Analysis of complications. Cancer 54:235–246

Pizzocaro G, Pisani E, Dormia E, Piva L, Maggioni A, Minervini G (1990) Neoadjuvant medium-dose methotrexate, cisplatin in category T3b-T4a (NOMO) bladder cancer. Prog Clin Biol Res 353:129–136

Radomski SB, Herschorn S (1992) Risk factors associated with perile prosthesis infection. J Urol 148:383–385

Rotman M, Macchia R, Silverstein M, et al. (1987) Treatment of advanced bladder carcinoma with irradiation and concomitant 5-fluorouracil infusion. Cancer 59:710–714

Rubin P, Wasserman TH (1988) International clinical trials in radiation oncology. The late effects of toxicity scoring. Int J Radiat Oncol Biol Phys 14:2

Schaeffer AJ, Grayhack JT, Merrill JM, Kies MS, Bulkley GJ, Shetty RM, Chmiel JS (1984) Adjuvant doxorubicin hydrochloride and radiation in stage D bladder cancer: a preliminary report. J Urol 131:1073–1076

Schmidt JD, Hawtrey CE, Buchsbaum HJ (1975) Transverse colon conduit: a preferred method of urinary diversion for radiation-treated pelvic malignancies. J Urol 113:308

Shipley WU, Rose MA, Perrone TL, Mannix CM, Heney NM, Prout GR Jr (1985) Full-dose irradiation for patients with invasive bladder carcinoma: clinical and histological factors prognostic of improved survival. J Urol 134:679–683

Skinner DG, Lieskovsky G (1988) Management of invasive and high-grade bladder cancer. In: Skinner DG, Lieskovsky G (eds) Diagnosis and management of genitourinary cancer. Saunders, Philadelphia, pp 295–312

Smith JA Jr, Whitmore WF Jr (1981) Salvage cystectomy for bladder cancer after failure of definitive irradiation. J Urol 125:643–645

Srougi M, Simon SD (1994) Primary methotrexte, vinblastine, doxorubicin and cisplatin chemotherapy and bladder preservation in locally invasive bladder cancer: a 5-year followup. J Urol 151:593–597

Stewart FA (1986) Mechanism of bladder damage and repair after treatment with radiation and cytostatic drugs. Br J Cancer Suppl 7:280–291

Swanson DA, von Eschenbach AC, Bracken RB, Johnson DE (1981) Salvage cystectomy for bladder carcinoma. Cancer 47:2275–2279

Villar A, Munoz J, Aguilo F, Arellano A, Cambray M, Serrallach N (1987) External beam irradiation for T1, T2–3 and T4 transitional cell carcinoma of the urinary bladder. Radiother Oncol 9:209–215

Wallace DM, Bloom HJG (1976) The management of deeply infiltrating (T3) bladder carcinoma: controlled trial of radical radiotherapy and radical cystectomy (first report). Br J Urol 48:587

Whitmore WF Jr, Batata M (1984) Status of integrated irradiation and cystectomy for bladder cancer. Urol Clin North Arn 11:681–691

Zincke H, Sen SE, Hahn RG, Keating JP (1988) Neoadjuvant chemotherapy for locally advanced transitional cell carcinoma of the bladder: do local findings suggest a potential for salvage of the bladder? Mayo Clin Proc 63:16–22

25 Treatment-Related Complications for Bladder Carcinoma: Radical Surgery Versus Bladder-Preserving Techniques

B.J. Costleigh, W.A. Longton, L.W. Brady, C.T. Miyamoto, J.E. Freire, B. Micaily, and F. Farzin

CONTENTS

25.1
Introduction

The morbidity and mortality of bladder carcinoma treatment are dependent upon which treatment modalities are employed. The treatment should be chosen to best fit the stage of disease. The standard treatment regimen for in situ or early-stage bladder cancer has been transurethral resection of the bladder tumor (TURBT). This treatment is given with or without intravesicular chemotherapy or BCG therapy for many years and is very tolerable with regard to morbidity of normal tissues.

B.J. Costleigh, MD, The Cancer Center at Kent General Hospital, Delaware, USA and Department of Radiation Oncology and Nuclear Medicine, Allegheny University Hospitals, Center City, Mail Stop 200, Broad & Vine Sts., Philadelphia, PA 19102-1192, USA
W.A. Longton, MD, L.W. Brady, MD, Professor, C.T. Miyamoto, MD, J.E. Friere, MD, B. Micaily, MD, F. Farzin, MD, Department of Radiation Oncology and Nuclear Medicine, Allegheny University Hospitals, Center City, Mail Stop 200, Broad & Vine Sts., Philadelphia, PA 19102-1192, USA

For muscle-invasive bladder carcinoma, the traditional standard of care has been cystectomy. In recent years, treatment of this tumor has evolved from the single-modality therapy to a multimodality treatment regimen including TURBT followed by combination chemoradiation in an attempt at bladder preservation. The trend is to reserve cystectomy for combined modality treatment failure.

In order to truly evaluate the new multimodality treatment methods, we need to examine the efficacy as well as the treatment morbidity and mortality and the effect on quality of life. As the treatment changes from a single local therapy which involves only pelvic morbidity, to a combination therapy, systemic as well as pelvic side-effects become evident. We will review the complications related to the different individual treatment regimens as well as combinations of various extents of surgery, radiation, and chemotherapy.

25.2
Treatment of Noninvasive Carcinoma

For early-stage carcinoma including Tis, Ta, and low-grade T1 lesions, TURBT with or without instillation of BCG/chemotherapy remains a very well tolerated treatment of choice. Complications from surgical intervention are directly related to the extent of the procedure. With TURBT and intravesicular therapy the patient usually retains normal bladder function. Side-effects are usually transient and local. They may include cystitis, dysuria, gross or microscopic hematuria, and incontinence. The intravesical therapy may cause a severe mucositis reaction of the bladder causing hematuria, dysuria, incontinence, or severe pain. There may be systemic absorption to various extents causing reactions such as malaise or bone marrow suppression in up to 20% of patients. TURBT and intravesical therapy can be repeated if needed with little in the way of consequences. However, with multiple repeated treatments of this nature, severe scarring may lead to symptomatic bladder contracture in up to 15% of patients, possibly necessitating cystectomy.

25.3
Surgery for Invasive Bladder Cancer

Until recently, radical cystectomy or, in a few cases, partial cystectomy has been the most effective treatment for invasive bladder carcinoma. However, while radical cystectomy alone can locally control disease in up to 90% of patients, it fails to cure more than 50%, in part because of rapidly occurring metastatic spread. In addition, radical cystectomy cannot be performed without risk of complications with subsequent poor quality of life due to the resulting morbidity. With cystectomy, the operative mortality is a concern, death occurring in 0%–5% of patients in modern series. The standard operative risks include small bowel, colon, or ureteral injury, urethral strictures, sepsis, fistula formation, and leg and genital edema. Since radical prostatectomy is part of a radical cystectomy, impotency can also occur in more than 95% of men. More importantly, the patient will be left with an ileostomy if radical cystectomy is performed, which may greatly impact on quality of life. However, new surgical procedures such as Walsh's potency-sparing procedure can spare potency in 30%–40% of patients. Also, construction of continent diversions with ileal or cecal pouches being anastomosed to the urethra, and use of the Valsalva maneuver to empty, permits near-normal voiding and substantial improvement of quality of life. However, these procedures can only be performed successfully by expert surgeons experienced in these new procedures. Even with these new procedures, the high distant metastasis rate is unchanged and will still result in the standard operative morbidity and mortality. Hence, we need to look for possible alternative modalities or combinations which not only will have equal or better results with regard to local control and disease-free survival, but also will have acceptable and preferably reduced morbidity while maintaining the patient's own functional bladder. Given that invasive carcinoma eventually develops in up to 50% of patients with noninvasive cancers, there is a need to explore the nonradical surgery techniques which can be tolerated despite the mucosal damage caused by previous TURBT and intravesicular therapy.

25.4
Radiation Therapy

When radiation is employed to manage bladder cancer, external beam irradiation (EBRT) and/or brachytherapy may be used. Each of these will account for different morbidity due to the differences in the dose distribution. Irradiation via brachytherapy demonstrates a much more rapid fall off in dose compared with EBRT. This is due to the diminished source-target distance seen with brachytherapy. Therefore, while brachytherapy may concentrate its morbidity of normal tissues in close proximity to the tumor site, EBRT may cause morbidity both in the immediate tumor area and in the surrounding tissues. Complication rates are dependent upon many factors. There is a correlation with increasing dose, dose per fraction, and radiation target volume. Bladder complications occur less often than bowel complications with the same dose due to a higher tolerance of the normal bladder tissue (7500 vs 7000 cGy, respectively, using standard 180- to 200-cGy fractions). Sophisticated treatment planning, e.g., using computerized axial tomography-guided three-dimensional treatment planning with conformal radiation, allows more precise targeting of the structures designated to receive the prescribed dose while the normal tissues are spared to a greater degree.

Patient- and tumor-related parameters must be considered. Certain medical conditions such as collagen vascular disease, hypertension, diabetes, diverticulitis, other gastrointestinal diseases, and previous abdominal or pelvic surgery may all act to enhance the radiation-induced morbidity. Larger tumors will have already caused damage to the bladder integrity and, hence, increase the risk as well. Increased risk of postradiation sequelae is evident if radiation is preceded by ulceration, infection, fibrotic changes from multiple TURBTs, or intravesicular instillations of chemotherapy or biologic therapy. While, in the relatively normal functioning treatment-naive bladder, the risk of major sequelae is greatly decreased.

25.4.1
Acute Toxicity

Radiation morbidity of normal structures can be classified as acute (early) when it occurs during or up to 3 months after radiation treatment. The severity is related to the total dose and overall treatment time.

It is also associated with the location and extent of the tumor and with treatment technique. Patients with tumors invading the trigone or located near the bladder neck are more likely to develop acute irritative symptoms than those with small lesions involving lateral walls.

The majority of patients treated with EBRT will experience acute side-effects related to the lower gastrointestinal and urinary tract. Early morbidity of the bladder with EBRT results from transient mucosal erythema usually beginning within 24h. This and the mild mucositis seen as inflammation and blanching of irritated mucositis at 3–4 weeks usually pass unnoticed. A decreased bladder capacity is noted due to the irritability. All these side-effects may worsen as the dose increases. Severe acute reactions are not common but can occur at cancericidal doses and usually subside within 3–4 weeks after EBRT has been completed. The resulting symptoms may include frequency, urge incontinence, and dysuria. Bladder mucosa desquamation is rare. Some degree of diarrhea and rectal or anal irritation is to be expected during the latter portion of the treatment course and these problems are usually easily controlled with appropriate conservative measures.

25.4.2
Late Complications

Chronic (late) morbidity is that which occurs 3 or more months after completion of radiation therapy. Such complications may not resolve or may occur intermittently on a long-term basis and are related to total dose and dose per fraction. Late reactions to the bladder result from many factors. Interstitial fibrosis and contracture in the heavily irradiated tissue, along with obliterative endarteritis and telangiectases, are seen. After many months, the epithelium appears thin, pale, and atrophic with possible local hyperplasia. The late reactions are similar to changes seen in other highly irradiated tissues. It is often difficult to differentiate these late effects from tumor recurrence, both clinically and by cystoscopic visualization. Late radiation toxicities can be manifested as painless hematuria, chronic increased frequency, bladder neck obstruction, and, in the most severe cases, intractable bleeding (2%) or a contracted bladder (4%). Chronic intestinal toxicity is manifested by persistent diarrhea, rectal bleeding, or bowel obstruction. Fistulas are uncommon in the absence of recurrent tumor or surgical intervention.

Fortunately, severe toxicity is rare with the use of modern treatment. Late morbidity is affected by the condition of the bladder and the surrounding tissues. The bladder, heavily treated by prior radiation with repeated transurethral surgery or intravesicular chemotherapy, is more likely to develop radiation cystitis. Up to 50% of the reported chronic complications are actually due to recurrent tumor rather than the radiation itself. Therefore, biopsy is needed if late sequelae occur.

Various morbidity scales are used to rate the severity of the complications secondary to irradiation. However, there are no standard scales. In general, minor complications (grades 1 and 2) are those requiring conservative medical management, while major side-effects (grades 3 and 4) are those requiring hospitalization, intense medical intervention, or surgical management.

25.5
External Beam Radiation Therapy

Therapeutic modalities other than radical surgery, such as definitive radiation therapy alone, achieve locally control in 30%–50% of patients. Again, there is a high distant metastasis rate equivalent to that with radical surgery.

The treatment volume for definitive EBRT includes the bladder as well as the pelvic structures for the first portion of definitive treatment. The tumor itself, neighboring bladder, and select peribladder tissues will receive full-dose radiation. The total dose of 65–70 Gy given for curative radiation therapy was developed historically because of normal tissue limitations. Since complications may occur in any irradiated tissues, radiation-related morbidity presents as a wide spectrum of clinical syndromes, with potential injury to any structure in the pelvis. The severe late morbidity for radiation therapy alone has been shown to be very acceptable. Overall, there is about a 0%–11% risk of chronic bowel or bladder morbidity after full-dose EBRT with standard fractionation (Table 25.1).

25.5.1
EBRT Studies

SHIELS et al. (1986) reported on 88 patients with a 12.5% total incidence of late bladder complications after definitive EBRT. Of these, 55% had persistent or recurrent tumor as per cystoscopy with biopsy, re-

Table 25.1. Late grade 3 and 4 complications after standard fractionated EBRT alone

	Total	Contracted bladder	Bowel
SHIELS et al. (1986)	5.7%	0	–
ABRATT et al. (1983)	0	–	0
LYNCH et al. (1992)	0	0	0
SHIPLEY et al. (1985)	11%	–	–

Table 25.2. Late grade 3 and 4 complications using altered fractionation radiation therapy

	Total	Contracted bladder	Bowel
ABRATT et al. (1983)	–	–	17%
Cox et al. (1988)	10%	–	–
HORWICH (1991)	–	20%	0
COLE et al. (1992)	0	–	0

sulting in a 5.7% overall chronic bladder morbidity due to radiation. None experienced contracted bladder severe enough to require cystectomy. No fistula formation was noted. Cystectomies were only performed for residual or recurrent disease.

ABRATT et al. (1983) retrospectively reviewed 69 patients treated definitively with radiation of varying fractionation regimens for T2 and T3 tumors. While 4 of 24 patients (17%) treated with 3.47 Gy per day to 48.6 Gy developed severe late bowel complications. No patients treated with standard fractionation experienced late bowel complications.

LYNCH et al. (1992) reported on the quality of life after radical radiotherapy for bladder cancer. Seventy-two patients treated with radical radiation therapy for muscle-invasive bladder cancer were compared to 55 patients with no history of prior urinary or bowel disease. No significant difference was noted in subjective complaints of urinary or bowel symptomatology. However, there was a mild trend toward increased symptoms in the irradiated group. Also, in patients requiring salvage cystectomy after radiation failure, there was an acceptable morbidity without a significantly higher complication rate compared to cystectomy performed on a radiation-naive bladder.

In a report by SHIPLEY et al. (1985) it was shown that delivering 1.80 Gy per day to a total of 65–70 Gy resulted in 11% of patients developing severe complications leading to incontinence or requiring surgical intervention.

Most reports using EBRT for bladder carcinoma do not describe resulting potency rates. However, extrapolating from EBRT data for prostate cancer, impotency rates due to radiation for bladder cancer should be approximately 20%.

25.5.2
Altered Fractionation Radiation Regimens

Altered fractionation schedules including hyperfractionation and accelerated fractionation are nicely tolerated without significantly increasing late morbidity risk (Table 25.2).

The Radiation Therapy Oncology Group (RTOG) hyperfractionation protocol tolerance of normal pelvic tissues was reported by Cox et al. (1988). Radiation was delivered in fractions of 1.2 cGy b.i.d. to a total whole pelvic dose of 5040 cGy with reduced volume fields to 6000, 6480 or 6960 cGy. The cumulative probability of these groups having a grade III or grade IV late complication was 10% at 24 months. In the 6960 cGy total dose group, the cumulative probability of grade III or IV late reactions was 11% at 24 months. In comparing patients treated with standard fractionation to 60 Gy, there was no suggestion of any deleterious effects from hyperfractionated radiation to the pelvis.

A study of accelerated fractionation for bladder cancer was reported by COLE et al. (1992). Patients were treated with 1.8–2.0 Gy b.i.d. with a wide field to 40–44 Gy and a bladder-only field to 54–64 Gy. As expected, grade II acute large bowel side-effects were seen in 52% of patients, grade III in 26%, grade IV in 8%, and grade V in 4%. With regard to the acute urinary side-effects, 30% had grade II, 17% had grade III, and none had grade IV or V. Late radiation morbidity in patients surviving more than 6 months was very low; 12% experienced grade I bowel toxicity and 12% and 18% had grade I and grade II urinary toxicity, respectively. There were no late skin effects.

In a study by HORWICH (1991) using accelerated fractionation, there was actually a lower incidence of acute bowel toxicity. Thirty percent of the patients had grade II gastrointestinal effects and there were no grade III effects. Grade II bladder toxicity was seen in 10% and grade III in 20%.

25.6
Photon Radiation Versus Neutron or Pi-meson Radiation Therapy

In an attempt to improve the outcome with radiation, alternative energies were tried. Unfortunately,

Table 25.3. Radiation-induced late complications: photon versus neutron radiation

	Bladder (%)		Bowel (%)	
	Neutron	Photon	Neutron	Photon
Duncan et al. (1986)	59	40	33	8
Russell et al. (1989)	45	10	38	25

Table 25.4. Comparison of brachytherapy, EBRT, and surgery: late grade 2–4 complications

	GI tract	Bladder	Ureter
Moderate-dose EBRT + brachytherapy	7%	0	0
High-dose EBRT	9%	21%	0
Moderate-dose EBRT	10%	1%	4%

this was also associated with a substantially increased incidence of late complications (Table 25.3) and such treatment should not be used in the treatment of bladder carcinoma.

Duncan et al. (1986) analyzed radiation-related morbidity in a trial of neutron therapy for bladder carcinoma. The acute reactions after photon therapy were significantly worse than with neutron therapy (severe bladder reactions occurred in 46% and 11% of patients, respectively). Severe acute bowel reactions were observed in 8.5% of patients after photons, compared with 3.8% after neutron therapy. However, severe late reactions were significantly worse after neutrons (59% vs 40% in the bladder and 33% vs 8% in the bowel).

Russell et al. (1989) also evaluated the use of neutron radiation therapy for bladder carcinoma. Late morbidity in normal tissues following neutrons exceeded those experienced after photon irradiation and led to an unexpectedly high rate of treatment-related morbidity and mortality (78% vs 38%). Specifically, the late bowel morbidity was 45% vs 10% and late bladder contracture was seen in 38% of patients treated with neutrons versus 25% of those treated with photons. This may be related to the neutron beam's poor depth dose characteristics and a lack of differential in radio-responsiveness to neutrons between bladder tumor and adjacent normal tissues. Also, in the photon group, morbidity was generally limited to one tissue while 45% of patients receiving neutrons had multiple organ toxicity. As a result of the higher neutron-associated morbidity, more treatment-related deaths were attributed to neutrons (36% vs 3%).

Studer et al. (1993) reported on the use of pi-meson in the treatment of bladder cancer. The side-effects during the treatment were not clinically significant. However, a steep dose-response curve for late side-effects was observed, with severe complications in 64% of patients who received 3600 cGy or more of the pi-meson treatment. Forty-eight percent of patients developed a contracted bladder, 90% of whom had been treated with a dose of 3600 cGy or

more. Only one patient who received a dose of 3600 cGy developed no side-effects.

25.7
Brachytherapy

Compared with EBRT, interstitial brachytherapy at the same dose can give a higher local complication rate. However, moderate-dose brachytherapy in conjunction with EBRT can be given safely and does not appear to have an increased risk of late morbidity (Table 25.4). There is a risk of ulceration of the bladder mucosa which is not generally seen with EBRT alone.

Grossman et al. (1993) reported on seven patients undergoing treatment of bladder cancer with iridium-192 implantation after EBRT (45 Gy with EBRT and 20 Gy with implant). Although there was no long-term bladder toxicity attributable to the radiation, 29% of patients had immediate and delayed postoperative complications, including prolonged urinary drainage from the implant site, wound dehiscence, and pulmonary embolism postoperatively. Diarrhea was seen in one patient.

Straus et al. (1988) reported on results after interstitial iridium-192 with EBRT in 14 patients. The severity and frequency of treatment complications were minimal. Grade III or IV morbidity was seen in 14%. Only one patient required cystectomy for a contracted bladder. Less severe complications included transient radiation cystitis (21%) and moderate scrotal and penile edema (7%).

Deneve et al. (1992) compared the results of interstitial brachytherapy with EBRT to those of EBRT with or without cystectomy for stage T1 and T2 carcinomas of the bladder. EBRT-related morbidity greater than grade I was seen in 28% of the definitive, high-dose radiation group, 9% of the moderate-dose EBRT with brachytherapy group, and 14% of the moderate-dose EBRT with cystectomy group. Among those treated with cesium-137 implantation, ulceration of the bladder mucosa was observed in

30% and bladder calculi in 17%. In patients treated with radiation and surgery, gastrointestinal complications were most pronounced. However, in the patients treated with only external radiation, bladder complications were most notable.

25.8
Radiation Therapy and Cystectomy

Due to the poor disease-free survival after radical cystectomy, particularly in those at high risk for recurrence, subsequent full-dose radiation is often employed. Conversely, radiation is often used prior to radical surgery to allow for pathologic downstaging for the more locally advanced bladder cancers. Combinations of high-dose radiation and radical surgery may increase the risk of chronic complications if given inappropriately. Using radiation with standard fractionation to a moderate total dose can easily be performed with minimal long-term side-effects (Table 25.5). Additional tolerance can be achieved if radiation and surgery are separated by at least 4 weeks. This has been well demonstrated through multiple reports.

The results of definitive and preoperative radiation therapy in 390 patients were reported by MAMEGHAN et al. (1991). Eighty-seven patients received preoperative radiation followed by cystectomy and 303 patients received definitive radiation. The cystectomy group received up to 5000 cGy, while the definitive radiation therapy group received 6500 cGy. Most patients experienced acute radiation reactions in the bladder and bowel which were easily controlled conservatively. Only 11 patients experienced grade II or III late complica-

tions. The severe complication rate in bladder and bowel, after definitive radiation therapy, was 1.2% and 4.1%, respectively. After preoperative radiation therapy and cystectomy, the severe bowel complication rate was 8%. This incidence of severe complications was considered acceptably low and patients treated definitively with radiation retained acceptable bladder function.

A comparison of preoperative radiation therapy regimens for bladder carcinoma was carried out by SPERA et al. (1987). Group 1 received 4000 cGy in 4 weeks prior to cystectomy. Group 2 received 2000 cGy in 1 week prior to surgery, and group 3 received 500 cGy on the day prior to surgery with or without postoperative radiation therapy. Upon evaluation of the morbidity, the incidence of both ureteroenteral strictures and stomal complications was found to be higher in the 2000-cGy group than in those patients treated with the other regimens (27% in the 2000-cGy group, 19% in the 4000-cGy group, and 4% in the 500-cGy group). The overall incidence of bowel complications was similar in all groups (11%–13%). The disease-free survival for the 4000 cGy in 4 weeks group was 63%. On the other hand, the disease-free survival for the 2000 cGy in 1 week group was 21%, with suboptimal late complication rates. As a result, the 2000 cGy in 1 week regimen should be avoided.

Combined preoperative and postoperative radiation was analyzed by MOHIUDDIN et al. (1985). Ninety-two patients were given a preoperative radiation dose of 500 cGy to the whole pelvis on the day of or before cystectomy. Patients with tumor size T2 or greater were given 4500 cGy in 5 weeks postoperatively. No complications were observed following low-dose preoperative radiation. The major compli-

Table 25.5. Severe bowel toxicity after combination EBRT and cystectomy

	% Complications
MAMEGHAN et al.	
High-dose EBRT	4
Moderate-dose EBRT + radical cystectomy	8
KONNAK and GROSSMAN (1985)	
High-dose EBRT + radical cystectomy	6
KOPELSON and HEANEY (1983)	
High-dose EBRT + TURBT/partial cystectomy	0
High-dose EBRT + radical cystectomy	67
FREIHA and FAYSAL (1983)	
High-dose EBRT + radical cystectomy	25
REISINGER et al. (1992)	
Radical cystectomy alone	8
Moderate EBRT + radical cystectomy	37

cations observed were the result of surgery and/or postoperative irradiation. The overall incidence of major complications was 15%. These essentially consisted of small bowel obstruction, anastomotic leaks, and peritonitis. For patients who did or did not receive postoperative adjuvant radiation, the complication rates were 17% and 16%, respectively.

KOPELSON and HEANEY (1983) reported on postoperative radiation therapy for muscle-invading bladder carcinoma. Of the seven patients alive after 2 years, two developed late small bowel complications including chronic diarrhea or obstruction. The risk of severe complications is related to the degree of the surgical procedure. The small bowel complications were seen in two of three patients who underwent radical cystectomy, while patients who underwent partial cystectomy or TURBT experienced no severe complications.

KONNAK and GROSSMAN (1985) reported on 18 salvage cystectomies following definitive radiation therapy failure for bladder carcinoma. Major early complications were seen in 28%, including rectal lacerations, small bowel obstruction, ureteral leak, ureterosigmoidostomy leak, myocardial infarction, and pelvic abscess. Late complications included ureteral stenosis in 11%, stomal stenosis in 6%, and small bowel obstruction in 6%.

FREIHA and FAYSAL (1983) reported on salvage cystectomy after radiation failure. All patients had failure or recurrence after 7000 cGy. The 40 cystectomies performed yielded a 15% mortality (5% operative and 10% postoperative). Complications were seen in 40% of patients. The early postoperative complications were the same as those encountered with any major surgery, including systemic sepsis, myocardial infarction, and pelvic abscesses. There was a 25% overall late postoperative complication rate which was related to surgery on irradiated bowel.

REISINGER et al. (1992) reported on combined pre- and postoperative adjuvant radiation therapy for bladder cancer. Patients received 500 cGy preoperatively on the day of or before cystectomy, with or without postoperative radiation to 40–45 Gy with conventional fractionation. Bowel obstructions developed in 8% of patients who received no postoperative radiation therapy versus 37% who did receive radiation. Genitourinary complications were similar in the two groups, 13% versus 10%, respectively. Although combined pre- and postoperative radiation therapy for favorable stages of bladder cancer is associated with a better than 50% 5-year survival rate, the bowel toxicity is unacceptably high.

25.9
Radiation Therapy and Intravesical Therapy

LAMM et al. (1989) reviewed 2602 radiation-naive patients for complications of intravesical BCG therapy, and found the most common side-effect to be self-limited, irritative voiding symptoms, including dysuria and frequency. Such symptoms occurred in 90% of patients. Other complications included hematuria requiring catheterization or transfusion in 1%, skin rash in 0.3%, ureteral obstruction in 0.3%, orchitis in 0.4%, bladder contracture in 0.2%, and arthritis or arthralgia in 0.5%. Fever greater than 103°F was reported in 2.9%, BCG pneumonitis or hepatitis in 0.7%, hypotension in 0.1%, and cytopenia in 0.1%.

Complications of mitomycin C include bladder irritation, which occurs in 10%–15% of patients and palmar or generalized rash. Bladder contracture has occasionally been reported after intravesicular mitomycin C. Significant systemic side-effects of mitomycin C, including bone marrow depression, were not observed, primarily due to the inability of the body to absorb this from the bladder.

Radiation therapy can induce late changes in the bladder mucosa and could theoretically alter the safety and morbidity of intravesically instilled agents. It was traditionally thought that the mucosal changes may interfere with the absorption or viability of the mechanism of action, metabolism, or elimination of the intravesicular agent. This was shown not to be the situation by PISTERS et al. (1991).

PISTERS et al. (1991) used intravesical BCG or mitomycin for recurrent in situ bladder carcinoma after external pelvic radiation. These results are similar to those reported by LAMM et al. (1989), with hematuria usually not occurring until after 6000 cGy. After BCG therapy, 90% of the patients had irritative voiding symptoms including frequency and dysuria; however, these symptoms resolved on their own after 2–3 days. Twenty-five percent developed gross hematuria, also resolving within 1–3 days without intervention, and one patient required catheterization for clot evacuation. Ten percent of the patients were symptomatic from bladder contracture after intravesical BCG. The most severe side-effect of BCG therapy was fever greater than 103°F reported in 15% of the patients. No sepsis, hepatitis, pneumonitis, cytopenia, or death was related to intravesical therapy and no side-effect was severe enough to cause discontinuation of the therapy regimen. No serious side-effects were noted in any patient receiving intravesical mitomycin after full-dose radiation.

ABRATT et al. (1991) treated muscle-invading bladder cancer with radiation with or without oral and intravesicular misonidazole. Two of 53 patients had grade III late bowel complications, both of whom were in the misonidazole arm. Also, both of these patients underwent salvage cystectomy and subsequently required colostomies for bowel obstruction, equating to a 9% late complication rate. An additional 9% in the misonidazole arm developed wound sepsis following salvage cystectomy. The overall complete response and 5-year survival rates were not improved with the use of oral and intravesicular misonidazole with radiation therapy. The use of unconventional radiation fractionation (misonidazole plus 12 Gy in two fractions over 2 weeks vs 20 Gy in ten fractions over 2 weeks) may have accounted for the increased bowel morbidity in the misonidazole arm. No patients had severe late bladder complications and no misonidazole-related toxicity was noted.

25.10
Systemic Chemotherapy

The most effective chemotherapy for bladder cancer is cisplatin. This has been shown to yield response rates of about 20%–40%, but a continuous complete response rate of only about 10%. Adding methotrexate to the regimen can allow for a 30% continuous complete response rate. Addition of some of the less effective drugs, such as adriamycin and vinblastine, may improve the complete response to a slightly greater degree. With such treatment, local recurrence or persistence continues to be a major problem. Unlike with radiation or surgery, morbidity from chemotherapy is usually systemic and is related to the number of drugs given and their intensity. Bone marrow suppression is of most concern and is seen to some degree in the majority of patients. Depending on which chemotherapeutic agent is used, organ-specific side-effects need to be considered. These include cardiac, renal, hepatic, and bladder effects. Cytotoxic chemotherapy is known to enhance the mucosal reaction and historically has been thought to limit the radiation tolerance. Limiting the dose of chemotherapy (i.e., 70–100 mg/m^2 for cisplatin) will allow for good efficacy while avoiding toxicity requiring decreased cycles of the chemotherapy or limitation of the radiation dose.

Cisplatin, when used alone, appears very tolerable. However, when other drugs are added, the systemic toxicity rises (Table 25.6). This was clearly demonstrated in randomized studies comparing single-agent cisplatin with combination regimens using cisplatin for advanced diseases.

Severe toxicity rates for cisplatin alone versus CisCA combination were reported by KHANDEKAR et al. (1985) to be 24% and 43% (8% fatal), respectively. Conversely, in the M.D. Anderson experience reported by LOGOTHETIS et al. (1985), CisCA appeared less toxic, with no fatalities. However, clinical hearing loss was seen in 11% and symptomatic neuropathy in 7%. An increase in mucositis (0% vs 20%) and grade 3/4 bone marrow depression (2% vs 27%) was seen when methotrexate was added to cisplatin (HILLCOAT et al. 1989). The use of MVAC (methotrexate, vinblastine, adriamycin, and cisplatin) with radiation therapy was reported by TANNOCK et al. (1989). It was found that this regimen was associated with severe toxicity. Neutropenia was seen in 90%, 41% of the patients experienced neutropenic sepsis, and 54% required hospitalization for management of toxic complications. The probability of requiring hospitalization tended to be greater for patients with metastatic or recurrent disease (58%) than for those receiving neoadjuvant or postoperative MVAC (37%). Pulmonary embolism was seen in 6%, and 2% experienced a deep vein thrombosis. One drug-related death from sepsis was noted. SOLOWAY et al. (1989,1993) reported the effects of MVAC chemotherapy with radical cystectomy for bladder carcinoma. The severe toxicity and mortality for perioperative chemotherapy were significant. Patients regularly required hospi-

Table 25.6. Systemic chemotherapy: grade 3 and 4 toxicity

	Cisplatin alone (%)	Cisplatin-based combination chemotherapy
KHANDEKAR et al. (1985)		
Overall	24	43
HILLCOAT et al. (1989)		
Hematologic	2	27
Mucositis	0	20
TANNOCK et al. (1989)		
Hematologic	–	41
SHIPLEY et al. (1987)		
Hematologic	4	–
Renal	1	–
CHAUVET et al. (1993)		
Hematologic	1	–
MGH update (1996)	0	13

talization because of nadir sepsis or severe leukopenia. Conversely, Memorial Sloan-Kettering Hospital reported good tolerance with an MVAC regimen, with a 12% rate of nadir sepsis. For patients who develop distant failure (particularly low-volume disease) after definitive therapy, MVAC may be beneficial. Although there is a limitation due to morbidity, tolerance is acceptable in light of the potential long-term benefits. However, caution is suggested in the widespread application of this regimen.

25.11
Radiation Therapy and Systemic Chemotherapy

There has been substantial recent investigation into the efficacy of combining chemotherapy and radiation therapy as the primary modality for invasive disease. This combination has multiple benefits. The chemotherapeutic agents alone can help reduce the risk of distant disease. However, cisplatin and 5-fluorouracil (5-FU) among others, may also act as radiosensitizers to offer a greatly increased probability of complete response (25% for cisplatin-based chemotherapy alone, 45% for EBRT alone, and 70% or more with chemoradiation, particularly after TURBT), with improved local control and survival compared to either modality alone. With chemotherapy and radiation having different morbidity, the combination, if delivered in an appropriate schedule, will allow for a low local morbidity which is possibly no higher than with radiation alone, particularly if CMV chemotherapy is used as opposed to the more toxic MVAC regimen. Also, a decrease in total dose of radiation or chemotherapy may not be needed.

Perhaps an effective chemoradiation regimen after maximum TURBT would lessen the need for routine use of radical surgery, thus allowing patients the chance to maintain their own functional bladder. Recent protocols using integrated and well-tolerated chemoradiation (Table 25.7) seem to show promise and confirm this hypothesis. The local control rate appears at least equal to that achieved by cystectomy, with improvement in survival rate. Moreover, 60%–70% of patients will also retain their own functional bladder.

In the First National Bladder Cancer Group report by SHIPLEY et al. (1987) on the use of single-agent cisplatin and full-dose radiation therapy, neutropenic sepsis was reported in only 4% of cases. Though a large proportion of cisplatin-treated pa-

Table 25.7. Severe late radiation-induced toxicity using bladder-sparing combined modality therapy

	Contracted bladder (%)	Bowel toxicity (%)
KACHNIC et al. (1996)	0	0
MGH update (1996)	0	–
DUNST et al. (1994)	1.6	–
RAGHAVEN et al. (1988)	0	–
TESTER et al. (1993)	1.4	1.4
HOUSSET et al. (1993)	0	0
ROTMAN et al. (1990)	–	5
RUSSELL et al. (1988)	0	2.5

tients (6%–30%) experienced a rise in serum creatinine, irreversible renal failure becomes uncommon with good hydration and was seen in only 1 of 70 patients. Patient acceptability is largely governed by the acute toxicity of cisplatin, in particular, emesis. The discomfort which such acute toxicity can cause is evident in a report by ROBERTS et al. (1991), in which the combination of cisplatin and methotrexate produced no life-threatening toxicities, yet 12% of patients refused any further treatment.

Results of combined radiation and cisplatin in 69 patients for locally advanced bladder carcinoma were reported by CHAUVET et al. (1993). Six patients did not receive full-dose radiation (60 Gy) to the bladder due to acute genitourinary toxicity. An additional 16.7% required a break in EBRT for more than 15 days due to acute toxicity. Seventy-eight percent of the patients received the planned two courses of cisplatin. Reasons for discontinuation of chemotherapy after the first course were transient elevation in the serum creatinine (6%), hematologic toxicity (1%), death from intercurrent disease (1%), decreased performance status (10%), and patient refusal (3%). One treatment-related death was noted. Most patients experienced manageable grade II nausea and vomiting. Late toxicity was infrequent. One percent of patients experienced ureteral stenosis. Grade II chronic proctitis and cystitis were seen in 3% and 6% of patients, respectively. Persistent increase in serum creatinine was seen in four patients. The complete response rate for cisplatin was 76%, which was comparable to rates previously reported in the literature.

KACHNIC et al. (1996) reported on the long-term tolerance to combined modality treatment for bladder consevation in female patients with invasive bladder carcinoma. The treatment regimen consisted of maximal TURBT followed by induction MCV chemotherapy, then cisplatin in conjunction with external beam radiation therapy. Of the 21 patients available for a subjective survey, none experienced new urinary incontinence or dysuria; 90% actually reported improved or unchanged bladder capacity and/or function. There was no reported bowel or sexual dysfunction. Overall, 67% of the female patients, including most of the long-term survivors, retained their bladder with excellent function.

In updated Massachusetts General Hospital results using neoadjuvant CMV and concomitant cisplatin with radiation, systemic complications were as before, bone marrow depression occurring in about 60%, irreversible renal failure in 2%, and acute mild bladder and bowel toxicity in about 60% and 35%, respectively. Severe methotrexate-induced mucositis was seen in 13%. This experience is very favorable, with no cystectomy required for severe bladder symptoms in 71 patients.

DUNST et al. (1994) reported that 3 of 192 patients required cystectomy for bladder contracture following concomitant radiation to 50 Gy and cisplatin. RAGHAVAN et al. (1988) reported that none of the 15 elderly patients developed bladder contracture or proctitis. In this study, it was shown that single-agent cisplatin at a dose of 80–100 mg/m^2 in conjunction with EBRT can be given to patients over 70 years of age with little trouble.

Results of an RTOG study using concomitant cisplatin and EBRT were reported by TESTER et al. (1993). One of 42 patients experienced acute grade 3 small bowel toxicity and none experienced grade 3 or higher bladder toxicity. Grade 1 or 2 chemotherapy toxicity was seen in most patients. However, 10% experienced reversible hematologic toxicity and 2% had reversible renal toxicity. Late complications were minimal as well. Only one patient experienced grade 3 or higher bladder and bowel toxicity. Conversely, 22 of the 28 patients did experience grade 1 or 2 late toxicity of the skin, bladder, rectum, small bowel, kidney, or neurological system.

HOUSSET et al. (1993) reported on the results of a prospective trial in which patients with invasive bladder carcinoma were treated with TURBT and neoadjuvant combined chemoradiation with 5-FU and cisplatin followed by cystectomy or additional chemoradiation. Grade I leukopenia and a slight rise in serum creatinine occurred in nearly all patients but required no dose reductions. No acute cardiovascular problems were noted. Acute radiation effects such as dysuria and diarrhea did occur to a small degree. No chronic effects such as bladder contracture or small bowel obstruction were seen. The conclusion was that chemoradiation therapy is easy to implement and is well tolerated even in elderly patients.

For those patients in whom cisplatin is medically contraindicated, reasonable local and systemic tolerance to combined therapy with radiation and 5-FU alone has been reported. ROTMAN et al. (1990) treated 20 patients with radiation and concomitant 5-FU with or without mitomycin. Acute side-effects, including diarrhea (95%), anorexia (15%), and mucositis (15%), occurred in virtually all patients but there was no need for treatment interruption or dose reduction in any patient. Late complications also occurred. Hemorrhagic cystitis was seen in 5%, moderate dysuria and cystitis in 10%, irritable bladder in 10%, diarrhea in 15%, and chronic proctitis requiring colostomy in 5%. Bladder preservation was achieved in 95% of patients and no hematologic complications were observed. RUSSELL et al. (1988) reported that 3 of 40 patients developed 5-FU-related coronary vasospasm and angina. There was one fatal diarrhea and sepsis case and there were no late bladder contracture or bowel complications.

If chemoradiation gives suboptimal results locally, radical cystectomy can still be performed. Most bladder-sparing protocols have a built-in check after moderate doses of radiation to look for a poor response. The results using radiation or systemic chemotherapy in conjunction with cystectomy show that these modalities can be safely combined, with a minimal increase in the incidence of morbidity compared to any modality alone, particularly with moderate-dose radiation. If a patient develops a symptomatic contracted bladder or recurrent invasive disease after completing a bladder-sparing regimen, cystectomy can still be performed after high-dose radiation, with only a mild increase in the risk of morbidity.

After bladder-sparing therapy, 20%–30% of patients may develop a superficial recurrence. There is a trend towards a more conservative management approach using TURBT and intravesicular agents rather than proceeding directly to cystectomy. As seen in Pister's evaluation, delivery of intravesicular therapy after EBRT can also be done safely without an increase in morbidity to any significant degree (PISTER et al. 1991).

25.12
Conclusion

Based on a review of the current literature, each patient needs to have their treatment regimen individualized to make the appropriate allowances for the host and tumor-related parameters. Radiation therapy can easily be used in patients undergoing chemotherapy and various extents of surgery, especially if good care is taken with regard to the delivery and dose of radiation. Combined modality therapy with radiation therapy and chemotherapy after maximal TURBT will yield excellent tolerance as well as control rates equaling those achieved with radical cystectomy. If the excellent results in respect of disease-free survival and overall survival continue, this method may replace radical cystectomy as the standard of care.

Attention to detail will optimize the cure or control rate while maintaining excellent quality of life. What needs to be realized in a patient's treatment regimen is that a patient cannot have complications unless he lives long enough to experience them. The worst complication in the management of bladder cancer is failure to cure or at least control the cancer. With this in mind, complications can be expected in any patient undergoing definitive treatment of any type. However, they need to be kept to a minimum. With the new radical surgical techniques, combination modalities, and bladder-sparing protocols, this is being accomplished.

References

Abratt RP, Craighead P, Reddi VB, et al. (1991) A perspective randomized trial of radiation with and without oral and intravesicular misonidazole for bladder cancer. Br J Cancer 64:968–970

Abratt RP, Tuker RD, Barnes DR (1983) Radical irradiation of T2 grade III and T3 bladder cancer, tumor response and prognosis. Int J Radiat Oncol Biol Phys 9:1213–1215

Chauvet B, Brewer W, Felix-Faure C, et al. (1993) Combination radiation therapy and cisplatin for locally advanced carcinoma of the urinary bladder. Cancer 72:2213–2218

Cole DJ, Durrant KR, Roberts JT, et al. (1992) A pilot study of accelerated fractionation in the radiotherapy of invasive carcinoma of the bladder. Br J Radiol 65:792–798

Cox JD, Guse C, Asbell S, et al. (1988) Tolerance of pelvic normal tissues to hyperfractionated radiation therapy: results of protocol 83-08 of the radiation therapy oncology group. Int J Radiat Oncol Biol Phys 15:1331–1336

DeNeve W, Lybeert LM, Goor C, et al. (1992) T1 and T2 carcinoma of urinary bladder: long term results with external, preoperative, or interstitial radiotherapy. Int J Radiat Oncol Biol Phys 23:299–304

Duncan W, Williams JR, Kerr GR, et al. (1986) An analysis of the radiation related morbidity observed in a randomized trial of neutron therapy for bladder cancer. Int J Radiat Oncol Biol Phys 12:2085–2092

Dunst J, Sauer R, Schrott KM, et al. (1994) A organ sparing treatment of advanced bladder cancer: a 10 year experience. Int J Radiat Oncol Biol Phys 30:261–266

Freiha FS, Faysal MH (1983) Salvage cystectomy. Urology 23:496–498

Grossman HB, Sandler HM, Perez-Tamayo C (1993) The treatment of T3a bladder cancer with iridium implantation. Urology 41:217–220

Hillcoat BL, Raghaven D, Matthews J, et al. (1989) A randomized trial of cisplatin versus cisplatin plus methotrexate in advanced cancer of the urothelial tract. J Clin Oncol 7:706–709

Horwich A (1991) Treatment of muscle-invasive (T2/T3) disease: the role of radiotherapy. In: Alderson AR, Oliver RTD, Hanham IWF, Bloom HJG (eds) Urological oncology dilemmas and developments. Wiley, Chichester, pp 137–144

Housset M, Maulard C, Chretien Y, et al. (1993) Combined radiation and chemotherapy for invasive transitional cell carcinoma of the bladder: a prospective study. J Clin Oncol 11:2150–2157

Kachnic LA, Shipley WU, Griffin PP, et al. (1996) Combined modality treatment with selective conservative for invasive bladder cancer: long term tolerance in the female patient. Cancer J Sci Am 2:79–84

Khandekar JD, Elson PJ, DeWys WD, et al. (1985) Comparative activity and toxicity of cis-diamminedichloroplatinum and combination of doxorubicin, cyclophosphamide and DDP in disseminated transitional cell carcinomas of the urinary tract. J Clin Oncol 3:539–545

Konnak JW, Grossman HB (1985) Salvage cystectomy following failed definitive radiation therapy for transitional cell carcinoma of the bladder. Urology 26:550–553

Kopelson G, Heaney JA (1983) Postoperative radiation therapy for muscle invading bladder carcinoma. J Surg Oncol 23:263–268

Lamm DL, Steg A, Boccon-Gibod L, et al. (1989) Complications of BCG immunotherapy: review of 2602 patients and comparison of chemotherapy complications. Prog Clin Biol 310:335–355

Logothetis CJ, Samuals ML, Ogden S, et al. (1985) Cyclophosphamide, doxorubicin and cisplatin chemotherapy for patients with locally advanced urothelial tumors with or without nodal metastases. J Urol 134:460–464

Lynch WJ, Jenkins BJ, Fowler CG (1992) The quality of life after radical radiotherapy for bladder cancer. Br J Urol 70:519–521

Mameghan H, Fisher RJ, Watt WH, et al. (1991) Management of invasive transitional cell carcinoma of the bladder. Cancer 69:2771–2778

Marks LB, Kaufman SD, Prout GR Jr, et al. (1988) Invasive bladder carcinoma, preliminary report of selective bladder conservation by transurethral surgery, up front MCV chemotherapy and pelvic irradiation plus cisplatin. Int J Radiat Oncol Biol Phys 15:877–882

Marks LB, Carroll TR, Dugan TC, et al. (1995) Response of urinary bladder, urethra and ureter to irradiation and chemotherapy. Int J Radiat Oncol Biol Phys 31:1257–1280

Mohiuddin M, Kramer S, Newall J, et al. (1985) Combined preoperative and postoperative radiation for bladder cancer. Cancer 55:963–966

Pisters LL, Tykochinsky G, Wajsman Z (1991) Intravesical BCG or mitomycin in the treatment of carcinoma in-situ of the bladder following prior pelvic radiation therapy. J Urol 146:514–517

Raghavan D, Grundy R, Greenaway T, et al. (1988) Preemptive chemotherapy prior to radical radiotherapy for fit septuagenarians with bladder cancer: age itself is not a contraindication. Br J Urol 62:154–159

Reisinger SA, Mohiuddin M, Mulholland SG (1992) Combined pre- and postoperative adjuvant radiation therapy for bladder cancer; a ten year experience. Int J Radiat Oncol Biol Phys 24:463–468

Roberts JT, Fossa SP, Richards SB, et al. (1991) Results of Medical Research Council phase II study of low dose cisplatin and methotrexate in the primary treatment of locally advanced transitional cell carcinoma of the bladder. Br J Urol 68:162–168

Rotman M, Aziz M, Porrazzo M, et al. (1990) Treatment of advanced transitional cell carcinoma of the bladder with irradiation and concomitant 5 FU infusion. Int J Radiat Oncol Biol Phys 18:1131–1137

Russell KJ, Boileau MA, Ireton RC, et al. (1988) Transitional cell carcinoma of the urinary bladder: histologic clearance with combined 5–FU chemotherapy and radiation therapy: preliminary results of bladder preservation study. Radiology 167:845–848

Russell KJ, Laramore GE, Griffin TW, et al. (1989) Neutron radiotherapy for treatment of carcinoma of the urinary bladder. Am J Clin Oncol 12:301–306

Shiels RA, Nissenbaum NN, Mark SR, et al. (1986) Late radiation cystitis after treatment for carcinoma of the bladder. S Afr Med J 70:727–728

Shipley WU, Rose MA, Perrone TL, et al. (1985) Full dose irradiation for patients with invasive bladder carcinoma: clinical and historical prognostic factors of improved survival. J Urol 134:679

Shipley WU, Prout GR, Einstein AB, et al. (1987) Treatment of invasive bladder cancer by cisplatin and radiation in patients unsuited for surgery. JAMA 258:931–935

Shipley WU, Zietman AL (1996) Bladder cancer: the combination of chemotherapy and irradiation in the treatment of patients with muscle invading tumors. ASTRO refresher course 203

Soloway MS, Ishikawa S, Taylor T, et al. (1989) MVAC or MVC for the treatment of advanced transitional cell carcinoma: metastasis, induction and adjuvant. J Surg Oncol 1:40–45

Soloway MS, Lopez AE, Patel J, et al. (1993) Results of radical cystectomy for transitional cell carcinoma of the bladder and the effect of chemotherapy. Cancer 73:1926–1931

Spera JA, Whittington R, Littman P, et al. (1987) A comparison of preoperative radiotherapy regimens for bladder carcinoma. Cancer 61:255–262

Straus KL, Littman P, Wein AJ, et al. (1988) Treatment of bladder cancer with interstitial iridium 192 implantation and external beam irradiation. Int J Radiat Oncol Biol Phys 14:265–271

Studer UE, Gerber E, Zimmermann A, et al. (1993) Late results in patients treated with pi-mesons for bladder cancer. Cancer 71:439–447

Tannock I, Gospodarowicz M, Connolly J, et al. (1989) MVAC chemotherapy for transitional cell carcinoma: the Princess Margaret Hospital experience. J Urol 142:289–292

Tester W, Porter A, Asbell S, et al. (1993) Combined modality program with possible organ preservation for invasive bladder carcinoma: results of RTOG protocol 85–12. Int J radiat Oncol Biol Phys 25:783–790

Zietman AL, Shipley WU, Kaufman DS (1993) The combination of cisplatin based chemotherapy and radiation in the treatment of muscle invading transitional cell cancer of the bladder. Int J Radiat Oncol Biol Phys 27:161–170

26 Special Considerations in the Management of Carcinoma in the Neurogenic Bladder

D.J.M.K. DE RIDDER, J. BINARD, and L. BAERT

CONTENTS

26.1
Introduction

Bladder cancer is more frequent in the spinal cord-injured population. The current literature concerning this subject is reviewed below; the incidence, pathology, diagnosis, and prognosis are discussed, along with some specific considerations regarding the treatment of bladder cancers in patients with spinal cord disease.

D.J.M.K. DE RIDDER, MD, Consultant Urologist, Department of Urology, UZ Gasthuisberg, University Hospitals of Leuven, Herestraat 49, B-3000 Leuven, Belgium
J.E. BINARD, MD, FRSC(C), Department of Urology, College of Medicine, University of South Florida, Tampa, FL 33612, USA
L. BAERT, MD, PhD, Professor and Chairman, Department of Urology, UZ Gasthuisberg, University Hospitals of Leuven, Herestraat 49, B-3000 Leuven, Belgium and Clinical Professor, Department of Urology and Radiation Oncology, University of Southern California, USC/Norris Comprehensive Cancer Center, 1441 Eastlake Avenue, Los Angeles, CA 90033, USA

26.2
Incidence of Bladder Cancer in Neurogenic Bladders

26.2.1
Spinal Cord Injury

In the general population of the European Community the incidence of spinal cord injury in males is 0.018% and in females 0.004% (ESTEVE et al. 1993). The incidence of bladder cancer is thought to be higher in spinal cord-injured (diseased) patients. This incidence ranges from 0.27% as reported by BICKEL et al. (1991) to 9.6% in the publication of KAUFMAN et al. (1977). In a larger series of more than 2000 spinal cord injury patients, an incidence of bladder cancer from 0.27% to 0.37% was reported. Combining all the data from these reports, an overall incidence of 0.66% in 13 357 patients is obtained. The most important publications on bladder cancer in spinal cord injury patients are listed in Table 26.1. In this group of patients early diagnosis is difficult due to the low sensitivity of cystoscopy and cytology. In addition bladder cancer in spinal cord-diseased patients is thought to be more aggressive and to result in higher mortality rates than those reported in the population with an intact spine. Bladder cancer is reported to be responsible for 0.3%–2.8% of the known deaths among this population (STONEHILL et al. 1996).

Besides the higher incidence of transitional cell carcinoma, the incidence of otherwise rare tumors such as squamous cell carcinoma and adenocarcinoma is also higher in neurogenic bladders.

26.2.2
Multiple Sclerosis

As in spinal cord injury, chronic bladder dysfunction in multiple sclerosis can lead to permanent catheterization and chronic infection. Moreover,

Table 26.1. Incidence of bladder cancer in spinal cord injury patients

Author	Total no. of patients	No. with cancer	No. with TCC	No. with SCC	No. with adenocarcinoma	No. of mixed tumors
Melzak (1966)	3 800	11 (0.29%)	7 (64%)	4 (36%)	0	2 (18%)
Kaufman et al. (1977)	62	6 (9.6%)	5 (83%)	6 (100%)	0	0
Broecker et al. (1981)	1 053	10 (0.9%)	4 (40%)	2 (20%)	0	0
El-Masri and Fellows (1981)	6 744	25 (0.37%)	13 (52%)	11 (44%)	0	5 (20%)
Locke et al. (1985)	25	2 (8%)	2 (100%)	0	0	0
Bejany et al. (1987)	478	11 (2.3%)	1 (9%)	9 (82%)	0	1 (9%)
Bickel et al. (1991)	2 900	8 (0.27%)	6 (75%)	2 (25%)	0	0
Yaqoob et al. (1991)	14	4 (28%)	1 (25%)	3 (75%)	0	0
Chao et al. (1993)	81	6 (7.4%)	4 (67%)	1 (16%)	1 (16%)	0
Stonehill et al. (1996)	>2 000	17 (<0.8%)	5 (29%)	10 (59%)	2 (12%)	0
Total	>13 357	89 (0.66%)	41 (46%)	48 (49%)	3 (3.4%)	8 (9%)

many patients with multiple sclerosis have been included in medical trials using cytotoxic medication such as cyclophosphamide, which has a probable carcinogenic effect. Nevertheless, the literature does not mention a higher incidence of bladder cancer in these patients. Our data accumulated since 1967, however, show an incidence of 0.29% in 2351 patients (De Ridder et al. 1997). This incidence of bladder cancer seems comparable to that found in spinal cord-injured patients.

26.3
Risk Factors

26.3.1
Spinal Cord Injury

Besides the well-known risk factors for development of bladder cancer, such as smoking and exposure to certain chemicals, additional risk factors have been identified by several investigators. These additional risk factors include: (a) long-term catheterization, (b) chronic bladder stones, (c) chronic cystitis, (d) nonfunctioning bladder, and (e) long-term immunosuppressive therapy. Chronic need for an indwelling catheter has been recognized by several authors as the most important risk factor for bladder cancer (Stonehill et al. 1996; Chao et al. 1993; Broecker et al. 1981; Kaufman et al. 1977; Jacobs and Kaufman 1978; El-Masri and Fellows 1981).

Indwelling catheterization for more than 10 years seems to induce squamous metaplasia (Broecker et al. 1981; Kaufman et al. 1977) which may eventually lead to squamous cell carcinoma (Stonehill et al. 1996). A study by Kantor et al. (1984) estimated the risk for developing bladder cancer in the

presence of a long-term catheter to be between 2% and 10%.

Besides the presence of the catheter itself, chronic infection and bladder stones are also proven important risk factors. The presence of a catheter and the presence of bladder stones were demonstrated to be statistically significant risk factors in a retrospective study by Stonehill et al. (1996). El-Masri and Fellows (1981) postulated the possible tumor-promoting role of nitrosamines, which are present in chronically infected urine. A possible link between resistant micro-organisms and urothelial changes is at present not well understood (Bejany et al. 1987).

A nonfunctioning bladder by itself seems to be another risk factor for the development of transitional cell carcinoma and squamous cell carcinoma (Moloney et al. 1981). Mucinous adenocarcinomas have been reported in nonfunctioning bladders by Young and Parkhust (1984) and Djavan et al. (1995).

Special attention needs to be given to patients in renal failure who are treated by chronic dialysis or renal transplant. Unusually high incidences of invasive bladder cancer with a very high mortality have been described in a series of 14 patients on renal replacement therapy by Yaqoob (1991). In these patients immunosuppression substantially increases the risk of bladder cancer.

26.3.2
Multiple Sclerosis and Other Autoimmune Disorders

Besides the above-mentioned risk factors such as long-term catheterization, bladder stones, and chronic infection, some patients with multiple sclerosis are exposed to additional iatrogenic risks for developing bladder cancer (DE RIDDER et al. 1997).

Immunosuppressive therapy has been used in the treatment of multiple sclerosis and other autoimmune disorders. Cyclophosphamide has been used extensively in these diseases. Other agents such as mitoxantrone and azathioprine are currently under investigation.

One case of a Buschke-Löwenstein tumor has been described in a patient treated with azathioprine for multiple sclerosis (WIEDEMANN et al. 1995). Also an isolated condyloma acuminatum of the bladder has been described by VAN POPPEL et al. (1986) in a patient with multiple sclerosis treated with cyclophosphamide.

An increased risk of bladder cancer has also been noted in patients receiving cyclophosphamide for rheumatoid arthritis (RADIS et al. 1995), non-Hodgkin's lymphoma (TRAVIS et al. 1995), Wegener's granulomatosis (STEIN et al. 1993), lupus nephritis (ORTIZ et al. 1992), or ovarian cancer (KALDOR et al. 1995) and in renal transplant patients (TUTTLE et al. 1988). The metabolite acrolein plays a role in the pathogenesis of the cyclophosphamide-induced hemorrhagic cystitis, but its role in the induction of secondary urinary tract malignancy is not well understood (CANNON et al. 1991).

The induction of bladder cancer through cyclophosphamide is dependent on the total cumulative dose. TRAVIS et al. (1995) studied a cohort of 6171 2-year survivors of non-Hodgkin's lymphoma and identified 48 patients with a secondary urinary tract tumor. For a cumulative dose of cyclophosphamide between 20 and 49 g, the absolute risk of cancer is increased. This increase consists in three additional bladder cancers per 100 patients after 15 years of follow-up. At a cumulative dose of 50 g or more the excess risk increases to seven excess bladder cancers per 100 patients. RADIS et al. (1995) estimated the relative risk of cancer at 1.5 for patients with rheumatoid arthritis treated with cyclophosphamide. The total dose of cyclophosphamide was higher in those patients who developed cancer. STEIN et al. (1993) reported on an increased incidence of squamous cell carcinoma of the bladder in patients with Wegener's granulomatosis treated with cyclophosphamide. They noted at least a ninefold increase in the incidence of lower urinary tract malignancy in patients with prolonged cyclophosphamide therapy.

In addition to the importance of the cumulative dose of cyclophosphamide in the induction of blad-

der cancer, the duration of follow-up is also of critical importance. Bladder cancer was reported up to 17 years after discontinuation of the cyclophosphamide treatment (RADIS et al. 1995; KALDOR et al. 1995; DE RIDDER et al. 1997).

The dose of cyclophosphamide used in patients with multiple sclerosis is usually limited. KORNHUBER et al. (1987) proposed a dose of 8 mg/kg with a total dose of 1.5–2 g per cycle. This means that in a lifetime at least 20 cycles would be required to reach the cumulative dose of 50 g. However, the use of higher cumulative doses of up to 95 ± 27 g has been reported (LATERRE et al. 1989; DE RIDDER et al. 1997). The use of cyclophosphamide for nonneoplastic diseases carries a substantial risk for secondary malignancies if a high cumulative dose is reached. Multiple sclerosis, especially in its advanced stage, by itself already carries an increased risk for the development of bladder cancer. To what extent cyclophosphamide or other immunosuppressive therapy adds to the existing risk cannot be speculated upon at this time. In view of the above data, patients receiving immunosuppressive therapy should be carefully followed to exclude the possibility of bladder carcinoma.

26.4
Anatomopathological Considerations

In the reported series of patients with neurogenic bladders who have bladder cancer (Table 26.1), the incidence of transitional cell carcinoma ranges from 9% to 100%. When data are combined, transitional cell carcinoma was present in 46% of all patients. Squamous cell carcinoma was present in 49% of all cases, with a range from 16% to 100% (Table 26.1). Adenocarcinoma of the bladder was present in 3.6% of patients.

Chronic infection and the presence of indwelling catheters may cause changes in the bladder transitional cell epithelium. The response of bladder epithelium to environmental stimuli is classified into three categories: (a) nonneoplastic proliferation, (b) metaplasia, and (c) neoplasia (MOSTOFI 1954). Metaplastic responses of the bladder epithelium include changes to columnar or squamous epithelium. These changes have been noted to occur with vitamin A deficiency, chronic chemical and/or mechanical irritation, chronic urinary tract infection, and radiation. Squamous metaplasia and cystitis glandularis are common responses to bladder irritation, but squamous cell carcinoma and adenocarcinoma account for only 5% of all bladder malignancies in the general population (BROECKER et al. 1981). In Egypt, parts of Africa, and the Middle East this number increases to 60% due to the known association with bilharzial infection owing to *Schistosoma haematobium* (EL-BOLKAINY et al. 1981).

Long-term indwelling catheterization is frequently associated with squamous metaplasia. BROECKER et al. (1981) showed a higher frequency of metaplasia in catheterized patients compared to patients treated with an external condom catheter. KAUFMAN et al. (1977) showed that the incidence of squamous metaplasia increased with the duration of catheterization. In this study KAUFMAN et al. report on one patient with invasive squamous cell carcinoma who only presented superficial changes in the bladder. The evidence of an association between squamous metaplasia and squamous cell carcinoma is only circumstantial, but the high incidence of coexistence of both in neurogenic bladders should trigger an aggressive investigation when squamous metaplasia is found on cystoscopy or cytology.

The same recommendation applies to cystitis glandularis and intestinal metaplasia as they may indicate the presence or anticipate the development of adenocarcinoma of the bladder. LIN et al. (1980) reported on three cases of cystitis glandularis, one of which was associated with adenocarcinoma. All three patients had neurogenic bladders. YOUNG and PARKHUST (1984) published a case of intestinal metaplasia, carcinoma in situ, and adenocarcinoma in a defunctionalized bladder. DJAVAN et al. (1995) described a case of adenocarcinoma of a defunctionalized bladder of a patient with prune-belly syndrome and one in a neurogenic bladder due to spinal cord injury. These authors discuss the possible origin of glandular tissue in the bladder. Besides chronic inflammation as a well-established causative factor, they mentioned the possibility of glandular tissue being derived from embryonic nests or persistent inclusions of intestine, displaced in the separation of the rectum from the urogenital sinus.

As with squamous cell carcinoma, BROECKER et al. (1981) noted an increased incidence of cystitis glanduralis in patients with an indwelling catheter when compared to those patients with an external condom catheter. These changes, however, are less frequent than squamous metaplasia. KAUFMAN et al. (1977) found a higher incidence of cystitis glandularis in patients catheterized for more than 10 years, compared to those with a shorter period of

catheterization. Some investigators have also reported premalignant leukoplakia in a few patients (BROECKER et al. 1981; KAUFMAN et al. 1977; LOCKE et al. 1985).

Few data have been published on the pathological stage of bladder tumors in spinal cord injury patients. In the important study of EL-MASRI and FELLOWS (1981), 22 of the 25 (88%) tumors were reported to be "invasive" without further specification. In a study of eight patients reported by BICKEL et al. (1991), five (62.5%) presented with stage pT3. All tumors in this report were grade II or III. In the study of 17 patients by STONEHILL et al. (1996), ten (59%) presented with a stage pT3 or higher. In the general population, however, only 30%–50% of bladder tumors are diagnosed in an invasive stage (CUTLER et al. 1982). In neurogenic bladders, another important difference from the general population is the presence of bladder diverticuli that are devoid of detrusor muscle. Diverticular cancers tend to have a higher recurrence rate and a high mortality secondary to the development of metastatic disease (SWEENEY et al. 1992). Thus, in patients with neurogenic bladders, a better and earlier diagnosis of bladder cancer is imperative.

26.5
Diagnosis of Carcinomatous Changes in Neurogenic Bladders

The classic symptom prompting further investigation for bladder cancer is hematuria. This is also true in spinal cord-injured patients. In this population several authors described hematuria as being the first symptom of bladder cancer in addition to chronic infection and bladder stones (STONEHILL et al. 1996; KAUFMAN et al. 1977; LOCKE et al. 1985; BEJANY et al. 1987).

The role of cytology in the diagnosis of bladder cancer in neurogenic bladders is uncertain. LOCKE et al. (1985) found cytology to be consistent with the diagnosis of carcinoma in 15 patients. They did not find false-negative or false-positive results in their patients. STONEHILL et al. (1996) diagnosed four patients with bladder cancer based on a positive cytology, although initial cystoscopy was nondiagnostic. KAUFMAN et al. (1977), BICKEL et al. (1991), and BEJANY et al. (1987) do not consider cytology as an important tool in the diagnosis of bladder cancer in this population.

Diagnosis of carcinoma on endoscopy is frequently difficult due to epithelial changes in the bladder induced by chronic irritation. BEJANY et al. (1987) found endoscopy to be nonspecific in 8 of 11 cancer patients. STONEHILL et al. (1996) had to perform random biopsies in four patients with negative cystoscopy and positive cytology. Most authors use cytology and cystoscopy as complementary tools in this specific situation. Random biopsies should be performed if there is any suspicion of cancer. BEJANY et al. (1987) proposed including ultrasound examination of the bladder and pelvis and computerized axial tomographic scan in the preventive follow-up. This recommendation was based on the finding that many patients present with local invasion or bulky tumors at the time of diagnosis.

The fact that so many of these tumors are diagnosed in advanced stages is partially due to the lack of specificity of cytology and endoscopy in this population. Another reason is probably the erroneous attitude of sparing disabled people from invasive investigations such as random biopsies. Also since many neurogenic bladders show signs of chronic inflammation or infection, repetitive biopsies with negative results for carcinoma are finally discontinued.

New developments in the noninvasive and semi-invasive diagnosis such as the recent bladder tumor antigen test (BTA test) and fluorescence detection of bladder carcinoma are promising but they still have to prove their usefulness in neurogenic bladders (D'HALLEWIN et al. 1994; D'HALLEWIN and BAERT 1996).

All authors agreed that a regular follow-up with a high degree of suspicion for bladder cancer is necessary. Yearly cystoscopy and cytology are imperative. Cystoscopy should be performed by a urologist experienced in the field of neurogenic bladders. Biopsy is warranted if suspected lesions are visualized or if there is a discrepancy between the basic investigations. Most patients with neurogenic bladders undergo at least annual ultrasound examination of the upper urinary tract. This should be combined with an ultrasound examination of the full bladder to exclude locally invasive and bulky tumors.

26.6
Prognosis of Bladder Cancer in Patients with a Neurogenic Bladder

Reports on survival of spinal cord-injured patients with bladder cancer are generally pessimistic. The existence of many cellular diverticuli, devoid of blad-der detrusor, may predispose to more rapid tumor penetration and tumor spread. In the general population it appears that the low rates of disease-free survival and 5-year survival (both <10%) are related more to early tumor dissemination than to local recurrence (MICIC and ILIC 1983; FAYSAL and FRIEHA 1981).

For spinal cord-diseased patients, the worst survival rates were reported by EL-MASRI and FELLOWS (1981), where 20 of the 25 patients died within 2 years after the initial diagnosis. The authors estimated that the mortality risk in their population was increased by a factor of 20. One has to realize that this study was an update of the older study of MELZAK (1966), which already contained 11 of these 25 patients. More recent studies are less pessimistic. However, the mortality rates remain high. Whether this is due to the advanced stage at the time of diagnosis or to the neurogenic bladder or to the differentiation of the tumor is not clear.

In their study, STONEHILL et al. (1996) found a median survival rate of 2 years. They calculated the disease-specific mortality to be 2.9%. LOCKE et al. (1985) presented data on two patients with squamous cell carcinoma who died from metastatic disease within 5 months of diagnosis. BEJANY et al. (1987) reported a slightly better survival in patients with squamous cell carcinoma versus patients with transitional cell carcinoma when corresponding stages were compared. They also noted urethral involvement in 55% of patients and could demonstrate an improvement in disease-free survival for cystectomy with urethrectomy compared to cystectomy alone. BICKEL et al. (1991), in their series of eight patients, found the survival to be comparable to the survival in patients with bladder carcinoma occurring in the general population.

The available data do not allow us to draw definitive conclusions concerning survival after treatment for bladder cancer in spinal cord-injured patients. In many series the exact pathological stages have not been well defined. The fact that many tumors are diagnosed in a locally advanced stage compromises the cure and survival rates. Some series contain older data gathered at a time when the treatment of the bladder cancer was not comparable to that in more recent series. Except for immuno-compromised spinal cord-injured patients, in whom an excessive mortality has been noted (YAQOOB et al. 1991), there is no strong evidence that survival in this population differs from the survival in the general population. The main problem remains the fact that the diagnosis is often made in late stages of the disease.

26.7
Prevention of Bladder Cancer

In addition to the usual preventive measures such as cessation of smoking and avoidance of carcinogenic chemicals, whenever feasible, indwelling catheters should be avoided. Low-pressure bladder storage and emptying without indwelling catheters can almost always be obtained with the available pharmaceutical or surgical interventions, and the use of external condom or intermittent catheterization (SELZMAN and HAMPEL 1993). So far, only one case of bladder cancer in a patient on intermittent catheterization has been published (SENE et al. 1990). Intermittent catheterization programs should be encouraged in rehabilitation centers. Continuous motivation of the individual patient, the patient's family, the general practitioner, and the nursing staff is necessary to ensure the continuation of this treatment. Recent developments such as the portable patient-controlled ultrasound device (PCI 5000, Bladdermanager) offers the patient improved continence control by volume-directed catheterization (BINARD et al. 1996; DE RIDDER et al. 1996a). Capsaicin instillations seem to be able to extend the use of intermittent catheterization in multiple sclerosis patients with refractory detrusor hyperreflexia (DE RIDDER et al. 1996b). These data will make intermittent catheterization more appealing, and thus avoidance of indwelling catheters even more often indicated. Regular monitoring and treatment of urinary tract infection, bladder stones, and residual urine will help in decreasing the risk factors for bladder mucosal changes and induction of eventual bladder tumors.

26.8
Treatment Options

The treatment of bladder cancer in spinal cord-injured patients is fully comparable to the treatment of bladder cancer in other patients. All therapeutic options are extensively discussed in other chapters of this book and are fully applicable to patients with spinal cord disease.

Special consideration should be given to manual dexterity, abdominal muscle tone and bowel continence when cystectomy and urinary tract recon-

struction are contemplated. For example, when surgical treatment is necessary the choice of the type of diversion should be thoroughly discussed with the patient. If a poor hand function is present or the progressive nature of the neurological disease, as in multiple sclerosis, predicts the loss of hand function, continent reservoirs are not to be used. If patients are able and willing to catheterize themselves continent reservoirs can be proposed. Otherwise the classic uretero-ileo-cutaneostomy or Bricker diversion is the diversion of choice.

26.9
Conclusions

Bladder cancer is more frequent in patients with spinal cord disease. Chronic irritation by indwelling catheters, bladder stones, and infection may eventually cause premalignant changes in the bladder epithelium. Squamous cell carcinoma and adenocarcinoma of the bladder are more frequent in spinal cord disease than in the general population. Most tumors are identified in a locally advanced stage, which leads to a higher mortality. Diagnosis of bladder cancer in these patients is frequently difficult. It is necessary for the clinician to be aware of the high incidence of carcinoma of the bladder in this patient population in order to make an early diagnosis. Surgical treatment should take the neurological condition into account, especially if a urinary diversion is to be constructed.

References

Bejany DE, Lockhart JL, Rhany RK (1987) Malignant vesical tumors following spinal cord injury. J Urol 138:1390–1392

Bickel A, Culkin DJ, Wheeler JS Jr (1991) Bladder cancer in spinal cord injury patients. J Urol 146:1240–1242

Binard JE, Persky L, Lockhart JL (1996) Intermittent catheterisation the right way (volume versus time directed). J Spin Cord Med 19:194–196

Broecker BH, Klein FA, Hackler RH (1981) Cancer of the bladder in spinal cord injury. J Urol 125:196–197

Cannon J, Linke CA, Cos LR (1991) Cyclophosphamide associated carcinoma of urothelium. Modalities for prevention. Urology 38:413–416

Chao R, Clowers D, Mayo ME (1993) Fate of the upper urinary tracts in patients with indwelling catheters after spinal cord injury. Urology 42:259–262

Cutler SJ, Heney NM, Friedell GH (1982) Longitudinal study of patients with bladder cancer: factors associated with disease recurrence and progression. In: Bonney WW, Prout GR (eds) Bladder cancer, AUA Monographs. Williams and Wilkins, Baltimore

De Ridder D, Van Poppel H, Baert L (1996a) From time dependent intermittent catheterisation to volume dependent catheterisation in multiple sclerosis patients, using the PCI5000. Spinal Cord (in press)

De Ridder D, Van Poppel H, Baert L (1996b) Intravesical capsaicin as treatment for detrusor hyperreflexia in multiple sclerosis: results in 41 patients. Neurourol Urodyn 15:376–377

De Ridder D, Van Poppel H, Demonty R, Baert L (1997) Cancer of the bladder in multiple sclerosis patients treated with cyclophosphamide. Submitted to the J Urol

D'Hallewin MA, Baert L (1996) Initial evaluation of the bladder tumor antigen test in superficial bladder cancer. J Urol 155:475–476

D'Hallewin MA, Baert L, Vanherzeele H (1994) In vivo fluorescence detection of human bladder carcinoma without sensitizing agent. J Am Paraplegia Soc 17:161–164

Djavan B, Litwiller SC, Milchgrub S (1995) Mucinous adenocarcinoma in defunctionalized bladders. Urology 46:107–110

El-Bolkainy MN, Mokhtar NM, Ghoneim MA, Hussein MH (1981) The impact of schistosomiasis on the pathology of bladder carcinoma. Cancer 48:2643

El-Masri WS, Fellows G (1981) Bladder cancer after spinal cord injury. Paraplegia 19:265–270

Estève J, Kricker A, Ferlay J, Parkin DM (1993) Facts and figures of cancer in the European Community. International Agency for Research on Cancer, Lyon, p 36, p 50

Faysal MH, Frieha FS (1981) Primary neoplasm in vesical diverticula: a report of 12 cases. Br J Urol 53:141

Jacobs SC, Kaufman JM (1978) Complications of permanent bladder catheter drainage in spinal cord injury patients. J Urol 119:740–741

Kaldor JM, Day NE, Kittelmann B, et al. (1995) Bladder tumors following chemotherapy and radiotherapy for ovarian cancer: a case control study. Int J Cancer 63:1–6

Kantor AF, Hartge P, Hoover RN, et al. (1984) Urinary tract infection and risk of bladder cancer. Am J Epidemiol 119:510–515

Kaufman JM, Fam B, Jacobs SC, et al. (1977) Bladder cancer and squamous metaplasia in spinal cord injury patients. J Urol 118:967–971

Kornhuber HH, Petru E, Schmähl D (1987) Zum Malignitätsrisiko bei Cyclophosphamid Therapie der Multiplen Sklerose. DMW 112:530

Laterre C, Sindic CJM, Heule H (1989) Oral cyclophosphamide treatment in multiple sclerosis. In: Gonsette R, Delmotte P (ed) Recent advances in multiple sclerosis therapy. Elsevier, Amsterdam, pp 147–150

Levine LA, Richic JP (1989) Urological complications of cyclophosphamide. J Urol 141:1063–1069

Lin JI, Tseng CH, Choy C, et al. (1980) Diffuse cystitis glandularis associated with adenocarcinomatous change. Urology 15:411–415

Locke JR, Hill DE, Walzer Y (1985) Incidence of squamous cell carcinoma in patients with long term catheter drainage. J Urol 133:1034–1035

Malek RS, Rosen JS, O'Dea MJ (1983) Adenocarcinoma of bladder. Urology 21:357

Melzak J (1966) The incidence of bladder cancer in paraplegia. Paraplegia 4:85–96

Micic S, Ilic V (1983) Incidence of neoplasm in vesical diverticula. J Urol 129:734

Moloney PJ, Fenster HN, McLoughlin MC (1981) Carcinoma in the defunctionalized tract. J Urol 126:260

Mostofi FK (1954) Potentialities of bladder epithelium. J Urol 71:705

Ortiz A, Gonzalez-Parra E, Alvarez-Costa G, Egido J (1992) Bladder cancer after cyclophosphamide therapy for lupus nephritis. Nephron 60:378–379

Radis CD, Kahl LE, Baker GL, et al. (1995) Effects of cyclophosphamide on the development of malignancy and on long term survival of patients with rheumatoid arthritis: a 20 year follow up. Arthritis Rheum 38:1120–1127

Robertson DAF, Low-Beer TS (1983) Long term consequences of arsenical treatment for multiple sclerosis. BMJ 286:605–606

Selzman AA, Hampel N (1993) Urological complications of spinal cord injury. Urol Clin North Am 20:453–464

Sene AP, Massey JA, McMahon RTF, et al. (1990) Squamous cell carcinoma in a patient on clean intermittent self catheterisation. Br J Urol 65:213

Stein JP, Skinner EC, Boyd SD, Skinner DG (1993) Squamous cell carcinoma of the bladder associated with cyclophosphamide therapy for Wegener's granulomatosis: a report of 2 cases. J Urol 149:588–589

Stonehill WH, Dmochowski RR, Patterson AL, Cox CE (1996) Risk factors for bladder tumors in spinal cord injury patients. J Urol 155:1248–1250

Sweeney P, Kursh ED, MI Resnick (1992) Partial cystectomy. Urol Clin North Am 19:707–708

Travis LB, Curtis RE, Glinelius B, et al. (1995) Bladder and kidney cancer following cyclophosphamide therapy for non Hodgkin lymphoma. J Natl Cancer Inst 87:524–530

Tuttle TM, Williams GM, Marshall FF (1988) Evidence of cyclophosphamide induced transitional cell carcinoma in a renal transplant patient. J Urol 140:1009–1011

Van Poppel H, Stessens R, De Vos R, Van Damme B (1986) Isolated condyloma acuminatum of the bladder in a patient with multiple sclerosis: etiological and pathological considerations. J Urol 136:1071–1073

Wiedemann A, Diekmann WP, Holtmann G, Kracht H (1995) Report of a case with giant condyloma (Buschke-Löwenstein tumor) localized in the bladder. J Urol 153:1222–1224

Yaqoob M, McClelland P, Bell GM, et al. (1991) Bladder tumors in paraplegic patients on renal replacement therapy. Lancet 338:1554–1555

Young RH, Parkhust EC (1984) Mucinous adenocarcinoma of bladder. Urology 24:192–195

27 Hyperthermia in Bladder Cancer

H. Goethuys, L. Baert, and Z. Petrovich

CONTENTS

27.1
Introduction

Hyperthermia is the application of heat to attain elevated tumor temperatures of 41°–46°C. It has been

H. Goethuys, MD, Senior Resident, Department of Urology, UZ Gasthuisberg, University Hospitals of Leuven, Herestraat 49, B-3000 Leuven, Belgium
L. Baert, MD, Professor and Chairman, Department of Urology, UZ Gasthuisberg, University Hospitals of Leuven, Herestraat 49, B-3000 Leuven, Belgium and Clinical Professor, Department of Urology and Radiation Oncology, University of Southern California, USC/Norris Comprehensive Cancer Center, 1441 Eastlake Avenue, Los Angeles, CA 90033, USA
Z. Petrovich, MD, FACR, Professor and Chairman, Department of Radiation Oncology, University of Southern California, USC/Norris Comprehensive Cancer Center, 1441 Eastlake Avenue, Los Angeles, CA 90033, USA

used most frequently in cancer therapy as an adjuvant to radiotherapy or chemotherapy and only sporadically as a monotherapy.

Experimental studies have shown that transitional cell carcinoma is sensitive to heating in combination with radiotherapy or chemotherapy. The challenge for modern technology is to develop a device capable of homogeneously heating a larger mass deep in the pelvis without causing substantial side-effects. This ideal device has yet to be developed. Several ways of heating the bladder are currently under investigation, including:

1. Deep regional hyperthermia
2. Intracavitary microwave/radiofrequency hyperthermia
3. Bladder irrigation with warm solutions

The currently available and potentially curative treatment modalities have a high incidence of tumor control in patients with superficial bladder tumors. However, obtaining a high probability of tumor control in patients with deeply invasive and bulky lesions remains a challenge to urologists. For these patients with large tumor volumes, the effective treatment combination still has to be established. In the past 20 years, hyperthermia has been used in combination with different treatment modalities in order to improve the probability of tumor control.

27.2
Experimental Studies

27.2.1
Studies In Vitro

The potential inhibitory effect of hyperthermia on various human bladder cancer cell lines, normal human bladder cells, and the murine MBT-2 bladder cancer cell line has been studied (Matzkin et al.

1992). These cell lines were exposed for 1 h to 43°C ± 0.5°C and compared with the unheated controls. Cell survival was assessed comparing the cell growth curve and colony formation. The human transitional cell carcinoma cell lines varied in their sensitivity to heat. MGH-U1 was found to be the most heat-sensitive cell line. The human A-1698, CUB-2, and UM-UC-3 lines and the murine MBT-2 line were relatively heat insensitive. Varying cytotoxic effects of hyperthermia on transitional cell carcinoma of the bladder were thus clearly established.

Using an in vitro colony-forming assay system, cytotoxic effects of the anticancer drugs adriamycin and peplomycin and the combined effect of hyperthermia and anticancer drugs on cultivated KK-47 cells were investigated by NITTA et al. (1988). When hyperthermia was combined with various concentrations of adriamycin ranging from 0.005 to 0.1 µg/ml, enhanced cell-killing effects were obtained at the concentrations of less than 0.02 µg/ml. There was, however, no increase in cell-killing effect at concentrations of more than 0.05 µg/ml of adriamycin. The combination of hyperthermia with peplomycin considerably enhanced the cell-killing effect, this enhancement increasing in accordance with the increase in the concentration of peplomycin. When hyperthermia was combined with various concentrations of adriamycin ranging from 0.005 to 0.1 µg/ml and bleomycin from 0.01 to 1.0 µg/ml, enhanced cell-killing effects were obtained at an adriamycin concentration of less than 0.02 µg/ml and with increasing concentrations of bleomycin (UCHIBAYASHI et al. 1993b). Using the cell lines T-24, MGH-U1, and KU-1, hyperthermia of 42°C enhanced the growth inhibitory effect of mitomycin C and cis-diamminedichloroplatinum (II), but did not influence the effect of doxorubicin (SAWAMURA et al. 1989).

At the dose of radiation and hyperthermia at 43°C required to produce 90% killing of a human bladder cancer cell line (MGU-2), it was demonstrated that those cells which initially survive radiation frequently show sustained growth delay and that their progeny may stop growing after a few generations of cell division. After an "equilethal" dose of hyperthermia there was a transient growth delay but there was no long-term loss of reproductive integrity in the surviving cells (MACKILLOP 1985). It has been clearly demonstrated that hyperthermia potentiates the cytotoxic action of irradiation (DEWEY et al. 1977).

27.2.2
Studies In Vivo

Hyperthermia of BC-50 bladder cancer cells in ACI/N rats had a marked cytotoxic effect on BC-50 transitional carcinoma cells in vitro. A significant difference was found between the effects of heat treatment at 41° and 42°C, indicating that the critical temperature for killing tumor cells was 42°C. Hyperthermia in combination with x-ray irradiation prolonged the survival of the rats (OGURA et al. 1981).

Most of the in vivo studies on hyperthermia in bladder cancer cell lines were performed with systemic chemotherapy. HAAS (1994) combined localized hyperthermia (43.5°C) of 60 and 90 min duration with systemic doxorubicin hydrochloride, cisplatin, cyclophosphamide, or mitomycin C to treat tumors implanted into the hind legs of C3H mice. Untreated tumors grew with an exponential rate and had a doubling time of 4 ± 1.5 days. Animals bearing such tumors survived for 25 ± 7 days. When the mice were treated with hyperthermia alone, there was no significant reduction in the growth rate and no improvement was noted in the survival time. Treatment with doxorubicin hydrochloride, cyclophosphamide, or mitomycin administered alone was likewise ineffective. The administration of cisplatin alone was able to induce only a minimal decrease in the growth rate. When the administration of chemotherapy was accompanied by hyperthermia, a significant synergistic effect was noted for doxorubicin hydrochloride, cisplatin, and cyclophosphamide ($P < 0.01$); only the mitomycin C and hyperthermia combination failed to improve survival and decrease the growth rate. The duration of the hyperthermia exposure influenced the degree of tumor response. Hyperthermia of 90 min duration resulted in a consistently greater decrease in tumor growth rate with doxorubicin hydrochloride, cisplatin, or cyclophosphamide than did 60 min of hyperthermia combined with the same agents. These results indicate that local hyperthermia combined with chemotherapy can induce tumor regression, decrease tumor doubling time, and improve the survival of the tumor-bearing animal (HAAS et al. 1985).

The combined effect of cis-diamminedichloroplatinum (II) and hyperthermia in the murine bladder tumor (MBT-2) was investigated by SHIMIZU (1988) following transplantation into the hind leg of a C3H/He mouse. The leg was submerged in a hot water bath immediately after the intraperitoneal administration of cis-diamminedichloroplatinum (II). The antitumor effects were evaluated from tumor volume. The cis-diamminedichloroplatinum (II) and hyperthermia (43°C) group showed remarkable tumor growth retardation.

The effects of a new recombinant human tumor necrosis factor (rTNF-S) on the growth of MBT-2 were studied by IIZUMI et al. (1989). The growth of MBT-2 was significantly inhibited by intratumoral injection of rTNF-S. Hyperthermia at a relatively low temperature enhanced the antitumor effect of rTNF-S.

Combined therapy with hyperthermia (43.5°C) and tumor necrosis factor (10^3 and 10^4 units) was also studied for the treatment of experimental bladder carcinoma KK-47 in athymic mice (AMANO et al. 1990). The animals were divided into control, hyperthermia alone, tumor necrosis factor alone, and combined therapy groups. The results of this study showed no significant difference between 10^3 units of tumor necrosis factor given intravenously and control but significant tumor regression in the hyperthermia alone group. Antitumor effects were significantly increased in mice receiving hyperthermia and 10^3 units tumor necrosis factor as compared with those receiving hyperthermia alone. Similar results were seen with 10^4 units of tumor necrosis factor given intravenously, though in the combination group of hyperthermia and tumor necrosis factor, eight mice of eight died 1–3 days following treatment. In those rodents receiving intratumoral injections, there was no difference between the tumor necrosis factor and control groups. The combination of tumor necrosis factor with hyperthermia had approximately the same antitumor effects as hyperthermia alone and therefore there was no synergistic effect. These results support on the suggestion that combination therapy with hyperthermia and systemic administration with the proper dose of tumor necrosis factor may produce synergistic anticancer effects in bladder cancer patients.

The effect of hyperthermia and intravesical chemotherapy has also been studied in an animal model (PREVOST et al. 1996). The microscopic changes in the bladder wall at two temperatures (43°C and 45°C) were studied with two different concentrations of mitomycin C (40 and 80 mg in 60 ml of serum). Hyperthermia was applied for 1 h with a flexible microwave applicator, operating at 915 MHz with an internal water cooling system. Immediately after the experiment the bladder was removed. No micro-

scopic changes were identified with hyperthermia at 43°C alone or in combination with either of the concentrations of mitomycin C. The urothelium was unchanged and only a moderate degree inflammation of the connective tissue was noted. However, at a temperature of 45°C, with or without the presence of mitomycin C, the investigators noticed the destruction of the urothelium, inflammatory changes, and hemorrhages in the connective tissue. The bladder muscle was not affected by this treatment.

These data provide strong evidence that transitional cell carcinoma is a heat-sensitive tumor and that radiosensitization or chemosensitization is possible. However, the bladder is a deep-seated pelvic organ, hampering a homogeneous therapeutic heating pattern with the presently available clinical hyperthermia equipment.

27.3
Deep Regional Hyperthermia

27.3.1
Introduction

The most common indication for hyperthermia in bladder cancer is bulky disease in the pelvis. In order to heat a large volume of tissue, deep regional hyperthermia has been used. However, it remains difficult to obtain and to maintain an average intratumoral temperature of 42°C or more. KAPP (1989) reported the maximum temperature obtained in his study to be between 42.2° and 43.9°C, with average temperatures ranging from 40.4° to 41.1°C. More than 50% of the recorded intratumoral temperature points were on average less than 41°C. With an annular phased array, PETROVICH et al. (1991) treated 53 patients with advanced tumors of the genitourinary tract. Tumor temperature was increased to more than 40°C for a sufficient length of time to accumulate thermal dose in only 28 (53%) of the patients, while in 25 (47%) the tumor temperature was less than 40°C and the thermal dose was 0.

Despite the preferential heating of the subcutaneous fat due to the high impedance for radiofrequency current, radiofrequency capacitive heating is the most commonly used method to heat deep-seated tumors in Japan. The success of this type of heating may be attributed to the relatively thin subcutaneous fat layer of the Japanese and it also may be due to superficial cooling. Intratumoral temperatures of 41.2°–47.8°C were reported by UCHIBAYASHI et al. (1992), with an average temperature of 44.2°C. The average intravesical temperature was 42.9°C. The maximum temperature in the tumors in the lateral and posterior wall of the bladder was higher than that in the tumors located in the trigone, dome, and bladder neck. The presence of intestinal gas or the pubic bone may be an important cause of the difficulty of raising the temperature.

27.3.2
Deep Regional Hyperthermia–Radiotherapy Combinations

Forty-three patients with deep-seated pelvic malignancies were treated at the University of Utah in a pilot study involving regional hyperthermia produced by the BSD-1000 hyperthermia system with the annular phased array applicator (SAPOZINK et al. 1986). Acute toxicity consisted primarily of pain within the aperture of the device (seen in 74% of patients), pain outside the aperture (33%), bladder spasm (26%), and systemic stress (25%). The most common power-limiting factors were pain (33%) and excessive heating of normal tissues (23%). In nine (21%) patients, there was no power-limiting factor. Treatment-related complications were uncommon and consisted of superficial second-degree burns (three patients), small bowel obstruction (one patient), and rectal fistula (one patient), all of which resolved with supportive nonsurgical therapy.

Detailed thermal mapping and thermal dosimetry were performed in 36 patients. Thermal dosimetry parameters were all rather disappointing; however, the protocol prioritized the prevention of complications, and patients with acute toxicity or other power-limiting factors were not pushed to achieve high thermal doses. "Concurrent radiation dose" and "number of satisfactory heat treatments" were highly and independently correlated with response ($P = 0.002$). Responders (median survival = 10 months) survived significantly longer (SAPOZINK et al. 1986)

Hyperthermia using the Thermotron RF-8 was performed in 19 patients with various forms of cancer (five bladder, three uterine, and three rectal cancers, four soft tissue tumors, two oral cancers, one biliary tract cancer, and one renal cell carcinoma) between April 1986 and December 1986 (TERASHIMA et al. 1987). They were irradiated with a daily dose of

1.5–2.0 Gy, 5 times a week, and hyperthermia was performed within 30 min after the irradiation once or twice a week. Intratumoral temperature was kept between 43°C and 45°C. A temperature of more than 41°C was maintained in most patients. Partial response, defined as 80% or more regression in tumor volume, was obtained in one bladder cancer patient. Side-effects were observed in all patients, including mild skin burn, nausea, and diarrhea. A rectovaginal fistula developed in one patient.

During a 6-year period, 53 patients with advanced tumors of the genitourinary tract were treated in phase I protocols with deep regional hyperthermia in combination with irradiation (83% of patients) or chemotherapy (11% of patients) (PETROVICH et al. 1991). Primary tumors included bladder tumors in 22 (41%) patients, prostate tumors in 20 (37%), kidney tumors in nine (17%), and ureter, testicle, or adrenal tumors in three (5%). The majority (77%) had had prior definitive therapy and had experienced treatment failure, and 11% had clinically important distant metastases. The deep regional hyperthermia was administered in a mean of four sessions. Among the 22 patients with transitional cell carcinoma of the bladder, only two had a partial response. The treatment tolerance was good in 79% of patients.

These three reported studies were all phase I studies performed in heterogeneous groups of patients. The reasons for the poor results obtained in treating bladder cancer patients are not clear. Although minor toxicity was common, severe complications were rare. The two American studies reported difficulty in obtaining hyperthermic (>42°C) intratumoral temperatures.

A recent Japanese phase I/II study (MASUNAGA et al. 1994), evaluated preoperative thermoradiotherapy in a group of 49 patients with T1–4N0M0 bladder cancer. Twenty-one patients were preoperatively treated by radiotherapy alone, with 4 Gy per fraction and three fractions per week to a total dose of 24 Gy (group 1). The other 28 patients were treated by the same radiotherapy regimen in combination with hyperthermia (group 2). Regional hyperthermia was administered for 35–60 min immediately after irradiation (two sessions per week to a total of four sessions), using an 8-MHz radiofrequency capacitive heating device. Group 2 was divided into two subgroups according to the obtained treatment temperature. The first subgroup (high) had an average intravesical temperature, $T_{average}$, of >41.5°C, while the second subgroup (low) had a $T_{average}$ of <41.5°C. The first subgroup (high) showed a significantly higher incidence of downstaging and tumor necrosis than both group 1 and the subgroup 2 (low). In addition, the incidence of local recurrence was lower and survival time was longer in group 2 than in group 1. This difference was, however, not statistically significant. In particular, the patients with T3–4 or grade 3 bladder cancer in group 2 had a longer average survival than those in group 1, although again this difference was not statistically significant.

27.3.3
Deep Regional Hyperthermia–Radiotherapy–Chemotherapy Combinations

The combination of regional hyperthermia, radiotherapy, and chemotherapy has been reported exclusively in the Japanese literature. ENDOW et al. (1990) reported treatment results in 311 patients (a heterogeneous group of tumors) with an overall response rate of 53%.

A multi-institutional study of clinical hyperthermia in deep-seated tumors was undertaken using 8-MHz radiofrequency capacitive heating devices (Thermotron RF-8) at seven medical centers (KAKEHI et al. 1990). Each medical center was designated to treat tumors of specific sites. A total of 177 patients treated from January 1985 to December 1988 were evaluated. Complete and partial responses were obtained in 71% of patients with urinary bladder cancer. Thermometry was performed using indirect measurement of the intracavitary temperature. An intracavitary temperature greater than 42°C was obtained in 73.7% of patients. The contribution of hyperthermia in improving the quality of life of patients under terminal care was also investigated. It was indicated that hyperthermia was one of the most effective treatment techniques in patients with advanced or inoperable tumors. In this study most of the discussion focused on the local control rate because the period of follow-up was only 3 years. Side-effects were observed in 37 (21%) patients. The side-effects of importance included fatty induration, pain during treatment, and local burns. However, no side-effects were severe enough to interrupt the course of treatment.

Eleven patients with invasive transitional cell carcinoma of the bladder were treated by UEDA et al. (1991) with hyperthermia, combined with hydroxypropyl cellulose (HPC)-adriamycin, or radiation therapy. The staging of these 11 patients was as follows: T2 in five (45%), T3 in three (27%), and T4 in

three (27%). Tumor grade was as follows: grade 2 in eight (73%) patients, grade 3 in two (18%), and grade 3 with anaplastic carcinoma admixture in one (9%). Pretreatment radiation therapy, transurethral resection, and chemotherapy were given in all patients. Among the 11 patients treated, complications were observed in eight (73%). Complications included cases of severe heart disease. Complete response was observed in four patients (36%), partial response in four (36%), no change in two (18%), and progressive disease in one (9%).

Despite these early positive reports obtained in small nonrandomized studies, NAITO et al. (1991), who included a control group, could not detect a significant difference in the studied outcomes. Sixty-three patients with bladder cancer that was of stage greater than T3b and/or nonresectable were analyzed with regard to treatment and prognosis. Of the 63 patients treated, 31 (49%) had nonresectable bladder cancer, 9 (14%) had T3b tumor, 15 (24%) had T4b tumor, 6 (10%) had M1 disease, and 4 (6%) had N4 disease. Twenty-four of the 31 patients with nonresectable disease received systemic chemotherapy, 8-MHz radiofrequency hyperthermia, radiation therapy, or a combination of these three modalities. The administration of this treatment resulted in a partial response in nine (32%) patients and a minor response in four (13%); seven patients (23%) had no change and two (6%) had progressive disease. In two additional patients treatment response was not evaluated. Seven of the 31 patients received no treatment. The 1- and 2-year survival rates with the above treatment and with no treatment were 27.7% and 16.7%, respectively, and 33.4% and 16.7%, respectively. There was no significant difference between the survival rates of the two groups. Thirty-two of the 63 patients underwent surgical treatment. In 17 patients, total cystectomy was carried out. Of these 17 surgically treated patients, nine received the above outlined preoperative treatment and eight received no preoperative therapy. The 1- and 2-year survival rates in the group receiving adjuvant therapy were 33.3% and 11.1%, respectively, while they were 66.7% and 66.7%, respectively, in the group which received surgical treatment alone. Survival of the two groups was not significantly different statistically. NAITO et al. (1991) concluded that anticancer treatment as given in their study, which included chemotherapy, hyperthermia, and radiation, did not enhance long-term survival.

NOGUCHI et al. (1992) investigated the additional effect of M-VAC (methotrexate, vinblastine, adriamycin, and cisplatin) on a combination of radiotherapy and hyperthermia, followed by surgery. A total of 17 patients received the combination of radiation, hyperthermia, and M-VAC therapy between January 1989 and July 1990. Of these 17 patients, 12 underwent cystectomy and 14 were evaluable for tumor response. The objective response rate was 64% (9/14), with four patients achieving a complete remission that was histologically confirmed. Treatment complications included nausea and vomiting in all patients, and 71% (12/17) of the patients developed leukopenia. However, these side-effects were not serious. No significant difference in the tumor response was detected between the radiation and hyperthermia only group and the radiation and hyperthermia plus M-VAC group. It has not yet been possible to evaluate the long-term results.

The advantage of administration of a preoperative combination of radiotherapy and chemotherapy in the management of patients with advanced transitional cell carcinoma remains to be proven. The role of hyperthermia in this combination is not clear, since most studies have included a relatively small number of patients who were treated in nonrandomized trials.

27.4
Intracavitary Radiofrequency Hyperthermia

27.4.1
Intracavitary Hyperthermia Combined with Intravesical Chemotherapy

COLOMBO et al. (1995) treated 44 patients with recurrent superficial transitional cell carcinoma of the bladder with a combination of microwave hyperthermia and mitomycin C at a does of 30 mg in 60 ml of distilled water. Hyperthermia was delivered by direct bladder wall irradiation by a 915-MHz applicator, built into a three-way 20-French transurethral catheter. Temperature was monitored by thermocouples at the bladder wall. Hyperthermia was delivered at a mean temperature of 42.5°C–44.5°C. Mild urgency and urethral burning were present during all hyperthermia sessions. This treatment was very well tolerated, with only 3.4% of patients showing poor treatment tolerance. Endoscopic and histologic evaluation proved that combined local hyperthermia and chemotherapy can induce necrosis in transitional cell carcinoma. The overall

response rate was 90.8%, which included, 70.4% complete and 20.4% partial responses. Four (9.2%) patients had no response. A prospective randomized study is scheduled to be performed in order to evaluate the effect of hyperthermia versus hyperthermia and chemotherapy.

27.4.2
Intracavitary Hyperthermia Combined with Intra-arterial Chemotherapy

BICHLER et al. (1989) applied transurethral microwave hyperthermia by a modified 24-French endoscope, operating at a frequency of 300–500 kHz. According to the Seldinger technique a catheter was placed through the femoral artery into the internal iliac artery and then downstream to the branch of the superior gluteal artery. An infusion of 10 mg mitomycin C in 15 ml (900 mg) Spherex was administered. The patient population consisted of six T3 and T4N0M0 patients and six with metastatic, T3–4N1M0–1 transitional cell bladder cancers. These patients were treated with combined intra-arterial cytostatic microsphere infusion and scheduled adjunctive transurethral radiofrequency hyperthermia. From the group of six patients with locally advanced tumors, three had complete remission and three had partial remission. These responses after the combined treatment were histologically evaluated following radical cystectomy.

27.5
Bladder Irrigation with Hyperthermic Solutions

27.5.1
The Effects of Hyperthermic Irrigation on the Bladder Wall

JACOB et al. (1982) performed electron microscopic studies of the normal bladder urothelium of elderly subjects treated by hyperthermic perfusions and showed that the tissue responded in every instance with desquamation. There was no evidence of cell death prior to desquamation, although various organelles underwent structural alterations. Mitochondria were especially prone to suffer varying degrees of damage. A short heat shock revealed differences in the initial response of the thick and thin regions of bladder urothelium known to occur in elderly subjects. After a long, fractionated treatment, regeneration was evident within 3 days after the end of treatment. Follow-up biopsies of the bladder revealed a hyperplastic urothelium within 10–12 weeks after the completion of therapy. The constituent cells showed signs of cytodifferentiation at this time, but it remains unknown when an ultrastructurally normal urothelium with characteristic cell layers would be restored. The results obtained with the various treatments in this study suggest that the stem cells in the epithelium are unaffected by the levels of hyperthermia employed and that their unimpaired proliferative capacity ensures regeneration of the urothelium.

27.5.2
Intravesical Hyperthermic Instillations

In a study by Uchibayashi et al. (1993a), 33 patients with malignant bladder tumors were treated by hyperthermic intravesical perfusion. The study group included 25 (76%) patients with superficial T1 tumors, four (12%) with T2 tumors, and four (12%) with T3 tumors. Physiologic saline solution containing 40 µg/ml of peplomycin with or without 2% ethanol was used as a perfusate. Perfusion was carried out for 2 h, 3 times per week and this regimen was repeated every other week, totaling six sessions in 3 weeks. Of the 33 patients treated, three (9%) achieved a complete response, five (15%) had a partial response (more than 50% tumor reduction), eight (24%) had a minimal response (25%–50% tumor reduction), and the remaining 17 (51%) patients showed no response. Complete, partial, and minimal responses were obtained only in patients with T1 tumors. The nonresponders included four patients with T2 and four with T3 lesions. Profuse hematuria from invasive tumor was markedly reduced after the treatment. A major side-effect recorded in this study was irritation of the bladder and urethra. The investigators concluded that their results indicated that hyperthermic perfusion with ethanol and peplomycin is clinically safe and may be useful for the management of superficial bladder tumors in elderly patients.

Another study (Nishimura et al. 1985) used hyperthermic irrigation of the bladder with bleomycin at 43°–44°C for 3 h. This treatment was given to 80 patients after transurethral resection had been performed for bladder cancer. Bleomycin 90 mg, in 3000 ml saline solution, was used to irrigate

the bladder for 10 days postoperatively. No severe side-effects were observed, though bladder irritability was reported in 58% of patients. Freedom from recurrence was calculated by the actuarial method in 54 patients with primary bladder cancer. The incidence of tumor control was 88.0% after 1 year, 73.3% after 2 and 3 years, and 63.5% after 4 years following treatment. Recurrence rate per 100 patient-months was 0.98. On the basis of these observations, it was concluded that hyperthermic irrigation with bleomycin is useful in the prophylaxis against recurrence of bladder cancer after local removal of the tumor.

27.5.3
Radiotherapy Combined with Intravesical Hyperthermic Irrigation

Kubota et al. (1984) reported on a patient with advanced urinary bladder cancer treated with a combination of radiation and radiofrequency hyperthermia, and intravesical irrigation with warm water. The tumor temperature was successfully maintained between 43°C and 44.6°C by external application of 13.56 MHz radiofrequency hyperthermia when the bladder was irrigated with heated saline (intravesical temperature: 43°C). Hyperthermia was performed for 30 min immediately after each course of external bladder irradiation, which consisted of 40 Gy, given twice a week at 400 cGy, for a total period of 5 weeks. Complete tumor regression was reported after the completion of the combination therapy.

In a study by Matsui et al. (1991), immediately following daily external irradiation (40 Gy/4 weeks), patients were irrigated with a solution of warmed saline (intravesical temperature, 42°–43°C) containing 30 µg/ml of bleomycin. Of a total of 56 patients, complete responses were observed in 25 (46%), and partial responses in 21 (37.5%) patients. Among the T2 and T3 patients, an 84% response rate was noted in combination therapy, whereas a 56% response rate was observed after radiation alone (50–70 Gy). The side-effects of the combination therapy were limited to reversible bladder irritation, and bladder capacity could be maintained within normal limits. These results suggest that combination therapy represents an effective conservative therapy for the management of bladder cancer (Matsui et al. 1991).

27.5.4
Intra-arterial Cisplatin Chemotherapy with Hyperthermic Bladder Irrigation

In a study by Jacobs et al. (1984), a total of six patients with bulky bladder cancers underwent combination therapy with hypogastric artery infusion of cisplatin and local bladder hyperthermia. Hyperthermia was given as a preoperative adjunct to radical cystectomy, heated water being circulated through a 24-French, three-way catheter by means of a pump. Pathologic examination of the specimens showed extensive tumor necrosis on the luminal side, with a gradient of tumor destruction to viable tumor on the serosal surface in four of the six bladders, while two specimens showed no tumor. Uninvolved portions of the bladders showed minor changes in the urothelium, submucosal edema, and no effect on detrusor muscle or perivesical fat. Analysis of tissue for cisplatin revealed uptake by the tumors and normal tissue. Systemic effects of cisplatin were not seen. Adjunctive preoperative hypogastric artery infusion of cisplatin is safe and well tolerated. Further study is required to determine the upper limits of safety of the regimen.

27.6
Conclusion

In vitro and in vivo experimental studies provide strong evidence that transitional cell carcinoma of the bladder is sensitive to heating. Hyperthermia may be a useful modality as an adjuvant treatment to chemotherapy and/or radiotherapy.

Attempts have been made to obtain local tumor control in superficial bladder cancer by hyperthermic instillations or intracavitary microwave hyperthermia, combined with local chemotherapy. If this treatment were to be proven successful in controlling superficial bladder cancer without transurethral manipulations, it would be a milestone in urologic oncology. Although the reported phase I studies were promising, further prospective randomized studies will have to objectively prove the benefit of this therapy.

The best prognostic factor for the achievement of local control in the management of bladder cancer is total tumor eradication at the time of surgery. Long-term survival rates of 50%–78% have been reported (Kapp 1989). After transurethral resection, the role of hyperthermia as an adjuvant treatment to preoperative radiotherapy needs to be evaluated.

Today local hyperthermia is gradually being investigated, and perhaps is coming to replace deep regional hyperthermia.

For locally advanced disease, the main question associated with the use of hyperthermia still remains relevant, namely how to heat homogeneously and maintain hyperthermic temperatures in a large volume in the pelvis without causing major side-effects. At this stage, only deep regional hyperthermia can, to a certain extent, meet these goals, although it is common knowledge that therapeutic temperatures are hard to obtain and maintain with this treatment mode.

References

Amano T, Kumini K, Nakashima K, Uchibayashi T, Hisazumi H (1990) A combined therapy of hyperthermia and tumor necrosis factor for nude mice bearing KK-47 bladder cancer. J Urol 144:370–374

Bichler KH, Fluchter SH, Steimann J, Strohmaier WL (1989) Combination of hyperthermia and cytostatics in the treatment of bladder cancer. Urol Int 44:10–14

Colombo R, Lev A, Da Pozzo LF, Freschi M, Gallus G, Rigatti P (1995) A new approach using local combined microwave hyperthermia and chemotherapy in superficial transitional bladder carcinoma treatment. J Urol 153:959–963

Dewey WC, Hopwood LE, Sapareto SA, Gerweck LE (1977) Cellular responses to combinations of hyperthermia and radiation. Radiology 123:464

Endow M, Suzuki H, Nakashima Y, et al. (1990) Curability of multidisciplinary treatment including combined hyperthermia, radiotherapy and chemotherapy. Gan No Rinsho 36:505–513

Haas GP, Klugo RC, Hetzel FW, Barton EE, Cerny JC (1985) The synergistic effect of hyperthermia and chemotherapy on murine transitional cell carcinoma. J Urol 132:828–833

Iizumi T, Yazaki T, Waku M, Soma G (1989) Immuno-chemotherapy for murine bladder tumor with a new human recombinant tumor necrosis factor (rTNF-S), VP-16 and hyperthermia. J Urol 42:386–389

Jacob J, Hindmarsh JR, Ludgate CM, Chisholm GD (1982) Observations on the ultrastructure of human urothelium: the response of normal bladder of elderly subjects to hyperthermia. Urol Res 10:227–237

Jacobs SC, McCellan SL, Maher C, Lawson RK (1984) Pre-cystectomy intra-arterial cisplatin with local bladder hyperthermia for bladder cancer. J Urol 131: 473–476

Kakehi M, Ueda K, Mukojima T, Hiraoka M, Seto O, Akanuma A, Nakatsugawa S (1990) Multi-institutional clinical studies on hyperthermia combined with radiotherapy or chemotherapy in advanced cancer of deep-seated organs. Int J Hyperthermia 6:719–40

Kapp DS (1989) Indications for the clinical use of deep local and regional hyperthermia in conjunction with radiation therapy. Strahlenther Onkol 165:724–728

Kubota Y, Takebayashi S, Asakura K, Oshima H (1984) Application of radiofrequency hyperthermia for treating advanced urinary bladder cancer – a case report. Gan No Rinsho 30:215–219

Mackillop WJ (1985) The non-lethal effects of ionizing radiation and hyperthermia on colony growth in a human bladder cancer cell line. Cancer Lett 27:315–322

Masunaga SI, Hiraoka M, Akuta K, et al. (1994) Phase I/II trial of preoperative thermoradiotherapy in the treatment of urinary bladder cancer. Int J Hyperthermia 10:31–40

Matsui K, Takebayashi S, Watai K, Kakehi M, Kubota Y, Yao M, Shuin T (1991) Combination radiotherapy of urinary bladder carcinoma with chemohyperthermia. Int J Hyperthermia 7:19–26

Matzkin H, Rangel MC, Soloway MS (1992) In vitro study of the effect of hyperthermia on normal bladder cell line and on five different transitional cell carcinoma cell lines. J Urol 147:1671–1674

Naito K, Hasegawa T, Ishida T, et al. (1991) A clinical survey of advanced bladder cancer: treatment of advanced and non-resectable bladder cancer. Hinyokika Kiyo 37:1601–1606

Nishimura K, Ogawa O, Yoshimura N, Nakagawa T, Sasaki M (1985) Effect of hyperthermic irrigation with bleomycin on prophylaxis of recurrence of bladder cancer. Hinyokika Kiyo 31:769–773

Nitta M, Hisazumi H, Nakajima K (1988) Combined cell killing effects of anticancer drugs and hyperthermia in vitro. Hinyokika Kiyo 34:1525–1528

Noguchi S, Kubota Y, Miura T, Shuin T, Hosaka M (1992) Use of methotrexate, vinblastine, adriamycin, and cisplatin in combination with radiation and hyperthermia as neo-adjuvant therapy for bladder cancer. Cancer Chemother Pharmacol 30(Suppl P):S63–S65

Ogura K, Kagawa S, Kurokawa K (1981) Effect of hyperthermia on experimental bladder tumors. Eur Urol 7:100–104

Petrovich Z, Emami B, Kapp D, et al. (1991) Regional hyperthermia in patients with recurrent genitourinary cancer. Am J Clin Oncol 14:472–477

Prevost B, Demetriou D, Mauroy B, Sozansky JB, Vanseymortier L, Delobelle-Deroide A, Chivé M (1996) Thermo-chemotherapy (mitomycin C). Experimental study on normal dog bladders: immediate post experimental effects. Hyperthermic Oncology 1996, Abstract Book 7th International Congress on Hyperthermic Oncology, Italy, April 9–13, 1996, volume II, pp 647–649

Sapozink MD, Gibbs FA Jr, Egger MJ, Stewart JR (1986) Regional hyperthermia for clinically advanced deep-seated pelvic malignancy. Am J Clin Oncol 9:162–169

Sawamura M, Odajima K, Nagakura K, Nakamura H (1989) Chemosensitivity testing on human bladder cancer cell lines, using MTT-assay. Nippon Hinyokika Gakkai Zasshi 80:1195–1202

Shimizu K (1988) Combination effects of CDDP and hyperthermia in mouse bladder tumor (MBT-2) Hinyokika Kiyo 34:627–632

Terashima H, Ishino Y, Nakata H, Norimura T, Tsuchiya T (1987) Combined radiotherapy and local external hyperthermia in advanced cancer – animal experiment and clinical study. Sangyo Ika Daigaku Zasshi 9:171–180

Uchibayashi T, Nakajima K, Hisazumi H, Mihara S, Yamamoto H, Koshida K (1992) Studies of temperature rise in bladder cancer and surrounding tissues during radiofrequency hyperthermia. Eur Urol 21:299–303

Uchibayashi T, Lee SW, Hisazumi H, et al. (1993a) Studies of combined treatment of radiofrequency hyperthermia with anticancer agents or irradiation for invasive bladder cancer. Hinyokika Kiyo 39:1209–1213

Uchibayashi T, Nakajima K, Hisazumi H, Nishino A, Miyoshi N (1993b) Hyperthermic intravesical peplomycin perfusion treatment for bladder cancer. Br J Urol 72:65–67

Ueda K, Sakagami H, Kato F, Mogami T, Ohtaguro K (1991) Current status of the conservative treatment of urinary bladder for invasive bladder cancer. Hinyokika Kiyo 37:1597–1599

28 Management of Patients with Metastatic Carcinoma of the Bladder

C.C.D. VAN DER RIJT and T.A.W. SPLINTER

28.1 Introduction

Survival in untreated patients with metastatic carcinoma of the bladder is poor, the median survival being 3 months (BABAIAN et al. 1980). The current therapy of choice is combination chemotherapy, which is given with palliative intent, although some long-term survivors have been reported after achieving a complete response on chemotherapy. No clinical trials have been performed on treatment with chemotherapy versus best supportive care. Nevertheless, results from studies on prognostic factors and from phase III clinical trials support a beneficial effect of chemotherapy on survival in metastatic urothelial cancer. In most studies, data on urothelial cancer from different localizations have been clustered, as no differences in prognosis seem to exist between them.

In practice, decisions on the employment of chemotherapy and the choice of the combination of chemotherapeutic agents have to be made for the individual patient. Knowledge on prognostic factors and toxicity profiles may help in this decision-making process.

C.C.D. VAN DER RIJT, MD, Rotterdam Cancer Institute, Groene Hilledijk 301, 3075 EA Rotterdam, The Netherlands
T.A.W. SPLINTER, MD, University Hospital Rotterdam, Dr. Molewaterplein 40, 3015 GD Rotterdam, The Netherlands

28.2 Prognostic Factors

Factors affecting the response to chemotherapy and survival have been studied for different treatment regimens. A better response was found for nodal (N+) than for metastatic (M+) disease (LOGOTHETIS et al. 1989, 1990a; JEFFERY and MEAD 1992; ROTH et al. 1994). Furthermore, survival was also better for N+ than for M+ disease with different cisplatin-containing regimens (LOGOTHETIS et al. 1990a; STERNBERG et al. 1989; BOUTAN-LAROZE et al. 1991; JEFFERY and MEAD 1992). Response rates were lower for metastases to liver and/or bone than for other metastatic tumor sites (OLIVER et al. 1986; MARU et al. 1987; STERNBERG et al. 1989; IGAWA et al. 1990; OGAWA et al. 1992; UEKI et al. 1992; LOEHRER et al. 1992), as were the survival rates (LOEHRER et al. 1992, 1994).

Multivariate analyses have been performed to study the importance of several prognostic factors and their possible joint interactions. Most of these analyses found the performance status of the patient to be an important prognosticator for survival (KHANDEKAR et al. 1985; GELLER et al. 1991; IGAWA et al. 1992; LOEHRER et al. 1992; SENGELOV et al. 1994). The importance of the site of metastases has been confirmed in some analyses by the selection of serum alkaline phosphatase (GELLER et al. 1991; SENGELOV et al. 1994) and a combined variable representing liver, bone, and/or lung metastases (LOEHRER et al. 1992) as poor prognostic factors. For patients treated with different chemotherapy regimens, the median survival was only 3.6 months when there was a poor performance score and an elevated serum alkaline phosphatase (SENGELOV et al. 1994). If there were lung, bone, and/or liver metastases in conjunction with a performance status <80% and recent weight loss, the survival on cisplatin-containing chemotherapy was only 4.2–4.4 months (LOEHRER et al. 1992). A much better median survival of about a year was found in patients with a good performance score and a normal serum alkaline phosphatase after treatment with chemotherapy (SENGELOV et al. 1994). Other factors which decrease survival rates may be former radiotherapy (KHANDEKAR et al. 1985; TRONER et al. 1987), former chemotherapy (IGAWA et al. 1991), and increased serum creatinine (SENGELOV et al. 1994).

28.3
Chemotherapy

28.3.1
Single-Agent Chemotherapy

Chemotherapeutic agents from the first generation, studied in metastatic urothelial cancer and reported by Yagoda, are summarized in Table 28.1. The most extensively studied drugs were cisplatin, methotrexate, and doxorubicin (YAGODA 1987). Cisplatin has long been considered the most active agent in transitional cell carcinoma, with a response rate in phase II studies of about 30%. Complete responses after cisplatin monotherapy have been rather uncommon, as is the case with the other first-generation chemotherapeutic agents. In later phase III studies, response rates on monotherapy with cisplatin were quite disappointing, with percentages ranging from 12% to 31% (SOLOWAY et al. 1983; KHANDEKAR et al. 1985; TRONER et al. 1987; HILLCOAT et al. 1989; LOEHRER et al. 1992). On the basis of the results of phase II studies, a dose of $70 \, mg/m^2$ every 3 weeks was suggested. However, in several phase III trials, doses were lower or were given with an interval of 4 weeks. Moreover, differences in patient selection between multicenter studies and single-institution studies might also have contributed to the lower response rates.

Methotrexate has been studied in low- and high-dose regimens. High-dose methotrexate, $100 \, mg/m^2$ or more, is given with leucovorin rescue. Higher doses of methotrexate may induce a higher response rate, but randomized studies have not been performed. Doxorubicin (adriamycin) and 5-fluorouracil have been studied in a large number of patients, with response rates of about 17%. The other chemotherapeutic agents with a potential effect have been studied in only small numbers of patients. The single-agent activities of vinblastine, vincristine, mitomycin C, and teniposide have been found to be less impressive, but all showed greater than 10% response rates.

28.3.2
Combination Chemotherapy Regimens

The combination of several chemotherapeutic agents with known single-agent activity in urothelial cancer was introduced in the 1980s. With combination chemotherapy, an increased complete response rate was aimed at to improve survival in metastatic urothelial cancer. Subsequent studies on different multiagent chemotherapy regimens indeed showed better survival rates for those who had responded on the therapy than for the nonresponders (HARKER et al. 1985; MARU et al. 1987; STOTER et al. 1987; STERNBERG et al. 1989; LOGOTHETIS et al. 1989; IGAWA et al. 1990; KOTAKE et al. 1992).

Several different combinations of chemotherapy have been studied. Most treatment regimens included cisplatin, as it seemed the most active compound in transitional cell carcinoma. The combinations of chemotherapy that have been studied most thoroughly are cisplatin with methotrexate, cisplatin with doxorubicin and cyclophosphamide, cisplatin with methotrexate and vinblastine, and a four-agent strategy composed of cisplatin, methotrexate, vinblastine and doxorubicin. Other combinations including 5-fluorouracil and teniposide have not been used as much.

28.3.2.1
Cisplatin and Methotrexate

As cisplatin and methotrexate seemed to be the two most active agents in urothelial cancer, a combination of the drugs seemed logical. Different investiga-

Table 28.1. Single-agent activity in urothelial tract tumors (from YAGODA 1987)

Drug	No.	%	CR + PR[a]
Cisplatin	320	30	25–350
Methotrexate			
All doses	236	29	23–35
High dose	57	45	32–50
Doxorubicin	248	17	12–23
5-Fluorouracil	105	15	12–19
Vinblastine	38	16	4–28
Vincristine	42	14	3–25
Mitomycin C	42	13	3–23
Teniposide i.v.	64	11	3–19
Cyclophosphamide	26	7	0–17
Bleomycin	79	5	0–10
Etoposide	47	2	0–4

[a] 95% confidence interval.

Table 28.2. Cisplatin plus methotrexate in advanced urothelial cancer

Author (year)[a]	Therapy	No.	Response	
			CR (%)	CR + PR (%) (95% conf. int.)
Phase II				
CARMICHAEL et al. (1985)	CDDP: 100 mg/m^2, d2 MTX: 200 mg/m^2, d1	19	21	68 (43–88)
OLIVER et al. (1986)	CDDP: 60–80 mg/m^2, d1 MTX: 60–80 mg/m^2, d1 30–50 mg/m^2, d10	20	15	45 (23–69)
STOTER et al. (1987)	CDDP: 70 mg/m^2, d1 MTX: 40 mg/m^2, d8 + 15	43	23	46 (31–62)
FOSSÅ et al. (1990)	CDDP: 50 mg/m^2, d1 MTX: 250 mg/m^2, d2	27	8	54 (33–75)
Phase III				
HILLCOAT et al. (1989)	CDDP: 80 mg/m^2, d1 MTX: 50 mg/m^2, d1 + 15	53	9	45 (32–60)

CDDP, Cisplatin; MTX, methotrexate.

[a] Cycles were given every 3 weeks by Carmichael, Oliver, and Stoter; every 2 weeks by Fossa; and every 4 weeks by Hillcoat.

tors studied the potential benefit of cisplatin plus methotrexate (Table 28.2); all used different treatment regimens. Methotrexate was used in low doses as well as in medium doses. Response rates (CR + PR) ranged between 45% and 68% in the phase II studies, which seemed consistently higher than the response to treatment with cisplatin alone. The largest phase II study, a multicenter one coordinated by the European Organization for Research and Treatment of Cancer (EORTC), was performed in 53 patients with metastatic bladder cancer, of whom 43 were evaluable for response. Methotrexate was used in a low dose of 40 mg/m^2, 7 and 14 days after the administration of cisplatin 70 mg/m^2. Leucovorin rescue was not required in the protocol. Toxicity was severe in this study, with mucositis grade 3/4 occurring in 28%, leukopenia in 30%, and severe thrombocytopenia in 17% of the patients. Only 17% of the patients could receive the therapy as scheduled. The complete response rate of 23% seemed promising (STOTER et al. 1987).

One multicenter phase III study on cisplatin and methotrexate has been performed by HILLCOAT et al. (1989). Following randomization, 55 patients were treated with cisplatin at a dose of 80 mg/m^2 every 4 weeks, and 53 patients were treated with the same dose of cisplatin, given on day 2, and two doses of methotrexate, 50 mg/m^2, on days 1 and 15, also every 4 weeks. The toxicity of the combination therapy was more severe, with 20% of the patients developing mucositis and 27% grade 3–4 bone marrow depres-

sion, as compared to 0% and 2%, respectively, of the patients treated with cisplatin alone. The response rate in the combination therapy arm (CR, 9%; CR + PR, 45%) did not differ significantly from that in the cisplatin arm (CR, 9%; CR + PR, 31%). There was also no significant difference in the survival (median survival of 8.7 and 7.2 months for the combination and for cisplatin alone, respectively). A definite conclusion on the value of cisplatin/methotrexate versus cisplatin chemotherapy is hampered, however, by the small sample size of the study. Furthermore, although not statistically different, more patients treated with the combination had metastases to the bone (38% vs 24%, respectively) and lungs (26% vs 15%, respectively).

28.3.2.2
Cyclophosphamide–Doxorubicin–Cisplatin Combination

Combination chemotherapy with cisplatin, cyclophosphamide, and doxorubicin [CAP (or CISCA)] was also introduced in the 1980s. As shown in Table 28.3, different dose schedules have been used in phase II studies, with response rates varying from 38% to 65%. The highest response rate of 65%, with a complete response in 36% of treated patients, came from M.D. Anderson Hospital in Houston, Texas (LOGOTHETIS et al. 1989). The study was a retrospective review of 97 patients treated with CISCA at a

Table 28.3. CAP in advanced urothelial tumors

Author (year)	Therapy	No.	Response	
			CR (%)	CR + PR (%)
Phase II				
TRONER and HEMSTREET (1981)	CDDP: 40 mg/m^2 Adria: 40 mg/m^2 Cyclo: 400 mg/m^2	34	9	38
MULDER et al. (1982)	CDDP: 40 mg/m^2 Adria: 40 mg/m^2 Cyclo: 400 mg/m^2	42	12	40
SCHWARTZ et al. (1983)	CDDP: 70 mg/m^2 Adria: 45 mg/m^2 Cyclo: 250 mg/m^2	28	7	46
LOGOTHETIS et al. (1989)	CDDP: 70–100 mg/m^2 Adria: 50 mg/m^2 Cyclo: 650 mg/m^2	97	36	65
Phase III				
KHANDEKAR et al. (1985)	CDDP: 60 mg/m^2 Adria: 40 mg/m^2 Cyclo: 600 mg/m^2	45	22	33
TRONER et al. (1987)	CDDP: 60 mg/m^2 Adria: 40 mg/m^2 Cyclo: 400 mg/m^2	43	5	21
MARU et al. (1987)	CDDP: 30–50 mg/m^2 Adria: 30–50 mg/m^2 Cyclo: 200–500 mg/m^2	96	0	13
LOGOTHETIS et al. (1990a)	CDDP: 100 mg/m^2 Adria: 50 mg/m^2 Cyclo: 650 mg/m^2	55	25	46

higher dose than in other phase II studies (Table 28.3). Of the 97 patients treated, 62 (64%) had locally advanced disease, and only 35 (36%) patients had distant metastases. The total response rate did not differ between the patients with locally advanced disease and those with visceral metastases (65% versus 63%, respectively), but the complete response seemed higher in the locally advanced group (36% versus 20%). Because of the retrospective nature of the study, no evaluation of toxicity was possible.

Two multicenter randomized studies were performed, comparing CAP chemotherapy with cisplatin alone. The Eastern Cooperative Oncology Group (ECOG) randomized 135 patients with metastatic urothelial cancer to receive either the combination cisplatin 60 mg/m^2, doxorubicin 40 mg/m^2, and cyclophosphamide 600 mg/m^2, or cisplatin 60 mg/m^2. Both regimens were given every 3 weeks. Treatment was stopped after three cycles in cases of stable disease or progression. The total response rate in the 45 evaluable CAP-treated patients did not dif-

fer significantly from that in the 48 evaluable cisplatin-treated ones (33% vs 17%, respectively), but the complete response rate was significantly higher in the group treated with CAP (22% vs 2%). No significant difference in survival could be proven, however, with a median survival of 7.3 months for CAP and 6.0 months for cisplatin alone (KHANDEKAR et al. 1985). The second randomized study on CAP versus cisplatin was performed by the Southeastern Cancer Study Group (SWOG) in 116 patients. Treatment regimens were similar to the ECOG study; only the cyclophosphamide dose was lower, 400 mg/m^2. Forty-three and 48 patients were evaluable for response in the CAP and cisplatin groups, respectively. The response rates did not differ significantly (21% vs 15%, with complete response in 5% vs 0%, for CAP and cisplatin, respectively). The median survival times were also quite similar: 29 and 21 weeks for CAP and cisplatin, respectively (TRONER et al. 1987). These randomized studies do not support a major benefit of treatment with CAP over monotherapy with cisplatin. However, the sample size of both studies was small and the statistical power, therefore, limited.

28.3.2.3
Cisplatin–Methotrexate–Vinblastine Combination

Combination chemotherapy with cisplatin, methotrexate, and vinblastine (CMV) was introduced in 1985 for the treatment of metastatic transitional cell carcinoma of the urinary tract (HARKER et al. 1985). The drugs were chosen because of their known single-agent activity. Sixty patients with metastatic disease were entered in a multicenter phase II trial. Cisplatin was infused in a dose of $100 \, mg/m^2$ on the second day. Methotrexate $40 \, mg/m^2$ and vinblastine $5 \, mg/m^2$ were given on days 1 and 8. After 22 patients were treated, however, doses were reduced to $30 \, mg/m^2$ and $4 \, mg/m^2$, respectively. This dose reduction became necessary because of excessive hematologic toxicity. Treatment was repeated every 3 weeks. In the 50 evaluable patients, the response rate was 56% ($n = 28$), with 28% ($n = 14$) attaining a complete response. Responses occurred in every metastatic tumor site. Response rates, however, were higher in patients with lymph node metastases than in those with liver and bone metastases. The median survival was 8 months. The toxicity of the scheme was noteworthy, with neutropenic fever occurring in 24% of patients, a rise in the serum creatinine to $>2.0 \, mg/100 \, ml$ occurring in 26%, and two patients, both treated with the higher doses of vinblastine and methotrexate, dying due to neutropenic sepsis.

In a smaller single-center study, similar treatment results were found with CMV chemotherapy (JEFFERY and MEAD 1992). In this study, cisplatin was given at a dose of 70 or $100 \, mg/m^2$. The doses of methotrexate and vinblastine were $30 \, mg/m^2$ and $4 \, mg/m^2$. Of the 33 evaluable patients, eight (24%) obtained a complete response and 11 (33%) a partial one, giving a response rate of 58%. Patients survived for a median of 7 months.

No randomized studies have been performed on CMV combination chemotherapy versus cisplatin alone. Because cisplatin was thought to be the most toxic agent, a recent randomized trial in 203 patients compared CMV with the combination of methotrexate and vinblastine alone (MEAD et al. 1996). No data on response rates were reported. However, progression-free survival, symptomatic progression-free survival, and overall survival were all significantly better for patients treated with CMV than for those treated with methotrexate and vinblastine. The survival benefit could be demonstrated despite six treatment-related deaths in the CMV group.

28.3.2.4
Methotrexate–Vinblastine–Doxorubicin–Cisplatin Combination

Combination chemotherapy with methotrexate, vinblastine, doxorubicin, and cisplatin (M-VAC) was introduced at Memorial Sloan-Kettering Cancer Center in New York by STERNBERG et al. (1988). The four agents were combined according to the scheme in Table 28.4. A group of 132 patients with advanced transitional cell carcinoma treated with M-VAC was reported in 1989 (STERNBERG et al. 1989). A large percentage, 83%, had distant metastases in the following sites: bone (26%), liver (11%), lungs (31%), and abdominal lymph nodes (60%). The clinical response rate in the 121 patients evaluable for response was as high as 70%, with 18% attaining a clinically complete response. Patients who achieved a marked response were urged to have surgery. Following surgical restaging and after resection of residual disease, the complete response rate was increased to 36% and the total response to 72%. The median duration of survival was 13.4 months, with a survival rate of 57% and 30% after 1 and 2 years, respectively. These excellent results, especially with respect to the response rates, were accompanied by significant toxicity. Fifty-eight percent of treated patients developed grade 3–4 leukopenia, with neutropenic sepsis in 25%. There were four (3%) drug-related deaths. The incidence of mucositis was 49%; it was grade 3–4 in 13%. The value of surgical resection of residual disease after a response to chemotherapy has not been investigated in randomized studies and is, therefore, still unproven.

Table 28.4. M-VAC chemotherapy (from STERNBERG et al. 1989)

	Dose (mg/kg)			
	Day 1	Day 2	Day 15	Day 22
Methotrexate	30		30	30
Vinblastine		2	2	2
Doxorubicin		30		
Cisplatin		70		

Table 28.5. M-VAC in advanced urothelial cancer

Author (year)	No.	Response		Survival	
		CR %	CR + PR %	Median (months)	1-yr (%)
Phase II					
STERNBERG et al. (1989)	121	18	70	13.4	57
TANNOCK et al. (1989)	30	13	40	10	34
CONNOR et al. (1989)	10	50	80	–	–
IGAWA et al. (1990)	58	17	57	8	55
IGAWA et al. (1991)	37	24	59	–	60
BOUTAN-LAROZE et al. (1991)	67	19	57	13	53
OGAWA et al. (1992)	14	7	57	–	–
KOTAKE et al. (1992)	86	15	49	9.8	–
UEKI et al. (1992)	29	14	62	–	48
Phase III					
LOGOTHETIS et al. (1990a)	55	35	65	14.4	69
LOEHRER et al. (1992)	126	13	39	12.5	50
LEE et al. (1992)	8	0	50	–	–
PIZZOCARO et al. (1991)	14	43	71	–	–

M-VAC has since become the most extensively studied combination chemotherapy regimen in phase II trials (Table 28.5). A wide range of response rates have been found, with clinically complete responses varying between 0% and 50%, both extremes found in very small studies. The larger studies, however, have not achieved complete response rates above 20%. Due to toxicity, especially bone marrow depression and mucositis, M-VAC can almost never be given as scheduled, with frequent deletions of interim chemotherapy on days 15 and 22, and/or frequent delay in starting the next cycle (TANNOCK et al. 1989).

Despite the toxicity of M-VAC, a phase III multicenter study has shown its superiority over cisplatin monotherapy (LOEHRER et al. 1992). The study randomized 269 patients to cisplatin alone, given at a dose of 70 mg/m^2 every 4 weeks, or M-VAC combination chemotherapy, given according to the Sternberg recommendations. Bone and liver and/or lung metastases were detected in 56% and 51%, respectively. The toxicity of M-VAC was indeed higher than for cisplatin, with grade 3–4 neutropenia occurring in 24% versus 1%, neutropenic fever occurring in 10% of the M-VAC-treated patients only, and severe mucositis also occurring only after M-VAC, at a frequency of 17%. The response rate in 126 evaluable patients treated with M-VAC was 39% (complete response in 13%). This response rate was significantly better than the 12% response rate (3% complete re-

sponse) in the 120 cisplatin-treated evaluable patients. Similarly, the median survival was significantly longer for the combined therapy group (12.5 vs 8.2 months). To correct for potential differences in prognostic factors between the two treatment arms, a multivariate analysis was performed. Adjusting for the prognostic factors (including performance status, weight loss, and metastases to the lung, liver, and/or bone), the difference in survival between M-VAC- and cisplatin-treated patients remained statistically significant. Although the study supported the use of M-VAC over cisplatin in advanced transitional cell cancer, the response rates were lower than anticipated, and especially lower than the results reported from Memorial Sloan-Kettering Medical Center. One factor contributing to these differences in response rate may be the definition of evaluability for response. In the Memorial Sloan-Kettering study, one treatment cycle had to be completed, whereas just 1 day of treatment was enough for response analysis in the phase III study. Differences in patient population may have contributed, too, but data on prognostic factors are lacking; the percentage of patients with only local nodal disease was unknown in the randomized study, as was the percentage of patients with nodal metastases in general. The relative numbers of patients with metastases to the liver, bone, and lungs, however, seemed similar between the two studies.

Because of the toxicity of M-VAC, a treatment regimen in which cisplatin and doxorubicin were substituted by carboplatin was developed (BELLMUNT et al. 1992). This treatment regimen, M-CAVI, consisted of methotrexate given at a dose of $30\,mg/m^2$ on days 1, 15, and 22, carboplatin at a dose of $300\,mg/m^2$ on day 2, and vinblastine at a dose of $3\,mg/m^2$ on days 2, 15, and 22. A response rate of 48% in 23 patients who could not tolerate cisplatin-based therapy seemed promising. However, a small randomized study in 47 patients comparing M-VAC with M-CAVI chemotherapy showed a statistically significant survival benefit for M-VAC (median survival time 16 months vs 9 months for M-VAC and M-CAVI, respectively) (BELLMUNT et al. 1996). The inclusion of cisplatin (with doxorubicin), therefore, seems essential for the best treatment effect.

28.3.2.5
Comparative Studies on Cisplatin Based Combination Chemotherapy

Just a few studies have been reported comparing different cisplatin-based combination regimens. The largest study, performed at the M.D. Anderson Cancer Center, randomized 110 patients with metastatic urothelial cancer between M-VAC and CISCA chemotherapy (LOGOTHETIS et al. 1990a). Patients were stratified by tumor dissemination and histology. The percentage of patients with visceral metastases was similar in the two treatment groups (47% for M-VAC and 49% for CISCA). One hundred and two patients were evaluable for response. M-VAC-treated patients responded significantly better than the patients treated with CISCA, with response rates of 65% and 46%, respectively. The survival was also significantly better for M-VAC versus CISCA, with a median survival time of 62.6 weeks versus 36.1 weeks and a 1-year survival rate of 69% versus 37%. No significant differences in toxicity were reported, but few results were given. There was a trend toward increased renal toxicity after CISCA, with a rise in serum creatinine level greater than $0.4\,mg/dl$ occurring in 41% of CISCA courses and in 17% of M-VAC courses. Leukopenic fever was reported in 14% and 5% of courses, respectively, with one toxic death in the CISCA group. Considering the results from this randomized study and the results from the phase III studies on CISCA versus cisplatin in advanced urothelial cancer, further use of CISCA combination chemotherapy for the treatment of metastatic bladder cancer is not recommended.

Two other randomized studies were performed on cisplatin-based combination therapy in advanced urothelial cancer, both of which included just a small number of patients. A study in 28 patients with advanced cancer of the urinary tract was aimed at detecting differences in toxicity between M-VAC and the combination of cisplatin with methotrexate (PIZZOCARO et al. 1991). M-VAC was given according to Sternberg (Table 28.4), with the omission of the administration of methotrexate and vinblastine on day 22. The cisplatin/methotrexate therapy was given every 3 weeks, with $300\,mg/m^2$ of methotrexate administered on day 1 and $100\,mg/m^2$ of cisplatin in a 24-h continuous infusion on day 4. Hematologic toxicity $\geq$ grade 2 was more frequent in the M-VAC-treated patients (85% in M-VAC vs 21% in cisplatin/methotrexate), but, due to the omission of the day 22 chemotherapy, was just grade 2 in most patients. Nausea and vomiting, mucositis, and nephrotoxicity were similar in both groups. The study was too small to detect significant differences in response and survival. Definite conclusions on toxicity, however, also cannot be drawn, as both treatment schedules differed from those used by other investigators (Tables 28.2, 28.4).

The other small controlled study on two cisplatin-based combination chemotherapy regimens randomized 19 patients to CMV or M-VAC therapy (LEE et al. 1992). Forty-five percent of the 11 patients treated with CMV responded, as did 50% of the eight patients treated with M-VAC. This study was clearly too small for help in clinical decision-making processes.

28.3.2.6
Long-Term Survivors

Several studies showed a small proportion of patients remaining alive and disease-free after cisplatin-based combination chemotherapy for follow-up periods of at least 2–3 years. Following the administration of CISCA chemotherapy about 30% of 35 patients attaining a complete response remained disease-free for more than 300 weeks of follow-up (LOGOTHETIS et al. 1989). Similarly, 4 out of the 17 patients with a clinical complete response after M-VAC did not relapse within a follow-up period of at least 3 years (STERNBERG et al. 1989). The phase III intergroup study comparing M-VAC combination chemotherapy with cisplatin alone identified prognostic factors for long-term survival (SAXMAN et al. 1996). In that study, 21 of 246 patients (8.5%)

survived for at least 3 years, and 11 (4.5%) for a minimum of 5 years. Of the 21 3-year survivors, just nine (43%) had been classified as clinically complete responders. Favorable prognostic factors included the following:

1. Localized disease
2. Good performance status
3. No weight loss
4. The presence of lymph node or pulmonary metastases without involvement of the bone or the viscera

28.3.2.7
Making a Choice on Cisplatin-Based Combination Chemotherapy

In conclusion, the available data on improvement of survival by chemotherapy in metastatic urothelial cancer are limited. The major reason is the lack of properly designed and performed phase III trials with adequate numbers of patients to show statistically significant survival differences of 25% or less. However, the few relatively large randomized trials have shown that M-VAC is superior to cisplatin alone and the CAP combination. The CMV combination was found to be superior to MV. Large comparative trials of M-VAC versus CMV, or cisplatin/ methotrexate have not been performed. Data from the use of M-VAC, CMV, or cisplatin plus methotrexate as neoadjuvant chemotherapy in a well-defined population of T3–4N0M0 bladder cancer patients followed by resection showed a similar pathologic complete response rate of approximately 25% for each of the three combinations (SPLINTER et al. 1992). Based on such data, it seems acceptable to conclude that combination chemotherapy with cisplatin and methotrexate improves the survival of patients with metastatic bladder cancer, and especially the survival of those with only lymphogenic and/or lung metastases. The value of the addition of vinblastine and/or doxorubicin is unproven, but there is a widespread feeling that M-VAC is superior. In the primary choice of treatment or no treatment of a patient with metastatic bladder cancer, performance status, kidney function, and sites of metastases should play a major role. The use of modern HT-3 antagonists as antiemetics and leucovorin rescue to prevent methotrexate-induced mucositis facilitates good tolerability of the cisplatin/ methotrexate combination even at old age. In our opinion, addition of vinblastine and adriamycin in-

creases the risk of bone marrow suppression and neurotoxicity and should, therefore, be restricted to patients less than 65 years of age.

28.3.3
New Treatment Strategies

28.3.3.1
Dose Escalation

Because of a potential relation between the delivered dose intensity of chemotherapy and the response to this treatment, dose escalation has been suggested to improve treatment results in urothelial cancer. As stated above, M-VAC seems one of the most effective chemotherapeutic regimens in transitional cell cancer. However, because of bone marrow depression, treatment often cannot be given as scheduled, leading to decreased dose intensity. With the use of colony-stimulating factors, several strategies have been tested to improve treatment results. When M-VAC, given in a classical dose scheme, was combined with recombinant granulocyte colony-stimulating factor (rhG-CSF), a full dose of the chemotherapy could be administered with less neutropenic fever and mucositis (GABRILOVE et al. 1988). However, the effect on repeated courses of chemotherapy was not studied with G-CSF. A study on consecutive cycles of M-VAC chemotherapy with colony-stimulating factors was performed with recombinant granulocyte-macrophage colony-stimulating factor (rhGM-CSF). Just the first two cycles could be given as scheduled with day 15 and day 22 treatments. By cycle 3 of treatment, no further benefit was apparent (MOORE et al. 1993). Colony-stimulating factors are also used with M-VAC given in escalated dose, using different treatment schedules. Conflicting results have been reported. LOEHRER et al. (1994) used a classical M-VAC scheme with regard to the treatment schedule, but with a 33% dose increase for each agent, in combination with rhG-CSF. They reported severe toxicity, with 23% of the patients dying because of adverse events. The benefit in response with dose escalation has been questioned by some (SCHER et al. 1993; SEIDMAN et al. 1993; LOEHRER et al. 1994), but supported by others (LOGOTHETIS et al. 1990b, 1992). To date, no definitive results have been reported on the benefit of M-VAC given in escalated doses. The results of a current randomized EORTC trial on M-VAC given in a classical scheme versus a 2-weekly, dose-escalated schedule with growth factor support are still awaited (STERNBERG et al. 1993).

28.3.3.2
New Agents

28.3.3.2.1
5-FLUOROURACIL (5-FU) WITH INTERFERON-α

In a group of 30 patients with metastatic urothelial cancer who had failed to respond to cisplatin-based polychemotherapy, a partial response rate of 30% was obtained with a combination of 5-FU and interferon-α. Most patients had nodal metastases (LOGOTHETIS et al. 1994). Further studies are ongoing to find effective combinations of 5-FU and interferon-α with other agents.

28.3.3.2.2
TAXANES

Paclitaxel 250 mg/m^2 followed by G-CSF has been studied in a phase II multicenter trial as first-line therapy in advanced urothelial cancer (ROTH et al. 1994). In a group of 26 patients, a promising response rate of 42% was achieved, with 27% of patients attaining a complete response. As with cisplatin-based therapy, the response rate was the highest in patients with lymph node metastases. The activity of paclitaxel as a single agent was also identified in a small study of nine patients with renal insufficiency or resistance to cisplatin, in which 56% responded partially (DREICER et al. 1996). Because of the promising activity of single-agent paclitaxel, a combination with other effective chemotherapeutic agents may improve treatment results in metastatic bladder cancer. Studies on different paclitaxel combinations are ongoing. Currently available results suggest a high activity of the combination with cisplatin, with 13 out of 18 patients (72%) achieving at least a partial response on this combination therapy (MURPHY et al. 1996). Paclitaxel plus carboplatin may be another beneficial treatment for urothelial cell cancer, with a response rate of 50% in a phase I study (VAUGHN et al. 1996). Results in respect of another taxane, docetaxel, are not yet available.

28.3.3.2.3
GEMCITABINE

Gemcitabine is a pyrimidine antimetabolite currently studied for its potential activity in different solid tumors. In a preliminary report from a phase I study, a potential benefit in metastatic bladder cancer was suggested (POLLERA et al. 1994). In a group of 15 patients, of whom 14 had been pretreated with M-VAC, a response was observed in four (27%) patients. Three of the responders had liver metastases.

The activity of gemcitabine in cisplatin-resistant bladder cancer was confirmed in a phase II study by the same investigators (DE LENA et al. 1996): among 25 evaluable patients, a response was found in 28%. Gemcitabine has also been studied as primary therapy for advanced urothelial cancer. Two recent phase II studies reported response rates of 38% and 56% in 21 and nine evaluable patients, respectively (MOORE et al. 1996; STADLER et al. 1995).

28.3.3.2.4
GALLIUM NITRATE

Another new agent for the treatment of metastatic urothelial cancer may be gallium nitrate. Giving the drug by continuous 24 h infusion may diminish its potential nephrotoxicity. Two studies were recently performed in transitional cell carcinoma patients already pretreated with cisplatin-based chemotherapy. In a small study in eight patients, gallium nitrate was given by continuous infusion 300 mg/m^2/day, for 7 days (SELIGMAN and CRAWFORD 1991). The response rate was 63%, with three (38%) patients attaining a complete response. In this group, four patients responded for at least 11 months. In another study, 40 cisplatin-resistant patients were given gallium nitrate in a phase I study (SEIDMAN et al. 1991). A response rate of 17% was found for treatment with doses of at least 350 mg/m^2/day on days 1–5 in a 3-week cycle. Future studies on combination therapy including gallium nitrate seem worthwhile; a combination regimen with ifosfamide has already been reported (see Sect. 28.3.3.2.5).

28.3.3.2.5
IFOSFAMIDE

Ifosfamide has also been demonstrated to exhibit promising single-agent activity in urothelial carcinoma (WITTE et al. 1993). Patients with advanced urothelial cancer and one prior chemotherapy regimen were treated with ifosfamide 3750 mg/m^2 on days 1 and 2. The dose was later changed to 1500 mg/m^2/day for 5 days because of excessive renal and CNS toxicity. Of the first 47 patients who were evaluable for response, four (8%) responded completely and six (13%) others achieved a partial response (response rate of 21%). Grade 3 or 4 renal and/or CNS toxicity was seen in 52% of the patients treated over 2 days and in 33% of the patients given the 5-day treatment regimen.

Ifosfamide has already been studied in combination regimens. A phase II trial studied the combination of vinblastine 0.11 mg/kg on days 1 and 2, ifosfamide 1200 mg/m^2/day for 5 days, and gallium nitrate 300 mg/m^2/day for 5 days (EINHORN et al. 1994). Twenty-seven patients with metastatic urothelial cancer were treated. Of these 27 patients, 18 (67%) achieved a response, with 11 (41%) complete and seven (26%) partial responses. Of the patients with a complete response, six had undergone surgery to achieve that result. The major toxicity turned out to be myelosuppression. Preliminary results from an ongoing study on the combination of ifosfamide, paclitaxel, and cisplatin are promising (McCAFFREY et al. 1996). Regression occurred in all of the first four evaluable patients. Ifosfamide has also been studied in combination with cisplatin, methotrexate, and vinblastine in 25 patients with metastatic urothelial carcinoma (DIMOPOULOS et al. 1996), a 64% response rate being observed. However, as yet no benefit of the use of this regimen, as compared with M-VAC therapy, has been established.

28.4
Conclusion

Despite a paucity of properly designed and performed phase III trials, it seems acceptable to conclude that cisplatin-based combination chemotherapy is beneficial in the treatment of metastatic urothelial cancer. Patients with a good performance score, no weight loss, and no metastases to the liver and the skeleton seem to respond best and benefit most. Current research is aimed at improving the therapeutic results. Two strategies are being investigated: dose escalation of currently used active drugs and the introduction of new compounds. The first step is to use them as single agents and later, probably more importantly, in combination regimens. Of the new drugs, the taxanes, gemcitabine, gallium nitrate, ifosfamide, and the immunomodulator interferon-α seem to be promising enough for further testing in combination regimes. Since combination chemotherapy in metastatic bladder cancer probably will remain a palliative treatment, future randomized phase III trials to investigate the optimal combination in terms of survival, tolerability, symptom relief, and costs will be of utmost importance.

References

Babaian RJ, Johnson DE, Llamas L, Ayala AG (1980) Metastases from transitional cell carcinoma of urinary bladder. Urology 16:142–144

Bellmunt J, Albanell J, Gallego OS, et al. (1992) Carboplatin, methotrexate, and vinblastine in patients with bladder cancer who were ineligible for cisplatin-based chemotherapy. Cancer 70:1974–1979

Bellmunt J, Ribas A, Bermejo B, et al. (1996) M-VAC versus M-CAVI (methotrexate, carboplatin, vinblastine) in advanced surgically incurable bladder cancer. Proc Am Soc Clin Oncol 15:265

Boutan-Laroze A, Mahjoubi M, Droz JP, et al. (1991) M-VAC (methotrexate, vinblastine, doxorubicin and cisplatin) for advanced carcinoma of the bladder. The French Federation of Cancer Centers Experience. Eur J Cancer 27:1690–1694

Carmichael J, Cornbleet MA, MacDougall RH, Allan SG, Duncan W, Chisholm GD, Smyth JF (1985) Cis-platin and methotrexate in the treatment of transitional cell carcinoma of the urinary tract. Br J Urol 57:299–302

Connor JP, Olsson CA, Benson MC, Rapoport F, Sawczuk IS (1989) Long-term follow-up in patients treated with methotrexate, vinblastine, doxorubicin, and cisplatin (M-VAC) for transitional cell carcinoma of the urinary bladder: cause for concern. Urology 34:353–356

De Lena M, Gridelli C, Lorusso V, et al. (1996) Gemcitabine activity (objective response and symptom improvement) in resistant stage IV bladder cancer. Proc Am Soc Clin Oncol 15:246

Dimopoulos MA, Kyriakakis Z, Kostakopoulos A (1996) Cisplatin, ifosfamide, methotrexate and vinblastine (CIMV) combination chemotherapy for metastatic urothelial cancer. Proc Am Soc Clin Oncol 15:255

Dreicer R, Gustin D, See WA, Williams RD (1996) Paclitaxel in advanced urothelial carcinoma: its role in patients with renal insufficiency and as salvage therapy. Proc Am Soc Clin Oncol 15:242

Einhorn LH, Roth BJ, Ansari R, Dreicer R, Gonin R, Loehrer PJ (1994) Phase II trial of vinblastine, ifosfamide, and gallium combination chemotherapy in metastatic urothelial carcinoma. J Clin Oncol 12:2271–2276

Fosså SD, Sager EM, Hosbach G, Waehre H, Ous S (1990) Cisplatin and medium dose methotrexate in advanced transitional cell carcinoma of the urinary tract. Scand J Urol Nephrol 24:199–204

Gabrilove JL, Jakubowski A, Scher H, et al. (1988) Effect of granulocyte colony-stimulating factor on neutropenia and associated morbidity due to chemotherapy for transitional-cell carcinoma of the urothelium. N Engl J Med 318:1414–1422

Geller NL, Sternberg CN, Penenberg D, Scher H, Yagoda A (1991) Prognostic factors for survival of patients with advanced urothelial tumors treated with methotrexate, vinblastine, doxorubicin, and cisplatin chemotherapy. Cancer 67:1525–1531

Harker WG, Meyers FJ, Freiha FS, et al. (1985) Cisplatin, methotrexate, and vinblastine (CMV): an effective chemotherapy regimen for metastatic transitional cell carcinoma of the urinary tract. A Northern California Oncology Group Study. J Clin Oncol 3:1463–1470

Hillcoat BL, Raghavan D, Matthews J, et al. (1989) A randomized trial of cisplatin versus cisplatin plus methotrexate in advanced cancer of the urothelial tract. J Clin Oncol 7:706–709

Igawa M, Ohkuchi T, Ueki T, Ueda M, Okada K, Usui T (1990) Usefulness and limitations of methotrexate, vinblastine, doxorubicin and cisplatin for the treatment of advanced urothelial cancer. J Urol 144:662–665

Igawa M, Ohkuchi T, Ueda M, Usui T, Kawanishi M (1991) Analyses of factors affecting the outcome of combination chemotherapy in patients with advanced bladder cancer. Eur Urol 20:12–15

Igawa M, Ohkuchi T, Ueda M, Usui T (1992) Factors affecting the outcome of patients with advanced urothelial cancer following chemotherapy with methotrexate, vinblastine, Adriamycin and cisplatin. Cancer Chemother Pharmacol 30(Suppl):S77–S80

Jeffery GM, Mead GM (1992) CMV chemotherapy for advanced transitional cell carcinoma. Br J Cancer 66:542–546

Khandekar JD, Elson PJ, DeWys WD, et al. (1985) Comparative activity and toxicity of cisdiamminedichloroplatinum (DDP) and a combination of doxorubicin, cyclophosphamide and DDP in disseminated transitional cell carcinoma of the urinary tract. J Clin Oncol 3:539–545

Kotake T, Akaza H, Isaka S, et al. (1992) Evaluation of systemic chemotherapy with methotrexate, vinblastine, Adriamycin, and cisplatin for advanced bladder cancer 30(Suppl):S85–S89

Lee M-H, Chen MT, Chen KK, et al. (1992) Cisplatin-based chemotherapy for the treatment of advanced transitional-cell carcinoma of the urinary tract – a preliminary report. Cancer Chemother Pharmacol 30(Suppl):S81–S84

Loehrer PJ, Einhorn LH, Elson PJ, et al. (1992) A randomized comparison of cisplatin alone or in combination with methotrexate, vinblastine, and doxorubicin in patients with metastatic urothelial carcinoma: a Cooperative Group Study. J Clin Oncol 10:1066–1073

Loehrer PJ, Elson P, Dreicer R, Hahn R, Nichols CR, Williams R, Einhorn LH (1994) Escalated dosages of methotrexate, vinblastine, doxorubicin, and cisplatin plus recombinant human granulocyte colony-stimulating factor in advanced urothelial carcinoma: an Eastern Cooperative Oncology Group Trial. J Clin Oncol 12:483–488

Logothetis CJ, Dexeus FH, Chong C, Sella A, Ayala AG, Ro JY, Pilat S (1989) Cisplatin, cyclophosphamide and doxorubicin chemotherapy for unresectable urothelial tumors: the M.D. Anderson experience. J Urol 141:33–37

Logothetis CJ, Dexeus FH, Finn L, Sella A, Amato RJ, Ayala AG, Kilbourn RG (1990a) A prospective randomized trial comparing MVAC and CISCA chemotherapy for patients with metastatic urothelial tumors. J Clin Oncol 8:1050–1055

Logothetis CJ, Dexeus FH, Sella A, Amato RJ, Kilbourn RG, Finn L, Gutterman JU (1990b) Escalated therapy for refractory urothelial tumors: methotrexate-vinblastine-doxorubicin-cisplatin plus unglycolylated recombinant human granulocyte-macrophage colony-stimulating factor. J Natl Cancer Inst 82:667–672

Logothetis C, Finn L, Amato R, Hossan E, Sella A (1992) Escalated MVAC +/– rhGM-CSF (Schering-Plough) in metastatic transitional cell carcinoma: preliminary results of a randomized trial. Proc Am Soc Clin Oncol 11:202

Logothetis CJ, Hossan E, Recondo G, et al. (1994) 5-Fluorouracil and interferon-α in chemotherapy refractory bladder carcinoma: an effective regimen. Anticancer Res 14:1265–1270

Maru A, Akaza H, Isaka S, et al. (1987) Phase III trial of the Japanese Urological Cancer Research Group for Adriamycin: cyclophosphamide, adriamycin and 5-fluorouracil in patients with advanced transitional cell carcinoma of the urinary bladder. Cancer Chemother Pharmacol 20(Suppl):S44–S48

McCaffrey J, Hilton S, Mazumdar M, et al. (1996) A phase II trial of ifosfamide, paclitaxel and cisplatin (ITP) in patients with advanced urothelial tract tumors. Proc Am Soc Clin Oncol 15:251

Mead GM, Crook AM, Russell JM, et al. (1996) An MRC randomised trial comparing MV (methotrexate and vinblastine) with CMV (cisplatin + MV) for metastatic transitional cell cancer. Proc Am Soc Clin Oncol 15:241

Moore MJ, Iscoe N, Tannock IA (1993) A phase II study of methotrexate, vinblastine, doxorubicin and cisplatin plus recombinant human granulocyte-macrophage colony stimulating factors in patients with advanced transitional cell carcinoma. J Urol 150:1131–1134

Moore MJ, Tannock I, Ernst S, Huan S, Murray N (1996) Gemcitabine demonstrates promising activity as a single agent in the treatment of metastatic transitional cell carcinoma. Proc Am Soc Clin Oncol 15:250

Mulder JH, Fosså SD, De Pauw M, Van Oosterom AT (1982) Cyclophosphamide, adriamycin and cisplatin combination chemotherapy in advanced bladder carcinoma: an EORTC phase II study. Eur J Cancer 18:111–112

Murphy BA, Johnson DR, Smith J, Koch M, DeVore R, Blanke C, Johnson DR (1996) Phase II trial of paclitaxel and cisplatin for metastatic or locally unresectable urothelial cancer. Proc Am Soc Clin Oncol 15:245

Ogawa T, Gotoh A, Takenaka A, et al. (1992) Clinical and pathological evaluations of methotrexate, vinblastine, Adriamycin and cisplatin chemotherapy for advanced urothelial cancers. Cancer Chemother Pharmacol 30(Suppl):S66–S71

Oliver RTD, Kwok HK, Highman WJ, Waxman J (1986) Methotrexate, cisplatin and carboplatin as single agents and in combination for metastatic bladder cancer. Br J Urol 58:31–35

Pizzocaro G, Milani A, Piva L, Faustini M, Spino E (1991) Methotrexate, vinblastine, Adriamycin and cisplatin versus methotrexate and cisplatin in advanced urothelial cancer. A randomized study. Eur Urol 20:89–92

Pollera CF, Ceribelli A, Crecco M, Calabresi F (1994) Weekly gemcitabine in advanced bladder cancer: a preliminary report from a phase I study. Ann Oncol 5:182–184

Roth BJ, Dreicer R, Einhorn LH, et al. (1994) Significant activity of paclitaxel in advanced transitional-cell carcinoma of the urothelium: a phase II trial of the Eastern Cooperative Oncology Group. J Clin Oncol 12:2264–2270

Saxman SB, Loehrer PJ, Propert K, et al. (1996) Long-term follow up of phase III intergroup study of M-VAC vs cisplatin in metastatic urothelial carcinoma. Proc Am Soc Clin Oncol 15:248

Scher HI, Geller NL, Curley T, Tao Y (1993) Effect of relative cumulative dose-intensity on survival of patients with urothelial cancer treated with M-VAC. J Clin Oncol 11:400–407

Schwartz S, Yagoda A, Natale RB, Watson RC, Whitmore WF, Lesser M (1983) Phase II trial of sequentially administered cisplatin, cyclophosphamide and doxorubicin for urothelial tract tumors. J Urol 130:681–684

Seidman AD, Scher HI, Heinemann MH, et al. (1991) Continuous infusion gallium nitrate for patients with advanced refractory urothelial tract tumors. Cancer 68:2561–2565

Seidman AD, Scher HI, Gabrilove JL, et al. (1993) Dose-intensification of MVAC with recombinant granulocyte colony-stimulating factor as initial therapy in advanced urothelial cancer. J Clin Oncol 11:408–414

Seligman PA, Crawford ED (1991) Treatment of advanced transitional cell carcinoma of the bladder with continuous-infusion gallium nitrate. J Natl Cancer Inst 83:1582–1584

Sengeløv L, Kamby C, Schou G, Von der Maase H (1994) Prognostic factors and significance of chemotherapy in patients with recurrent or metastatic transitional cell cancer of the urinary tract. Cancer 74:123–133

Soloway MS, Einstein A, Corder MP, Bonney W, Prout GR, Coombs J (1983) A comparison of cisplatin and the combination of cisplatin and cyclophosphamide in advanced urothelial cancer. A national bladder cancer collaborative group A study. Cancer 52:767–772

Splinter TAW, Scher HI, Denis L, et al. (1992) The prognostic value of the pathological response to combination chemotherapy prior to cystectomy in patients with invasive bladder cancer. J Urol 147:606–608

Stadler W, Kuzel T, Raghavan D, Levine E, Vogelzang N, Dorr FA (1995) A phase II study of gemcitabine in the treatment of patients with advanced transitional cell carcinoma. Proc Am Soc Clin Oncol 14:241

Sternberg CN, Yagoda A, Scher HI (1988) M-VAC (methotrexate, vinblastine, adriamycin and cisplatin) for advanced transitional cell carcinoma of the urothelium. J Urol 139:461–469

Sternberg CN, Yagoda A, Scher HI, et al. (1989) Methotrexate, vinblastine, doxorubicin, and cisplatin for advanced transitional cell carcinoma of the urothelium. Efficacy and patterns of response and relapse. Cancer 64:2448–2458

Sternberg CN, De Mulder PHM, Van Oosterom AT, Fossa SD, Giannarelli D, Soedirman JR (1993) Escalated M-VAC chemotherapy and recombinant human granulocyte-macrophage colony stimulating factor (rhGM-CSF) in patients with advanced urothelial tract tumors. Ann Oncol 4:403–407

Stoter G, Splinter TAW, Child JA, et al. (1987) Combination chemotherapy with cisplatin and methotrexate in advanced transitional cell cancer of the bladder. J Urol 137:663–667

Tannock I, Gospodarowicz M, Connolly J, Jewett M (1989) M-VAC (methotrexate, vinblastine, doxorubicin and cisplatin) chemotherapy for transitional cell carcinoma: the Princess Margaret Hospital experience. J Urol 142:289–292

Troner MB, Hemstreet GP (1981) Cyclophosphamide, doxorubicin, and cisplatin (CAP) in the treatment of urothelial malignancy: a pilot study of the Southeastern Cancer Study Group. Cancer Treat Rep 65:29–32

Troner M, Birch R, Omura GA, et al. (1987) Phase III comparison of cisplatin alone versus cisplatin, doxorubicin and cyclophosphamide in the treatment of bladder (urothelial) cancer: a Southeastern Cancer Study Group Trial. J Urol 137:660–662

Ueki O, Hisazumi H, Uchibayashi T, et al. (1992) Methotrexate, vinblastine, doxorubicin, and cisplatin for advanced urothelial cancer. Cancer Chemother Pharmacol 30(Suppl):S72–S76

Vaughn DJ, Malkowicz SB, Zoltick B, et al. (1996) Paclitaxel plus carboplatin in advanced carcinoma of the urothelium: a well-tolerated outpatient regimen. Proc Am Soc Clin Oncol 15:240

Witte R, Loehrer P, Dreicer R, Williams S, Elson P (1993) Ifosfamide in advanced urothelial carcinoma: an ECOG trial. Proc Am Soc Clin Oncol 12:230

Yagoda A (1987) Chemotherapy of urothelial tract tumors. Cancer 60:574–585

29 National Differences in the Management of Bladder Cancer

H.-P. HEILMANN

CONTENTS

29.1
Introduction

The treatment of bladder cancer is very similar in Western Europe and the United States. Nevertheless, certain differences in treatment approach can be identified between countries. Within Europe, the preferred specific treatment protocols in France, Spain, and other south European countries are somewhat different from those in the north European countries such as the United Kingdom, Germany, the Benelux countries, and the Scandinavian countries. Comparing European countries and the United States, on the other hand, there are certain differences in attitude toward the use of surgical techniques and radiation therapy.

29.2
Differences in Surgical Techniques

29.2.1
Transurethral Resection

The first treatment used in the management of superficial bladder cancer (pTcis III, pTa, pT1) is

H.-P. HEILMANN, MD, Professor of Radiation Oncology, Head of the Hermann-Holthusen-Institute for Radiotherapy, St. George's Hospital, Lohmühlenstrasse 5, D-20099 Hamburg, Germany

transurethral resection (TUR) or fulguration. In the United States, most frequently a single resection is performed, with repeated resection being performed on an "as needed" basis. In Germany, by contrast, in pT1 cases it is standard practice to perform two TURs with a 1-week interval between them in order to obtain better information on deep-lying structures. Furthermore, in the United States pathologists more often examine nine or ten cell layers, resulting in a higher incidence of pTcis III than in Germany. This makes it difficult to compare treatment series in the two countries.

29.2.2
Cystectomy with Neobladder

Cystectomy followed by bladder reconstruction is the principal approach used in the curative treatment of muscle-invasive bladder cancer. The alternative management entails bladder preservation. In the United States, there is little enthusiasm for the bladder-preserving protocols; the main treatment method for muscle-invasive bladder cancer is cystectomy, followed by an ileal conduit Bricker pouch (BRICKER 1950).

There are, however, newer surgical alternatives to the ileal conduit. In the United States, continent cutaneous diversions, such as the Kock pouch (KOCK et al. 1988) and the Indiana pouch (ROWLAND et al. 1987) have been developed. In Germany, the "ileum neobladder" [Hautmann pouch (HAUTMANN 1991)] and, more recently, the Mainz pouch (LAMPEL et al. 1995; FISCH et al. 1993) are the most popular surgical techniques used in bladder reconstruction. In the Mainz pouch technique, the ascending colon, the ileum, and the appendix are used to drain the urine via the umbilicus. This technique has also now been employed in the United States.

29.3
Treatment of Superficial and Muscle-invasive Tumors

29.3.1
Treatment of Superficial Bladder Cancer

As mentioned above, the treatment of patients with superficial bladder cancer (pTcis, pTa, pT1) consists in TUR or fulguration. The overall 5-year survival rate for patients with superficial bladder cancer is about 70% (CATALONA 1992). Cystectomy is performed in patients with multifocal pT1 III and pTcis III tumors and in those with symptomatic, diffuse, unresectable papillary tumors or those with carcinoma in situ that does not respond to intravesical therapy. The international trend is to combine this treatment with adjuvant treatment protocols, usually intravesical, in order to reduce the recurrence rate.

The following adjuvant intravesical treatments are currently available in clinical practice:

- Immunotherapy (BCG)
- Chemotherapy (thiotepa, etoglucid, mitomycin C, and doxorubicin)
- Intravesical interferon treatment
- Photodynamic therapy
- Laser therapy

Most treatment protocols employ BCG or intravesical chemotherapy. In the United States, BCG is the preferred treatment for patients with superficial bladder cancer. This is applied frequently due to the high rate of carcinoma in situ found by American pathologists as discussed above.

In Europe, intravesical BCG therapy is a standard treatment for patients with pTcis III, but there are several ongoing trials and retrospective studies on different chemotherapeutic protocols. Treatment results with doxorubin have been published by several groups (LUKKARINEN et al. 1991; VAN DER MEIJDEN et al. 1992; OOSTERLINCK et al. 1993; SCHWAIBOLD et al. 1994a, b; BOUFFIOUX et al. 1995), and have usually been favorable. A direct comparison of intravesical chemotherapy outcomes with those obtained in BCG patients is very difficult due to differences in the patient populations selected for European and American trials.

Only PAVONE-MACALUSO et al. (1993) from Italy have compared intravesical treatment with doxorubicin and BCG in a randomized trial. In this trial, results were very similar in terms of tumor control and the incidence of relapse. In the United States,

however, in a large, multi-institutional Southwest Oncology Clinical Group trial, doxorubicin was shown to be significantly less effective than intravesical BCG in the treatment of patients with carcinoma in situ and for prophylaxis against tumor recurrence (MORI et al. 1988).

The second chemotherapeutic agent widely used in Europe for intravesical therapy is mitomycin C. In a single-center retrospective study, HULAND and co-workers from Hamburg, Germany, found favorable outcomes in patients treated with mitomycin C (HULAND et al. 1984). Subsequently, in a large prospective randomized multicenter study which included 419 patients (HULAND et al. 1990; SCHWAIBOLD et al. 1994a), favorable results were reported with mitomycin C in comparison to a control group. The incidence of long-term recurrence was about 10% for the mitomycin C-treated patients. Studies with mitomycin C in the United States have yielded controversial results (CATALONA 1992).

There have been only a few publications on the use of other chemotherapeutic agents. In a large EORTC trial on the effect of pyridoxine, no difference in treatment outcome was observed between pyridoxine and control group patients (NEWLING et al. 1995). A large British trial demonstrated no advantage of adjuvant intravesical treatment with thiotepa (Medical Research Council Working Party 1994). In the Netherlands, MULDERS et al. (1994) found BCG, chemotherapy, and even radiotherapy to be equally effective in preventing tumor recurrences.

As NEWLING (1990) stated, all agents used for intravesical chemotherapy are about equally effective. There is, however, a big difference in the cost of treatments, and chemotherapeutic agents are normally much more expensive than BCG.

KRIEGMAIR et al. (1994) from Germany and D'HALLEWIN and BAERT (1995) from Belgium have published their experiences with photodynamic therapy, and BEER et al. (1989) reported preliminary results with Nd: YAG laser treatment. None of these treatment modalities, however, are in wide use. Similarly, interferon intravesical therapy is only infrequently applied.

29.3.2
Treatment of Muscle-Invasive Tumors

Cystectomy with bladder reconstruction is the standard treatment for advanced bladder carcinoma in the United States as well as in Europe. Nevertheless, there are some differences in the use of cystectomy. In Europe, the Edinburgh center (DUNCAN and QUILTY 1986) published a large retrospective analysis of 963 patients treated with radiation therapy for muscle-invasive bladder cancer. A comparison with cystectomy series is not possible because of the selection of poor prognostic cases for radiotherapy. Another series of 319 patients with invasive bladder cancer not suitable for cystectomy and therefore treated by radiotherapy was reported from Sweden (JAHNSON et al. 1991). The reported corrected 5-year survival rate in T1 tumors was 57%.

Bladder preservation protocols with chemo-radiotherapy were reported from Austria (with adriamycin) (JAKSE and FROMMHOLD 1988) and Germany (DUNST et al. 1994). The Erlangen group reported favorable results in a relatively high percentage of patients. Bladder function could be preserved by using combination treatment consisting of cisplatin and radiation therapy. A similar treatment approach has been used in the United States, being advocated primarily by Shipley and co-workers (SHIPLEY et al. 1987; PROUT et al. 1991; GOSPODAROWICZ et al. 1995) (see Chap. 17 for details).

On the other hand, preoperative radiotherapy followed by cystectomy was once very popular in the United States. An interim report of the Southwest Oncology Group (CRAWFORD et al. 1987), however, showed no statistically significant difference between preoperative irradiation followed by cystectomy and cystectomy without radiotherapy. Preoperative radiotherapy therefore may not be uniformly effective in patients with invasive bladder cancer, and as a result the frequency of application of this treatment modality has diminished.

Another approach to improve treatment results in invasive bladder cancer is neoadjuvant chemotherapy, especially with the M-VAC (methotrexte, vinblastine, adriamycin, and cisplatin) protocol. The disadvantages of neoadjuvant chemotherapy are somewhat similar to those of preoperative radiation therapy, i.e., patients may experience substantial treatment morbidity which excludes them from consideration for cystectomy. Patients who do not respond to chemotherapy, on the other hand, experience a delay prior to potentially curable surgical treatment.

Recently, prospective trials from Spain (MARTINEZ-PINEIRO et al. 1995) and Germany (STOECKLE et al. 1995) have reported favorable results of neoadjuvant chemotherapy. The use of neoadjuvant chemotherapy in patients with muscle-invasive tumor remains controversial. The reported clinical trials have demonstrated a better prognosis for responders to chemotherapy, but no apparent survival benefit.

29.4
Review of the International Literature

The publications on the treatment of bladder cancer are numerous, the overwhelming majority of papers deriving from the United States, Germany, the United Kingdom, Italy, and France (Fig. 29.1). As mentioned above, the treatment protocols used in these reports do not vary substantially between countries.

Unfortunately, it is nearly impossible to compare the results of different publications. In almost every report, the evaluation of the data on tumor remission, recurrence rates, disease-free intervals, median survival time, survival rates (corrected or crude), and complication rates has been performed in a different manner, not allowing for an objective evaluation of the data. Additionally, important data on the criteria used for evaluation of success, failure and defining sequelae frequently have not been included in the reports.

In view of the above problems, only prospective randomized trials allow for an objective comparison

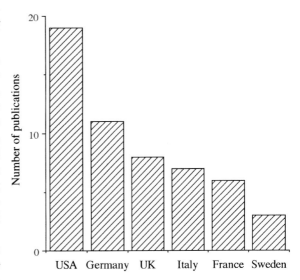

Fig. 29.1. Number of publications reported in the past few years on the management of bladder cancer in the United States and in several European countries

Table 29.1. Publications with 100 cases or less

No. of cases	Country	Year of publication	Author	Superfial/invasive
7	USA	1993	Grossman	
12	Italy	1995	Ferlazzo	Superficial
12	UK	1995	Kunkler	
13		1996	Rosenbaum	Muscle invasive
17	France	1994	Di Palma	
19	Germany	1995	Nost	Muscle invasive
21	USA	1994	Vikam	Muscle invasive
22	Denmark	1987	Havsteen	
23	Germany	1994	Kriegmair	Superficial, Rez
23	Japan	1995	Mizoguchi	Muscle invasive
23	Netherlands	1995	Van Gils-Gielen	CIS
24	France	1994	Pfister	Muscle invasive
24	UK	1992	Cole	Muscle invasive
25	Austria	1995	Mack	Superficial
25		1996	Vallancien	Superficial
26		1995	Pfister	Superficial
29	USA	1994	Rotman	B1–D2
29		1994	Thanos	Superficial
32	France	1993	Haab	CIS
33	Italy	1993	Cruciani	
39		1991	Al Khalifa	Superficial
40		1994	Moonen	Muscle invasive
42	Germany	1991	Kalble	Superficial
42	USA	1991	Kaufman	Muscle invasive
43	UK	1994	Talic	CIS
45	France	1993	Wetzel	Superficial
46	Japan	1994	Ueda	Transitional cell
47	Isreal	1989	Pavlotsky	Superficial
47	USA	1993	Tester	
48	Japan	1987	Washida	Superficial
50	Italy	1995	Pasadoro	Superficial
50	Scandinavia	1991	Bernstein	Muscle invasive
52	Germany	1991	Schreiter	Muscle invasive
55	Austria	1987	Handl Zeller	
55	Italy	1992	Magrini	Superficial
58	Belgium	1993	Kirkove	Muscle invasive
58	South Africa	1991	Abratt	
60	Italy	1994	Tombolini	
60	Italy	1994	Tombolini	
61	USA	1992	Herr	Superficial
64	UK	1994	Price	Muscle invasive
68	Finland	1995	Rintala	?
69	France	1993	Chauvet	Advanced
70	Switzerland	1991	Studer	Muscle invasive
70	USA	1987	Shipley	Muscle invasive
73	Spain	1989	Ojea	
75		1991	Lukkarinen	Superficial
78	Germany	1994	Kalble	Superficial
86	USA	1992	Cookson	Superficial
89	UK	1995	Vrouvas	
91	USA	1992	Rifkin	
92	USA	1991	Tester	
94	Norway	1992	Fossa	Muscle invasive
96	Sweden	1996	Holmang	
100	USA	1987	Catalona	Superficial

of outcomes between different treatment groups. Unfortunately, however, even the results of most randomized trials are not comparable due to the use of dissimilar treatment protocols in various studies.

Reviewing the international literature, it is obvious that a lot of reported prospective trials, as well as retrospective results, provide limited information because of the small number of patients treated and the relatively short follow-up time. Publications with less than 100 cases (Table 29.1) are frequently not very helpful in providing meaningful data.

In summary, there are many differences in the management of bladder cancer, but the national differences appear not to be very important.

29.5
The View of Expert Physicians on the Management of Bladder Cancer, from a Personal Perspective

The international literature provides information on what doctors recommend for their patients who have bladder cancer, but it is also of interest, how physicians would themselves want to be treated, were they to have cancer. MOORE and co-workers (1988) mailed a questionnaire describing six clinical scenarios of genitourinary cancer to urologists and radiation and medical oncologists who practiced genitourinary oncology in Britain, Canada, and the United States. In each scenario, the doctor was asked to consider himself as a patient with bladder, prostate, or kidney cancer, and to select his own treatment. Accompanying each scenario were one or two clinical trials for which the physician could be eligible. Every participant was asked to state whether he would agree to be randomized into a trial, and, if he refused the randomization, to state his reasons. The results were very interesting:

1. There were major differences of opinion as to the preferred management for each clinical scenario.
2. Choice of treatment was influenced more by specialty training or geographic location than by the results of previous trials (which were available to all).
3. British urologists tended to be less aggressive than their North American colleagues with respect to the use of radical surgery and chemotherapy.
4. Acceptance of clinical trials ranged from 3%–60%.
5. Agreement to accept clinical trials was quite poor even when they were designed to compare the most popular options for management.

Preferences for the management of superficial bladder cancer were:

1. Follow-up only (cystoscopies): 40%
2. Intravesical therapy (BCG or chemotherapy): 47%
3. Other treatment: 13%

The differences in the preferred treatment options of urologists of different nationalities were striking

Table 29.2. Treatment options for superficial bladder cancer preferred by urologists in the United States, Canada, and Great Britain (from MOORE et al. 1988)

Selected management	Britain	Canada	USA
Follow-up (cystoscopies only)	74%	47%	16%
Intravesical therapy (BCG, chemotherapy)	22%	50%	68%
Other treatment	4%	3%	16%

Table 29.3. Treatment options for muscle-invasive bladder cancer preferred by urologists in the United States, Canada, and Great Britain and by medical oncologists and radiation oncologists (from MOORE et al. 1988)

Selected treatment	All	Urologists			Medical oncologists	Radiation oncologists
		Britain	Canada	USA		
Cystectomy alone	32%	11%	53%	60%	29%	4%
Radiotherapy + cystectomy	22%	15%	32%	8%	18%	39%
Radiotherapy alone	14%	44%	0%	0%	0%	31%
Chemotherapy + cystectomy	12%	4%	5%	20%	25%	8%
Other	20%	26%	10%	12%	29%	19%

(Table 29.2). British urologists were most conservative, and American urologists most aggressive; Canadian experts voted equally for aggressive and less aggressive treatment options (47%–50%).

There were also substantial differences in opinion over the management of muscle-invasive bladder cancer. Among British urologists, 44% preferred to be treated by radiotherapy, whereas none of the American or Canadian urologists and none of the medical oncologists preferred this treatment modality (Table 29.3).

Consequently, there were far greater national differences in the personal views of doctors than in the treatment recommendations found in the international literature. Of special interest is the attitude of physicians toward clinical trials. In spite of the creed "only prospective randomized trials give correct answers," which is repeated in every paper which claims to be up-to-date, obviously there is a deep skepticism among physicians and urologists whether randomized trials really give the best results for the individual patient!

29.6
Conclusions

There are major differences in the treatment of both superficial and muscle-invasive bladder cancer, but these differences are not primarily national in character. In the United States intravesical BCG treatment is preferred for cases of superficial cancer, while in Europe BCG is commonly used but intravesical chemotherapy is preferred.

In the United States and in continental Europe, radical cystectomy is the standard treatment for muscle-invasive cancer. In the United States, for a long time preoperative radiotherapy before cystectomy was used, but it is infrequently used today. In the United Kingdom and Sweden, large series of patients treated with definitive radiotherapy have been reported. In Austria and Germany, combined chemotherapy–radiotherapy protocols with adriamycin and cisplatin have been developed with the aim of preserving bladder function. The Erlangen protocol has now been advocated elsewhere in Europe and also in the United States.

In bladder reconstruction, the Bricker pouch is the "gold standard" all over the world, though some newer bladder reconstruction techniques have been developed in the United States and in Sweden and Germany.

In contrast to the relatively small national differences in the treatment modalities used in the management of bladder cancer, the preferred personal treatment options of urologists, medical oncologists, and radiation oncologists in the United Kingdom, Canada, and the United States are very different. British urologists are the most conservative, while the American urologists are most radical in their personal treatment decisions. Interestingly, the willingness of doctors to take part as a patient in prospective randomized trials was low in all three countries.

References

Beer M, Jocham D, Beer A, Staehler G (1989) Adjuvant laser treatment of bladder cancer: 8 years' experience with the ND-YAG laser 1064 NM. Br J Urol 63:476–478

Bouffioux C, Kurth KH, Bono A, Oosterlinck W, Kruger CB, De Pauw M, Sylvester R (1995) Intravesical adjuvant chemotherapy for superficial transitional cell bladder carcinoma: results of 2 European Organization for Research and Treatment of Cancer randomized trials with mitomycin C and doxorubicin comparing early versus delayed instillations and short-term versus long-term treatment. European Organization for Research and Treatment of Cancer Genitourinary Group. J Urol 153:934–941

Bricker EM (1950) Bladder substitution after pelvic evisceration. Surg Clin North Am 30:1511

Catalona WJ (1992) Urothelial tumors of the urinary tract. In: Walsh PC, Retik AB, Stamey TA, Vaughan ED (eds) Campbell's urology, 6th edn. Saunders, Philadelphia, pp 1094–1158

Crawford ED, Das S, Smith JA (1987) Preoperative radiation therapy in the treatment of bladder cancer. Urol Clin North Am 14:781

D'Hallewin MA, Baert L (1995) Long term results of whole bladder wall photodynamic therapy for carcinoma in situ of the bladder. Urology 45:763–767

Duncan W, Quilty PM (1986) The results of a series of 963 patients with transitional cell carcinoma of the urinary bladder primarily treated by radical megavoltage x-ray therapy. Radiother Oncol 7:299–310

Dunst J, Sauer R, Schrott KM, Kühn R, Wittekind C, Altendorf-Hofmann AA (1994) Organ-sparing treatment of advanced bladder carcinoma: a 10-year experience. Int J Radiat Oncol Biol Phys 30:261–266

Fisch M, Wammack R, Steinbach F, Muller SC, Hohenfellner R (1993) Sigma-rectum pouch (Mainz pouch II). Urol Clin North Am 20:561–569

Gospodarowicz MK, Quilty PM, Scalliet P, et al. (1995) The place of radiation therapy as definitive treatment of bladder cancer. Int J Urol 2(Suppl 2):41–48

Hautmann RE (1991) The ileal neobladder. Acta Urol Belg 59:227–240

Huland H, Klöppel G, Otto U, et al. (1990) Comparison of different schedules of cytostatic intravesical installations in patients with superficial bladder carcinoma. First evaluation of a prospective multicenter study with 419 patients. J Urol 144:68

Huland H, Otto U, Droese M, Klöppel G (1984) Long-term mitomycin installation after transurethral resection of superficial bladder carcinoma: influence of recurrence, progression and survival. J Urol 132:27–33

Jahnson S, Pedersen J, Westman G (1991) Bladder carcinoma – a 20-year review of radical irradiation therapy. Radiother Oncol 22:111–117

Jakse G, Frommhold H (1988) Radiotherapy and chemotherapy in locally advanced bladder cancer. Eur Urol 14:45

Kaufaman DS, Shipley WU, Heney NM, et la. (1991) The integration of transurethral surgery, chemotherapy and radiation with bladder sparing in patients with invasive bladder cancer: an update of prognostic factors in a prospective trial (meeting abstract). Proc Annu Meet Am Soc Clin Oncol 10:A516

Kock NG, Ghoneim MA, Lycke KG (1988) Urinary diversion to the augmented and valved rectum: preliminary results with a novel surgical procedure. J Urol 140:1375

Koiso K, Shipley W, Keuppens F, et al (1995) The status of bladder-preserving therapeutic strategies in the managment of patients with muscle-invasive bladder cancer. Int J Urol 2(Suppl 2):49–57

Kriegmair M, Waidelich R, Baumgartner R, Lumper W, Ehsan A, Hofstetter A (1994) (Photodynamic therapy of superficial bladder cancer. An alternative to radical cystectomy?) Die photodynamische Therapie (PDT) des oberflachlichen Harnblasenkarzinoms. Eine Alternative zur radikalen Zystektomie? Urologe [A] 33:276–280

Lample A, Hohenfellner M, Schultz-Lampel D, Thuroff JW (1995) In situ tunneled bowel flap tubes: 2 new techniques of a continent outlet for Mainz pouch cutaneous diversion. J Urol 153:308–315

Lukkarinen O, Paul C, Hellstrom, P, et al (1991) Intravesical epirubicin with and without verapamil for the prophylaxis of superficial bladder tumors. Scand J Urol Nephrol 25:25–28

Martinez-Pineiro JA, Gonzalez-Martin M, Arocena F, et al. (1995) Neoadjuvant cisplatin chemotherapy before radical cystectomy in invasive transitional cell carcinoma of the bladder: a prospective randomized phase III study. J Urol 153:964–973

Medical Research Council Working Party on Urological Research (1994) The effect of intravesical thiotepa on tumor recurrence after endoscopic treatment of newly diagnosed superficial bladder cancer. A further report with long-term follow-up of a Medical Research Council randomized trial. Medical Research Council Working Party on Urological Cancer, Subgroup on Superficial Baladder Cancer. Br J Urol 73:632–638

Moore MJ, O'Sullivan B, Tannock IF (1988) How expert physicians would wish to be treated if they had genitourinary cancer. J Clin Oncol 1736:1736–1745

Mori K, Lamm KL, Crawford DE (1988) A trial of bacillus Calmette-Guérin vs. adriamycin in superficial bladder cancer: a Southwest Oncology Group Study. Urol Int 41:254

Mulders PF, Hoekstra WJ, Heybroek RP, Schapers ER, Verbeek AL, Oosterhof GO, Debruyne FM (1994) Prognosis and treatment of T1G3 bladder tumors. A prognostic factor analysis of 121 patients. Dutch South Eastern Bladder Cancer Study Group (see comments). Eur J Cancer 30A:914–917

Newling D (1990) Intravesical therapy in the management of superficial transitional cell carcinoma of the bladder: the experience of the EORTC GU Group. Br J Cancer 61:497–499

Newling DW, Robinson MR, Smith PH, et al. (1995) Tryptophan metabolites, pyridoxine (vitamin B6) and their influence on the recurrence rate of superficial bladder cancer. Results of a prospective, randomized phase III study performed by the EORTC GU Group. EORTC Genito-Urinary Tract Cancer Cooperative Group. Eur Urol 27:110–116

Oosterlinck W, Kurth KH, Schrodr F, Sylvester R, Hammond B (1993) A plea for cold biopsy, fulguration and immediate bladder instillation with epirubicin in small superficial bladder tumors. Data from the EORTC GU Group Stury 30863. Eur Urol 23:457–459

Pavone-Macaluso M, Tripi M, Ingargiola GB, Corselli G, Pavone C, Serretta V (1993) Current views on intravesical treatment and chemoprophylaxis of superficial bladder cancer. The present role of epirubicin and doxorubicin. J Chemother 5:207–211

Prout GR Jr, Shipley WU, Kaufman DS, Giffin PP, Heney NM (1991) Interval report of a phase I–II study utilizing multiple modalities in the treatment of invasive bladder cancer. A bladder-sparing trial. Urol Clin North Am 18:547–554

Rowland RG, Mitchell ME, Bihrle P (1987) Indiana continent urinary reservoir. J Urol 137:1136

Schwaibold H, Klingenberger HJ, Huland H (1994a) Langzeitergebnisse einer intravesikalen Rezidivprophylaxe mit Mitomycin C und Adriamycin bei Patienten mit oberflächlichem Harnblasenkarzinom. Urologe [A] 33: 479–483

Shipley WU, Prout GR Jr, Einstein AB, et al (1987) Treatment of invasive bladder cancer by cisplatin and radiation in patients unsuited for surgery. JAMA 258:931–935

Stoeckle M, Meyenburg W, Wellek S, et al. (1995) Adjuvant polychemotherapy of nonorgan-confined bladder cancer after radical cystectomy revisited: long-term results of a controlled prospective study and further clinical experience. J Urol 153:47–52

van der Meijden AP, Kurth KH, Oosterlinck W, Debruyne FM (1992) Intravesical therapy with adriamycin and 4-epirubicin for superficial bladder cancer: the experience of the EORTC GU Group. Cancer Chemother Pharmacol 30(Suppl):S95–S98

Subject Index

List of Contributors

Alex F. Althausen, MD
Department of Urology
Massachusetts General Hospital
Harvard Medical School
Boston, MA 02114
USA

Hassan Aziz, MD
Department of Radiation Oncology
SUNY Health Sciences Center at Brooklyn
450 Clarkson Avenue
Brooklyn, NY 11203
USA

Luc Baert, MD, PhD
Professor and Chairman
Department of Urology
UZ Gasthuisberg
University Hospitals of Leuven
Herestraat 49
B-3000 Leuven
Belgium

and

Clinical Professor
Department of Urology and Radiation Oncology
University of Southern California
USC/Norris Comprehensive Cancer Center
1441 Eastlake Avenue
Los Angeles, CA 90033
USA

Christina M. Bender, PhD
Department of Biochemistry and Molecular Biology
Urologic Cancer Research Laboratory
University of Southern California
USC/Norris Comprehensive Cancer Center
1441 Eastlake Avenue
Los Angeles, CA 90033
USA

Joseph E. Binard, MD, FRSC(C)
Department of Urology
College of Medicine
University of South Florida
Tampa, FL 33612
USA

S. Birkenhake, MD
Universitäts-Strahlenklinik
Universitätsstrasse 27
D-91054 Erlangen
Germany

Bernard H. Bochner, MD
Fellow, Urologic Oncology
Department of Urology
University of Southern California School of Medicine
USC/Norris Comprehensive Cancer Center
1441 Eastlake Avenue
Los Angeles, CA 90033
USA

C. Bouffioux, MD
University Hospital Sart Tilman - B35
B-4000 Liege
Belgium

Stuart D. Boyd, MD
Professor, Department of Urology
University of Southern California
USC/Norris Comprehensive Cancer Center
1441 Eastlake Avenue
Los Angeles, CA 90033
USA

Luther W. Brady, MD
Professor, Department of Radiation Oncology
and Nuclear Medicine
Allegheny University Hospitals, Center City
Mail Stop 200, Broad & Vine Sts.
Philadelphia, PA 19102-1192
USA

M. Brausi, MD
B. Ramazzini Hospital, Via S. Giacoma
I-41012 Capri (Modena)
Italy

Fabio Calabrò, MD
Department of Medical Oncology
San Raffaele Scientific Institute
Via E. Chianesi 53
I-00144 Rome
Italy

Joseph Cirrone, MD
Department of Radiation Oncology
SUNY Health Sciences Center at Brooklyn
450 Clarkson Avenue
Brooklyn, NY 11203
USA

Kwang Choi, MD
Department of Radiation Oncology
SUNY Health Sciences Center at Brooklyn
450 Clarkson Avenue
Brooklyn, NY 11203
USA

BRIAN J. COSTLEIGH, MD
The Cancer Center at Kent General Hospital Dover, Delaware

and

Department of Radiation Oncology
and Nuclear Medicine
Allegheny University Hospitals, Center City
Mail Stop 200, Broad & Vine Sts.
Philadelphia, PA 19102-1192
USA

RICHARD J. COTE, MD
Associate Professor of Pathology and Urology
Department of Pathology
University of Southern California
USC/Norris Comprehensive Cancer Center
1441 Eastlake Avenue
Los Angeles, CA 90033
USA

N. DE GRAEFE, MD
Department of Urology
UZ Gasthuisberg
University Hospitals of Leuven
Herestraat 49
B-3000 Leuven
Belgium

DIRK J.M.K. DE RIDDER, MD
Consultant Urologist
Department of Urology
UZ Gasthuisberg
University Hospitals of Leuven
Herestraat 49
B-3000 Leuven
Belgium

MARIE-ANGE D'HALLEWIN, MD
Consultant, Department of Urology
UZ Gasthuisberg
University Hospitals of Leuven
Herestraat 49
B-3000 Leuven
Belgium

JÜRGEN DUNST, MD
Professor, Direktor der Universitäts-Strahlenklinik
Dryanderstrasse
D-06097 Halle/Saale
Germany

ABDEL-AZIZ ELGAMAL, MD, PhD
Consultant Urologist and Research Associate
Department of Urology
UZ Gasthuisberg
University Hospitals of Leuven
Herestraat 49
B-3000 Leuven
Belgium

FARZANEH FARZIN, MD
Department of Radiation Oncology
and Nuclear Medicine
Allegheny University Hospitals, Center City
Mail Stop 200, Broad & Vine Sts.
Philadelphia, PA 19102-1192
USA

SILVIA C. FORMENTI, MD
Associate Professor
Department of Radiation Oncology and Medicine
University of Southern California
USC/Norris Comprehensive Cancer Center
1441 Eastlake Avenue
Los Angeles, CA 90033
USA

F.S. FREIHA, MD
Professor and Chief, Urologic Oncology
Department of Urology
Stanford University Medical Center
300 Pasteur Drive, Room S-287
Stanford, CA 94205
USA

JORGE E. FREIRE, MD
Department of Radiation Oncology
and Nuclear Medicine
Allegheny University Hospitals, Center City
Mail Stop 200, Broad & Vine Sts.
Philadelphia, PA 19102-1192
USA

HANS GOETHUYS, MD
Senior Resident, Department of Urology
UZ Gasthuisberg
University Hospitals of Leuven
Herestraat 49
B-3000 Leuven
Belgium

HANS-PETER HEILMANN, MD
Professor of Radiation Oncology
Head of the Hermann-Holthusen-Institute for Radiotherapy,
St. George's Hospital
Lohmühlenstrasse 5
D-20099 Hamburg
Germany

NIALL M. HENEY, MD
Department of Urology
Massachusetts General Hospital
Harvard Medical School
Boston, MA 02114
USA

W. HÖLTL, MD
Department of Urology
Krankenanstalt Rudolfstiftung
Juchgasse 25
A-1030 Wien
Austria

W. IJZERMANN, MD
Urological University Clinic
Aachen Technical University of Rheinisch-Westfalen (RWTH)
Pauwelstraße 30
D-52055 Aachen
Germany

GERHARD JAKSE, MD, PhD
Professor and Chairman
Urological University Clinic
Aachen Technical University of Rheinisch-Westfalen (RWTH)
Pauwelstraße 30
D-52055 Aachen
Germany

PETER A. JONES, PhD
Professor of Biochemistry and Molecular Biology
Urologic Cancer Research Laboratory
University of Southern California
USC/Norris Comprehensive Cancer Center
1441 Eastlake Avenue
Los Angeles, CA 90033
USA

P. JUNG, MD
Urological University Clinic
Aachen Technical University of Rheinisch-Westfalen (RWTH)
Pauwelstraße 30
D-52055 Aachen
Germany

DONALD S. KAUFMANN, MD
Medical Oncology Unit
Department of Medicine
Massachusetts General Hospital
Boston, MA 02114
USA

R. KÜHN, MD, Privat-Dozent
Urologische Universitätsklinik
Maximiliansplatz 5
D-91054 Erlangen
Germany

K.-H. KURTH, MD
Department of Urology
Academic Medical Center
Meibergdreef 9
1005 AZ Amsterdam
The Netherlands

GARY LIESKOVSKY, MD
Department of Urology
University of Southern California School of Medicine
USC/Norris Comprehensive Cancer Center
1441 Eastlake Avenue
Los Angeles, CA 90033
USA

YOLANDE LIEVENS, MD
Resident in Radiotherapy
Department of Urology
UZ Gasthuisberg
University Hospitals of Leuven
Herestraat 49
B-3000 Leuven
Belgium

WALLACE A. LONGTON, MD
Department of Radiation Oncology
and Nuclear Medicine
Allegheny University Hospitals, Center City
Mail Stop 200, Broad & Vine Sts.
Philadelphia, PA 19102-1192
USA

RICHARD MACCHIA, MD
Department of Urology
SUNY Health Sciences Center at Brooklyn
450 Clarkson Avenue
Brooklyn, NY 11203
USA

D. MACK, MD
Departmen of Urology
Landeskrankenanstalten
Müllner Hauptstraße 48
A-5020 Salzburg
Austria

P. MARTUS, MD, Privat-Dozent
Institut für Medizinische Dokumentation und Statistik der Universität
Waldstrasse 6
D-91054 Erlangen
Germany

BIZHAN MICAILY, MD
Department of Radiation Oncology and Nuclear Medicine
Allegheny University Hospitals, Center City
Mail Stop 200, Broad & Vine Sts.
Philadelphia, PA 19102-1192
USA

CURTIS T. MIYAMOTO, MD
Department of Radiation Oncology and Nuclear Medicine
Allegheny University Hospitals, Center City
Mail Stop 200, Broad & Vine Sts.
Philadelphia, PA 19102-1192
USA

E.C.M. OOMS, MD
Head of department of Pathology
Westeinde Ziekenhuis
Lijnbaan 32
Postbus 432
NL-2501 CK Den Haag
The Netherlands

RAYMOND H. OYEN, MD, PhD
Associate Professor, Department of Radiology
UZ Gasthuisberg
University Hospitals of Leuven
Herestraat 49
B-3000 Leuven
Belgium

ZBIGNIEW PETROVICH, MD, FACR
Professor and Chairman
Department of Radiation Oncology
University of Southern California
USC/Norris Cancer Center
1441 Eastlake Avenue
Los Angeles, CA 90033
USA

RONALD K. ROSS, MD
University of Southern California
USC/Norris Comprehensive Cancer Center
1441 Eastlake Avenue
Los Angeles, CA 90033
USA

MARVIN ROTMAN, MD
Professor and Chairman
Department of Radiation Oncology
SUNY Health Sciences Center at Brooklyn
450 Clarkson Avenue
Brooklyn, NY 11203
USA

ROLF SAUER, MD
Professor
Direktor der Universitäts-Strahlenklinik
Universitätsstrasse 27
D-91054 Erlangen
Germany

K. M. SCHROTT, MD
Professor
Direktor der Urologischen Universitätsklinik
Maximiliansplatz 5
D-91054 Erlangen
Germany

ALAN SCHULSINGER, MD
Department of Radiation Oncology
SUNY Health Sciences Center at Brooklyn
450 Clarkson Avenue
Brooklyn, NY 11203
USA

DAVID SCHWARTZ, MD
Department of Radiation Oncology
SUNY Health Sciences Center at Brooklyn
450 Clarkson Avenue
Brooklyn, NY 11203
USA

WILLIAM U. SHIPLEY, MD
Head, Genitourinary Oncology Unit
Department of Radiation Oncology
Massachusetts General Hospital
Boston, MA 02114
USA

EILA C. SKINNER, MD
Assistant Professor
Department of Urology
University of Southern California
USC/Norris Comprehensive Cancer Center
1441 Eastlake Avenue
Los Angeles, CA 90033
USA

DONALD G. SKINNER, MD
Professor and Chairman
Department of Urology
University of Southern California
USC/Norris Comprehensive Cancer Center
1441 Eastlake Avenue
Los Angeles, CA 90033
USA

TED A.W. SPLINTER
University Hospital Rotterdam
Dr. Molewaterplein 40
3015 GD Rotterdam
The Netherlands

JOHN P. STEIN, MD
Assistant Professor
Department of Urology
University of Southern California
USC/Norris Comprehensive Cancer Center
1441 Eastlake Avenue
Los Angeles, CA 90033
USA

CORA N. STERNBERG, MD, FACP
Chief, Department of Medical Oncology
San Raffaele Scientific Institute
Via E. Chianesi 53
I-00144 Rome
ITALY

R. SYLVESTER
Data Center EORTC
B-1000 Brussels
Belgium

WALTER VAN DEN BOGAERT, MD
Professor in Radiotherapy
Department of Radiotherapy
UZ Gasthuisberg
University Hospitals of Leuven
Herestraat 49
B-3000 Leuven
Belgium

MARIETTE VAN DEN HEUVEL, MD
Resident in Urology
Department of Urology
UZ Gasthuisberg
University Hospitals of Leuven
Herestraat 49
B-3000 Leuven
Belgium

ADRIAN P.M. VAN DER MEIJDEN, MD, PhD
Department of Urology
Bosch Medical Center
P.O. Box 90153
5200 ME 's-Hertogenbosch
The Netherlands

CARIN C.D. VAN DER RIJT
Rotterdam Cancer Institute
Groene Hilledijk 301
3075 EA Rotterdam
The Netherlands

HERMAN VANHERZEELE, PhD
Department of Applied Sciences
Vrije Universiteit Brussel
Pleinlaan 2
B-1050 Brussels
Belgium

ERIC VAN LIMBERGEN, MD, PhD
Professor in Radiotherapy
Department of Urology
UZ Gasthuisberg
University Hospitals of Leuven
Herestraat 49
B-3000 Leuven
Belgium

Hein Van Poppel, MD, PhD
Professor in Urology, Department of Urology
UZ Gasthuisberg
University Hospitals of Leuven
Herestraat 49
B-3000 Leuven
Belgium

Luc Vanuytsel, MD
Professor in Radiotherapy
Departments of Urology and Radiotherapy,
UZ Gasthuisberg
University Hospitals of Leuven
Herestraat 49
B-3000 Leuven
Belgium

R. Van Velthoven, MD
S. Institut Bordet
Rue Héger Bordet
B-1000 Brussels
Belgium

R. W. Veldhuizen, MD
Departent of Pathology
Westeinde Ziekenhuis
Lijnbaan 32
Postbus 432
NL-2501 CK Den Haag
The Netherlands

C. Wittekind, MD
Professor
Direktor des Pathologischen Instituts der Universität Leipzig
Liebigstrasse 6
D-04103 Leipzig
Germany

Mimi C. Yu, PhD
University of Southern California
USC/Norris Comprehensive Cancer Center
1441 Eastlake Avenue
Los Angeles, CA 90033
USA

Antony L. Zietman, MD
Genitourinary Oncology Unit
Department of Radiation Oncology
Massachusetts General Hospital
Boston, MA 02114
USA

MEDICAL RADIOLOGY
Diagnostic Imaging and Radiation Oncology

Titles in the series already published

MEDICAL RADIOLOGY
Diagnostic Imaging and Radiation Oncology

Titles in the series already published

Print and Binding: Kösel GmbH & Co., Kempten

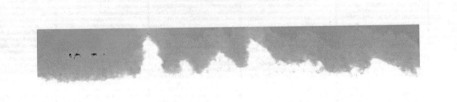